Differential Diagnosis for Primary Care

For Elsevier

Senior Commissioning Editor: Sarena Wolfaard
Associate Editor: Claire Wilson
Project Manager: Elouise Ball
Design Direction: George Ajayi
Illustration Buyer: Gillian Murray
Illustrator: Hardlines

Differential Diagnosis for Primary Care

A HANDBOOK FOR HEALTH CARE PRACTITIONERS

SECOND EDITION

Jennifer R Jamison
MBBCh PhD EdD DPH DTM&H FACNEM FICC (h)
Professor of Primary Care, Division of Health Sciences, Murdoch University, Perth, Western Australia

Foreword by

Stefan Pallister
DC DipHA
Foundation Professor, Head of Chiropractic, Murdoch University, Perth, Western Australia

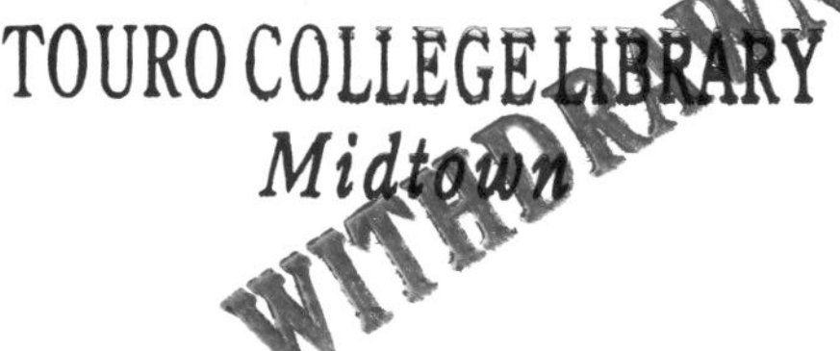

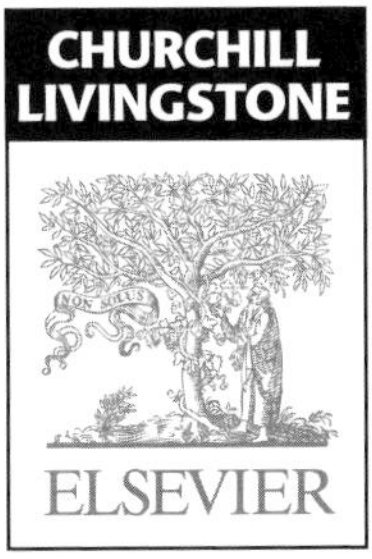

EDINBURGH LONDON NEW YORK OXFORD PHILADELPHIA ST LOUIS SYDNEY TORONTO 2006

MT

CHURCHILL
LIVINGSTONE
ELSEVIER

First Edition 1999
Second Edition 2006

ISBN 0443 102872
ISBN 9780 443102875

British Library Cataloguing in Publication Data
A catalogue record for this book is available from the British Library

Library of Congress Cataloging in Publication Data
A catalog record for this book is available from the Library of Congress

Notice
Neither the Publisher nor the Author assume any responsibility for any loss or injury and/or damage to persons or property arising out of or related to any use of the material contained in this book. It is the responsibility of the treating practitioner, relying on independent expertise and knowledge of the patient, to determine the best treatment and method of application for the patient.

Printed in China

The publisher's policy is to use **paper manufactured from sustainable forests**

5/22/07

Contents

Foreword

"Introductions inhibit pleasure, they kill the joy of anticipation, they frustrate curiosity"

Harper Lee in the foreword of *To Kill a Mocking Bird*

It has been a pleasure and a privilege to write this foreword to the second edition of Professor Jennifer Jamison's "Differential Diagnosis for Primary Care".

Differential diagnosis is a critical clinical skill that challenges both students and clinicians. Historically, students would struggle with establishing a differential diagnosis because diseases were often studied as isolated entities. Studying individual diseases and their attendant signs and symptoms encouraged rote learning and discouraged the consideration of clusters of signs and symptoms and their significance over a number of diseases.

The emphasis on the patient's presenting complaints is most welcome as it embraces the patient-centred model of care. This probably reflects Professor Jamison's long involvement in research projects that have concentrated on health promotion and the wellness model, always with the best interests of the patient first and foremost. Such an emphasis is a healthy one for our students who will be the clinicians of the future and it bodes well for the continuing development of patient-centred healthcare.

The text is well constructed with a useful first part that introduces the reader to the principles of diagnosis and the principles of drug therapy. The two case studies following the conclusion of Part I are excellent as they provide a clear demonstration of diagnostic decision-making; the first is a patient complaining of chest pain, the second a patient with no complaints but requesting a check-up. The balance between potentially life-threatening and apparently innocuous is evident and particularly well presented.

Part 2 of the text covers 58 different patient complaints, conveniently listed alphabetically and ranging from abdominal pain to wheezing. Flowcharts for each complaint compliment the text, which is presented in user-friendly point form. This approach, which is extremely clear and concise, will facilitate learning and retention.

Part 3 provides additional information related to other signs and symptoms associated with each of the differential diagnoses. It is detailed and comprehensive.

The final Cases and Questions section sets out a number of challenging scenarios relating to each of the 58 patient complaints. For students these will provide examples of clinical presentations yet to come, whilst for the clinician they will stimulate review of presentations previously experienced.

Professor Jamison's text will be welcomed by students and clinicians as a valuable addition to their professional libraries. She deserves our congratulations for the considerable time and effort she has made to develop and enhance the excellent material contained in the first edition.

Stefan Pallister 2006

Preface

Differential diagnosis is an exercise in problem solving. The patient provides the clues. The clinician detects aberrations in behavior and physiology, records signs and symptoms and searches for recognized patterns. Nosology provides the backdrop for labeling the condition. As in the first edition, Part 3 of the text lists common diseases, Part 2 provides algorithms for analyzing symptoms and Part 1 outlines approaches to solving clinical problems. The second edition differs from the first in that it uses technology to make the whole process more user-friendly. The CDROM offers students an interactive learning experience and the clinician a readily accessible information resource.

As always, it is the patient's presenting complaint that provides the trigger to differential diagnosis. Included on the CDROM are case studies, one or more for each of the 57 signs/symptoms listed in Part 2. By attempting to diagnose each case the student becomes actively engaged in an intellectually stimulating exercise that prepares them for their future practice. Instead of merely acquiring information, the student is enabled to apply knowledge in clinically relevant scenarios. The case studies provide an authentic learning experience.

For the clinician, the CDROM provides a handy resource. Instead of going to Part 2 of the text and then manually turning to Part 3 to locate further details of conditions that need to be considered, clicking on the relevant condition on the CDROM provides immediate access to a description of the suspect condition. Comparing this information with additional data gathered from the patient provides information upon which possible diagnoses can be confirmed or excluded. Consideration of signs and symptoms listed in Part 3 also provides hints for targeting further patient examination or investigation.

A further improvement in the second edition is the inclusion of practice tips. It is hoped these clinical gems will be helpful to both students and clinicians.

This text is the result of some 30 years of teaching. My thanks to all those students whose constructive criticisms have helped produce a work which I trust will provide readers with an enjoyable learning experience while contributing to a sound foundation for primary practice. Special thanks to my father, Dr Harry Jamison, for his critique and proof reading of the manuscript.

Jennifer R. Jamison

The principles and purpose of diagnosis

CHAPTER 1

The principles of diagnosis: from black box to glass bowl

PART ONE

CHAPTER CONTENTS

Clinical diagnosis involves collecting information about the presenting patient and comparing this with blueprints of disease. A correct diagnosis is most likely when the information on the patient has been accurately and completely gathered and when it matches the characteristics of a generally accepted disease picture.

THE PHASES OF DIAGNOSTIC DECISION-MAKING

Practitioners follow a definite series of steps in order to progress from the patient's presenting complaint to a working and, finally, a definitive diagnosis. The steps in making a diagnosis are thus to:

- *Detect an abnormality.* Any deviation from normal function or structure suggests disease. An important principle in diagnosis is to detect abnormalities early. Early diagnosis and therapy often result in a better patient outcome. Disease is detected early by:

- screening or case finding, which involves identifying covert or asymptomatic disease
- using diagnostic tests that are sensitive (i.e. give few false-negative results).

- *Match the presenting problem with known diseases.* Disease management is often specifically determined by the diagnostic label. The accuracy of diagnostic labeling is increased when:
  - a diagnosis is based on a number of signs and symptoms
  - diagnostic tests that are highly specific (i.e. seldom give false-positive results) are used.
- *Determine a working diagnosis.* A working diagnosis is an interim diagnosis. The principle of using a working diagnosis is to create an interim management protocol while the diagnosis is being confirmed through gathering additional information by:
  - the use of more invasive tests or examination procedures
  - monitoring the response to a therapeutic trial. If the patient responds to specific therapy the definitive diagnosis is made retrospectively.
- *Make a definitive diagnosis.* The definitive diagnosis provides the trigger for selecting appropriate therapy.

This chapter explores the above process and attempts to clarify various stages of diagnostic decision-making.

THE PHILOSOPHY OF DIAGNOSTIC DECISION-MAKING

Disease is biologically based and is diagnosed by detecting deviations of structure or function in one or more organ system. Conventional thinking in western healthcare is dominated by notions of reductionism, mechanism, and determinism.

Reductionism. A reductionist philosophy suggests that systematic breakdown of complex phenomena into their more simple component parts is a sound basis for understanding the complex system. By understanding how each organ system works, and learning to recognize the characteristics of malfunction of each organ system, the practitioner can diagnose disease in presenting patients.

Mechanism. A mechanistic approach explains phenomena on the basis of physical or biological causes. Objective information is regarded with more respect than are subjective data. When making a diagnosis, signs are regarded as more clinically important than symptoms (patient complaints). As the patient's symptoms are not amenable to independent objective measurement, signs are regarded as more impartial evidence of change. Signs are detected by the practitioner, either directly or through the use of special investigations. Two levels at which distortions may arise from diagnostic testing are:

- *data collection* – standardization of data-collection techniques is an important strategy for increasing objectivity
- *data interpretation* – previous learning and personal clinical experience influence the diagnostician's judgement at this stage.

Determinism. A deterministic perspective assumes that outcome is predictable. The underlying idea is knowing in order to control. A unilinear cause–effect relationship presumes a predictable link between cause and effect. Causes are those noxious stimuli without which disease would not have occurred. In its simplest form, a single cause may be sufficient stimulus for disease. The notion of a unilinear cause–effect relationship is popular in diagnostic thinking. In reality, outcome is more often determined by interaction between various stimuli and the ability of the individual to adapt.

THREE THEMES IN DIAGNOSTIC DECISION-MAKING

Knowledge of the natural history of disease provides the basis upon which the three themes in diagnosis rest. All three themes may emerge when making a single diagnosis. The three themes underlying diagnosis are pattern recognition, probability reasoning, and causal thinking.[1]

Pattern recognition involves identifying and comparing the patient's presentation with a known disease picture. When confronted by a patient, the diagnostician searches for and describes the various characteristics of the patient's complaint. The patient's signs and symptoms are then compared with patterns of disease that have been previously classified and labeled. Once a disease has been labeled or diagnosed, a treatment that matches the label can be initiated.

Probability reasoning takes cognisance of the relative possibility of a particular disease given the patient's presentation. The likelihood that a disease has been given a correct label is increased when a number of diagnostic criteria have been met, the diagnostic tests used rarely give false-positive results, and the condition is prevalent. Pattern recognition increases the probability of an accurate diagnosis.

Causal thinking seeks to identify the factor(s) or triggers responsible for the condition. By knowing and eliminating the cause, disease can be prevented. By understanding how a particular stimulus triggers an adverse response, the natural history of a disease may be described. The natural history of disease describes the physiological and pathological changes that occur and which serve as markers of disease. The earlier such changes are detected, the greater the chance of successfully interrupting disease progression.

These themes are routinely applied in everyday practice. The influence of unilinear cause–effect thinking results in diagnosticians making a concerted effort to explain all clinical findings on the basis of single pathology. In practice, use of a single theme may be insufficient. Dual pathology can be encountered. A radiograph may show cervical osteoarthritis which is not responsible for the neck stiffness experienced by the patient. Cervical osteoarthritis is almost universal in persons aged over 40 years, and is frequently asymptomatic. The patient whose magnetic resonance imaging (MRI) scan shows disc protrusion may have an unrelated cause of backpain. Cholecystography may show stones which, when removed, do not alter the patient's 'gallstone' dyspepsia. Good clinical practice employs all three themes in diagnostic decision-making.

PATHOGENESIS: FROM HEALTH TO DISEASE

The natural history of a disease describes the pathophysiological changes from health to disease or death. It provides the basis upon which diagnostic criteria can be identified and disease diagnosed. The prognosis, or outcome, of disease depends on the nature of the noxious stimulus and on the constitution of the individual. The natural history of a fatal disease, or one with an extremely poor prognosis, comprises:

- exposure to a noxious stimulus
- interaction between the stimulus and the individual's genetic composition and internal environment
- covert disease characterized by progressive
  - inability of the individual to adapt to increased demands
  - biochemical changes
  - histological changes
- overt disease presenting clinically with
  - symptoms
  - signs
- complications of disease
- death.

At each stage of the process (Fig. 1.1), detectable biological changes mark the transformation from health to disease. In the early phases of disease development such changes are small and can only be detected at a chemical or cellular level. At a later phase, the outcome of disease pathogenesis is overt and associated with signs and symptoms. Clinical evidence of overt disease includes the patient's awareness of 'something being wrong', their symptom experience, and the diagnostician's detection of signs of structural change and/or organ dysfunction. The earlier a change is detected, the greater the likelihood that the process can be reversed and health restored.

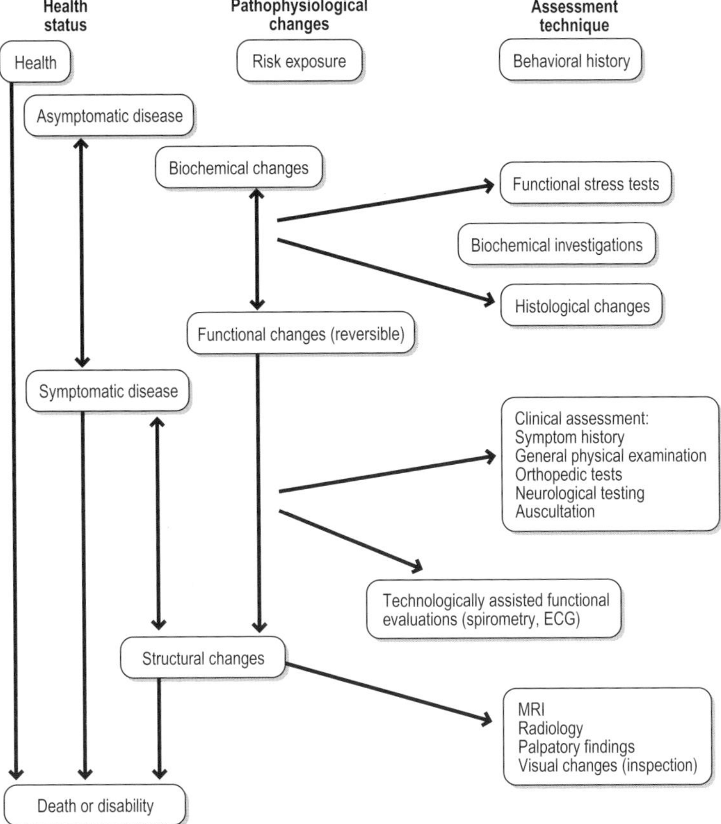

Figure 1.1 **Diagnosis and the natural history of disease.**

INFORMATION SOURCES FOR DIAGNOSTIC DECISION-MAKING

A correct diagnosis is important both because therapy is determined by diagnosis and because an incorrect diagnosis implies a missed diagnosis. The diagnostic label is used to determine treatment, and therapy is invariably associated with side-effects. While the benefits of appropriate therapy outweigh the inconvenience of side-effects, the adverse effects of incorrect therapy have a cost–benefit ratio that approximates infinity. In addition to an incorrect diagnosis being a trigger for inappropriate therapy, it also implies that the patient's condition has not been recognized and, therefore, is not being treated. In such instances unrecognized disease may progress while inappropriate intervention is pursued. Such delays in commencing therapy may mean that a preventable condition is transformed into irreversible disease.

In order to make a confident diagnosis, practitioners rely on various sources of information. Within diagnostic reasoning, the weakest information is anecdotal information provided by the patient about how he or she feels. Symptoms are subjective experiences that are influenced by a diversity of factors, including culture, and previous personal experience of the sick role and of the presenting condition. Diagnosticians like to verify the patient's complaint, and they do so by:

- history-taking
- physical examination
- using special investigations to evaluate the working diagnosis.

On history-taking, an attempt is made to identify whether the patient's complaints are consistent with the symptom pattern of a known disease. Nondirective questioning using open questions is most helpful in the early stages. The diagnostician's knowledge of the patient's presenting complaint is refined by checking whether the patient has symptoms similar to diseases that are prevalent for an individual of that gender, in that age group, or living in that community. A list of possible diagnoses is formulated on the basis of the patient's history.

On physical examination, clues identified during history are actively pursued and physical evidence is sought to confirm a condition suggested by the patient's history. Physical examination refines the list of possible diagnoses developed from history-taking and tests each option as an interim working diagnosis. The diagnostician particularly searches for signs of:

- the most probable diseases given the history
- serious diseases that are consistent with the history.

As special investigations are more invasive than physical examination they are selectively used to convert the preferred working diagnosis into a single definitive diagnosis. Special investigations include:

- laboratory investigations, such as hematology and blood chemistry
- imaging, ranging from radiological investigations to ultrasound and MRI
- biopsy, where tissue is removed and examined histologically
- a therapeutic trial (when the diagnosis is uncertain, monitoring the patient's response to therapy may be used as a strategy for arriving at a definitive diagnosis).

The usefulness of diagnostic tests

In order to increase the probability of a correct diagnosis, the procedures undertaken during physical examination and those requested as special investigations should be reliable, valid, sensitive, specific, and have an acceptable predictive value.[1,2]

Reliability refers to the reproducibility and consistency of a test. Reliability is usually expressed as a number between 0 and 1, with 0 indicating no reliability and 1 equating to perfect

Box 1.1
Sensitivity

- A sensitive test gives positive results when the disease is truly present; it seldom has false-negative results
- Sensitive tests are important when apparently healthy people are screened for disease

Sensitivity = $a/(a + c) \times 100$

	'Truth about the disease'	
Test result	Disease present	Disease absent
Positive	a	b
Negative	c	d
Total	$a + c$	$b + d$

reliability. The closer a test's reliability is to 1, the more precise is the resultant diagnosis. Test reproducibility requires a clear test protocol that specifies:

- *Conditions under which the test is performed.* Tests should be undertaken under prescribed circumstances that can be routinely replicated.
- *Interpretation of findings.* Findings would be interpreted within a known range of observer variation.

Reliability is influenced by the stability of a test or procedure measured in different settings, i.e. by different examiners (inter-examiner reliability) or by the same examiner at different times (intraexaminer reliability). High interexaminer or intraexaminer (observer) reliability does not automatically confer clinical value. If the prevalence of the disorder being examined is high, the possibility of finding a positive test by chance is also high. For a test to be of clinical value it must also be valid.

Validity reflects the accuracy of a test, it assesses the degree to which a test measures what it is designed to measure. Examiner reliability and clinical validity may not correlate. For example, muscle strength correlates poorly with suspected disease, yet when allowing for agreement within one full grade, interexaminer reliability is 90%, intraexaminer reliability is 95%. High reliability does not confer validity. However, tests that are sensitive and specific are valid indicators of disease.

A *sensitive* test is one which is positive in individuals with the disorder (Box 1.1). A sensitive test seldom gives false-negative results, and therefore is particularly important when screening for covert disease.

A *specific* test is one that is negative in individuals who do not have the disorder. It seldom gives false-positive results (Box 1.2). Tests with high specificity are particularly important when making a definitive diagnosis as this becomes the basis for therapy.

Box 1.2
Specificity

- A specific test is one that has negative results when the disease is absent; it seldom has false-positive results
- Specific tests are used to confirm the selection of a diagnostic label before therapy is initiated

Specificity = $d/(b + d) \times 100$

	'Truth about the disease'	
Test result	Disease present	Disease absent
Positive	*a*	*b*
Negative	*c*	*d*
Total	$a + c$	$b + d$

Box 1.3
Predictive value

- The positive predictive value is the number of occasions a positive test signifies disease. It is the ability of a positive test to predict the presence of disease (i.e. the likelihood that the disease is present). The predictive value of a test is influenced by the prevalence of the condition in the population in which it is used
- The negative predictive value is the number of occasions a negative test correctly indicated the absence of disease. It is the post-test likelihood of a negative test result in persons without disease

Positive predictive value = $d/(c + d)$
Negative predictive value = $a/(a + b)$

	'Truth about the disease'	
Test result	Disease present	Disease absent
Positive	*a*	*b*
Negative	*c*	*d*
Total	$a + b$	$c + d$

A positive *predictive value* is the likelihood that a positive test is a 'true' positive result; a negative predictive value is the likelihood that a negative test is a 'true' negative result. A test may have a high sensitivity and/or specificity but still have a low predictive value, because this index is a measure of the likelihood of a disease in a particular population. It takes into consideration the idiosyncrasies of the population being tested and is not determined solely by test parameters (Box 1.3). The positive predictive value is a measure of those people with a positive report who actually have the disease. If the number of people tested who actually have the disorder is very low, the predictive value of a positive test is also low, even if a sensitive and specific test has been used. Predictive values vary as a function of sensitivity, specificity, and prevalence.

Box 1.4
Likelihood ratio

$$\text{Likelihood ratio} = \frac{\text{True-positive rate}}{\text{False-positive rate}} = \frac{\text{Sensitivity}}{1 - \text{Specificity}}$$

Box 1.5
A case study of prevalence, predictive value and likelihood ratio

Framework

- Biopsy is the gold standard for prostate cancer
- Sensitivity of rectal examination is 71.4%, specificity is 94%
- Rectal examination is the investigation procedure.

For a population in which the prevalence of prostate cancer is 50%:

- the positive predictive value of a craggy prostate on rectal examination is 92%
- the negative predictive value is lower (around 77%).

For a population with a disease prevalence of 0.025%:

- the positive predictive value drops to less than 1%
- the negative predictive value is almost 100%.

The probability of the condition being present following a negative test decreases as the prevalence of the condition decreases. The probability that disease is truly present following a positive finding rises as the prevalence increases.

In either population:

- the likelihood ratio of prostate cancer in a positive rectal examination is 6.27
- the odds of finding prostate cancer at surgery in a patient with a craggy prostate on rectal examination are 6.27.

The *likelihood ratio* is a measure of the sensitivity and specificity of the text being used. *Odds ratios* provide information about the test and are useful for predicting disease in populations in which the nuances of the natural history of the disease are unknown. *Predictive values* require and consider population-specific information.

Likelihood ratios are similar to positive predictive values insofar as they provide information about the possibility that a positive test and the target disease are present. Unlike predictive values, disease prevalence does not influence likelihood ratios. The likelihood of disease being present is the ratio between the true-positive rate and the false-positive rate (Box 1.4). Sensitivity and specificity are essentially independent of prevalence. Likelihood ratios depend on the characteristics of the test and are independent of the population being tested. As likelihood ratios take into consideration the strength of the original mode of data collection (nominal, ordinal, or interval), they add an extra dimension to computing the probability of disease given a positive test. A case study is provided in Box 1.5.

The reality of clinical reasoning

Many tests and examination procedures have not been subject to rigorous scientific scrutiny. In fact, although many routinely used diagnostic tests have been demonstrated to be reliable, they have not been compared with a gold standard and may not be valid. While some tests have been demonstrated to give a certain level of accuracy through a properly designed study or series of studies, others are based on expert knowledge of structure and function and have never been tested for reliability or validity.

One strategy for addressing such a discrepancy in clinical testing is to undertake a number of tests and then use sequential positive and/or negative findings to narrow down the list of possible diagnoses. Basing a definitive diagnosis on a number of findings rather than a single test addresses some, but not all, of the potential problems associated with diagnostic tests. Other problems encountered include:

- the use of indirect measurements, which are extrapolated and interpreted
- variability of presentation attributable to
  - patient differences
  - patients presenting at different stages in the natural history of the condition
- the skill and experience of the examiner
- the bias of the examiner
- the practicality of the test in terms of
  - financial cost
  - invasiveness (this influences patients' acceptance)
- the placebo effect.[3]

A DIAGNOSTIC MODEL

Using hypertension as an example, a diagnostic model incorporating the three themes of diagnosis is presented. When the diagnostician is confronted with a patient with hypertension the phases of diagnosis are as follows:

- *Labeling of the disorder.* This requires knowledge of the diagnostic criteria, or pattern, which leads to designation of the label 'hypertension'. Diagnosing the disorder, in addition to involving a search for patterns of signs and symptoms, uses probability reasoning. The more reliable and valid the tests used when detecting the diagnostic criteria, the greater the likelihood of a correct diagnosis.
- *Identification of any complications resulting from the condition diagnosed.* The search for particular signs and symptoms is based on knowledge of the natural history of the disease. Probability reasoning, cause–effect thinking, and a search for patterns of disturbed physiology or pathological responses are used. In the case of hypertension, a search for target-organ

damage includes paying particular attention to the cardiovascular and renal systems.

- *Making a causal assessment.* This can be explored from two perspectives. Both the trigger causing raised blood pressure and the consequences of hypertension are relevant to patient assessment. The trigger causing raised blood pressure may be unknown (essential hypertension), or hypertension may be secondary to drugs, renal, or endocrine problems. By finding the stimulus that initiated a persistently raised blood pressure, treatment can be directed towards removing the cause rather than merely modifying its clinical effects. On the other hand, hypertension is a recognized risk factor for ischemic heart disease. As risk is cumulative, it is also prudent to screen patients with hypertension for other cardiovascular risk factors.

The natural history of the condition

Hypertension is a progressive disease. After 20 years' follow-up, 80% of those with borderline hypertension progress to hypertension, compared with only 45% of persons with normal blood pressure.[4] A raised blood pressure carries a risk, irrespective of whether it is the systolic or diastolic pressure that is elevated. A systolic blood pressure of 135 mmHg is equivalent in risk to a diastolic pressure of 90 mmHg; after middle age a systolic pressure of 160 mmHg is more risky than a diastolic pressure of 95 mmHg.[5] Although persons with hypertension are usually asymptomatic, some 35% of cases do have a throbbing occipital headache, which is worst in the morning.

Hypertension increases with age. The risk of target-organ damage in persons with untreated hypertension increases with the duration and severity of the condition. Target-organ damage in hypertensive patients presents as:

- Left ventricular failure. Complaints of breathlessness, particularly orthopnea and/or paroxysmal nocturnal dyspnea, should be investigated further by examining for enlargement of the left ventricle, a fourth and/or third heart sound, and bilateral crackles at the base of both lungs.
- Headaches and vertigo in mild hypertension. In malignant hypertension, cerebral manifestations include: hypertensive encephalopathy, nausea, severe headache, and transient disturbances of speech, vision, sensation and/or paresis. Disorientation and convulsions may occur.
- Proteinuria. Renal damage occurs late in benign, and early in malignant, hypertension. Patients with macroalbuminuria and hypertension are at increased risk of a major new cardiovascular event such as an infarction or stroke.[6]
- Hypertensive retinopathy. Grade I hypertensive retinopathy presents as narrowing of the arterioles (silver and copper wiring), grade II as arteriovenous nipping, and grade III as exudates and hemorrhages. In cases of malignant

hypertension, grade IV hypertensive retinopathy with papilledema is encountered. Other eye problems include:
- retinal branch vein occlusions at arteriovenous crossings
- central retinal vein occlusion in chronic hypertension (severe and frequently permanent loss of vision may result).

- Vascular complications of hypertension include:
  - rupture of aneurysms (e.g. Berry aneurysm)
  - dissecting aortic aneurysms
  - acceleration of atherosclerosis.

There is a linear rise in mortality with increasing levels of both systolic and diastolic blood pressure above 110/70 mmHg.[7] In practice, mild hypertension is responsible for over 50% of the excess mortality attributable to hypertension. A reduction of a population's systolic blood pressure by 9 mmHg is estimated to achieve a 7% overall reduction in mortality, a 9% reduction in stroke mortality, and a 14% reduction in ischemic heart disease.[8] Reducing blood pressure has an immediate impact on the risk of stroke, but it is estimated that it will take 5 years before the effect on ischemic heart disease is noted.

Making the diagnosis

As hypertension can cause progressive organ damage in persons who feel well, screening for raised blood pressure in asymptomatic people is routinely undertaken. Accurate diagnosis is imperative when diagnosing disease in apparently 'healthy' people. Ideally, a diagnosis is made using tests that are reliable and valid. In addition to an appreciation of its natural history, a diagnosis of hypertension requires:

- a set of diagnostic criteria for patient labeling
- a protocol for recording blood pressure.

Probability reasoning is the basis upon which the diagnostic criteria and the protocol for recording blood pressure have evolved.

A prerequisite to uniform diagnosis is a set of diagnostic criteria. Errors in diagnosis can be made when clinical findings are interpreted differently. It is therefore imperative that clinical findings are translated using a common scale. Widely accepted criteria for interpreting blood pressure readings include:[9]

- Normotension: systolic pressure less than 140 mmHg and diastolic pressure less than 90 mmHg
- Borderline hypertension: systolic pressure 140–159 mmHg and/or diastolic pressure of 90–94 mmHg
- Definite hypertension: systolic pressure of 160 mmHg or greater and/or diastolic pressure of 95 mmHg or greater
- Mild hypertension: systolic pressure 160–179 mmHg and/or diastolic pressure 95–104 mmHg
- Significant hypertension: blood pressure > 142/92 mmHg in a 16–18-year-old, > 136/86 mmHg in a 13–15-year-old, > 126/82 mmHg in a 10–12-year-old

- Malignant hypertension: diastolic pressure exceeds 120 mmHg and target organ damage (vascular disease) is detectable
- Isolated systolic hypertension: diastolic pressure less than 90 mmHg and systolic pressure exceeding 160 mmHg.

Hypertension may either be combined systolic/diastolic or isolated systolic. The need for a set of diagnostic criteria applies regardless of the test being interpreted. In the case of muscle testing, the equivalent system of guidelines for standardizing the clinician's interpretation of muscle strength is:

- a complete range of motion against gravity with full resistance, which is regarded as normal and graded 5
- a complete range of motion against gravity with some resistance, which is regarded as good and graded 4
- a complete range of motion against gravity, which is regarded as fair and graded 3
- a complete range of motion with gravity eliminated, which is regarded as poor and graded 2
- evidence of slight contractility with no joint motion, which is categorized as a trace and graded 1
- no evidence of contractility, which is categorized as zero and graded 0.

Patients with a grade 0 or 1 are said to be paralyzed, those with a grade 2 or 3 are said to have paresis.

Another prerequisite for the uniform diagnosis of hypertension is to comply with the approved protocol when recording blood pressure.[10,11] Diligent adherence to a precise protocol reduces the risk of an inaccurate diagnosis. By precisely following the protocol the reproducibility of a finding is increased. The reliability of a clinical result depends on it having been detected using a standard protocol. Interexaminer reliability increases when protocols for detecting signs are clearly specified. The protocol for accurate blood pressure evaluation incorporates consideration of the instrument, cuff size and application, patient preparation, and criteria for reading and establishing the blood pressure level. The procedure for taking a blood-pressure measurement includes:

- Instrument selection:
  - the mercury instrument remains accurate over time; aneroid instruments are more likely to be inaccurate
  - automatic blood pressure devices are not suitable for screening; a mercury sphygmomanometer should be used.
- Cuff selection and use with respect to:
  - Size: standard cuffs can be used in adults with arm circumference of 30 cm or less. The length of the cuff must be a minimum of 80% of the patient's midarm circumference, and its width must be a minimum of 40% of the patient's midarm circumference

PART ONE

- Position: place the bladder over the brachial artery
- Application: firm, neither tight nor loose
- Inflation: inflate at a medium pace; ensure that no bladder herniation occurs
- Deflation: deflate at an even rate of 2 mmHg per second.

- Patient preparation, such as:
  - avoidance of smoking and/or consuming 'caffeinated' food or drink for 120 minutes before assessment
  - comfortable seating
  - allowing for 5 minutes' rest before taking the reading.
- Taking the reading by recording:
  - Palpatory systolic pressure. A reading is taken of the pressure at which cuff inflation obliterates the radial pulse. Before reinflating the cuff, wait 30 seconds.
  - Auscultatory systolic pressure. Inflate the cuff to 30 mmHg above the palpatory systolic pressure and auscultate over the antecubital fossa while deflating the cuff. The systolic pressure at the appearance of the first Korotkoff sound is recorded.
  - Diastolic pressure. Continue to deflate the cuff at 2–5 mmHg per second after registering the systolic pressure. Record the disappearance of the Korotkoff sound. Sounds may be heard down to zero inflation in hyperdynamic states such as pregnancy or aortic incompetence. In these instances the diastolic pressure is recorded at muffling of the Korotkoff sound.
- Establishing the reading by:
  - Taking the blood pressure of both arms. A difference of 5–10 mmHg between arms is within normal limits. The arm with the highest level is used for subsequent readings. The blood pressure recorded is the mean of the lowest two readings in the arm registering the highest level.
  - Averaging two or more readings. If the first two readings differ by more than 5 mmHg, additional readings should be taken.

In addition to following the above protocol, diagnosticians need actively to avoid confounding variables. Practitioner variables frequently leading to erroneous blood-pressure readings include:

- Failure to exclude changes in posture in:
  - pregnant women
  - the elderly
  - those with orthostatic hypotension
  - those on antihypertensive therapy.
- Failure to allow a time lapse or period of relaxation in persons who are:
  - anxious, stressed
  - in pain
  - cold
  - aroused through recent exertion.

- Failure to detect:
  - an arrhythmia
  - an auscultatory gap (avoided by doing a palpatory systolic pressure)
  - indistinct Korotkoff sounds.
- Technique errors:
  - placing the cuff above or below the heart
  - taking column reading above or below eye level
  - rounding the reading upwards.

Patient variables leading to false-positive readings include:

- an underlying anxious personality
- the first visit to a new practitioner
- isometric exercise or discomfort while blood pressure is being taken.

Inaccurate diagnosis and its consequences

Contrary to the preferred approach of pattern recognition, which is based upon a number of signs and symptoms, diagnosis in hypertension is based upon detection of a single sign. A false-negative result, due to failure to detect and recognize an auscultatory gap, and a false-positive result, due to 'white coat hypertension', are consequently well-recognized phenomena.

The consequence of a false-negative diagnosis is unnecessary persistence of the underlying disease. Treatment of all grades of hypertension reduces the risk of stroke, renal disease, congestive heart failure, and ischemic heart disease.[12–14]

The consequence of a false-positive diagnosis is unnecessary therapy. In addition to lowering blood pressure, antihypertensive agents have other effects. All agents used to treat hypertension have side-effects. Diuretics may cause hyperuricemia, glucose intolerance, hypokalemia, hyperlipidemia, and/or impotence. Sympathetic nervous system depressants such as beta blockers may have a negative inotropic effect, and cause fatigue, bronchospasm, and/or hyperlipidemia. Adrenergic inhibitors, on the other hand, may cause dizziness, headache, orthostatic hypotension, weakness, palpitations, and incontinence in older women. Vasodilators such as hydralazine may cause fluid retention, reflex tachycardia, and postural hypotension. Calcium-channel blockers may cause headaches, dizziness, palpitations, and fluid retention. Angiotensin-converting enzyme (ACE) inhibitors may cause profound hypotension, hyperkalemia, headache, cough, dizziness, and fatigue. As a result of erroneous diagnosis, 10–15% of patients diagnosed with hypertension become normotensive.[15] To minimize unnecessary distress due to the adverse effects of antihypertensive therapy, criteria indicating the need for drug therapy have been identified. These include:

- A newly diagnosed patient with a blood pressure greater than 180/105 mmHg.

- A patient on nondrug therapy:
  - whose blood pressure remains above 160/95 mmHg and has an additional risk factor for coronary artery disease such as smoking, hypercholesterolemia, or diabetes, or has evidence of target organ damage
  - whose blood pressure remains above 160/100 mmHg and has no other risk factors present
  - who develops evidence of target-organ damage such as left ventricular failure, a very irregular pulse, chest pain suggestive of angina, hematuria and/or albuminuria, or a severe headache.
- A patient with a history of renal disease whose diastolic blood pressure remains above 90 mmHg.
- A diabetic of less than 60 years of age whose diastolic pressure remains above 90 mmHg.
- A pregnant patient with a blood pressure in the range 140–149/90–99 mmHg.

While a strategy for actively seeking criteria to justify drug therapy may reduce the risk of unnecessary drug therapy, it carries little psychological benefit for an individual who has acquired a 'sick' label based upon a diagnostic test.

Causal diagnosis

Although uncomplicated hypertension eludes the diagnostic principle of using numerous signs and symptoms in diagnosis, it is amenable to causal assessment. Causal diagnosis seeks to identify the particular reason why the presenting patient has raised blood pressure. Although the majority of patients have primary hypertension for which no cause can be identified, about 5% of patients with true hypertension have an identifiable cause. Clinical clues to secondary hypertension are:

- the onset of raised blood pressure in young or elderly people, especially if diastolic blood pressure exceeds 105 mmHg
- abrupt onset
- advanced fundal change
- accelerated or malignant hypertension
- an abdominal bruit
- resistance to appropriate therapy
- clinical manifestations of endocrine abnormality
- proteinuria.

More specifically, secondary hypertension may be attributable to:[16]

- Drugs. Nonsteroidal anti-inflammatory agents, steroids (corticosteroids, androgens and estrogens), alcohol, thyroid preparations, amfetamines, epinephrine, nasal decongestants and other cold remedies, and caffeine are all possible triggers. The hypertensive effect of alcohol and oral contraceptives seems to be additive.
- Renovascular disease. A renal cause should be suspected in individuals who:

  - are under 30 or over 50 years of age and present with a sudden onset of hypertension
  - have a sudden deterioration in their blood pressure status
  - have a history of hematuria, flank pain, dysuria, or an abdominal bruit. Renal masses are consistent with polycystic kidneys.
- Hyperaldosteronism. Check for muscle cramps, weakness, nocturia, and polyuria.
- Pheochromocytoma. Search for tachycardia, palpitations, headaches, tremor, excess sweating, and weight loss.
- Cushing's syndrome. Look for trunkal obesity, glucosuria, a moon face, easy bruising, muscle wasting, and weakness.
- Myxedema. In the elderly, myxedema may present initially with hypertension.
- Coarctation of the aorta. Aortic narrowing should be suspected in patients who have weak or delayed femoral pulses (radiofemoral delay), and have hypertensive readings in the upper and normotensive readings in the lower limbs. Evidence of a pulsatile collateral circulation should be sought. Check for a midsystolic murmur.

In patients with secondary hypertension a diagnosis of hypertension is incomplete. In these cases raised blood pressure is evidence of underlying disease and therapy must seek to treat the cause and not just the complication of the disease. Only in instances when the underlying condition is refractory to therapy is it sufficient to manage the patient by limiting treatment to lowering the raised blood pressure.

The recognition and treatment of the primary cause is an important principle that pervades diagnosis. In a hypothyroid patient with carpal tunnel syndrome, release of pressure on the median nerve may relieve the patient's symptoms, but it does not address the underlying problem. Replacement of thyroid hormone is required in the management of this patient. In a patient with pallor and a low hemoglobin, anemia is an inadequate diagnosis. The cause of the anemia needs to be identified and treated.

CONCLUSION

The principles of diagnosis are to:

- Make an accurate diagnosis. This is most likely when:
  - the diagnosis is based upon a number of signs and symptoms
  - using tests with high sensitivity and specificity
  - identifying a pattern of signs and symptoms that matches a known disease.
- Use the diagnostic label as the basis for patient management.

Using hypertension as an example, the hazards associated with diagnosis resting on a single sign were identified. Confident diagnoses are made upon detecting a number of signs and symptoms. Hypertension was also used to demonstrate the potential for doing harm when:

- An incorrect diagnosis is used as a guide for therapy – unnecessary therapy has no benefit and is likely to have adverse effects
- A diagnosis is missed – when treatable disease is permitted to progress unchecked, complications of the underlying condition develop and unnecessary suffering results.

The hypertension example also demonstrated the necessity to adhere to procedural guidelines when detecting signs. Protocols for detecting signs should be implemented in order to maximize reliability and validity and should be followed for best results. Accurate diagnosis is the basis of appropriate therapy.

A case study demonstrating diagnostic decision-making

A 45-year-old male presents complaining of chest pain. Examination findings are: blood pressure is 140/80, pulse – 75/min, regular, good volume, respiration – 13/min.

Clinical decision 1: Is this an emergency?

How would you manage this situation:
(a) Refer for urgent intervention – hospital referral
(b) Continue data collection

Answer

(a) Disagree. Refer for urgent intervention – hospital referral.
(b) Continue data collection as vital signs are satisfactory.

Clinical decision 2: What is the source of the pain?

In order to determine the source of the chest pain you consider:
(a) Structures in the chest
(b) The nature of the pain arising from each of these structures:
- location/radiation
- character – crushing, burning, stabbing, aching
- periodicity/frequency
- intensity – patient perception, change in autonomic nervous system
- aggravating and relieving factors
- associated findings – change in organ function.

With the above template in mind you take the following patient history:

Doctor: Do you have the pain now?
Patient: No.
Doctor: Tell me about your pain.
Patient: When I get the pain it feels like a vice around my chest.

Case study continues

Doctor: How long does it last?
Patient: Not long. Less than 5 minutes, but it's severe.
Doctor: What produces the pain?
Patient: I get it when I'm running. I have to stop and wait till the pain goes.
Doctor: Are there other occasions when you get the pain?
Patient: I sometimes get the pain when I am arguing with my teenage son.
Doctor: Have you ever had the pain when you are relaxed?
Patient: That is what happened this morning. I was sitting reading the paper with a cup of coffee and a cigarette and I got the pain. That's why I came in today.
Doctor: Is there anything that relieves the pain?
Patient: Just rest.
Doctor: Can you point to the part of your chest where the pain is worst?
Patient: It's in the middle of my chest.
Doctor: Do you get pain anywhere else?
Patient: I sometimes get pain down my left arm.
Doctor: Do you notice anything else when you get the pain?
Patient: I feel weak and sweaty when the pain is very bad.

The nature of the pain suggests that the anatomical source of the patient's pain is the:
(a) Esophagus
(b) Heart
(c) Vessels
(d) Pleura
(e) Trachea
(f) Muscles
(g) Ribs/vertebrae
(h) Skin

Answer (b) Heart

Clinical decision 3: What is the most common cause of pain from this source?

Using probability reasoning the most likely diagnosis is:
(a) Angina
(b) Myocardial infarction
(c) Atherosclerotic heart disease
(d) Psychogenic chest pain
(e) Esophageal spasm

Answer

(a) Agree. Angina
(b) Disagree. In myocardial infarction the pain lasts longer but ECG and cardiac enzymes should be requested to definitely exclude this condition.
(c) Disagree. Atherosclerotic heart disease is associated with recurrent chest pain but an arrhythmia is common.
(d) Disagree. Psychogenic chest pain is not precipitated by exercise and should only be diagnosed when pathology has been excluded.

Case study continues

(e) Disagree. Crushing retrosternal chest pain is precipitated by eating in cases with esophageal spasm.

Clinical decision 4: What is the pathophysiology of the suspected condition?

What is the natural history of angina? Does the patient have predisposing factors? Is there any evidence of complications?

The clinical consultation proceeds to see if the patient has any known risk factors for ischemic heart disease:

Doctor: Do you smoke?
Patient: 25 cigarettes a day.
Doctor: What about alcohol?
Patient: A couple of glasses a day of wine with my evening meal.
Doctor: What is your usual diet?
Patient: I like take away pizza, fried food, meat, cream, chips, salted nuts.
Doctor: Do you have heart disease in your family?
Patient: My father had a heart attack and died at the age of 49. Nobody else in the family has a heart problem.

Physical examination:

Height: 6 ft; weight: 70 kg; BMI: 21
Pulse: regular 75/min
BP: 140/80

Special investigations:

Fasting blood lipids: Total blood cholesterol was 6.5 mmol/l; LDL 5.5 mmol/l and triglycerides 1.9 mmol/l.
The patient is at increased risk of ischemic heart disease due to:
(a) A family history
(b) His BMI
(c) Hypercholesterolemia
(d) Hypertriclyceridemia
(e) Hypertension
(f) Smoking

Answer

(a) Agree. His father's early death suggests he may have a genetic predisposition.
(b) Disagree. Overweight people are at increased risk.
(c) Agree. Hypercholesterolemia. The therapeutic goal is a total blood cholesterol no more than 5.5 mmol/l, a low density lipoprotein (LDL) cholesterol below 3.0 mmol/l and an HDL well above 1 mmol/l.
(d) Disagree. Hypertriclyceridemia. Fasting triglycerides over 2.0 mmol/l is a marker of increased coronary heart disease risk.
(e) Disagree. His blood pressure is normal.
(f) Agree. Smoking increases the risk of coronary artery disease by at least 1.7-fold. It increases the risk of coronary artery spasm. Spasm is a particular risk for the critical event, i.e. it is a factor that precipitates a heart attack.

Case study continues

Having identified the patient has a family history and at least two of the major lifestyle risk factors for ischemic heart disease, the consultation turns to ascertaining whether there is evidence of any complications arising from the patient's angina.

Chest auscultation: Heart: No gallop. No pulse deficit. Heart regular.
Lungs: No basal crepitations.

Special investigations: Cardiac enzymes: normal, including rapid cardiac troponin.
ECG: Pain occurred while having the ECG. Transient ST segment elevation was recorded. The pain was relieved by nitroglycerine.

Based on the patient's history, physical examination and special investigations the definitive diagnosis is:
(a) Stable angina
(b) Nocturnal angina
(c) Decubitus angina
(d) Spasm angina
(e) Acute coronary insufficiency

Answer (d) Spasm angina

Clinical decision 5: How should this patient be managed? Intervention involves reducing the risk of a heart attack due to coronary occlusion attributable to:

- Spasm. Quit smoking immediately. See http://www.jamisonhealth.com. 300–1000 IU vitamin E or 1–3 grams vitamin C daily improve endothelium-dependent vasodilatation.
- Thrombosis. 200–400 IU vitamin E daily inhibits platelet adhesion. 35 grams of cold-water fish, a glass of red wine and/or 2 corms of garlic daily also reduce the risk of clot formation.
- Atheromatous plaque. Reduce oxidized cholesterol. A lifestyle change to regular exercise a diet high in fresh fruit and vegetables, whole grains and low in animal fats. Include fish and soy. Two serves of soy products, e.g. 200 g tofu + 2 cups soy milk or 1 cup soy flour daily lowers cholesterol.

A case study demonstrating the principles of screening

Mary Jones presents asking for a check-up. This 30-year-old woman says she is perfectly well and has really made the appointment because she wants to be 'on the books' should she become ill at some future time. She has no family or personal history that gives grounds for concern. She is a nonsmoker and drinks around 3 glasses of red wine each day.

Select the screening procedures you believe should be routinely performed on an apparently healthy patient:

Case study continues

(a) Total serum cholesterol
(b) Body mass index (BMI)
(c) Mammography
(d) Papanicolaou smear
(e) Blood pressure reading
(f) Digital examination for rectal cancer

Answer

(a) Agree. Total serum cholesterol readings are indicated every 4 years in adults under the age of 50 years. Older adults also require an HDL determination.
(b) Agree. Health risk increases when the BMI exceeds 25. The formula for calculation is BMI = weight (kg)/height (m^2). Acceptable body weight is a BMI of 20–25. Overweight persons have a BMI of over 25 but less than 30. Obesity is diagnosed when the BMI is 30 or over.
(c) Disagree. Mammography is only recommended for high-risk patients under the age of 50 years. Professional breast examination is recommended for all women over 20 years of age. Monthly breast self-examination is recommended for all women. Menstruating woman should perform breast self-examination a few days after the end of their menstrual period. Postmenopausal women can select any day of the month, provided they establish a routine. See http://www.jamisonhealth.com for details on how to perform breast self-examination and information on patient guidelines for seeking professional advice.
(d) Agree. Papanicolaou smears are recommended for sexually active women up to the age of 70 years. The first two smears should be performed annually; thereafter smears at 3-yearly intervals suffice.
(e) Agree. Hypertension is a silent killer. Persons who feel well can be walking around with blood pressure raised to levels that cause irreversible target organ damage. A blood pressure reading above 140/90 mmHg on three or more serial readings is diagnostic of hypertension in healthy adults 25–40 years of age.
(f) Disagree. Annual screening for colorectal cancer by digital rectal examination is recommended from the age of 40 years. Annual fecal occult blood tests are recommended for asymptomatic patients over the age of 50 years followed by one flexible proctosigmoidoscopy examination at 55 years of age.

Results *Mary's total blood cholesterol, breast examination, Pap smear and BMI are all within normal limits. Her blood pressure is however of some concern.*

Please indicate whether and, where appropriate, why accurate determination of Mary's blood pressure requires attention to:

Case study continues

(a) Selection of the type of baumanometer used
(b) Cuff selection
(c) Palpated systolic pressure
(d) Blood pressure in both arms
(e) Patient comfort

Answer (a–e) agree.

You chat to Mary for several minutes making sure she is relaxed before taking her blood pressure again. This time in her right arm. You carefully adhere to the blood pressure protocol and note the following:

BP right arm: 150/93.
You repeat the reading: BP right arm 148/94; 149/93.

You compare this to the reading in the left arm: BP 145/92; 146/93.

Your final determination and interpretation of Mary's blood pressure on this occasion is:
(a) 150/94 – Mild hypertension
(b) 145/92 – Normotension
(c) 149/93 – Normotension
(d) 145/92 – Mild hypertension
(e) 149/93 – Mild hypertension

Working diagnosis (e) 149/93 – Mild hypertension

In the light of your diagnosis you:
(a) Discharge Mary and tell her she is 'on your books' as a patient.
(b) Suggest she return for further evaluation of her blood pressure.
(c) Place her on antihypertensive therapy.
(d) Suggest she cut down her wine intake to no more than 2 glasses, or preferably 1 glass daily.
(e) Suggest she decreases her sodium intake and increases her potassium intake by eating more fruit and vegetables and avoiding salty and processed foods.

Answer
(a) Disagree. Further care is required both to establish the diagnosis, exclude a treatable cause and screen for the early onset of complications.
(b) Agree. Before initiating therapy, particularly drug therapy, further evaluation of her blood pressure is desirable. When therapy is initiated on the basis of a single sign it is important that the diagnosis is based on a specific test that is accurately performed.

Case study continues

(c) Disagree. Antihypertensive medication has side-effects. Before placing a patient on medication an accurate measurement and interpretation of the blood pressure level is essential. At this level of hypertension drug therapy is not indicated.
(d) Agree. Suggest she cut down her wine intake to no more than 2 glasses, or preferably 1 glass daily. The consumption of alcohol by women should not exceed 2 glasses (20 grams) of alcohol per day on a regular basis, or 140 grams per week. More than 20 grams of alcohol daily tends to raise blood pressure.
(e) Agree. Suggests she decreases her sodium intake and increases her potassium intake by eating more fruit and vegetables and avoiding salty and processed foods. This dietary recommendation benefits blood pressure and general health.

Before ending the consultation you check to see if Mary has secondary hypertension by:
(a) Confirming she isn't troubled by headaches and palpitations
(b) Urinanalysis
(c) Asking about her drug intake
(d) Check the blood pressure in her lower limbs
(e) Ask if her sleep is disturbed by having to pass urine at night.

Answer
(a) Agree. Headaches and palpitations may indicate pheochromocytoma.
(b) Agree. Proteinuria suggests renal disease.
(c) Agree. Many drugs including NSAIDs, steroids, caffeine and cold remedies may raise blood pressure.
(d) Agree. Patients with coarctation of the aorta have normal blood pressure in their lower limbs, raised blood pressure in the upper limbs and a delay between the radial and femoral pulse on palpation.
(e) Agree. Nocturia is found in renal disease and in hyperaldosteronism.

As you expected there is no evidence of secondary hypertension. Your working diagnosis is essential hypertension. You have Mary make an appointment to confirm your diagnosis and make a note in her file to remind you to exclude target organ damage. When Mary returns for her next appointment you confirm she has mild hypertension and although complications are not currently anticipated, you check her target organs for damage to ensure you have a baseline for future reference:

(a) Left ventricular failure
(b) Congestive cardiac failure
(c) Retinopathy
(d) Renal bruits
(e) Ascites

Case study continues

Answer (a) Agree. Systemic hypertension is a cause of left-sided failure.
(b) Disagree. Congestive cardiac failure is a consequence of pulmonary hypertension. Cor pulmonale is right heart failure due to lung disease.
(c) Agree. However hypertensive retinopathy is not likely at Mary's current level of hypertension.
(d) Disagree. Renal bruits may indicate stenosis of the renal artery and are a cause not a consequence of hypertension.
(e) Disagree. Ascites is a consequence of portal hypertension.

You tell Mary you want to keep an eye on her blood pressure, suggest further lifestyle changes and make an appointment to see her in 3 months time to review the need for drug therapy.

REFERENCES

1 Jamison J R 1991 Diagnostic decision making in primary practice. In: Lawrence D, Forsman S (eds) Seminars in chiropractic. Vol 2(1). Williams & Wilkins, Baltimore, MD
2 Souza T 1994 Which orthopedic tests are really necessary? Advances in Chiropractic 4:101–158
3 Jamison J R 1996 The placebo in clinical care. Advances in Chiropractic 3:319–343
4 Sagie A, Larson M G, Levy D 1993 The natural history of borderline systolic hypertension. New England Journal of Medicine 329:1912–1917
5 Applegate W B 1992 The relative importance of focusing on elevations of systolic vs diastolic blood pressure: a definitive answer at last. Archives of Internal Medicine 152:1969–1971
6 Agewall S, Wikstrand J, Ljungman S et al 1995 Does microalbuminuria predict cardiovascular events in nondiabetic men with treated hypertension? American Journal of Hypertension 8:337–342
7 Kannel W B, Gordeon T, Schwartz M J 1971 Systolic versus diastolic blood pressure and the risk of coronary artery disease: the Framingham Study. American Journal of Cardiology 27:335–346
8 Cranswick R 1988 Hypertension and the heart. Patient Management 12:45–55
9 Stamler J, Rose G, Stamler R et al 1989 Intersalt study findings: public health and medical care implications. Hypertension 14:570–577
10 Fraser A 1989 Measurement of blood pressure. Australian Family Physician 18:355–357
11 Hunyor S N, Kewal N K 1985 Screening for high blood pressure – do's and don'ts. Patient Management July:91–101
12 Phillips P A 1993 Initial and long-term monitoring of hypertension. General Practitioner 1:217–220
13 Kannel W B 1987 Hypertension. Current Therapeutics January:87–106
14 Colquhoun D 1993 Hypertension and heart disease. Australian Family Physician 22:679–687
15 Moser M, Black H, Stair D 1987 The dilemma of mild hypertension. Current Therapeutics 28:29–43
16 Tallis G, Judd S 1996 Case studies in endocrine hypertension. Australian Family Physician 25:331–344

CHAPTER

2 The principles of drug therapy

PART ONE

CHAPTER CONTENTS

A clinical response may be the result of spontaneous remission or regression to the mean, or to a nonspecific or a specific therapy. Spontaneous remission is the predicted outcome given the natural history of a self-limiting disease. A nonspecific or placebo outcome may be anticipated to produce marginal gains in a wide variety of conditions. Specific therapy may, however, be expected to produce substantial improvement in a limited number of conditions. While nonspecific therapy may enhance well-being in most patients, the usefulness of specific therapy is limited to those conditions for which it achieves a particular physiological change.

The success of specific therapy is determined by a correct diagnosis, the efficacy of the therapy, and the prevalence and nature of side-effects. As the therapy selected is based on the diagnosis, an incorrect diagnosis results in inappropriate therapy. A wrong diagnosis is the basis of bad clinical care. A wrong diagnosis can exacerbate the patient's illness by:

- *Omission.* The patient's condition may worsen due to failure of the clinician to halt the progression of the disease by failing to use the best available treatment.
- *Commission.* Prescribing the wrong therapy results in inappropriate modification of the patient's physiology or biochemistry and exposes the patient to unnecessary

side-effects. Taking the wrong drug can cause illness; even taking the right drug therapy can have unwanted side-effects. The likelihood of adverse consequences is reduced by an accurate diagnosis and by using drugs that specifically interact at a limited number of biochemical sites. The more selective the drug, the fewer the side-effects and the more imperative the need for a correct diagnosis.

The basis of good patient care is an accurate diagnosis.

DRUG THERAPY

Drugs are chemical agents that have been produced to alter the pathophysiological environment of the patient. While the ritual of the clinical consultation ensures that all drugs have some nonspecific impact, drug therapy is most effective when used to produce a specific functional change. As drugs inevitably have a potent physiological impact, continuous monitoring of the patient's response is recommended. This includes:[1]

- an attempt to explain, within a biologically plausible framework, any clinical changes detected following introduction of the therapy
- evaluation of the timeframe between therapy and clinical change
- some assessment of patient compliance or adherence to any management regimen.

The drug intervention model prefers to err on the side of caution.

Every drug prescriber should want to know the range of possible adverse effects of the medicines he or she prescribes. One needs to know the probability of such effects being related to the medicine, the possible severity and duration of the effects, and how frequently they occur to decide, in each therapeutic situation, the risk to benefit balance.[2]

All drugs have adverse reactions or side-effects. These unwanted outcomes may be attributable to:

- Direct drug toxicity due to an
  - overdose
  - unavoidable consequence of the mechanism of drug action.
- Drug interactions. Drugs may interact and thus
  - potentiate the clinical response (e.g. aspirin and warfarin enhance a bleeding tendency)
  - neutralize overall drug efficacy (e.g. the anticoagulant effect of warfarin is impaired by vitamin K administration).
- Individual susceptibility. This may present as:
  - intolerance: the usual pharmacological reaction occurs at a low dose

  - idiosyncrasy: particular individuals have unusual and unpredictable reactions
  - allergy: an immunologically mediated response may make a drug unsafe in hypersensitive individuals
  - pseudoallergy: a reaction that mimics allergy in the absence of an immune response.
- Disease-induced susceptibility. Abnormalities of drug metabolism or excretion may be encountered in disease states.

Adverse effects may be immediate or delayed (e.g. teratogenicity, malignancy). Confirmation that an immediate clinical outcome is attributable to a particular drug may be sought by withdrawing the therapy and monitoring the clinical change. If the intervention is causative then the clinical change should weaken or disappear. Reintroduction of a causative therapy should once again precipitate the clinical change.

MECHANISM OF DRUG THERAPY

Drug therapy seeks to restore the patient's health status by:

- Modifying the host's response to the disease process through mechanisms such as:
  - Pathophysiological responses. Exaggeration or inappropriate stimulation of physiological responses can have deleterious effects. Drugs can limit potentially deleterious host responses to physical, chemical, or microbial stressors. Drugs can be used to: alter the responsiveness of cell membrane receptors; inhibit enzyme activation of inflammatory responses; or neutralize toxic metabolic products such as free radicals.
  - The autonomic nervous system. The balance between the parasympathetic and sympathetic nervous system can be altered by using drugs that mimic neurotransmitters, block receptors, or inhibit enzyme breakdown of neurotransmitters.
- Eliminating the agent responsible for the disorder by
  - preventing multiplication of and allowing the body to eliminate infective organisms
  - destroying a pathogenic bacterium.

DRUG PRESCRIPTION

Once the efficacy of an intervention has been established and awareness of adverse effects has been achieved, then the cost–benefit ratio of using any particular intervention can be ascertained. It is the utility of one intervention compared with another, given a particular patient's circumstances, that guides the clinician in determining which intervention is preferred in a specific situation.

Optimal drug prescription takes cognisance of the effects of various drug formulations with regard to efficacy and safety in diverse circumstances. Changes to the structure of a compound can markedly modify safety and efficacy. Attempts to reduce the adverse effects of pharmaceuticals include measures such as the following:[3]

- *Producing 'new' drugs.* Different formulations may have diverse clinical actions and be less prone to cause indirect side-effects. Niacin at a therapeutic dose of about 3 g/day reduces blood cholesterol, but causes flushing, gastric irritation, and pruritus.[4–6] Niacinamide causes vasodilatation, but does not have these side-effects. Niacinamide, however, also fails to reduce elevated serum cholesterol levels.
- *Modifying the form in which a drug is ingested.* Aspirin is manufactured in enteric-coated, soluble, and sodium salicylate forms in order to reduce the risk of gastrointestinal bleeding and dyspepsia.
- *Timing the medication in relation to the ingestion of food and drink.* Nonsteroidal anti-inflammatory drugs (NSAIDs) and alcohol should not be taken together. NSAIDs should be taken with meals or with an antacid before eating.
- *Modifying the dose and frequency of drug ingestion.* High doses of water-soluble vitamins delivered in a bolus may saturate the active transport mechanism, and passive diffusion can contribute to nutrient absorption. Maximum bioavailability of water-soluble nutrient supplements appears to be achieved when preparations release their contents rapidly and achieve a maximum concentration at the intestinal mucosa. Both drug efficacy and side-effects may be affected.
- *Modifying the structure of the pharmaceutical to limit its activity to a target site.* Etodolac, a new structurally distinct NSAID, is believed to inhibit prostaglandin synthesis in a tissue-specific fashion. Cyclooxygenase-1 (cox-1) is the isoform responsible for physiological protection of stomach mucosa, regulation of renal blood flow, and sodium excretion, and is involved in platelet aggregation. Cyclooxygenase-2 (cox-2) is produced following tissue damage and is mediated via cytokines involved in the inflammatory response. It stimulates the synthesis of prostaglandins from arachidonic acid. Inhibition of cox-2 should reduce inflammation. Newer NSAIDs selectively inhibit cox-2. Prostaglandin depletion in gastric mucosa appears to be avoided, as the prostaglandin produced in the stomach is produced by cox-1. A cox-2-selective inhibitor would be expected to inhibit some prostaglandin synthesis without exhibiting ulcerogenic activity.

Intervention with pharmacologically active agents requires a knowledge of the dose at which a therapeutic effect can be achieved and how this dose differs from that at which toxicity emerges. The larger the difference between a therapeutic and toxic dose, the smaller the risk of an inadvertent overdose. Drug intervention also requires some appreciation of the active principle in a pharmaceutical product, and how the delivery and activity of this chemical may be modified by alterations in its chemical environment. In some cases an understanding of the mechanism underlying the pharmaceutical's mode of action may be helpful in detecting and predicting untoward effects.

MODIFYING THE TONE OF THE AUTONOMIC NERVOUS SYSTEM

The autonomic nervous system is composed of parasympathetic and sympathetic components. Acetylcholine is the neurotransmitter in the parasympathetic nervous system. Acetylcholine is the neurotransmitter at the ganglion of the sympathetic nervous system, while norepinephrine is the transmitter at the post-ganglionic effector site. Specific receptors in the neuroeffector organ take up the neurotransmitter. Drugs may modify the effect of the autonomic nervous system by blocking these receptors or by masquerading as the neurotransmitter. Drugs that stimulate receptors and mimic endogenous transmitters are termed *agonists*.[7] Drugs that block receptors and inhibit endogenous transmitters are termed *antagonists*. Their effect is determined by their site.

Drug interaction with the sympathetic nervous system

The activity of the sympathetic nervous system can be influenced by drugs acting at receptor sites. Two major groups of receptors, α- (α_1 and α_2) and β- (β_1 and β_2) adrenergic receptors, take up and respond to norepinephrine. Both α- and β-adrenergic receptors affect diverse organ systems. Organ function is often affected by the balance or mixture of α- and β-adrenergic receptors in an organ. The combined action of α- and β-adrenergic receptors in the gut decreases bowel motility and increases sphincter tone.

α-Adrenergic receptors in

- blood vessels cause vasoconstriction
- the pancreas decrease insulin and glucagon release
- the liver enhance glycogenolysis
- the uterus cause contraction
- the skin stimulate sweating.

The action of adrenergic receptors within a particular group may be subdivided further. β-Adrenergic receptors can be divided into at least two groups:

- β_1-Receptors predominate in the myocardium and the cardiac conducting system. Stimulation of β_2-receptors causes:

  - Tachycardia: stimulation increases the rate and force of myocardial contraction. Repeated agonist stimulation of cardiac β_1-receptors reduces the clinical effect.
  - Lipolysis: adipose lipids are mobilized and enter the bloodstream.
  - Decreased digestion.
  - Decreased gastrointestinal motility.
  - Renin release. Subsequent angiotensin II formation and vasoconstriction cause an increase in renal blood flow.
- β_2-Receptors predominate in airways, blood vessels, uterus, and skeletal muscle. Stimulation of β_2-receptors causes:
  - Airway bronchodilatation. Repeated agonist stimulation of airway β_2-receptors does not result in down-regulation of the receptor responsiveness.
  - Vasodilatation.
  - Uterine relaxation.
  - Muscle tremors.
  - Glycolysis, gluconeogenesis, increased insulin secretion.
  - Lipolysis and hypokalemia.

β_2-Receptor stimulation benefits patients with bronchospasm. β_2-Receptor agonists are used in asthma therapy. The potential clinical benefits of β_2-receptor agonists (sympathomimetics) in asthma include:

- bronchodilatation
- inhibition of inflammatory mediator release (membrane stabilization reduces mediator release from mast cells)
- modulation or normalization of mucus production
- modulation of mucociliary transport (ciliary activity is increased)
- inhibition of microvascular damage
- inhibition of cholinergic transmission (parasympathetic stimulation enhances bronchoconstriction and mucus production).

However, β_2-receptors are not limited to airways. Drugs used to stimulate β_2-receptors inevitably have a number of unwanted effects. Side-effects may be due to:

- Direct stimulation of β_2-receptors in tissue other than the lung. Unwanted effects of using β_2-agonists in asthma treatment are dose related and include:
  - tachyarrhythmias, vasodilatation, and prolongation of the QT interval in the electrocardiogram (ECG)
  - anxiety, agitation, tremor, and headache
  - muscle cramps and elevated creatinine kinase
  - hyperglycemia, hypokalemia, lactacidemia, and hypophosphatemia.
- Associated inadvertent β_1-receptor stimulation. This is most likely to occur when the drug (agonist) is used in high doses.

In selecting a particular agonist to treat asthma, the relative receptor activity of the drug is taken into consideration. The relative β_2/β_1-receptor activity of isoprenaline is 1, of salbutamol is 650, of fenoterol is 200, of fromoterol is 500, and of salmeterol is 50 000.

In addition to stimulating receptors by mimicking the transmitter, drugs may be used to prevent the neurotransmitter reaching the receptor. Sympatholytics or adrenergic antagonists acting at the level of α_1-receptors cause:

- vasodilatation and hypotension
- pupil constriction
- increased intestinal motility and secretion
- glycogen synthesis, thereby decreasing blood glucose
- impotence
- enhanced micturition.

A major clinical use for α_1-receptor blockers is the treatment of high blood pressure. Phenoxybenzamine, phentolamine, and prazosin are α_1-receptor antagonists used in the control of hypertension and peripheral vascular disease. Common adverse effects are nasal congestion, postural hypotension, and lack of energy. β_1-Receptor blockers are used to control hypertension, but through a different mechanism. β_1-Receptor antagonists:

- decrease heart rate and stroke volume and, therefore, cardiac output
- increase gut motility and secretions
- inhibit renin release and, therefore, decrease blood pressure.

β_1-Receptor antagonists such as atenolol, esmolol, and metoprolol are used in the treatment of hypertension. Acebutolol, pindolol, propranolol, and timolol are nonselective β-blockers and, consequently, have more side-effects. Common side-effects include dizziness, lethargy, insomnia, cardiogenic shock, and circulatory disorders. β_1-Receptor antagonists are also used to treat cardiac disease, migraine, and thyrotoxicosis.

Drug interaction with the parasympathetic nervous system

Drugs can also be used to modulate parasympathetic nervous activity. Two types of cholinergic receptor have been identified: nicotinic receptors, which are located centrally, in autonomic ganglia, and the neuromuscular junction of skeletal muscles; and muscarinic receptors, which are widespread centrally and peripherally.

Stimulation of nicotinic receptors results in:

- behavior changes with increased relaxation and a sense of well-being
- increased autonomic tone
- increased skeletal muscle tone

- release of epinephrine and norepinephrine from the adrenal medulla.

Adverse effects of stimulation of nicotine receptors include cardiovascular stimulation, headaches, nausea, and insomnia. Nicotinic antagonists are used to:

- control hypertension by inducing vasodilatation of systemic blood pressure
- achieve profound muscle relaxation (suxamethonium, a nicotinic antagonist, is used when intubating patients during anesthesia).

Muscarinic receptors are located at the postganglionic effector site of glands and in smooth and cardiac muscle. Three types of muscarinic receptor have been identified:

- M_1 receptors are located predominantly in the brain and mediate higher cerebral function. A decrease in M_1 receptors is found in Alzheimer's disease and other dementias. M_1 receptor agonists enhance cognition and increase gastric acid secretion.
- M_2 receptors are found in the myocardium, where they trigger a decrease in the rate (negative chronotropic) and force (negative inotropic) of cardiac contraction.
- M_3 receptors are found in visceral smooth muscle and exocrine glands. Stimulation of M_3 receptors results in:
  - miosis or pupil constriction
  - an increased rate of aqueous fluid drainage from the anterior chamber of the eye
  - relaxation of gastrointestinal sphincters
  - increased gastrointestinal motility
  - increased secretion of digestive juices
  - promotion of micturition and defecation
  - increased insulin resistance, enhanced glycogenesis, and gluconeogenesis
  - lacrimation
  - bronchoconstriction and increased bronchial mucus production
  - vasoconstriction in the skin and external genitalia
  - vasodilatation in skeletal muscle
  - sweating.

Muscarinic agonists, such as acetylcholine, bethanechol, carbochol, and pilocarpine, are used to treat:

- glaucoma and mydriasis
- constipation and other intestinal disorders with diminished motility
- urinary retention
- tachycardia.

Adverse effects include pupillary constriction, diarrhea, urinary incontinence, bronchoconstriction, and sweating. These drugs should not be used in persons with urinary or intestinal obstruction.

The concentration of acetylcholine at receptor sites can also be increased by inhibiting the breakdown of this transmitter. Cholinesterase inhibitors, such as neostigmine and physostigmine, are used in the treatment of glaucoma and conditions affecting the neuromuscular junction (e.g. motor neuron disease).

Muscarinic antagonists (anticholinergic agents) include atropine, hyoscine, mebeverine, and many others. Anticholinergic agents are used as:

- antispasmodics, to counter gastrointestinal spasm
- antiarrhythmics, to counteract bradycardia
- antiasthmatics, to suppress bronchial mucus production and enhance bronchodilatation
- antiemetics, because their central action counteracts motion sickness
- gastric acid secretion suppressants in patients with peptic ulcer syndrome.

MODULATING PATHOPHYSIOLOGICAL RESPONSES

Pathophysiological responses may be modified by drugs acting on a diversity of mechanisms. Three important pathophysiological mechanisms that are the target for drug intervention are:

- the allergic response
- inflammation
- production and quenching of free radicals.

Modifying an allergic response

Histamine is plentiful in lung, skin, and intestinal mucosa. It is found in an inactive bound form in platelets, mast cells, and basophils. Histamine:

- causes vasodilatation
- increases vascular permeability
- enhances gastric acid secretion.

In classic allergy, the cross-linkage of two immunoglobulin E (IgE) molecules on the mast cell membrane releases histamine and other mediators from the mast cell. Histamine achieves its effect through binding to cell receptors. Drugs which are used to prevent the clinical effects of histamine exert their effect by successfully competing with histamine for cell receptors. The greatest successes of antihistamines are in the treatment of allergic rhinitis, urticaria, and atopic eczema. Antihistamines may also be used in asthma therapy. As histamine is only one of a number of chemicals involved in the mediation of allergic reactions, antihistaminics improve, but do not totally prevent, the clinical manifestations of allergy.

The effectiveness of antihistamines is therefore determined by:

- The ability of the drug to reach and block the receptor before it is occupied by histamine. All antihistamines are, consequently, most appropriately used in a prophylactic manner.[8,9]
- The specificity and fit of the drug and the histamine receptor on the cell membrane.

There are three types of histamine receptor:

- H_3 receptors have a modulating function in the brain.
- H_2 receptors are plentiful in the parietal cells of the stomach. A major clinical effect of stimulating H_2 receptors is acid production in the stomach. Stimulation of H_2 receptors results in:
  - gastric acid secretion
  - mucus secretion
  - increased cyclic adenosine monophosphate (cAMP)
  - inhibition of lymphokine release, basophil histamine release, neutrophil enzyme release, eosinophil migration, and T-lymphocyte mediated cytotoxicity.

Blocking H_2 receptors by antihistamines with a specific H_2 blocking action is useful for treating peptic ulcers. By selectively targeting cell receptors side-effects are minimized. The H_2 blocking action of these drugs can even counteract the ulcerogenic effect of NSAIDs and achieve healing of peptic ulcers in these patients. Intervention with one drug can enhance the safe use of a second drug. Antihistamines with a specific H_2 blocking action include cimetidine (Tagamet), ranitidine (Zantac), and famotidine (Amfamox, Pepcidine).

- H_1 receptors mediate the allergic response. H_1 receptors are found mainly in smooth muscles and the exocrine glands of the respiratory tree. Stimulation of H_1 receptors results in:
  - increased vascular permeability leading to edema and pruritus
  - smooth-muscle constriction leading to bronchospasm, abdominal pain, and vomiting
  - irritant receptor stimulation resulting in itching, pain, and sneezing
  - prostaglandin generation
  - increased cyclic guanosine monophosphate (cGMP)
  - a positive chronotropic effect manifest as an increased heart rate.

Older 'classic' histamines lacked specificity. This resulted in them having a diversity of side-effects. In addition to their H_1 blocking action, they have:

- An anticholinergic effect with resultant:
  - drying of secretions (this side-effect is useful in rhinitis, but the associated dry mouth can be unpleasant)
  - elevation of intraocular pressure resulting in blurred vision (these drugs are contraindicated in narrow angle glaucoma)
  - urinary retention in prostatic hypertrophy (any sign of prostatism is a contraindication to use of these drugs).
- An antiserotoninergic effect.
- A local anesthetic effect.
- A membrane stabilizing effect (this reduces the allergic response).
- A depressant effect on the central nervous system, leading to:
  - sedation (drowsiness is a major problem, and alcohol consumption while on these drugs is proscribed)
  - impaired psychomotor performance.
- Other side-effects, including:
  - gastrointestinal upsets (abdominal discomfort, nausea, constipation, and diarrhea)
  - rarely, neutropenia and agranulocytosis.

In view of these unwanted effects, a new generation of antihistamines was developed which bound avidly to H_1 receptors. The H_1 receptors blocking antihistamines, in contrast to the older antihistamines, are:

- nonsedating
- lack anticholinergic effects
- lipophobic (they have no psychomotor effect, as they do not cross the blood–brain barrier)
- more anti-inflammatory (blocking H_1 receptors decreases release of inflammatory mediators from cells during antigen challenge).

By refining the drug–receptor fit an improved therapeutic effect is achieved with fewer side-effects. These drugs are, however, more expensive.

Both H_1 and H_2 receptors are found in the brain and cardiac muscle. Stimulation of both H_1 and H_2 receptors results in:

- vasodilatation (hypotension)
- headache
- flushing.

Headaches, dizziness, and hypotension can be a problem.

Combination preparations of antihistamines with adrenergic agents may also be purchased over the counter as, for example, decongestants. Potential side-effects of such preparations are palpitations, tachycardia, weakness, mydriasis, and insomnia. Combinations of antihistamines, adrenergic agents, and an antipyretic/analgesic agent may be found in certain cold remedies. Potential adverse effects include sedation, urinary retention (prostatism), and glaucoma.

Modifying inflammation

A diversity of drugs are used to modify the inflammatory response. In addition to their anti-inflammatory effects, NSAIDs are used for their analgesic, antipyretic, and antithrombotic effects. The analgesic and anti-inflammatory effects of NSAIDs are dose dependent, rapid in onset, and reversible.

The clinical effectiveness of NSAIDs is influenced by:[10]

- *The ability to concentrate the drug in an area of inflammation.* This depends on the ionization constant (p*K*a) of the preparation, which determines the distribution of a drug in tissue. NSAIDs are all weakly acidic. The p*K*a of NSAIDs is 3–5; that is, at a pH of 3–5 half of the NSAID is ionized and half is un-ionized. The un-ionized drug is more lipid soluble than the ionized drug, and consequently un-ionized drugs penetrate lipid membranes more easily. In an acidic environment there is relatively more un-ionized drug to diffuse across the cell membrane. Once inside the cell there is proportionately less un-ionized drug and the drug is 'trapped' inside the cell. The extracellular fluid of the synovium is relatively acidic, and the intracellular environment of the synovial tissue is relatively alkaline. Relatively more un-ionized NSAID is found in the synovial fluid. The un-ionized drug is lipid soluble and diffuse across the cell membrane. Once inside the synovial cell, the relatively alkaline environment enhances ionization and intracellular trapping of the drug. Acidic NSAIDs concentrate in areas of relative acidity, such as inflamed joints, the renal medulla, and the gastric mucosa.
- *The dose of the drug used.* The dose of aspirin used is a determinant of both its clinical efficacy and its toxic effect. Aspirin toxicity is strongly dose related: 0.73 for 651–2600 mg/day, 1.08 for 2601–3900 mg/day, and 1.91 for more than 3900 mg/day.[11] The toxicity index for aspirin is 1.37, as compared with 1.87–2.9 for selected NSAIDs. Toxicity for plain aspirin is 1.36, for buffered aspirin 1.1, and for enteric-coated aspirin 0.92. The dose required for clinical efficacy of aspirin is as follows:[12]
  - For cardiovascular complications, 75–325 mg/day. A dose of 75–80 mg/day appears to have a maximum effect on platelet adhesiveness. At these doses selective inhibition of thromboxane can prolong the bleeding time for up to 5 days
  - For cerebrovascular problems, more than 325 mg/day
  - For analgesia, 300–600 mg/day, with peak effect at doses of 2.0–5.0 g/day. The analgesic effect lasts for about 4 hours
  - For an anti-inflammatory effect, 900–3600 mg/day. The optimal anti-inflammatory effect is achieved at a plasma level of 1.1–2.2 mmol/l (150–300 mg/l). The anti-inflammatory effect lasts much longer than the analgesic effect.

- *Their ability to modify prostaglandin synthesis.* Prostaglandins, PGE and $PGF_2\alpha$, thromboxane A_2, and prostacyclin are an integral part of the inflammatory reaction. Prostaglandins
  - are directly proinflammatory, increasing vascularity and permeability
  - facilitate mediators such as bradykinin and histamine, which further potentiate the pain, vascularity, and permeability of the lesion.

NSAIDs have been found to be potent inhibitors of cyclooxygenase, the enzyme that converts arachidonic acid to prostaglandins. Aspirin differs from other NSAIDs in that it irreversibly acetylates cyclooxygenase. The ability of platelets to synthesize the vasoactive agent thromboxane A_2 is eliminated by a single aspirin dose. This makes aspirin the NSAID of choice for prevention of coagulation. Mechanisms other than inhibition of cyclooxygenase have also been postulated to explain the clinical effects of NSAIDs:[13]

- Inhibition of lipoxygenase, the enzyme involved in formation of the inflammatory leukotrienes.
- Inhibition of polymorph functions, such as the release of
  - free radicals
  - lysosomal enzymes
  - polymorph migration.
- The ability of aspirin to inhibit the activity of NF-κB, a factor needed for transcription of some genes associated with inflammation in general and replication of the human immunodeficiency virus (HIV) in particular.[14] The dose of aspirin required to achieve this anti-inflammatory effect is higher than that required to inhibit prostaglandin synthesis. The transcription factor activates genes for several cytokines, an interferon, and a tumor necrosis factor. The dose needed is compatible with clinical treatment levels.

In addition to their antipyretic, anti-inflammatory, and analgesic effects, NSAIDs may have a role as a chemopreventive agent in colon cancer. In rat models of colon carcinogenesis, cyclooxygenase inhibitors, such as indometacin, prioxicam, and sulindac, have exhibited chemopreventive effects. The mechanism is as yet unknown. One possible mechanism may be via an inhibitory effect on prostaglandin synthesis, causing suppression of cell proliferation or stimulation of the immune response. Certain eicosanoids stimulate or inhibit cell proliferation, enhance or retard tumor cell metastasis, and depress the immune response. Sulindac has also been shown to produce a sulfide metabolite when acted upon by anaerobes in the colon; the end-product causes regression of adenomatous polyps. Sulindac reduces the size and number of rectal polyps in individuals with familial polyposis. When sulindac administration is discontinued, the tumors recur, and resumption of sulindac treatment causes regression.

The beneficial effects of aspirin on gastrointestinal cancer are still under investigation, but an aspirin on 4 days per week or more ('regular use') over more than 12 months has been associated with a 40% reduction in the incidence of colorectal and stomach cancers.[15] Various reports suggest that aspirin may reduce death rates from colorectal cancer in persons who, over 10 years, take aspirin 16 times a month or more, compared with nonusers. A study in the USA found that 22 000 people who took aspirin every other day over 5 years had their risk of colorectal cancer reduced by no more than 20%. In 1991, the American Cancer Society suggested that, of 600 000 people, those who took aspirin more than 15 times a month for at least 12 months, 40% are less likely to die of colorectal cancer. A similar finding was a 50% decreased risk in an English study. A prospective mortality study of 662 424 adults found death rates through 1988 from colorectal cancer decreased with more frequent use of aspirin. The risk of colorectal cancer was halved in a woman who had taken 4–6 aspirin tablets each week over a 20-year period. A hospital-based case-control study found a 50% reduction in colorectal cancer with regular use of NSAIDs of at least 4 days a week for a minimum of 3 months. People who take aspirin or other NSAIDs (e.g. ibuprofen) appear to be at a significantly lower risk of colorectal cancer. Recently, several groups have reported the detection of a proliferation-associated gene cyclooxygenase (cox-2).[16] This form of prostaglandin is different to that required by gastric mucosa (cox-1). Development of a drug that selectively inhibits the cox-2 form of cyclooxygenase responsible for prostaglandin synthesis in the colon may offer effective chemoprevention against colon cancer, with minimal gastric side-effects. Adverse effects of NSAIDs may be attributed to the following factors:

- *The physiological consequences of prostaglandin synthetase inhibition.* Alteration of prostaglandin production impairs their normal function, including:[17,18]
  - Modulation of acid production and mucosal blood flow in gastric mucosa. Prostaglandins stimulate secretion of bicarbonate and mucus, and thus protect the mucosa from luminal acid and pepsin. Prostaglandin E_2 inhibits acid secretion and accelerates ulcer healing. The form of cyclo-oxygenase responsible for prostaglandin synthesis in the stomach appears to be cox-1. Inhibition of cox-1 by NSAIDs leads to gastric ulceration. NSAIDs may also precipitate protective glycoproteins. The most frequent of all serious adverse reactions associated with NSAID therapy involves the upper gastrointestinal tract. The total risk of gastro-intestinal ulceration, including dyspepsia, gastritis, bleeding,

and perforation, is 1–2% of patients who take NSAIDs for 3 months, and increases to 2–5% for patients who take NSAIDs for 12 months. The odds ratio for chronic gastric ulcers of at least 12 months' duration is assessed as 4.7 for NSAIDs, 6.9 for cigarette smoking, and 16.4 for over-the-counter aspirin. Recent research suggests that selective targeting of specific forms of cyclooxygenase production may provide a solution.[16]
  - Autoregulation of renal blood flow. Prostaglandins affect glomerular filtration, modulation of renin release, tubular ion transport, and water exchange. High doses of NSAIDs taken over a prolonged period are associated with progressive decline in renal function. Damage attributable to analgesic nephropathy is irreversible. The clinical outcome of prostaglandin inhibition on the kidney includes fluid retention, hyperkalemia, interstitial nephritis, and hypertension.
  - A vasodilator effect in the liver. NSAIDs concentrate liver enzymes and may precipitate hepatitis.
- *An idiosyncratic reaction.* An individual may have an unpredictable untoward response. At doses as low as 1 or 2 tablets, aspirin may cause allergic reactions in sensitive individuals. The idiosyncratic response may present as lacrimation, rhinorrhea and, occasionally, bronchospasm.
- *Dose-related side-effects.* In the case of aspirin, a dose below 300 mg/day is rarely associated with toxicity, while a dose above 900 mg/day frequently induces gastrointestinal bleeding.
- *Production of reactive intermediate metabolites.* Aspirin owes at least part of its pharmacological activity to its metabolites.

General guidelines for the use of NSAIDs and other drugs are as follows:[19,20]

- Avoid the use of particular drugs in persons at increased risk of toxic side-effects from that drug.
- Start therapy with a low initial dose.
- Use the lowest feasible maintenance dose. In certain cases, other drugs or nutrients may facilitate dose reduction. The dose of a NSAID required to achieve a therapeutic effect may be reduced by the judicious use of fish oil.[21,22]
- Minimize the risks of toxicity by
  - not combining drugs with similar toxicity
  - avoiding behaviors that potentiate toxic effects (e.g. cigarette smoking while on NSAIDs)
- Consider extra precautions in:
  - the elderly
  - pregnancy
  - patients with renal or hepatic insufficiency (avoid, depending on drug excretion by compromised organ).
- Exercise caution when prescribing drugs that interact (e.g. NSAIDs and anticoagulants).

- Monitor progress with respect to
  - the benefit the patient is deriving from the intervention
  - the development of unwanted or toxic effects.
- Modify the drug dose or change the drug when necessary.

Neutralizing free radicals

Oxygen, even in its stable ground state, is a highly reactive element that readily accepts electrons. Oxygen is a good oxidizing agent. When oxygen accepts an electron, superoxide (a free radical) is formed. Normal biochemical processes in which oxygen is associated with free-radical production include aerobic metabolism, phagocytic oxidation, and cytochrome P450 detoxification. Free-radical generation is a result of natural cell metabolism, and this is exaggerated in any hypermetabolic state or disease process involving inflammation.

A free radical is defined as any species capable of independent existence that contains one or more unpaired electrons. Free radicals can donate electrons in chemical reactions. About 95% of the oxygen involved in oxidative metabolism forms stable compounds. The 5% which ends up in unstable compounds must be quickly metabolized in order to avoid cell damage. Free-radical pathology may occur if one of these fragments exists long enough to react independently. Free radicals react with

- Polyunsaturated fats in lipid membranes.
- Amino acid residues in enzymes and structural proteins. The (*S*)-amino acids (e.g. cysteine, methionine) and amino acids containing aromatic rings (e.g. histidine, tyrosine, tryptophan) are particularly susceptible.
- Purine and pyrimidine bases in DNA and RNA.

At a cellular level, free-radical-induced pathology results in changes in cell metabolism and permeability, as demonstrated by changes in:

- Membrane transport.
- Surface receptors, including those which interact with hormones, antigens, and antibodies.
- Immunocompetent cells (the function and numbers of helper, suppressor, and killer cells is modified).
- Prostanoid synthesis.
- Metabolite structure. Apolipoprotein B100, when altered by the reactive products of lipid peroxidation, is recognized by scavenger receptors on macrophages, which then phagocytose low-density lipoprotein (LDL) and produce foam cells – the underlying lesion in atherosclerosis.

The body has a natural free-radical neutralization system, which rapidly detoxifies highly reactive molecular oxygen by converting free radicals to less-reactive species. The primary defense mechanism depends on enzymes including superoxide dismutase, glutathione, and glutathione peroxidase. The secondary defense system depends largely on vitamins and can also be influenced by minerals. The secondary defense mechanism can be successfully boosted by appropriate dietary selection and nutritional supplementation. Important vitamin antioxidants include:

- *Vitamin C.* In low doses, vitamin C acts as a coenzyme facilitating the hydroxylation of proline and lysine; at higher doses it acts as an antioxidant, quenching free radicals and helping to regenerate vitamin E. Vitamin C is a powerful water-soluble reducing agent. Vitamin C is the first antioxidant to be consumed when fresh human plasma is exposed to the gas phase of cigarette smoke. Smokers may benefit by taking 3–5 g of vitamin C for each packet of cigarettes smoked. Megadose vitamin C supplementation has, however, been implicated in the distortion of laboratory results, with subsequent impairment of clinical judgment.[23,24] Depending on the reagents used, clinical urinalysis may produce false-positive or false-negative results for glycosuria in persons taking vitamin C supplements. Vitamin C may also produce persistently false-negative stool guaiac or hemoccult tests in persons with bowel cancer.
- *Vitamin E.* Vitamin E is the major lipid-soluble antioxidant. It neutralizes lipid radical and interrupts lipid radical chain reactions. The potency of vitamin E is modified by structural change. If the biological activity of various forms of vitamin E is compared in international unit (IU) equivalents per milligram, then D-α-tocopherol has a value of 1.49, D-β-tocopherol a value of 0.75, and D-α-tocotrienol a value of 0.45.[25] In doses of 800 IU or more, vitamin E appears to decrease oxidative stress associated with exercise, as measured by decreased excretion of lipid peroxidation products.[26] It has also been suggested that vitamin E in doses of 400 IU reduces platelet adhesion, and that smokers may benefit from taking 800 IU/day vitamin E. Men who take more than 60 IU/day vitamin E have a relative risk of 0.64 for an ischemic cardiac event compared with men who take 7 IU/day.[27] Free radicals released from arterial endothelial and smooth-muscle cells lead to oxidation of LDLs. Oxidized LDL is taken up by receptors on macrophages that do not have an affinity for native LDL. Foamy macrophages are found in atherosclerotic plaques. Oxidized LDL is chemotactic for monocytes, and further endothelial damage occurs. A spectrum of carotenoids and vitamin E isoforms are required to protect LDL.
- *β-Carotene.* Unlike retinol, β-carotene is a water-soluble antioxidant. It neutralizes singlet oxygen. Lycopene, the principal carotenoid of tomatoes, is an even more effective singlet oxygen quencher than β-carotene. A number of case-control studies suggest that β-carotene has a protective effect against cancer of the lung, colon, and stomach.

- An increased risk of ischemic heart disease and stroke have consistently been found at low plasma concentrations of antioxidants,[28] and dietary antioxidants may exert their protective effect against carcinogenesis.[16]

INACTIVATING A CAUSATIVE ORGANISM

In addition to modifying human physiology, drugs can be used to modify the pathogenicity of microbes. Antimicrobial agents may be bacteristatic or bactericidal. Bacteristatic antimicrobials impair the metabolism and multiplication of the organism, and depend on the host's immune response to eliminate the organism. Bactericidal antibiotics kill or lyze the organism. The principles underlying the use of antimicrobial agents are:

- *Differential toxicity*. The aim is to produce an antimicrobial agent that is toxic to the organism but not the host. This may be achieved by using an antimicrobial agent which:
  - Acts upon an enzyme unique to the organism. Bacteria contain an enzyme that converts *p*-aminobenzoic acid to folic acid. Sulfonamides block this enzyme. As humans lack this enzyme, sulfonamides can impair bacterial metabolism without affecting the metabolism of the host's cell.
  - Impairs protein synthesis at the level of the ribosome. The ribosomes of mammalian and bacterial cells differ. Chloramphenicol and tetracyclines impair bacterial protein synthesis without impairing protein synthesis by the host's cells.
  - Acts upon the organism's cell wall. Fungi incorporate a particular sterol, which is not found in humans, into their cell membrane. Blocking introduction of this sterol weakens the cell structure of the fungus but not the host cell. Penicillin, by similarly interfering with the molecular structure of the bacterial cell wall, causes bacterial lysis.

Treatment of viral infections is more difficult than treatment of bacterial infections, as viral structural components are chemically indistinguishable from mammalian nucleic acid.

- To concentrate the drug in its active form at the site of the infection. Ion concentration and pH may need to be taken into consideration.
- Selecting a drug to which the organism is susceptible. Organisms may be resistant to a drug due to the organism:
  - being impermeable
  - producing an enzyme that inactivates the drug
  - changing its structure so that the drug can no longer attach to its biochemical site of action.

- *To expose the patient to the drug for a period which exceeds the lifecycle of the organism.* The duration of therapy is shortest with actively multiplying organisms. Infections caused by *Escherichia coli*, an organism with a short generation time, are usually cured in days rather than weeks. Infections caused by *Mycobacterium tuberculosis*, an organism with a longer generation time, require treatment for months and sometimes years. Furthermore, clinical cure is not necessarily synonymous with microbial elimination. Treatment for fungal infections should be continued after apparent clinical cure, in order to eliminate the organism.

CONCLUSION

Drug therapy lends itself to treatment of the disease rather than management of the patient. Although highly successful in the control of certain conditions, due to the nature of their action drugs are often associated with the development of unwanted effects. Even when clinically indicated, drug therapy may have adverse effects. The benefit of therapy for each patient therefore needs to be weighed up against the probability of an adverse reaction. Consequently, a prerequisite to responsible drug therapy is accurate diagnosis.

REFERENCES

1 Jamison J R 1991 Drugs in chiropractic clinical practice. Journal of Manipulative Physiological Therapeutics 14:255–261

2 Edwards I R 1987 Adverse drug reaction monitoring. Current Therapeutics July:47–53

3 Moll J M H 1987 NSAIDs in clinical practice. Current Therapeutics March:133–155

4 Roncari D A K 1977 A practical guide to hyperlipidaemic disorders. Modern Medicine 45:53–61

5 Crouch M A 1988 Should cholesterol lowering drugs be used routinely to treat moderate hypercholesterolaemia. Journal of Family Practice 26:665–675

6 Allgower C A 1977 Management of hyperlipidaemias. Journal of the American Chiropractic Association 11(suppl):107–109

7 Thompson P J, Watkins D N 1994 β-agonists. Current Therapeutics 35:11–17

8 Walls R 1992 Antihistamines: where, when and which one? Modern Medicine, Australia September:44–55

9 Katelaris C 1993 Nonsedating antihistamines. Australian Family Physician 22:1649–1653

10 Brooks P, Girgis L 1995 Nonsteroidal anti-inflammatory drugs. Current Therapeutics 36:31–39

11 Fries J F, Ramey D K, Singh G et al 1993 A re-evaluation of aspirin therapy in rheumatoid arthritis. Archives of Internal Medicine 153:2465–2471

12 Hung J, Joyce D A 1994 An aspirin a day. Current Therapeutics 35:11–15

13 Day R O 1988 Mode of action of non-steroidal anti-inflammatory drugs. Medical Journal of Australia 148:195–199

14 Kopp E, Gosh S 1994 Inhibition of NF-κB by sodium salicylate and aspirin. Science 265:956–958

15 Thun M J, Namboodiri M M, Calle E E, Flanders W D, Heath C W 1993 Aspirin use and risk of fatal cancer. Cancer Research 53:1322–1327

16 Heizisouer K J, Block G, Blumberg J et al 1994 Summary of the Round Table Discussion on Strategies for Cancer Prevention: diet, food, additives, supplements, and drugs. Cancer Research 54(suppl): 2044s–2051s

17 Brooks P M 1988 Side-effects of non-steroidal anti-inflammatory drugs. Medical Journal of Australia 148:248–251

18 Chapman G D 1988 A perspective on the cost-effectiveness and risks of non-steroidal

anti-inflammatory drug therapy. Medical Journal of Australia 149:346–349

19 Australian Gastroenterology Institute, Arthritis Foundation of Australia and Australian Rheumatology Association Joint Statement 1992 Nonsteroidal anti-inflammatory drugs (NSAIDs) and the upper gut. Modern Medicine, Australia July:105–107

20 Chapman G D 1988 Therapeutic usage of the non-steroidal anti-inflammatory drugs. Medical Journal of Australia 149:203–213

21 Lau C S, Morley K D, Belch J J F 1993 Effects of fish oil supplementation on non-steroidal anti-inflammatory drug requirement in patients with mild rheumatoid arthritis – a double-blind placebo controlled study. British Journal of Rheumatology 32:982–989

22 Skoldstam L, Borjesson O, Kjallman A et al 1992 Effect of six months of fish oil supplementation in stable rheumatoid arthritis. A double-blind, controlled study. Scandinavian Journal of Rheumatology 21:178–185

23 Smith D, Young W W 1977 Effect of large-dose ascorbic acid on the two drop clinitest determination. American Journal of Hospital Pharmacy 34:1347–1349

24 Jaffee R M, MacLowney J D 1975 False negative stool occult blood tests caused by ingestion of ascorbic acid. Annals of Internal Medicine 83:824–826

25 Ogunmekan A O, Hwang P A 1988 Vitamin E therapy – facts and fancies. International Clinical Nutrition Review 8:69–74

26 Meydani M 1992 Protective role of dietary vitamin E on oxidative stress in ageing. Age 15:89–93

27 Rimm E, Stampfer M J, Ascherio A et al 1993 Vitamin E consumption and the risk of coronary heart disease in men. New England Journal of Medicine 328:1450–1456

28 Gey K F, Moser U K, Jordan P, Stahelin H B, Eichholzer M, Ludin E 1993 Increased risk of cardiovascular disease at suboptimal plasma concentrations of essential antioxidants: an epidemiological update with special attention to carotene and vitamin C. American Journal of Clinical Nutrition 57(5 Suppl): 787S–797S

PART

2

The differential diagnosis of patients' complaints

CHAPTER 3

Introduction

CHAPTER CONTENTS

This section has been designed to help novice diagnosticians find their way through the maze of signs and symptoms encountered in primary practice. Questions and flowcharts have been used as triggers to alert the clinician to some of the more prevalent and serious diagnostic options.

The chapters are arranged in alphabetical order according to the patient's complaint. In certain cases medical terms have been used; for example, dysuria is used as a chapter heading instead of discomfort or burning on passing urine, and similarly dysphagia is used rather than difficulty with swallowing. If you are uncertain of a term, refer to the glossary on page 655. The strategy employed relies on:

- Identifying a number of important questions that need to be asked given the presenting patient's complaint. The indications for referral have often assumed the reader does not have access to prescription drugs. The appropriateness of the referral listing to the reader's clinical practice varies depending on their professional qualification.
- Utilizing flowcharts to arrange clinical data into diagnostic streams (Fig. 3.1). More than 58 flowcharts have been developed to provide pathways for analyzing prevalent symptoms. More than one flowchart may be developed for a single symptom.

Taking the presenting complaint of the patient as a starting point, the differential diagnosis of symptoms and signs is considered. In each instance a number of questions are used to guide the diagnostician through a series of possible diagnoses. Once the flowchart suggests a particular diagnosis, the reader should turn to Part 3 to obtain further information on other signs and symptoms. The better the match between the patient's signs and symptoms and the condition, the higher the probability that a diagnostic option is correct.

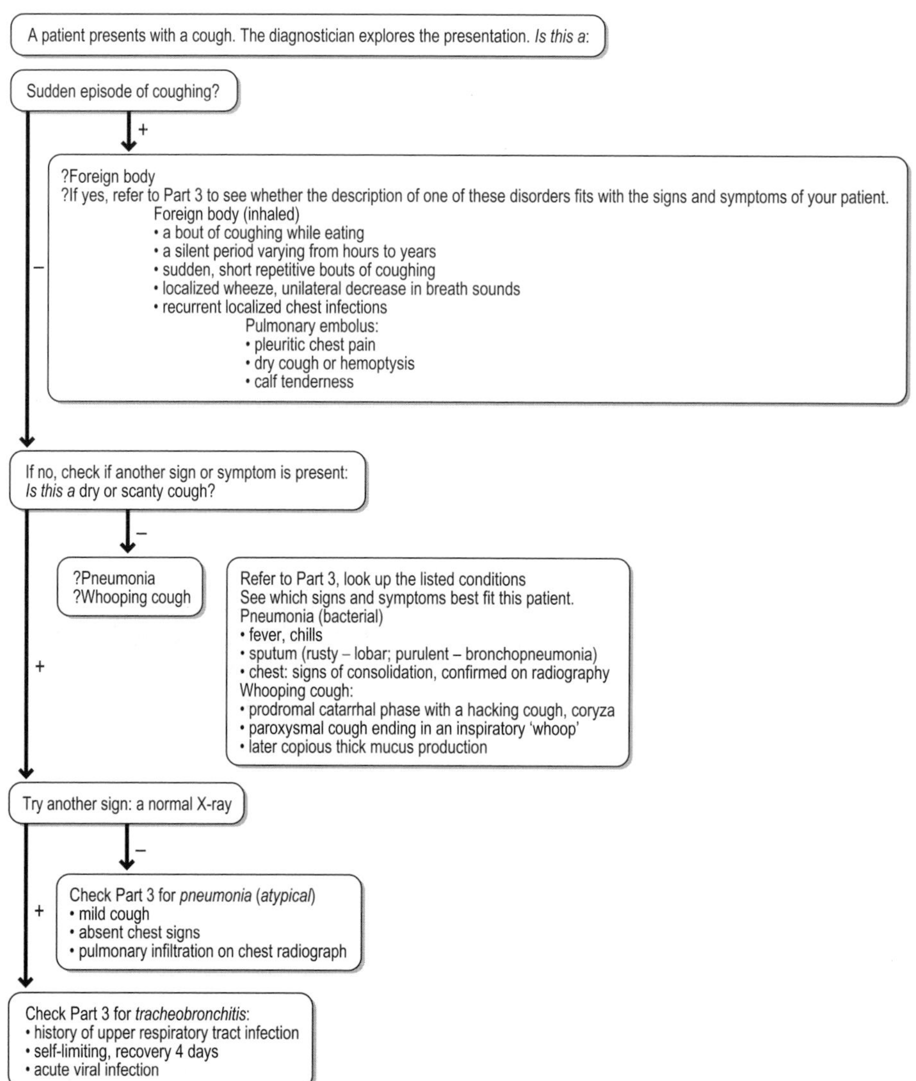

Figure 3.1 **Using the flowcharts.**

It should be noted that the list of options is not comprehensive and only the more serious and most prevalent conditions have been included. Furthermore, it should be emphasized that the presentation of a condition and failure to conform within the framework provided does not necessarily exclude the diagnosis.

Parts 2 and 3 are both arranged in alphabetical in order to facilitate easy reference. Figure 3.1 outlines the approach used. The underlying model is to take the patient's complaint and ask if a second sign or symptom is present:

PART TWO

- If *yes*, a possible diagnosis is suggested. The clinical features of the suggested diagnosis are listed in Part 3. Other signs and symptoms being experienced by the patient should be compared with the features of the disease given in Part 3. A good match suggests a correct working diagnosis; a poor match suggests another diagnosis should be sought.
- If *no*, another sign or symptom is listed. If the patient has this second clinical feature a possible diagnosis is suggested. The clinician should refer to Part 3 and check the disease description against the total clinical picture of the patient.

The process is repeated until a good fit is obtained between a disease and the patient's presentation.

FURTHER READING

Goroll A H, May L A, Mulley A G 1995 Primary care medicine. J B Lippincott, Philadelphia

Griffith H W, Dambro M R 1994 The 5 minute clinical consult. Lea & Febiger, Philadelphia

Hodgkin K 1978 Towards earlier diagnosis in primary care. Churchill Livingstone, Edinburgh

Isselboch H J, Adams R D, Bromwald E et al 1988 Harrison's principles of internal medicine. McGraw Hill, New York

Murtagh J 1996 General practice. MacGraw Hill, Sydney

Abdominal pain

CHAPTER CONTENTS

PART TWO

Is urgent referral indicated?

Acute abdominal pain plus abdominal distension suggests an active intra-abdominal disorder (Fig. 4.1). Clinical indications for urgent referral include:

- Prostration.
- Atrial fibrillation and abdominal pain.
- A risk of dehydration. Patients have:
  - intractable vomiting
  - a decreased urinary output.
- Shock. Intra-abdominal bleeding should be suspected in patients who have more than one of the following:
  - collapse at toilet
  - are light-headed
  - are pale and sweating
  - have hypotension
  - have tachycardia.
- Peritoneal irritation. Peritonitis should be suspected in patients with:
  - progressive abdominal distension
  - progressively worsening pain. Pain becomes: constant; sharp or lancinating; well localized
  - rebound tenderness and guarding
  - pain which is aggravated by movement
  - sudden, temporary, relief of abdominal pain.

The nature of the pain is also helpful in determining a working diagnosis in patients with evidence of shock or peritonitis (Table 4.1).

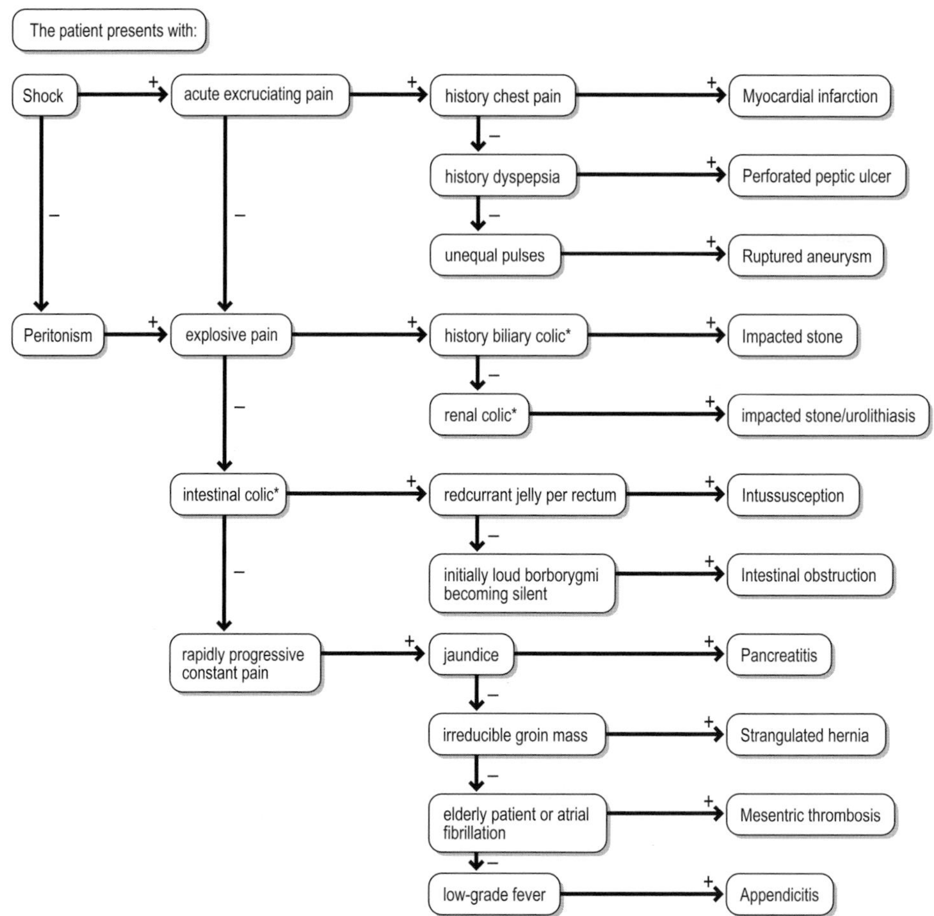

Figure 4.1 **Abdominal pain.**

Table 4.1
The diffferential diagnosis of colic*

Site of spasm	Intensity	Interval
Large bowel	Moderate (+)	Pain waves at 6–10 min
Small bowel	Severe (++)	Pain waves at 3–5 min
Biliary	Very severe (+++)	Constant pain for 20–360 min
Renal	Intense (++++)	Loin to groin radiation every 10 min

*See Figure 4.1

What is the source of the abdominal pain?

Abdominal pain is largely a clinical diagnosis. In cases of abdominal pain, it is always necessary to:

- do a rectal examination
- examine the scrotum (testicular disease and hernias may both be sources of abdominal pain).

Table 4.2
Somatic pain

Source	Localization	Nature	Comments
Skin (superficial pain)	Clear, well defined	Sharp	Pain is associated with minor irritation
Muscles, joints (deep pain)	Poorly localized	Dull ache	Referred to associated dermatome. Occasionally, hyperesthesia and/or muscle spasm in structures with common innervation
Parietal peritoneum	Varies depending on site of irritation	Sharp, severe	Overlying rigidity and hyperesthesia

The diagnosis and prognosis are influenced by the cause of the pain. The character of abdominal pain provides a clue to its origin. Abdominal pain that arises from a somatic source should be suspected when the pain is:

- aggravated by posture or movement
- unrelated to visceral activity
- follows injury
- localized and fairly intense.

The nature and particular presentation of somatic pain varies depending on the source (Table 4.2). The skin has a rich supply of sensory nerves and presents with well-defined pain. In contrast, the pain from muscle and joints is poorly defined. Pain from parietal peritoneum is well localized at the site of the irritation when the overlying structure is the anterior abdominal wall. This clear localization to the site of irritation does not apply with irritation of the peritoneum overlying the:

- Central diaphragm: pain refers to the shoulder via the phrenic nerve.
- Peripheral diaphragm: pain refers to the subcostal region via the lower thoracic spinal nerves.
- Pelvic peritoneum: pain refers to the perineum via the sacral nerves.
- Posterior abdominal wall below the transverse colon: pain refers to the front of the abdomen.
- Posterior abdominal wall on the right side of the transverse colon: pain refers to the umbilical region.
- Posterior abdominal wall on the left side of the transverse colon: pain refers to the hypogastric region.

In contrast to pain that arises from the skin, musculoskeletal system, and peritoneum, visceral pain arises from the male genitalia, abdominal or pelvic organs, and their associated mesentery. Ischemia, muscle spasm, chemical irritants, and distension of a

Table 4.3
Recognizing somatic and visceral pain

	Somatic pain	Visceral pain
Nature	Constant	Intermittent
Localization	Varies; often well defined	Poorly localized, diffuse
Associated findings	Presentation, including the character of the pain, depends on source of somatic pain	Pain is often referred and associated with disturbances of myotomal, dermatomal, autonomic, and visceral function
Pain adaptation	Fair	Poor, very slow

hollow organ all elicit visceral pain. Individuals seldom become tolerant to visceral pain. Somatic and visceral pain are compared in Table 4.3.

Visceral pain is often referred. Referred pain is:

- Usually sharp and well localized
- Is experienced in predictable sites. Pain may be referred according to embryological development. Structures arising from the:
  - Foregut (i.e. lower esophagus, stomach, duodenum, liver, gallbladder, bile duct, and pancreas) refer to the epigastrium. Other findings associated with upper abdominal pain that suggest a foregut problem are anorexia, nausea, and vomiting.
  - Midgut (i.e. small intestine, Meckel's diverticulum, terminal ileum, appendix, and cecum) refer to the periumbilical region. Anorexia, nausea, and vomiting are also associated with midgut problems.
  - Hindgut (i.e. large bowel, sigmoid colon, and rectum) refer to the suprapubic region. Lower abdominal pain associated with blood, mucus, and an alteration in bowel habit suggests a hindgut problem.

Other characteristic referral patterns are:

- The pancreas, kidney/ureter, and aorta referring pain to the back. Low backache associated with a vaginal discharge, dyspareunia, or a menstrual disorder suggests a lesion of the female genital tract.
- The spleen and gallbladder refer pain to the shoulder.
- The kidney and/or urinary tract may refer pain to the groin or tip of the penis. Pain in the loin, groin, or suprapubic area that is associated with frequency, dysuria, or hematuria suggests a renal or urinary tract problem.

As inflammation of a viscus spreads to involve the overlying parietal peritoneum, pain may move from its referred site to overlie the involved organ (e.g. the periumbilical pain of acute appendicitis moves to the right iliac fossa).

Other clinical findings associated with visceral pain are:

- Hyperesthesia due to dermatomal involvement.
- Muscle spasm due to myotomal involvement.
- The influence of the organ involved and the nature of the pathological process:
  - obstruction to hollow muscular organs present with cramping intermittent (colicky) pain
  - irritation of organs results in pain described as gnawing, burning, boring.
- A disturbance of visceral function:
  - vomiting
  - diarrhea
  - constipation.
- Exaggerated autonomic nervous reflexes:
  - sweating
  - vasomotor changes (hypotension, changes in heart rate)
  - nausea.

What is the likely diagnosis?

Pain location is a helpful starting point in differential diagnosis (Fig. 4.2).

Does the patient need to be referred?

All patients with abdominal pain should be referred if an organic cause for the visceral pain is suspected. In general, when vomiting precedes pain consider medical referral, and when pain precedes vomiting make a surgical referral.

In a patient with abdominal pain, findings that suggest referral may be prudent include:

- A raised temperature.
- The passage of blood per rectum (red or black) or hematemesis.
- Persistent vomiting.
- Dark or bright red vaginal bleeding.
- Pain:
  - which lasts for more than 4 hours
  - with diarrhea which lasts for more than 24 hours
  - which is severe, localized, and related to meals
  - which disturbs sleep
  - with faintness.
- Chronic or recurrent abdominal pain associated with one or more of the following:
  - anemia
  - significant weight loss
  - chronic diarrhea
  - nocturnal diarrhea or pain
  - chronic constipation
  - steatorrhea.

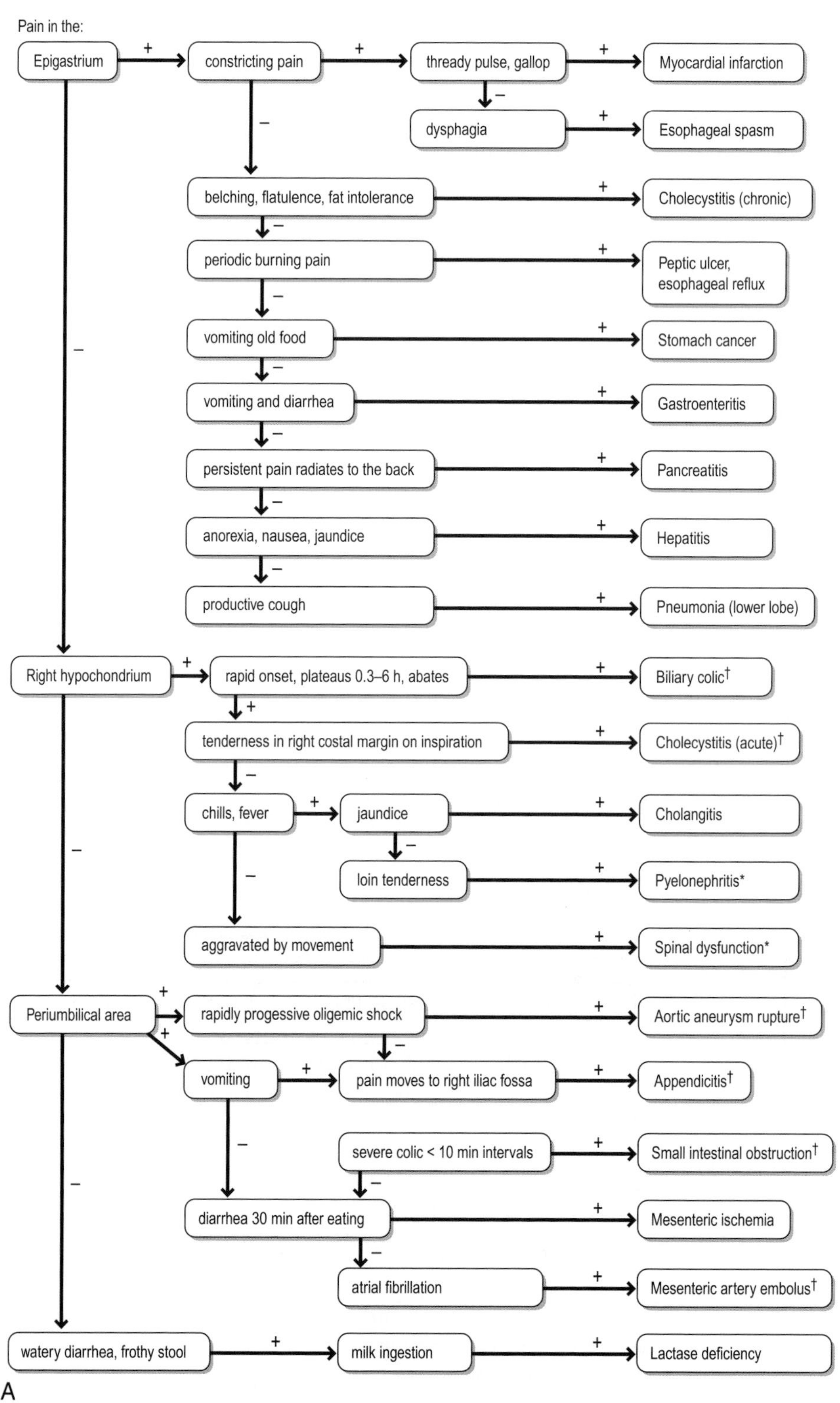
Pain in the:
Epigastrium
+
constricting pain
+
thready pulse, gallop
+
Myocardial infarction
–
dysphagia
+
Esophageal spasm
–
belching, flatulence, fat intolerance
+
Cholecystitis (chronic)
–
periodic burning pain
+
Peptic ulcer, esophageal reflux
–
vomiting old food
+
Stomach cancer
–
vomiting and diarrhea
+
Gastroenteritis
–
persistent pain radiates to the back
+
Pancreatitis
–
anorexia, nausea, jaundice
+
Hepatitis
–
productive cough
+
Pneumonia (lower lobe)
–
Right hypochondrium
+
rapid onset, plateaus 0.3–6 h, abates
+
Biliary colic†
+
tenderness in right costal margin on inspiration
+
Cholecystitis (acute)†
–
chills, fever
+
jaundice
+
Cholangitis
–
loin tenderness
+
Pyelonephritis*
–
aggravated by movement
+
Spinal dysfunction*
–
Periumbilical area
+
rapidly progessive oligemic shock
+
Aortic aneurysm rupture†
–
+
vomiting
+
pain moves to right iliac fossa
+
Appendicitis†
–
severe colic < 10 min intervals
+
Small intestinal obstruction†
–
diarrhea 30 min after eating
+
Mesenteric ischemia
–
atrial fibrillation
+
Mesenteric artery embolus†
–
watery diarrhea, frothy stool
+
milk ingestion
+
Lactase deficiency
A

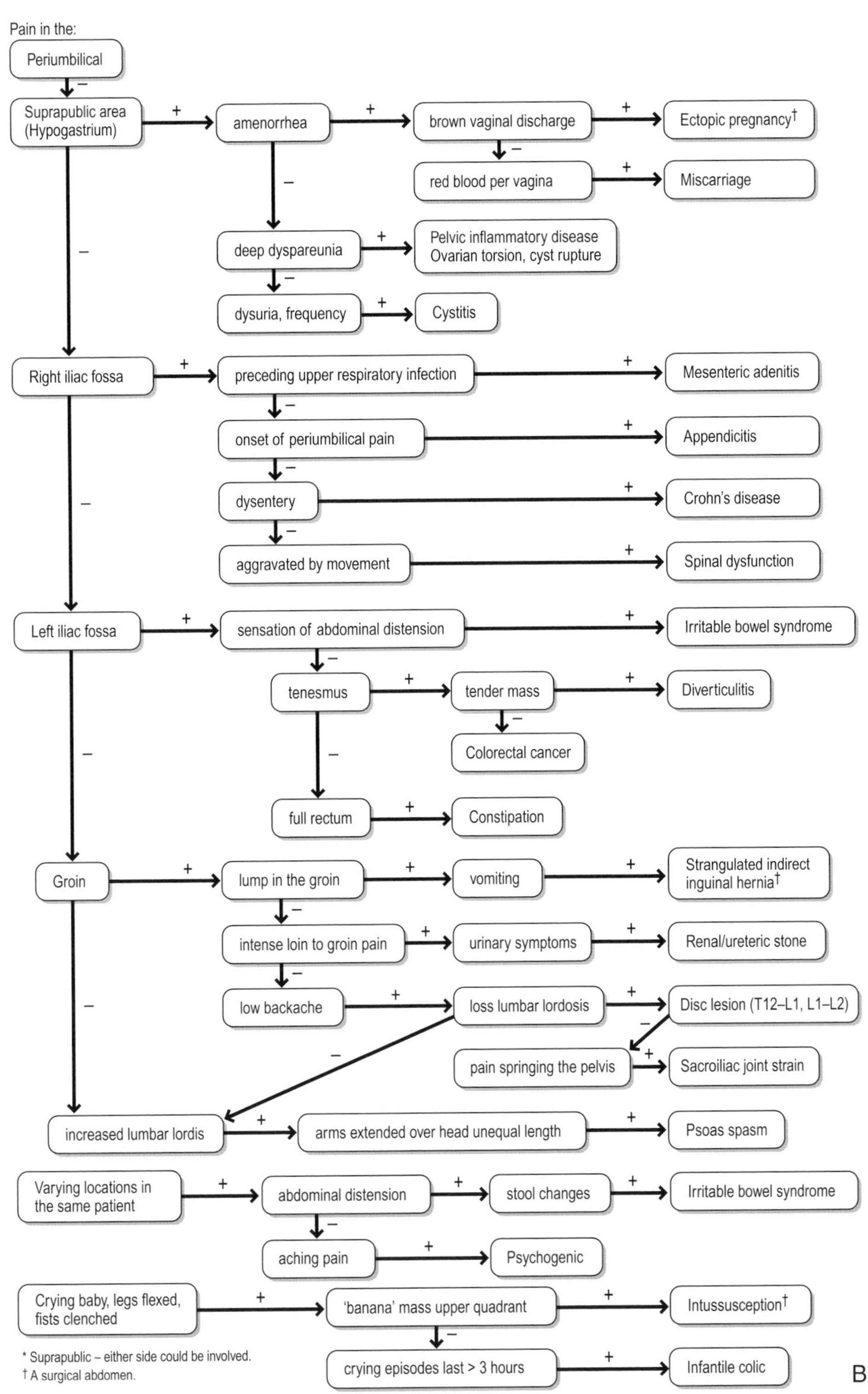

Figure 4.2 **Abdominal pain.**

PART TWO

B

In the differential diagnosis of recurrent or chronic abdominal pain, referral for screening by ultrasound is useful in the diagnosis of suspected:

- Gallstones. Patients with epigastric pain, severe enough to cause sweating, which starts several hours after a rich meal and radiates to the back may have their gallstones confirmed with ultrasound.
- Retroperitoneal problems including:
  - pancreatic cancer (symptoms are steadily and slowly progressive)
  - abdominal aneurysm.
- Pelvic pathology (e.g. ovarian cancer, ectopic pregnancy).

In patients with chronic or recurrent abdominal pain, endoscopy is another option. Gastroscopy is recommended in patients with:

- epigastric pain, relieved by food
- dysphagia
- anorexia
- vomiting or hematemesis
- melena.

Colonoscopy should be considered in patients with:

- crampy lower abdominal pain
- a change in bowel habit
- abdominal distension
- rectal bleeding
- a family history of polyps or cancer.

If indications for referral of chronic or recurrent abdominal pain are present and ultrasound and endoscopy are negative, the most likely lesion is one of the following:

- pancreatic cancer
- ovarian cancer
- small bowel tumor
- Crohn's disease
- mesenteric ischemia
- metabolic disorders (e.g. lactase deficiency)
- porphyria
- heavy metal poisoning.

PART TWO

FURTHER READING

Corazziari E 2004 Definition and epidemiology of functional gastrointestinal disorders. Best Pract Res Clin Gastroenterol 18(4):613–131

Holten K B, Wetherington A, Bankston L 2003 Diagnosing the patient with abdominal pain and altered bowel habits: is it irritable bowel syndrome? Am Fam Physician 67(10):2157–2162

Hugh T B 1995 The investigation and management of recurrent or chronic abdominal pain. Modern Med 38:126–132.

Mackay S, Dillane P 2004 Biliary pain. Aust Fam Physician 33(12):977–981

Oberndorff-Klein Woolthuis A H, Brummer R J, de Wit N J, Muris J W, Stockbrugger R W 2004 Irritable bowel syndrome in general practice:

an overview. Scand J Gastroenterol Suppl (241):17–22

Old J L, Dusing R W, Yap W, Dirks J 2005 Imaging for suspected appendicitis. Am Fam Physician 1;71(1):71–78

Unwin R J, Capasso G, Robertson W G, Choong S 2005 A guide to renal stone disease. Practitioner 249(1666):18, 20, 24

Anorectal pain

CHAPTER CONTENTS

What is the nature of the anal discomfort?

Anal discomfort may present as:

- A sharp searing pain. Tearing of the anal verge due to the passage of a constipated stool is likely.
- A dull pressure. Hemorrhoids are a possible cause.
- A throbbing. Complicated hemorrhoids or an anal abscess should be suspected.
- An itch. Anal irritation can result from skin disorders or an anal discharge associated with prolapsed mucosa, a fistula, or sphincter incontinence.

Anal discomfort may be associated with:

- A bloody discharge. The nature of bleeding may suggest a diagnosis. Blood may be found:
  - In the toilet pan. Bright red blood suggests internal hemorrhoids.
  - On toilet paper. Bright red blood suggests hemorrhoids, a fissure, anal cancer, or warts.
  - On underwear. If only blood is present check for:
    anal cancer
    an ulcerated perianal hematoma.

If blood and mucus are present, suspect:

  - advanced hemorrhoids
  - rectal prolapse
  - anal prolapse
  - a prolapsed polyp
- Mixed with feces. Colitis, proctitis, and cancer need to be investigated.

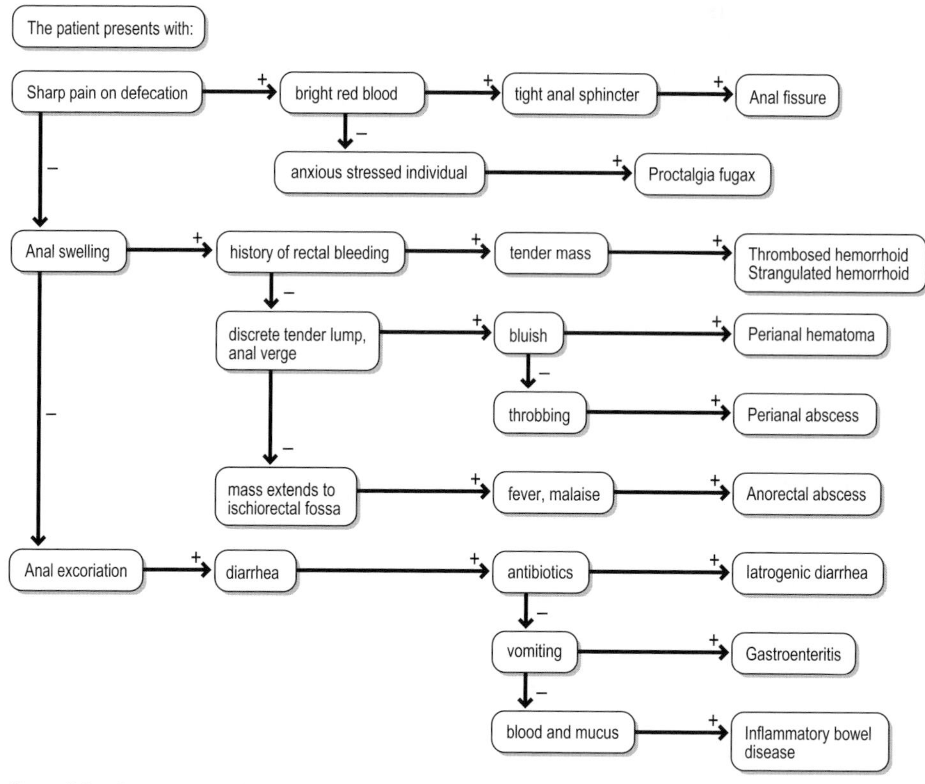

Figure 5.1 **Anorectal pain.**

- A lump. Lumps may be:
  - Prolapsing or retractable. Possible causes are:
    hemorrhoids (second and third degree)
    rectal prolapse
    a prolapsed polyp.
  - Persistent. Check for:
    a fourth-degree hemorrhoid
    anal cancer
    perianal warts, hematomas, or abscesses.

What is the likely diagnosis?

See Figure 5.1.

Does the patient need to be referred?

The following are the referral criteria for patients with anorectal pain:

- Persistent constipation due to uncontrolled pain.
- Suspected underlying colorectal cancer.
- Incontinence.
- Diagnostic uncertainty.
- Persistent infection.

FURTHER READING

Mazza L, Formento E, Fonda G 2004 Anorectal and perineal pain: new pathophysiological hypothesis. Tech Coloproctol 8(2):77–83

Wald A 2001 Anorectal and pelvic pain in women: diagnostic considerations and treatment. J Clin Gastroenterol 33(4):283–288

Wald A 2001 Functional anorectal and pelvic pain. Gastroenterol Clin North Am 30(1):viii–ix, 243–251

CHAPTER 6

Anxiety

CHAPTER CONTENTS

PART TWO

Is the patient anxious?

Anxiety is a sensation akin to fear. Persons with acute anxiety experience physical, emotional, and cognitive changes. Anxiety may be acute or chronic.

Patients should be screened for evidence of acute distress by searching for physical, emotional, and cognitive evidence of stress (Box 6.1).

Persons habitually exposed to stimulation that exceeds their optimal level of function may demonstrate signs and symptoms consistent with chronic stress. Chronic anxiety is evidenced by failure to cope with persistent stress (Box 6.2).

What is the nature of the patient's anxiety?

The clinical presentation of anxiety is influenced by the initiating stimulus and the individual's perception of that stimulus, their psychological coping skills, and their overall psychophysiological health status. Anxiety may be: physiological, pathophysiological, or psychopathological.

Physiological anxiety. Anxiety is a normal response to an unusual situation. Physiological anxiety may be used as a stimulus to achievement. Healthy anxiety can be used to facilitate adaptation to demanding situations. Persons who learn to control their anxiety can harness this energy for productive purposes.

Pathophysiological anxiety. This is a consequence of physical disease. It is important to discriminate between the psychophysiological changes associated with anxiety and the signs and symptoms of a disease process.

Psychopathological anxiety. Morbid anxiety serves no useful purpose once established and is maladaptive. Links between chronic anxiety and physical dysfunction have long been postulated. Although a causal link between stress and disease has yet

Box 6.1
Assessing the impact of acute stress

Physical evidence of stress. Check for:
- Trembling hands
- Butterflies in the stomach
- Tight shoulder, head, lower back
- Restless: foot tapping, key jiggling, cannot relax
- An exaggerated startle response
- Stuttering or speaking very fast, falling over words
- Easily fatigued
- Frequent minor ailments:
  - sleep problems
  - hatband headache
  - back pain
  - loss of libido
  - stomach upsets

Emotional lability. Check for:
- Tearfulness
- Impulsive behavior
- Irritability, short temperedness, edginess
- Hostility, aggressiveness
- Feelings of being a failure
- Feelings of frustration
- Apathy or agitation
- Sadness, depression
- Withdrawal, disinterest
- Emotional outbursts with little provocation
- Significant interpersonal conflict, argumentativeness

Cognitive evidence of stress. Check for:
- Memory problems, forgetfulness
- Indecisiveness
- Flitting from one idea/activity to another
- A tendency to make mistakes or get muddled
- Mental blocks
- Foggy, disorganized thinking
- Procrastinating, unable to plan ahead, unable to manage time
- Working longer hours, unable to relax, finding no time for enjoyment

to be established, interactive biological signaling has been clearly demonstrated between psychosocial stress and immune function. Morbid anxiety may be classified as:

- *Generalized anxiety.* Anxiety pervades the individual's lifestyle and is unrelated to particular persons or events. Autonomic changes associated with anxiety in turn lead to changed body sensations. Awareness of changed body sensations can,

Box 6.2
Checking for evidence of chronic stress

Features include:
- Becoming rigid or inflexible in an effort to maintain control
- Needing sleeping tablets or tranquilizers
- Needing alcohol or other drugs
- Losing contact with friends
- Having flare-ups of stress-related illnesses:
  - asthma
  - psoriasis
  - irritable bowel
  - ulcers
  - headaches
- Being depressed
- Always feeling anxious
- Overeating or a loss of appetite with weight changes

in turn, lead to anxiety. Once initiated, a cycle of increasing anxiety can be perpetuated.
- *A phobia.* Fear is linked to specific situations. The intensity of fear is out of proportion to any realistic threat.
- *A panic attack.* Episodes of intense incapacitating fear are experienced.
- *Post-traumatic stress.* Persons who have been exposed to a particularly stressful event persistently relive the event.
- *Neurotic behavior patterns.* Maladaptive lifestyle patterns are typified by anxiety and defense-orientated avoidance behavior. The maladaptive behavior reduces anxiety in the short term. In the long term the behavior may disrupt the individual's life. Repeated handwashing or checking that the door is locked are examples of disruptive behavior in obsessive–compulsive neurosis.

What is the likely diagnosis?

Anxiety is experienced and expressed in physical and psychological dimensions. While the initiating stimulus to anxiety may be in either dimension, the inevitable interaction between psychosocial stress and physical function may cloud the clinical presentation. In order to provide appropriate therapy for an overtly anxious patient, it is important to differentiate whether physical signs and symptoms have a psychogenic or physical origin (Fig. 6.1).

Diagnosis of presenting signs and symptoms in anxious patients results in consideration of the conditions listed in Figure 6.2.

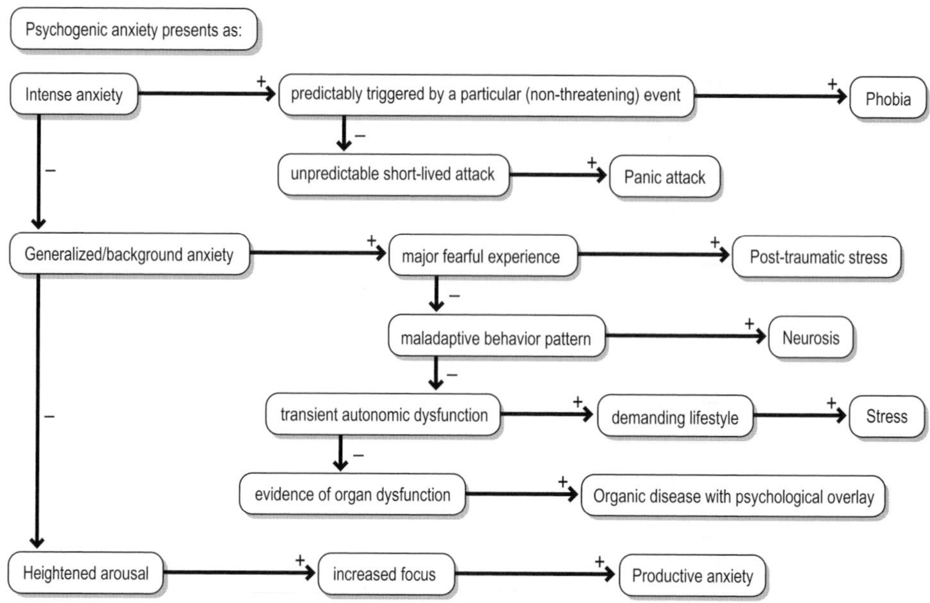

Figure 6.1 **Psychogenic anxiety.**

Does the patient need to be referred?

Referral should be considered when:

- anxiety is debilitating
- assistance is required in the diagnosis or management of organic disease
- functional patients may benefit from development of improved coping skills.

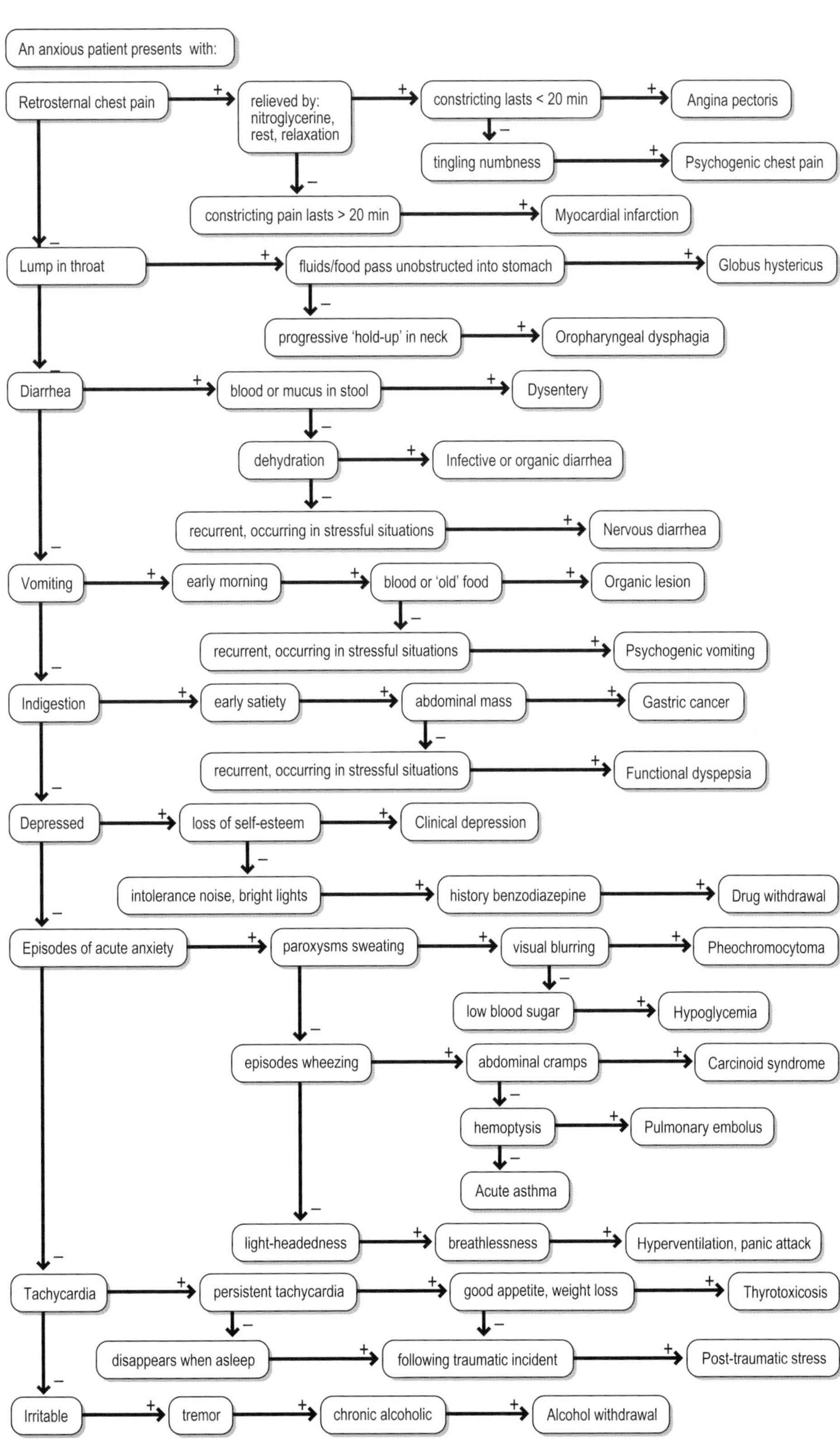

Figure 6.2 **Anxiety.**

PART TWO

FURTHER READING

Ballenger J C, Davidson J R, Lecrubier Y, Nutt D J 2001 A proposed algorithm for improved recognition and treatment of the depression/anxiety spectrum in primary care. Prim Care Companion J Clin Psychiatry Apr;3(2):44–52

Chavira D A, Stein M B, Bailey K, Stein M T 2004 Child anxiety in primary care: prevalent but untreated. Depress Anxiety 20(4):155–164

Gale C, Oakley-Browne M 2004 Generalised anxiety disorder. Clin Evid Dec;(12):1437–1459

Kelly M N 2005 Recognizing and treating anxiety disorders in children. Pediatr Ann 34(2):147–150

Kemper K J, Danhauer S C 2005 Music as therapy. South Med J 98(3):282–288

Marmot M 2005 'Status, anxiety and health or my anxiety is bigger than yours': review of status anxiety. Int J Epidemiol 34(2):493–496

Kiecolt-Glaser J K, Glaser R 1995 Psychoneuroimmunology and health consequences: data and shared mechanisms. Psychosom Med 57(3):269–274

O'Brien C P 2005 Benzodiazepine use, abuse, and dependence. J Clin Psychiatry 66 Suppl 2:28–33

Van den Bergh B R, Mulder E J, Mennes M, Glover V 2005 Antenatal maternal anxiety and stress and the neurobehavioral development of the fetus and child: links and possible mechanisms. A review. Neurosci Biobehav Rev 29(2):237–258.

Backache

CHAPTER CONTENTS

PART TWO

Is urgent referral indicated?

Patients with backache should be immediately referred in cases of a suspected cauda equina or unstable vertebral fracture.

Cauda equina presents with:

- Pain:
  - in the low back, thighs, and legs
  - relief is associated with assuming a flexed spinal position.
- Sensory changes to the:
  - buttocks (numbness of the buttocks is described as saddle anesthesia)
  - paresthesia to the thighs
  - backs of legs, soles of feet.
- A motor deficit:
  - weakness or paralysis of the leg
  - foot drop
  - calf atrophy.
- Visceral dysfunction:
  - bowel incontinence
  - bladder incontinence or retention.

A vertebral fracture is suggested by:

- Pain that is:
  - aggravated by activity, coughing, sneezing, straining, or standing
  - relieved by rest.
- Marked restriction of movement.

- Muscle spasm.
- Deformity.

Instability of a vertebral fracture is suggested by pain which:

- is rapidly relieved by lying down
- readily recurs on standing.

What is the nature of the backache?

A major differentiation in primary practice is to discriminate between musculoskeletal, visceral, and psychological causes of backache. In practice, the dominant presentation is simple back pain due to either muscle or ligament strain or dysfunction of the intervertebral joints. Although recurrences are common, at least half of patients with simple back pain will recover spontaneously in 14 days, and over three-quarters will recover without treatment in 28 days. It is helpful to determine if backache is attributable to:

- A musculoskeletal cause due to:
  - a mechanical problem (mechanical back pain is attributed to spinal dysfunction involving the facet joints and/or disruption of the intervertebral disc)
  - an inflammatory process
  - a neoplastic lesion.
- A visceral or organic lesion.
- Psychogenic causes. Chronic pain inevitably has a psychological impact. Psychological dysfunction can, however, also be the cause of pain.

Musculoskeletal backache may occur with or without a history of overt trauma. *Mechanical backache* is modified by movement and activity. *Simple backache* attributable to ligamentous sprain, muscular strain, or a mechanical problem usually:

- Is unilateral.
- Has an ill-defined onset, unless related to overt trauma.
- Is related to posture. Pain is:
  - aggravated by movement, sitting, coughing, or straining
  - relieved by rest, a change in position, heat.
- Lasts for hours.
- Does not prevent continued exercise.
- Is worst in the evenings, particularly after physical exertion.
- Has a history of many years.
- Varies with the underlying lesion:
  - muscular strain presents as a superficial steady local pain
  - radicular pain is sharp and stabbing
  - facet joint syndrome presents with pain of sudden onset, muscle spasm, and protective lateral deviation.

Other findings that may be present include:

- Interference with sleep.
- Associated physical phenomena:

- spinal muscle spasm
- restriction of movement.
- Associated neural phenomena:
  - shooting pains, paresthesia (patients with nerve root pain use a finger to point out an area of sharp, shooting pain)
  - motor weakness, foot drop.
- Referred pain. Referred back pain is experienced as an aching, deep pain. Patients use a hand to describe the pain as occurring over a general diffuse or patchy area.

In cases in which *overt trauma* is recalled, the nature of the injury provides useful diagnostic information:

- Falling in the seated position predisposes to:
  - a fractured coccyx
  - an acute disc prolapse.
- A violent twisting force predisposes to:
  - a fractured transverse process
  - a fractured spinous process.
- A less severe twisting force predisposes to:
  - a muscular tear with apophyseal joint injury
  - an isolated muscular tear.
- Lifting excessively heavy weights predisposes to:
  - posterior longitudinal ligament injury
  - interspinous injury
  - disc injury.
- Lifting and twisting with a flexed spine predisposes to:
  - apophyseal joint injury
  - intervertebral disc prolapse.
- Direct force applied to the back predisposes to:
  - soft tissue injury
  - vertebral fracture.
- Crushing force applied to the spine predisposes to:
  - compression fractures.

Inflammatory causes of backache are characterized by stiffness. Backache that is inflammatory in origin is frequently associated with:

- Pain and stiffness that is:
  - insidious in onset
  - aggravated by rest and relieved by exercise
  - worst at night and early morning
  - aching or throbbing in nature
  - persists for more than 30 minutes after getting up in the morning.
- Morning stiffness that is severe and prolonged.
- Pain that tends to be localized; may be bilateral or alternating in low backache.
- One or more positive laboratory investigation:
  - raised erythrocyte sedimentation rate (ESR)

- evidence of immunologically mediated inflammation: HLA B27 antigen; rheumatoid factor; antinuclear antibodies.

Continuous pain suggests inflammation associated with infection or malignancy.

Neoplasia causes bone pain that is unremitting and becomes progressively worse. Backache due to neoplasia should be excluded in patients who complain of:

- Pain which:
  - is continuous and unrelenting
  - is experienced at night
  - is present on waking
  - had an insidious onset
  - is rapidly increasing
  - is unrelieved by rest
  - fails to respond to treatment
  - presents as: a local boring deep ache; *or* can be referred (radicular pain involving more than one nerve root should be regarded as highly suggestive)
  - is aggravated by movement.
- Localized tenderness over the vertebrae.
- Relentless progression of neurological signs.

Associated findings include:

- Weight loss.
- Fatigue and malaise.
- Fever.
- One or more positive laboratory investigation, such as:
  - a raised ESR
  - a raised alkaline phosphatase
  - Bence–Jones proteinuria (this is diagnostic of myeloma).
- A positive bone scan. Consider a primary malignancy in the lung, breast, prostate, thyroid, kidney/adrenal, and melanoma. In the case of an osteoid osteoma, a benign tumor, pain is aggravated by alcohol and relieved by aspirin.

A cardinal feature of *psychogenic pain* is its indefinite nature and the inconsistency of its symptom pattern with recognized causes of backache. Psychogenic backache tends to be present with:

- Pain which:
  - has a vague onset
  - has an indefinite character (a constant acute or chronic ache may be described)
  - is bilateral, often diffuse, pain (is ill-defined with respect to its site, at best it is vaguely localized)
  - has an inappropriate radiation
  - has an inconsistent duration and seldom, if ever, wakes the sleeping patient

  - has a degree of severity out of all proportion to any identifiable lesion
  - is refractory (fails to respond to a diversity of interventions).
- Tenderness to palpation. Such tenderness is, however, not consistent with any recognized lesion, with respect to either its distribution or it severity.
- Pain modification. Pain is:
  - provoked by any and all movements
  - aggravated by mood, anxiety
  - relieved by alcohol, relaxation.
- Nonanatomical distribution of:
  - hyperesthesia or anesthesia.
- Hyperactive/brisk reflexes.
- Anxiety and/or depression. Patients tend to seek acceptance, demonstrate practitioner dependence, and deny emotional problems.

Visceral backache does produce symptom patterns consistent with known disorders. Visceral causes of backache should be suspected when there is evidence of organ system dysfunction. Visceral backache is characterized by:

- Localized pain with appropriate pain radiation.
- Periods when pain is absent.
- Tenderness consistent with recognized pain patterns.
- An axial loading test that does not cause pain. The axial loading test is performed by placing both hands on the erect (seated or standing) patient's head and pressing down firmly.
- Findings that favor involvement of a particular organ system:
  - cardiac origin:
    a gripping pain which is precipitated by exertion, prevents continued exercise; the onset of pain can be pinpointed to a specific time
    palpitations
    syncope
    dyspnea
  - gastrointestinal origin:
    attacks of pain which are related to meals, of variable duration (often hours)
    chronic symptomatology of varying intensity associated, in upper gastrointestinal lesions, with indigestion, regurgitation, dysphagia, and in lower intestinal lesions with a change in bowel habit, blood, or mucus in the stool
  - genital origin (female):
    low or sacral backache
    a vaginal discharge
    a history of dyspareunia
    menstrual disorders
  - renal or urinary origin:
    loin, groin, or suprapubic pain

urinary frequency and/or urgency
dysuria
hematuria.

What is the likely diagnosis?

See Figure 7.1.

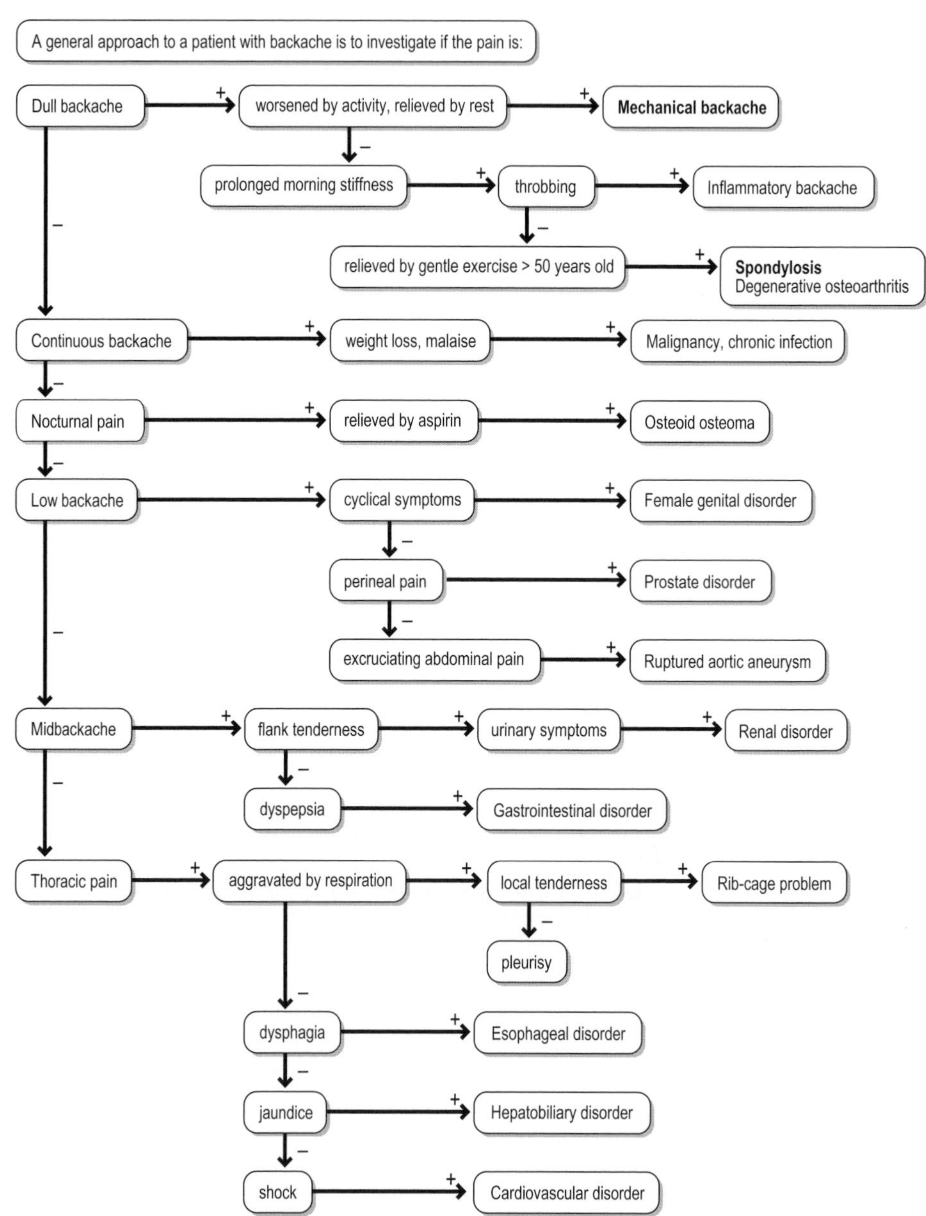

Figure 7.1 **Backache.**

What is the likely diagnosis in low backache?

See Figure 7.2.

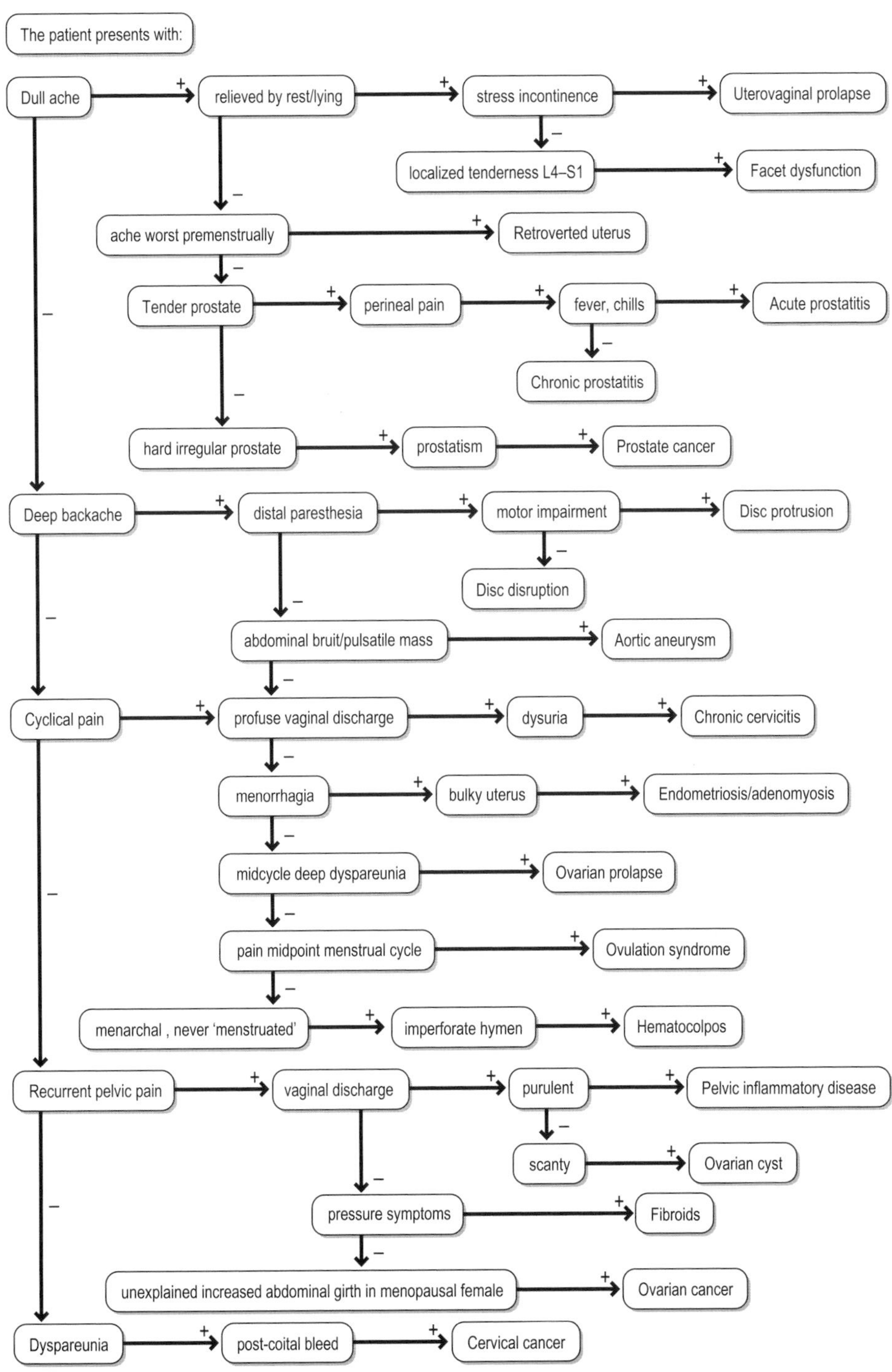

Figure 7.2 **Low back pain.**

What is the likely diagnosis in thoracic or midback pain?

See Figure 7.3.

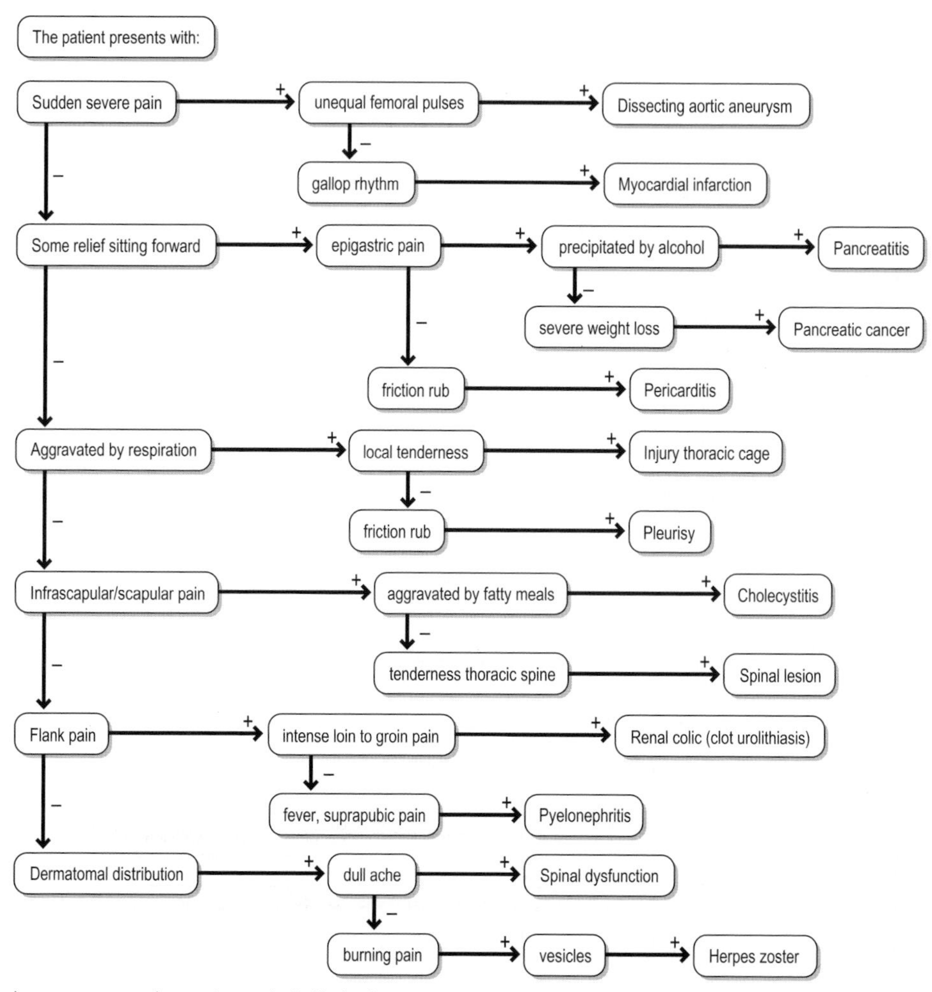

Lung cancer may rarely present as mechanical back pain

Figure 7.3 **Midback pain.**

What is the likely diagnosis in neck pain?

See Figure 7.4.

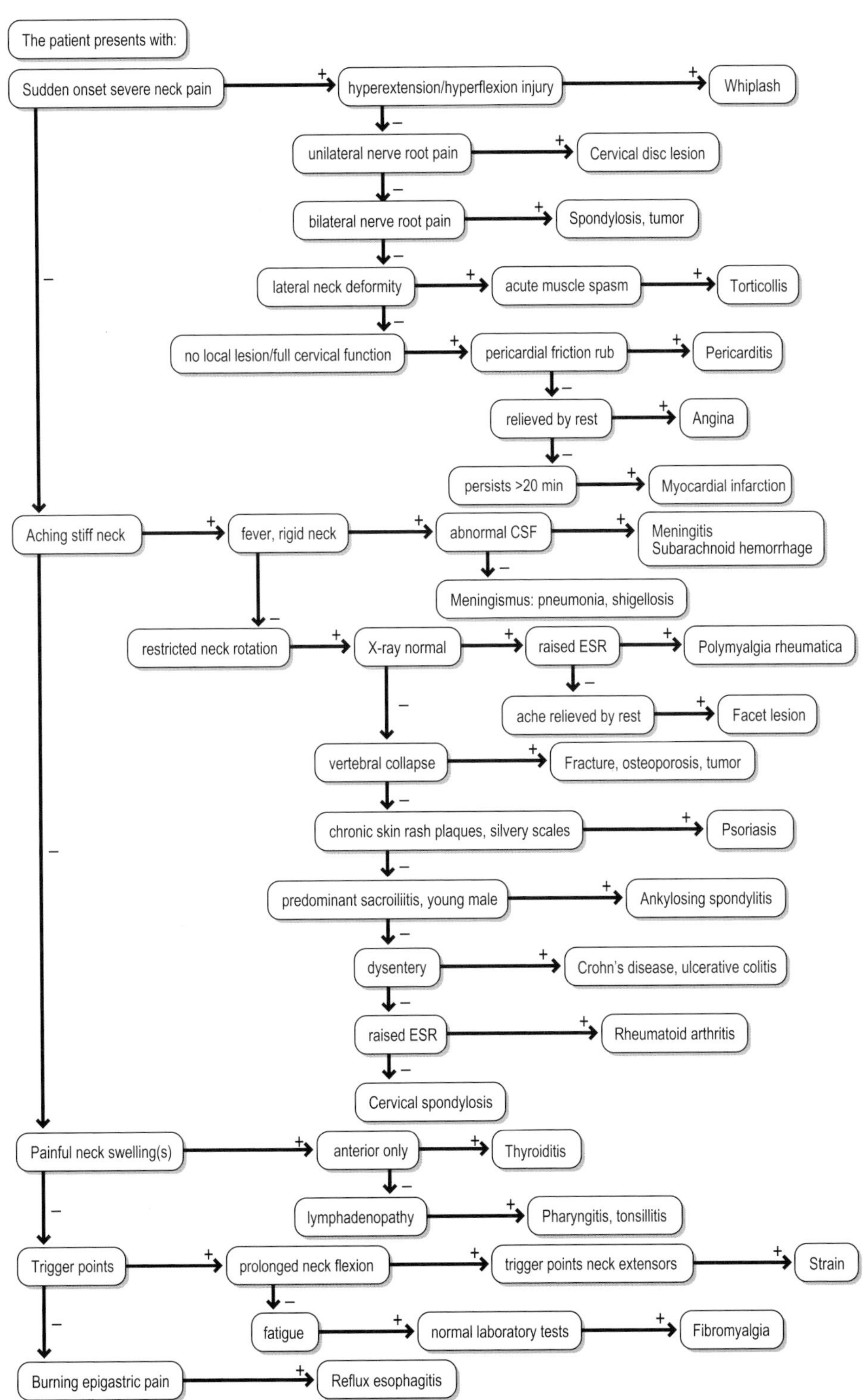

CSF: cerebrospinal fluid, ESR: erythrocyte sedimentation rate

Figure 7.4 **Neck pain.**

Does the patient need to be referred?

Conditions in which referral for special investigations, surgery, or drug therapy are indicated in a patient with backache include a:

- Suspected fracture. Suggestive findings are:
  - a history of trauma
  - pain aggravated by activity and relieved by rest
  - radiculopathy
  - radiographic changes.
- Suspected inflammatory condition. Suggestive findings are:
  - an insidious onset
  - aching or throbbing pain
  - pain and stiffness that is exacerbated by rest and relieved by exercise, and worst at night and in the early morning (morning stiffness is severe and prolonged).
- Suspected systemic condition. Suggestive symptoms are:
  - fatigue
  - malaise
  - weight loss.
- Suspected malignancy. Suggestive symptoms are:
  - back pain in older persons
  - unrelenting back pain that is not relieved by rest
  - rapidly increasing pain
  - constitutional symptoms (weight loss, fever, malaise).
  - a history of cancer treatment, especially for a primary lesion in the lung, breast, prostate, thyroid, kidney, adrenals, or a malignant melanoma.
- Suspected benign tumor. An osteoid osteoma may present with backache.

Conservative therapy without further investigations is indicated in patients under 50 years of age who present with:

- low back pain
- no sciatica
- a normal neurological examination
- no history of cancer
- no present signs or symptoms of a systemic disorder.

There is a 99% probability of a musculoskeletal cause in such patients.

An ESR and radiography are indicated prior to therapy in patients over 50 years of age who present with:

- low back pain
- no sciatica
- systemic signs:
  - fever
  - weight loss
  - hematuria
  - a history of cancer.

There is a 1–10% probability of systemic disease in these patients.

Provided there is no evidence of urinary retention, saddle anesthesia, or bilateral neurological abnormalities, even patients with low back pain and sciatica may be treated conservatively and given trial therapy.

FURTHER READING

Carragee E J 2005 Clinical practice. Persistent low back pain. N Engl J Med 352(18):1891–1898

Hagen K B, Jamtvedt G, Hilde G, Winnem M F 2005 The updated Cochrane review of bed rest for low back pain and sciatica. Spine 30(5):542–546

Hayden J A, van Tulder M W, Tomlinson G 2005 Systematic review: strategies for using exercise therapy to improve outcomes in chronic low back pain. Ann Intern Med 142(9):776–785

Jackson J L, Browning R 2005 Impact of national low back pain guidelines on clinical practice. South Med J 98(2):139–143

Manek N J, MacGregor A J 2005 Epidemiology of back disorders: prevalence, risk factors, and prognosis. Curr Opin Rheumatol 17(2):134–140

Old J L, Calvert M 2004 Vertebral compression fractures in the elderly. Am Fam Physician 69(1):111–116

Resnik L, Dobrykowski E 2005 Outcomes measurement for patients with low back pain. Orthop Nurs 24(1):14–24

van Tulder M, Koes B 2004 Low back pain (acute). Clin Evid 12:1643–1658

van Tulder M, Koes B 2004 Low back pain (chronic). Clin Evid 12:1659–1684

Blackouts

CHAPTER CONTENTS

Is there loss of consciousness?

The first step in diagnosis is to clarify the nature of the patient's 'blackout'. When patients complain of blackouts they may mean:

- a temporary loss of consciousness
- a memory lapse or blanks (see *Confusion and confused behavior*, p. 117)
- a 'funny turn' (see *Dizziness*, p. 157).

A good starting point in diagnosing blackouts is to explore the patient's level of consciousness before, during, and after the attack. The level of consciousness may be described as:

- *Alert.* Alert patients readily respond to the environment. People with 'funny turns' may experience dizziness but still be fully conscious and able to respond to commands.
- *Lethargic.* This implies drowsiness other than that of normal sleep.
- *Confused.* Patients present with impaired perception, poor attention, defective memory, and dulled awareness of their surroundings.
- *Delirium.* Confusion is accompanied by hallucinations or false perceptions.
- *Stupor.* A somnolent state in which the patient may be momentarily aroused by painful stimuli or questions. Reflexes are preserved.
- *Blackout.* This implies a brief loss of consciousness.
- *Coma.* This implies a more prolonged loss of consciousness. Comatosed patients fail to respond to stimuli, lose their deep and superficial reflexes, and become incontinent. Patients in a coma are more likely to present in a hospital than in primary practice.

Once it has been established that the patient has experienced a transitory loss of consciousness, a description of the blackout is helpful. Useful diagnostic information is gathered by asking the patient and observers to describe:

- events or sensations preceding the loss of consciousness
- the attack
- the recovery period.

Blackouts are largely attributable to cardiovascular causes or neurological causes.

Cardiovascular causes. Cerebral hypoxia due to impaired perfusion can result in a temporary loss of consciousness. An increased vascular capacity or reduced cardiac output can result in impaired cerebral perfusion. Cardiac output may be reduced by hypovolemia or changes in the heart rate, such as bradycardia or a heart beat irregularity. An imbalance of the autonomic nervous system with parasympathetic dominance can increase the volume or capacity of the vasculature. Cardiovascular syncope is clinically characterized by:

- a prodrome of
  - sweating
  - nausea
  - visual changes
- a syncopal phase of
  - muscle weakness
  - mental confusion
- a recovery phase that is
  - rapid
  - characterized by immediate awareness.

Neurological causes. Neurological blackouts are often associated with an alteration in the electrical activity of the brain. Compared with syncope, patients with seizures are more likely to:

- experience motor changes (e.g. jerking, twitching, staring)
- experience a slower recovery period (confusion or memory loss may be pronounced during the recovery period)
- demonstrate electroencephalogram (EEG) changes during the attack.

Certain types of seizure may be associated with disturbed consciousness rather than a loss of consciousness.

Is emergency resuscitation indicated?

See Figure 8.1.

The *recovery position* aims to prevent inhalation of saliva or stomach contents. The patient is placed:

- midway between lying on one side and their stomach
- with the upper limb, which is not in contact with the floor, flexed, and the hand placed under the head
- with the head turned to one side

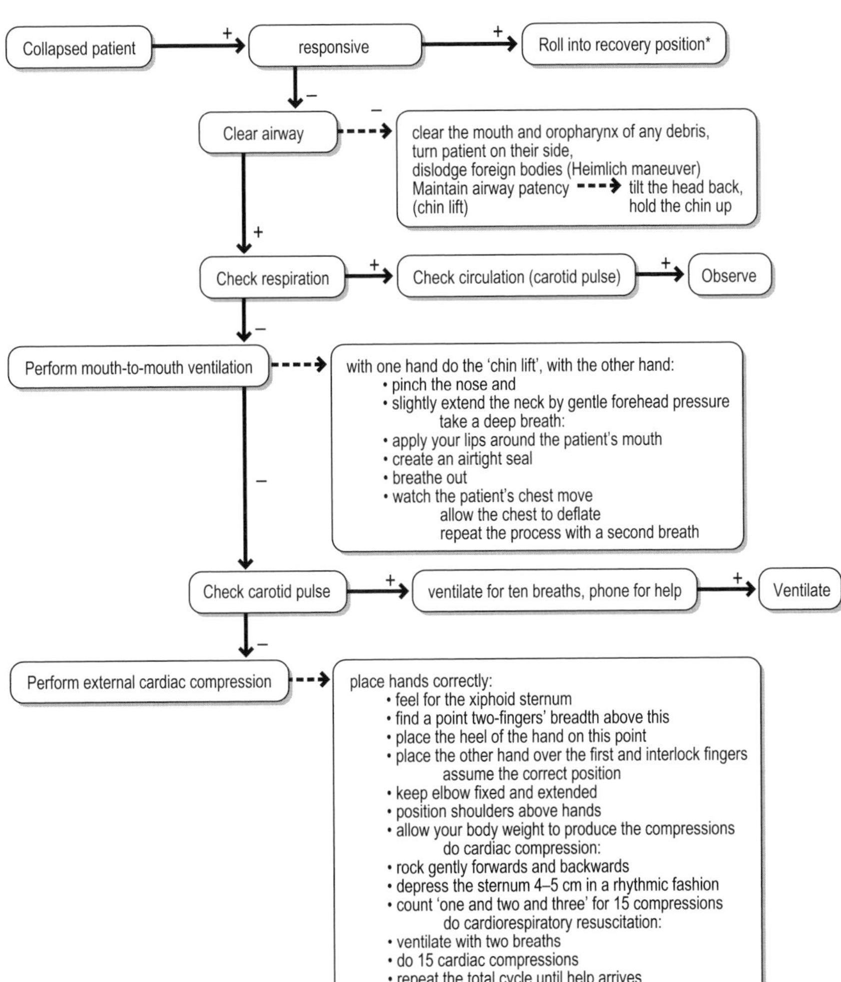

Figure 8.1 **Resuscitation.**

- with the lower limb, which is not stretched along the floor, flexed at the hip, with the knee and foot resting on the floor on the same side as the face.

The *Heimlich maneuver* attempts to dislodge foreign bodies obstructing the upper airway by raising the intrathoracic pressure. It is performed by

- kneeling astride the supine patient
- placing a fist on the epigastrium and covering the fist with the other hand
- thrusting both hands up beneath the costal margin.

What is the likely cause?

See Figure 8.2.

PART TWO

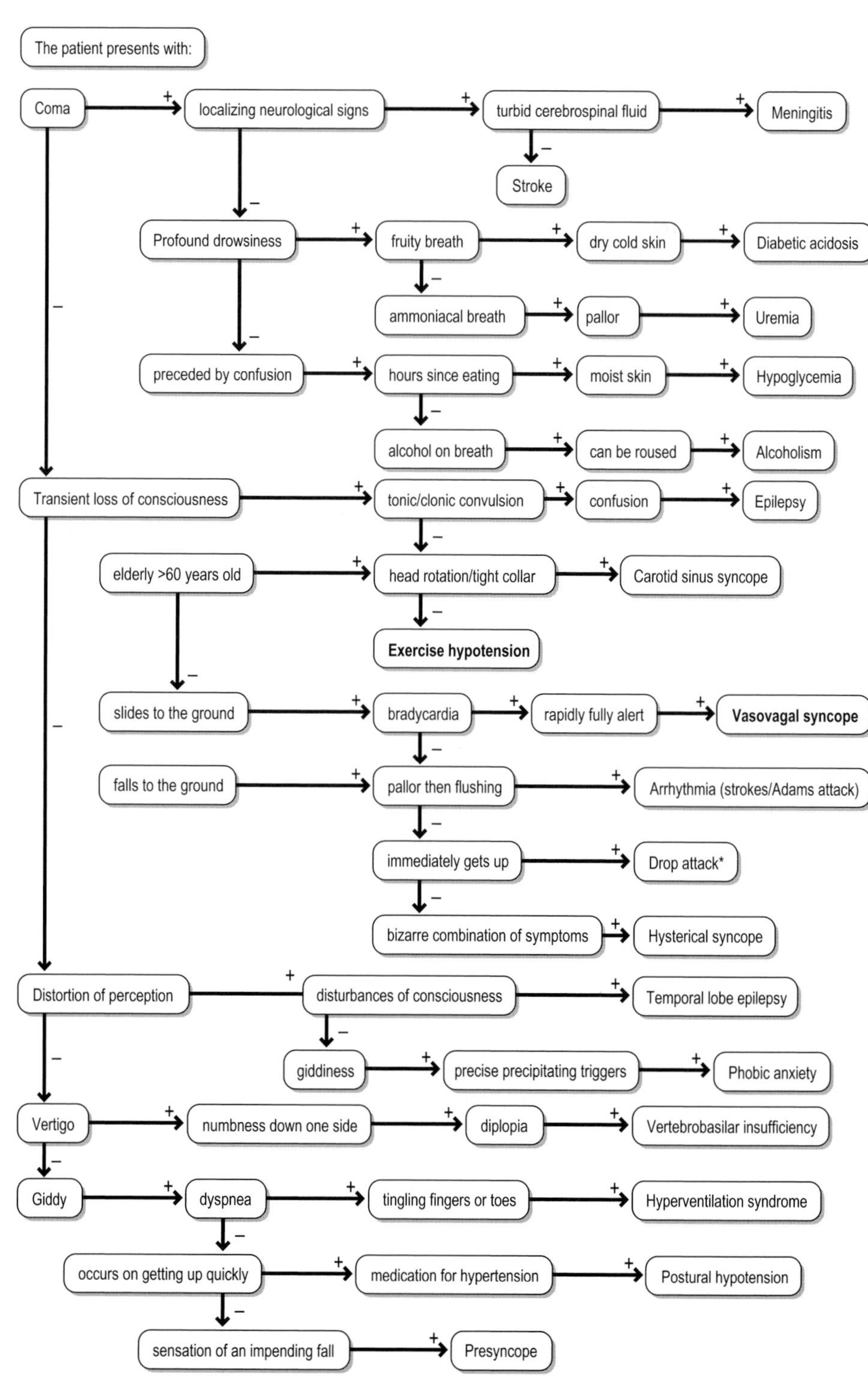

Figure 8.2 **Loss of consciousness.**

Does the patient need to be referred?

Patients in a coma require hospital admission. All patients with blackout should be referred if they have:

- unexplained transient loss or disturbance of consciousness
- undiagnosed or untreated vertigo
- require specific treatment outside your scope of practice.

FURTHER READING

Alboni P, Brignole M, Menozzi C, Raviele A, Del Rosso A, Dinelli M, Bettiol K, Bottoni N, Solano A 2004 Clinical spectrum of neurally mediated reflex syncopes. Europace 6(1): 55–62

Brignole M 2005 Neurally-mediated syncope. Ital Heart J 6(3):249–255

Tang A W 2003 A practical guide to anaphylaxis. Am Fam Physician 68(7):1325–1332

White A M 2003 What happened? Alcohol, memory blackouts, and the brain. Alcohol Res Health 27(2):186–196

Wohrle J, Kochs M 2003 Syncope in the elderly. Z Gerontol Geriatr 36(1):2–9

Bleeding from the bowel

CHAPTER CONTENTS

Is there blood in the stool?

Blood in the stool may be overt or occult. Depending on the volume of blood lost and the site of the lesion, bleeding from the gastrointestinal tract may present as:

- *Red blood.* Red blood suggests bleeding between the colon and the anus. In addition to its color, the relationship of blood in the stool to fecal matter provides clues to the anatomical site of the lesion. Red blood which:
  - coats but is not mixed with the stool suggests anal or rectal bleeding
  - is mixed with mucus suggests a rectal, or a descending or sigmoid colon lesion
  - is mixed with the stool suggests bleeding above the sigmoid colon
  - is associated with an unformed stool consistent with intestinal hurry may be due to a massive gastrointestinal hemorrhage (duodenal ulceration is found in one-third, erosive gastritis in one-quarter, and gastric ulcers in one-sixth of massive gastrointestinal bleeds).
- *A black tarry stool.* Black blood (melena) suggests loss of at least 60 ml of blood from the upper gastrointestinal tract. The tarry appearance of the stool is attributable to the conversion of hemoglobin into hematin by hydrochloric acid in the stomach.
- *Occult blood.* Small bleeds not visible to the naked eye may be detected during screening using occult blood tests. Such patients do not present complaining of blood in the stool. If symptomatic, their complaint is more likely to reflect the anemia which may result from chronic blood loss.

As occult blood is only detected using special tests criteria have been identified to actively screen for blood in the stool.

What is the likely diagnosis?

See Figure 9.1.

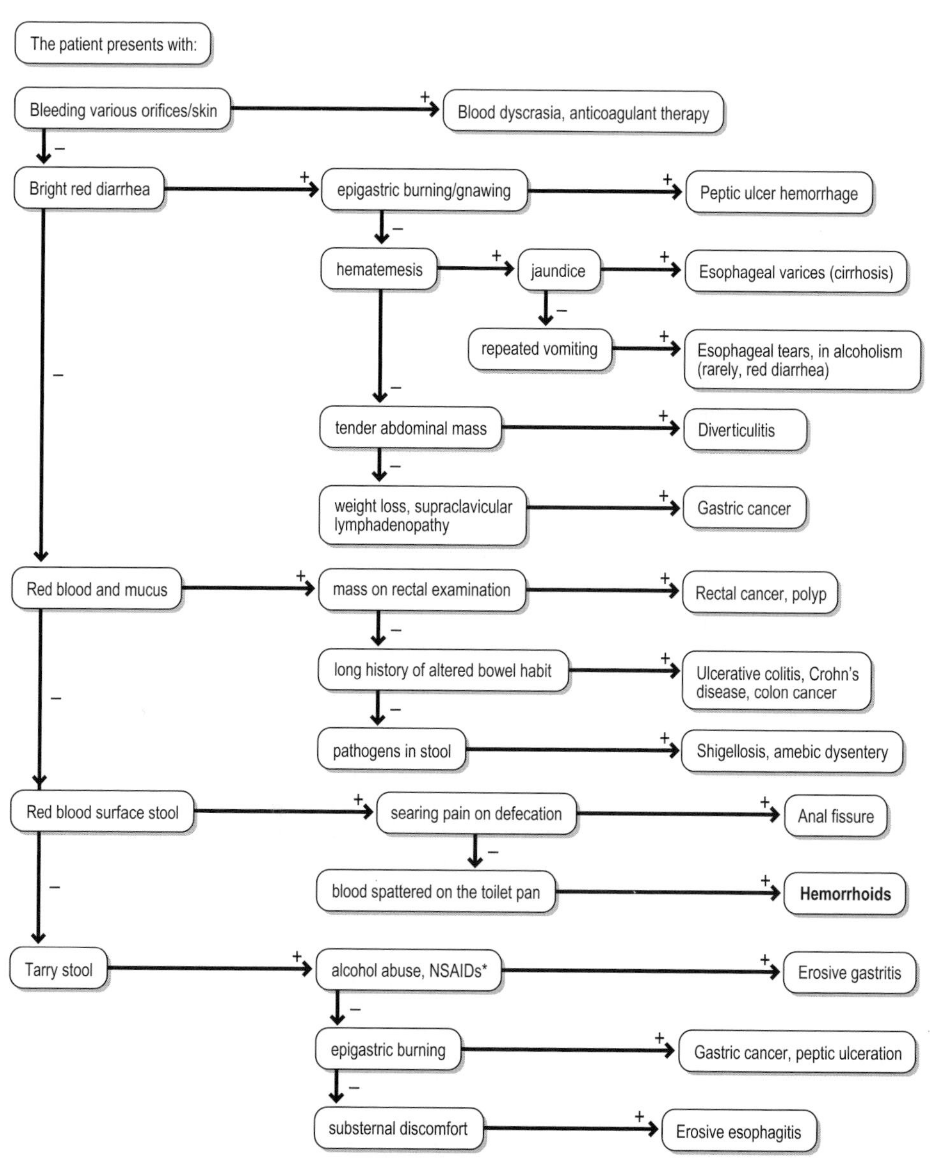

Figure 9.1 **Blood in the stool.**

Does the patient need to be referred?

Investigation to establish a definitive diagnosis is required in cases of bleeding from the gastrointestinal tract, including:

- Passing red blood per rectum.
- Melena. Urgent referral is indicated in patients with melena and evidence of shock:
  - pallor
  - light-headedness, fainting
  - cold, clammy extremities
  - sweating
  - tachycardia
  - hypotension.
- A positive occult blood test. In view of the prevalence of colorectal cancer, patients with a positive occult blood test are investigated using a combination of:
  - barium enema
  - flexible fiberoptic sigmoidoscopy
  - colonoscopy
  - colonoscopic polypectomy.

FURTHER READING

Hamilton W, Sharp D 2004 Diagnosis of colorectal cancer in primary care: the evidence base for guidelines. Fam Pract 21(1):99–106

Husain A, Triadafilopoulos G 2004 Communicating with patients with inflammatory bowel disease. Inflamm Bowel Dis 10(4):444–450; discussion 451

Manning-Dimmitt L L, Dimmitt S G, Wilson G R 2005 Diagnosis of gastrointestinal bleeding in adults. Am Fam Physician 71(7):1339–1346

Melmed G Y, Lo S K 2005 Capsule endoscopy: practical applications. Clin Gastroenterol Hepatol 3(5):411–422

Mitchell S H, Schaefer D C, Dubagunta S 2004 A new view of occult and obscure gastrointestinal bleeding. Am Fam Physician 69(4):875–881

CHAPTER 10

Breathlessness

CHAPTER CONTENTS

What is the nature of the patient's dyspnea?

Dyspnea is defined as subjective shortness of breath or the conscious awareness of the need for an increased respiratory effort. Dyspnea may be categorized as:

- *Blockpnea.* The patient has a subjective sensation of air not getting completely into the lungs.
- *Platypnea.* This is breathlessness that occurs only in the upright position.
- *Trepopnea.* Breathing difficulties are experienced in the left lateral decubitus position. Unilateral lung disease should be suspected.
- *Tachypnea.* This describes rapid breathing.
- *Orthopnea.* This term describes dyspnea that occurs when lying flat. It is found in persons who already have considerable limitation of exercise and is also a symptom of left ventricular failure. Early evidence suggestive of left-sided heart failure is patients finding lying more comfortable when they are propped up on a number of pillows. Recumbency leads to increased venous return. In patients with a failing left ventricle, blood pools in the lungs, decreasing lung compliance and vital capacity. Vital capacity may be further reduced in the recumbent position by relative elevation of the diaphragm, especially if the liver is enlarged.
- *Paroxysmal nocturnal dyspnea.* This is episodic dyspnea. It is precipitated by prolonged lying down and relieved by standing up. Dyspnea causes the patient to wake up. Cardiac asthma and acute pulmonary edema are causes of paroxysmal dyspnea.

- *Exertional dyspnea.* Shortness of breath is precipitated by exercise. Exertional dyspnea, defined as excessive breathlessness for the amount of exercise performed, is graded as follows:
  I no dyspnea on climbing stairs or walking uphill
  II breathlessness on climbing stairs or hills
  III breathlessness when walking fast on the flat
  IV breathlessness when walking more than 100 m on the flat
  V breathlessness when dressing, washing, or walking a few meters.
- *Dyspnea at rest.* This is the most severe form of dyspnea.

In general medical practice, for every 10 cases of dyspnea attributable to a trivial cause there is likely to be one patient with a serious cause of breathlessness.

Is the dyspnea functional or organic?

In view of their different prognoses, it is important to differentiate between organic and psychogenic causes of dyspnea. Clues to diagnosing the hyperventilation syndrome include:

- breathlessness that is worst at rest
- walking that is not impaired by dyspnea
- a sensation of being unable to take a deep satisfying breath
- being breathless all the time
- paresthesia may develop as a result of hyperventilation.

In patients with organic causes of dyspnea, it is helpful to remember that:

- Structural changes may be detected on a radiograph of the lung.
- Functional changes may be detected on spirometry.
- Patients may have acquired behaviors that provide some relief of their dyspnea, such as:
  - Sitting or standing in a forward-leaning position. Patients with chronic causes of dyspnea may stand leaning on a windowsill or counter, or they may sit leaning, with forearms resting on their thighs or knees.
  - Breathing through pursed lips. Increasing the intraluminal pressure may decrease the tendency of the terminal bronchioles to collapse, and reduce the sensation of breathlessness. This strategy also tends to reduce the rate of respiration.
- The onset and progression of dyspnea varies with the cause:
  - In heart disease dyspnea is worst on lying down.
  - In metabolic disorders: acidosis is associated with deep slow respiration and air hunger; alkalemia is associated with shallow respiration.
  - In respiratory disease an early symptom is exertional dyspnea.

Two important groups of respiratory disorder that cause dyspnea are:

- *Restrictive lung disease.* Movement of the chest walls or lung expansion is difficult. Reduced lung compliance may be encountered in lung fibrosis, cardiac failure, or neuromuscular disorders.

- *Obstructive airways disease.* Moving air through the airways is difficult.
  - Upper respiratory tract obstruction causes noisy respiration, stridor, and use of accessory muscles. Croup is an example.
  - Small airways disease causes patients to experience difficulty in breathing out. These patients have vesicular respiration with prolonged expiration. Wheezes and rhonchi are common. Emphysema and chronic bronchitis are examples.

Spirometry is helpful in discriminating between obstructive and restrictive lung disease. Four basic lung volumes measured by spirometry are:

- *Tidal volume.* The volume inhaled and exhaled with a normal breath at rest. Usually around 500 ml.
- *Inspiratory reserve volume.* Air inhaled from a position of quiet inspiration to full inspiration. Usually about 3100 ml.
- *Expiratory reserve volume.* Air exhaled from a position of quiet expiration to full expiration. Usually about 1200 ml.
- *Residual volume.* The volume of air left in the lungs after maximal exhalation. Normally around 1200 ml.

The *functional residual volume* is the sum of the residual volume and the expiratory reserve volume. The *vital capacity* is the sum of the expiratory reserve volume, the tidal volume, and the inspiratory reserve volume. The *forced expiratory volume* (FEV_1) is the volume expired in 1 second. The *forced vital capacity* (FVC) is the total volume expired (see Table 10.1).

What is the likely cause?

See Figure 10.1.

Does the patient need to be referred?

Dyspnea at rest is an indication of severity. Referral should be considered in dyspneic patients who have a:

- respiratory rate > 30/min
- pulsus paradoxus > 15 mmHg
- tachycardia > 120/min
- dyspnea when sitting

Table 10.1
Spirometry in health and disease

	Normal	**Obstructive airways disease**	**Restrictive lung disease**
FEV_1	3.8 l	2.5 l	1.4 l
FVC	4.8 l	4.5 l	1.7 l
FEV_1/FVC	80%	55%	82%

FEV_1, forced expiratory volume; FVC, forced vital capacity.

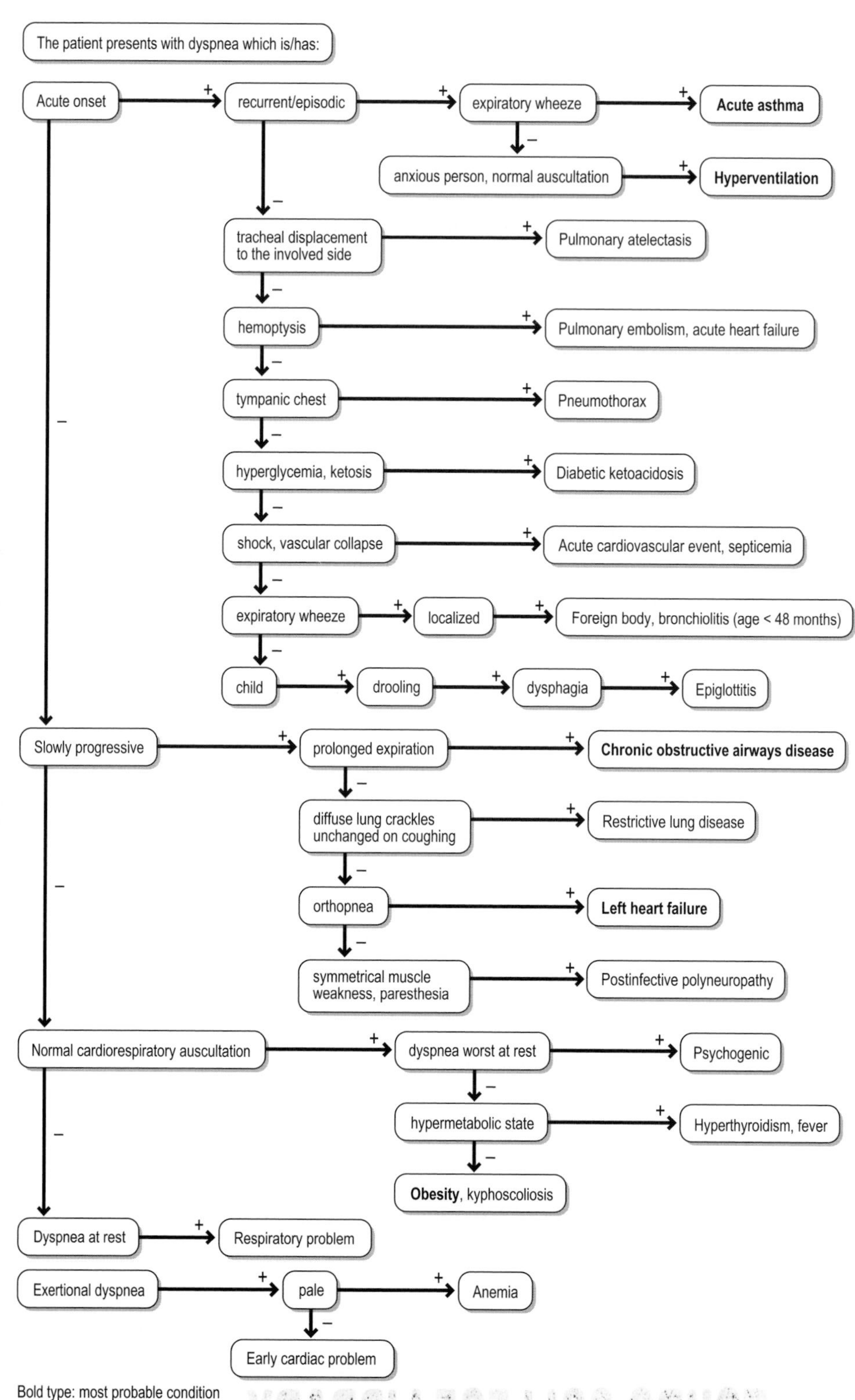

Bold type: most probable condition

Figure 10.1 **Dyspnea.**

- inability to talk in uninterrupted sentences
- cyanosis.

Early medical intervention in the following cases of breathlessness may avert serious consequences:

- Airway obstruction: asthma, upper airways obstruction.
- Parenchymal lung disease: infiltration, interstitial fibrosis.
- Pleural disease: pneumothorax, infectious pleurisy.
- Pulmonary vascular disease: pulmonary embolism, vasculitis.
- Cardiac disease: congestive heart failure.

A systematic approach to management involves:

- identifying the cause
- assessing the degree of disability
- documenting precipitating and relieving factors.

FURTHER READING

Barreiro T J, Perillo I 2004 An approach to interpreting spirometry. Am Fam Physician 69(5):1107–1114

Dosh S A 2004 Diagnosis of heart failure in adults. Am Fam Physician 70(11):2145–2152

Ebell M H 2004 Suspected pulmonary embolism: Part I. Evidence-based clinical assessment. Am Fam Physician 69(2):367–369

Karnani N G, Reisfield G M, Wilson G R 2005 Evaluation of chronic dyspnea. Am Fam Physician 71(8):1529–1537

Mintz M 2004 Asthma update: Part I. Diagnosis, monitoring, and prevention of disease progression. Am Fam Physician 70(5):893–898

Vallance G, Thomson N C 2004 Asthma: ten myths debunked. Practitioner 248(1664):844–847

Zoorob R J, Campbell J S 2003 Acute dyspnea in the office. Am Fam Physician 68(9):1803–1810

Bruising and easy bleeding

CHAPTER CONTENTS

What is the nature of the excess bleeding or easy bruising?

Bleeding into the skin causes purplish discoloration termed *purpura*. *Petechiae* are small purpura of less than 2 mm diameter; *ecchymoses* are large purpura. Local trauma and systemic conditions may result in bruising.

Persons prone to easy bruising or prolonged bleeding may have deficiencies affecting the vessel wall, platelets, or blood coagulation factors. Normal hemostasis requires:

- vascular constriction to diminish blood flow
- formation of a platelet plug
- local blood coagulation.

Bleeding time evaluates all these elements. It is normally less than 6 minutes.

The major mechanisms underlying systemic bleeding disorders (Table 11.1) are:

- Coagulation abnormalities. These present with:
  - delayed bleeding (oozing follows the initial hemostasis, which was achieved by platelets)
  - abnormal prothrombin and activated partial thromboplastin time.
- *Vascular defects*. These present clinically with:
  - easy bruising and bleeding into the skin
  - mucous membrane bleeding
  - normal investigations.
- Platelet abnormalities. These present as:
  - early bleeding following trauma
  - bleeding into mucous membranes
  - petechiae.

Table 11.1 **Differentiating bleeding disorders**

	Underlying defect type	
Bleeding manifestations	**Coagulation**	**Platelet**
Petechiae and bruises	–	++++
Epistaxis	+/–	++
Menorrhagia	+/–	++
GIT bleed (melena)	+	+
Hemarthrosis	++++	–
Bleeding into tissues	++++	–
Dental/postoperative bleed:		
Onset	Delayed	Immediate
Volume	Profuse	Ooze

GIT, gastrointestinal tract.

Platelet abnormalities may be due to defective platelet function (thrombasthenia) or reduced platelet numbers (thrombocytopenia). There is a correlation between symptoms and the platelet count:

- <20 × 10^9/l: spontaneous bruising or ecchymoses following minor trauma.
- 20–40 × 10^9/l: bruising follows minor trauma, and purpura develop using the capillary resistance test. In the Hess test inflation of a baumanometer cuff is used to test capillary resistance. The development of purpura or petechiae distal to the cuff indicate increased capillary fragility.
- >40–60 × 10^9/l: bruising only occurs following significant trauma.

Bleeding may present as:

- hemorrhagic shock with hypotension and tachycardia
- a coagulation defect with hemarthosis and hematomas
- a platelet defect with petechiae, purpura, and epistaxis
- chronic blood loss with pallor.

Blood loss of less than 500 ml does not result in circulatory changes, except in the elderly and those with cardiovascular disease or anemia. Blood loss in excess of 500 ml may result in oligemic or hypovolemic shock. (See *Shock*, pp. 587–588.)

What is the likely diagnosis?

See Figure 11.1.

Does the patient need to be referred?

Further investigation is indicated when there is suspicion of:

- a hemostatic disorder
- an underlying malignancy.

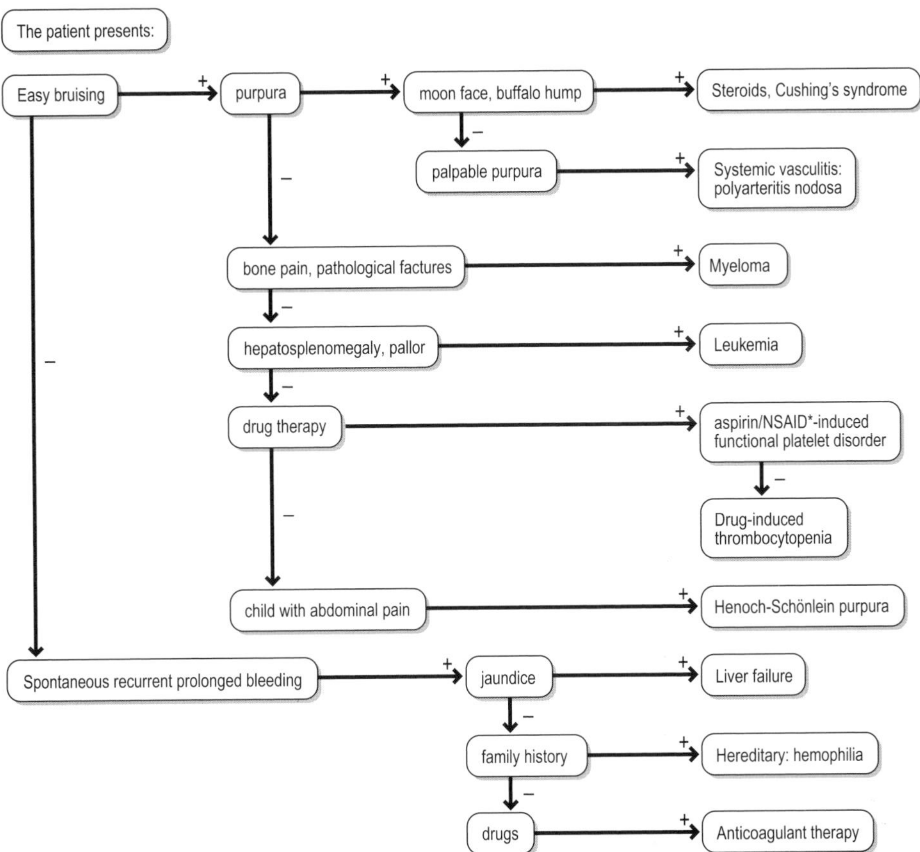

*NSAID: nonsteroidal anti-inflammatory drug

Figure 11.1 **Bruising and bleeding.**

FURTHER READING

Allen G A, Glader B 2002 Approach to the bleeding child. Pediatr Clin North Am 49(6):1239–1256

Kouides P A 2002 Evaluation of abnormal bleeding in women. Curr Hematol Rep 1(1):11–18

Teitel J M 2000 Clinical approach to the patient with unexpected bleeding. Clin Lab Hematol Suppl 1:9–11; discussion 30–32

CHAPTER 12

Chest pain

CHAPTER CONTENTS

Is the chest pain life-threatening?

Life-threatening disorders causing chest pain are most likely to arise from the cardiovascular system. Syncope and chest pain is a potentially ominous combination, and the cause of hypotension in such patients requires clarification (Fig. 12.1).

Criteria suggesting the need for urgent hospital referral include patients with:

- crushing retrosternal chest pain which lasts for more than 20 minutes with or without radiation to the jaw or arm
- suspected angina which fails to respond to nitrite spray within 90 seconds
- sudden onset of stabbing chest pain accompanied by rapidly progressive dyspnea and tracheal displacement

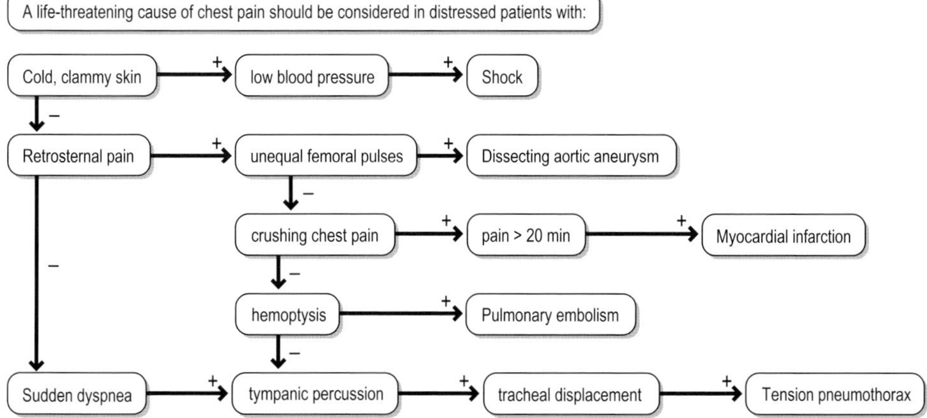

Figure 12.1 **Life-threatening chest pain.**

- acute onset of chest pain and dyspnea with hemoptysis or calf tenderness
- severe midline chest pain which radiates to the abdomen and legs and is associated with unequal femoral pulses.

What are the major sources of chest pain?

The most prevalent causes of chest pain are anxiety, musculoskeletal conditions, and myocardial hypoxia. In general terms, chest pain may be attributable to psychogenic, somatic, or visceral causes. All these possibilities need to be actively excluded in any patient complaining of chest pain. The clinical prognosis and management in each case is vastly different. It is consequently important to initially discriminate between the three major sources of pain.

Chest pain that is aggravated by anxiety or fatigue, described as continuous or stabbing, and lasts several hours or days is likely to be psychogenic in nature. Although the location varies, psychogenic chest pain is often experienced in the left submammary region. Radiation is uncommon. Hyperventilation can result in the patient experiencing a tingling numbness. The possibility of psychogenic pain needs to be considered when:

- The onset, character, and site of pain are vague or poorly defined. Psychogenic chest pain may be described as a sharp constant retrosternal pain, which lasts for several hours. The character of the pain may be altered by persistent hyperventilation, resulting in numbness or tingling which may radiate to the mouth, hands, and fingers.
- The pain:
  - is aggravated by anxiety
  - is relieved by alcohol, relaxation, and nitroglycerine
  - persistently fails to respond to a diversity of interventions
  - has no consistent relationship to exercise.
- The degree of pain intensity and duration is grossly inconsistent with any identifiable lesion.
- 'Severe' pain does not disturb the patient's sleep.

In all cases, the pain is real to the patient, regardless of whether it is primarily attributed to psychogenic, somatic, or visceral causes by the clinician. Furthermore, pain is exacerbated by fear and anxiety. All patients therefore require careful assessment in order that appropriate intervention is undertaken. As psychogenic causes of pain are less likely to have a poor short-term prognosis and various visceral causes of pain may be fatal, it is important to actively exclude visceral causes of pain before diagnosing psychogenic pain. A general principle is that diagnosis of psychogenic pain should only be made when visceral and musculoskeletal causes have been excluded. The propensity for psychogenic factors to exacerbate the pain of visceral and somatic conditions should also never be overlooked.

The working diagnosis of chest pain of *musculoskeletal origin* is facilitated by detection of local tenderness and pain that is reproduced on palpation of the thoracic cage or spine. The prognosis is good insofar as musculoskeletal causes of chest pain are seldom, if ever, fatal and many resolve spontaneously, albeit after some time. Musculoskeletal pain is often:

- Ill-defined in onset and may refer anywhere on the chest wall.
- Experienced as a dull ache which lasts for hours or days.
- Persistent, with a long history of many years.
- Precipitated by movement.
- Aggravated by certain postures, damp, cold weather, and activity. Pain is worst in the evenings, particularly after physical exertion.
- Relieved following rest, a change in position, heat, manipulation, and/or aspirin.
- Associated with physical phenomena: muscle spasm and restriction of movement.
- Associated with neural phenomena: sensory and motor changes.
- Tolerable, permitting continued exercise despite the persistence of pain.

Chest pain of musculoskeletal origin is frequently due to vertebral dysfunction of the lower cervical or upper thoracic spine. Facet and/or costovertebral joint dysfunction and disc prolapse of the lower cervical spine also deserve special consideration.

Unlike musculoskeletal causes of chest pain, spontaneous resolution of chest pain due to respiratory and/or cardiovascular disease is relatively uncommon. *Visceral causes* of pain:

- are often clear-cut in onset
- are usually associated with changes in the normal function of that organ
- may last for minutes or hours
- vary in nature from crushing to burning and intensity from mild to excruciating.

Although the most common causes of chest pain are benign conditions with a good prognosis, several serious visceral conditions are also prevalent. It is therefore important to identify the particular organ system involved. Visceral chest pain may arise from the heart and great vessels, the gastrointestinal tract, or the respiratory system. Each of these organ systems may cause retrosternal pain. Consideration of the nature, severity, radiation, and duration of retrosternal pain is particularly helpful in the differential diagnosis. Associated findings that suggest impaired function of an organ system also provides useful diagnostic clues.

Findings that favor pain of *cardiovascular origin* include:

- Deep retrosternal chest pain which radiates. Chest pain of visceral origin frequently arises from myocardial hypoxia. Myocardial hypoxia, which results in temporary pain and is

relieved by rest, differs from myocardial ischemia and necrosis, in which pain is more persistent and is unrelieved by, and can occur at, rest. The crushing pain of myocardial ischemia may radiate to the inner arm (left particularly), jaw, neck, between the shoulder blades, and epigastrium. The pain of myocardial infarction lasts for more than 15–20 minutes, while the pain of angina usually lasts 5 minutes or less. In contrast to myocardial ischemia, psychogenic chest pain is sharp and longer lasting. While the pain of cardiac ischemia radiates up to the jaw, the tearing midline pain of a dissecting aneurysm radiates down to the abdomen anteriorly and legs posteriorly. Acute pericarditis, although it may mimic myocardial ischemia, presenting with a crushing deep retrosternal pain that radiates to the back, more commonly is pleuritic in nature and is aggravated by deep inspiration.
- Pain that is precipitated by exertion and prevents continued exercise.
- Pain the onset of which can be pinpointed to a specific time.
- Progressive exertional dyspnea and orthopnea.
- Evidence of distress, including palpitations and syncope.
- Constitutional and/or behavioral factors, such as:
  - male gender
  - postmenopausal female
  - hypercholesterolemia
  - smoking
  - hypertension.

Findings that favor pain of *gastrointestinal origin* include:

- A pain which radiates. Retrosternal esophageal pain due to spasm radiates to the back and is crushing in nature. In contrast, gastroesophageal reflux causes burning retrosternal pain which radiates to the jaw.
- Attacks related to meals.
- Attacks of variable duration, often lasting for hours.
- Chronic symptomatology of varying intensity.
- A history of indigestion, regurgitation, dysphagia.

Findings that favor pain of *respiratory origin* include:

- Pain aggravated by deep inspiration or coughing. Pulmonary embolism usually causes retrosternal pain. Pleural involvement in pneumonia or following pulmonary infarction causes a sharp stabbing chest pain.
- A cough, which may be dry or productive.

Compared to other causes of chest pain, respiratory (pleuritic) chest pain rarely radiates.

Figure 12.2 considers the presentation of chest pain caused by different systems.

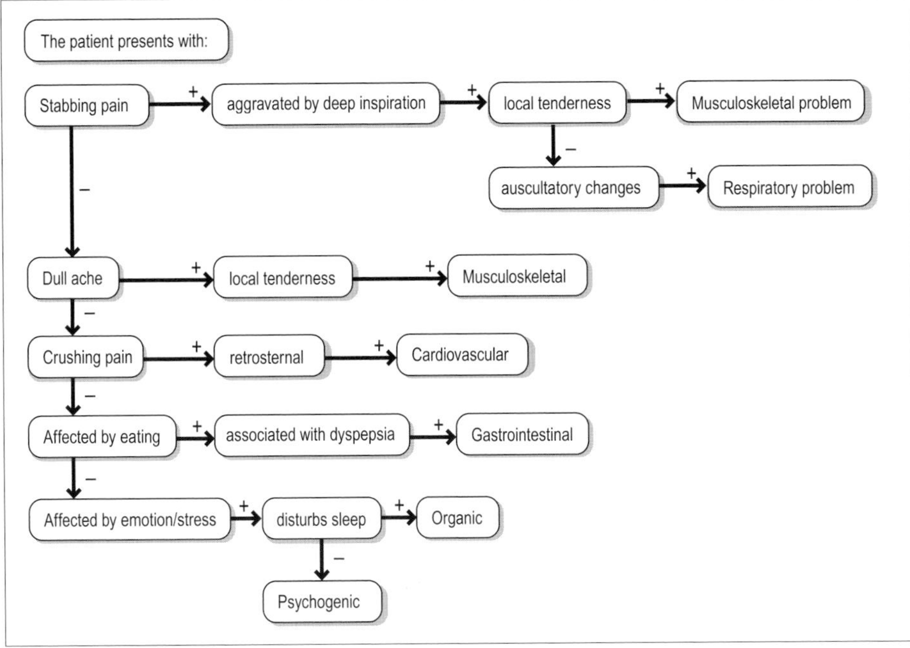

Figure 12.2 **Probable source of chest pain, by organ system.**

What is the likely diagnosis?

See Figure 12.3.

Does the patient need to be referred?

Patients who would benefit from referral for functional assessment, definitive diagnosis, or specialized treatment include those:

- At risk of myocardial damage:
  - suspected myocardial infarction
  - unstable angina
  - acute coronary insufficiency.
- With suspected:
  - pulmonary embolic disease
  - pneumothorax
  - aneurysm
  - gallbladder disease.
- Who fail to respond to treatment.
- Requiring therapy outside your scope of practice.

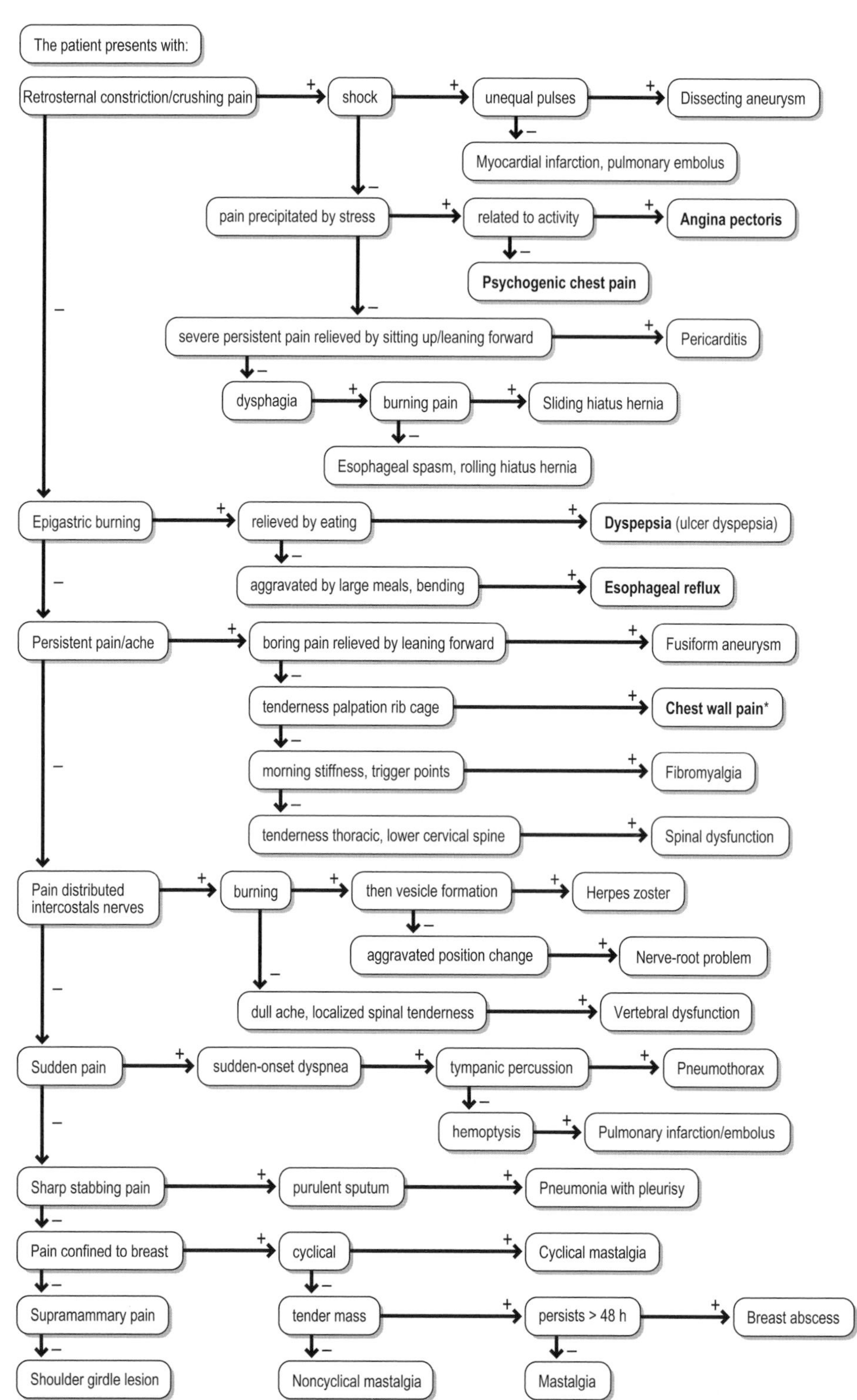

Bold type: most probable condition.
*Chest wall pain attributable to any of the following: fractured rib, sternalis syndrome, xiphoidalgia, costosternal/costochondral syndrome.

Figure 12.3 **Chest pain.**

FURTHER READING

Chesebro J H 2004 Acute coronary syndromes: pathogenesis, acute diagnosis with risk stratification, and treatment. Am Heart Hosp J 2(4 Suppl 1):21–30

Heading R C 2004 Review article: diagnosis and clinical investigation of gastro-esophageal reflux disease: a European view. Aliment Pharmacol Ther 20 Suppl 8:9–13

Katerndahl D 2004 Panic plaques: panic disorder and coronary artery disease in patients with chest pain. J Am Board Fam Pract 17(2):114–126

Kawano H, Ogawa H 2005 Endothelial function and coronary spastic angina. Intern Med 44(2):91–99

Mant J, McManus R J, Oakes R A, Delaney B C, Barton P M, Deeks J J, Hammersley L, Davies R C, Davies M K, Hobbs F D 2005 Systematic review and modelling of the investigation of acute and chronic chest pain presenting in primary care. Health Technol Assess 8(2):iii, 1–158

Raj P P 2004 Visceral pain. Agri 16(1):7–20

CHAPTER 13 Clubbing

CHAPTER CONTENTS

Does the patient have clubbing?

Clubbing is an overgrowth of the vascular nail bed tissue and is characterized by:

- A loss of the normal angle between the base of the nail and the cuticle. This is observed by holding the finger parallel to the eye and viewing the horizontal finger from the side.
- An increased longitudinal and lateral curvature of the nail.
- Fluctuation or sponginess of the nail bed.

In extreme cases the terminal phalanx may look like a drumstick.

To detect clubbing, the finger should be viewed in profile in two planes.

What is the likely cause?

The most common causes (Fig. 13.1) are chronic cardiorespiratory disorders (e.g. cyanotic congenital heart disease, lung cancer) or chronic infection (e.g. bacterial endocarditis, bronchiectasis, lung abscess).

Does the patient need to be referred?

Patients need to be referred if:

- undiagnosed disease is suspected
- the patient requires therapy outside your scope of practice.

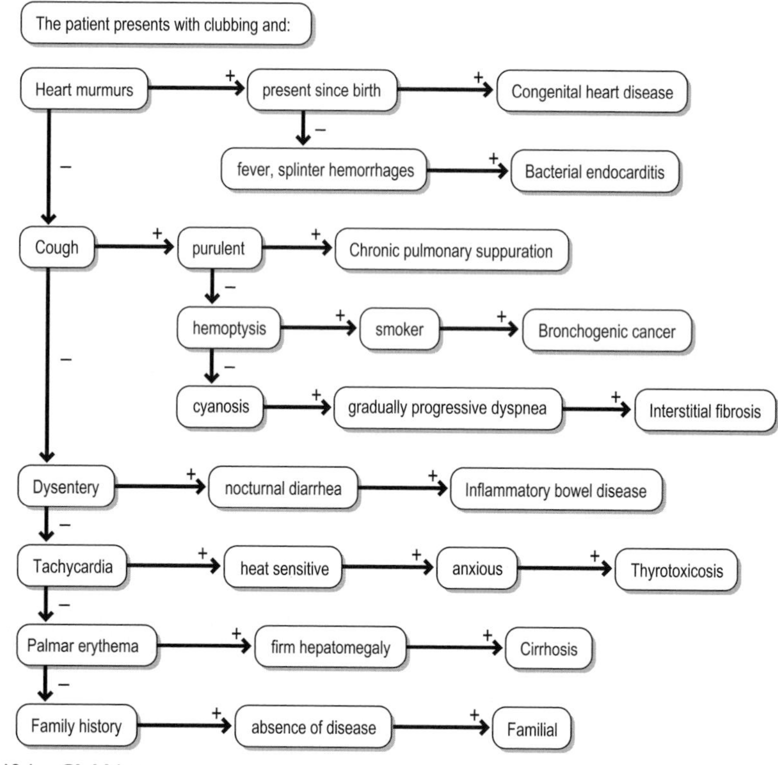

Figure 13.1 **Clubbing.**

FURTHER READING

Hamilton W, Sharp D 2004 Diagnosis of lung cancer in primary care: a structured review. Fam Pract 21(6):605–611.

CHAPTER

14 Confusion and confused behavior

CHAPTER CONTENTS

PART TWO

What is the nature of the patient's cognitive problem?

Confused behavior may result from a change in cognitive function. Cognition is the process of 'knowing', it refers to the mental functions of perception, thinking, and memory.

A mental status examination provides the data required to ascertain the patient's confused state. A mental status examination usually explores the patient's:

- *Level of consciousness* (see Ch. 8). Patients are assessed for alertness, drowsiness, and fluctuating consciousness. In comatose patients the level of consciousness is determined by evaluating:
  - Eye opening: eyes may remain closed or open spontaneously or in response to speech or a painful stimulus.
  - Verbal response: talking to the patient may indicate orientation, confusion, use of inappropriate words, incomprehensible sounds, or elicit no response.
  - Motor response: check for responses to commands and pain. Pain may provoke normal or abnormal flexion, a localized, generalized, or no response.
  - Pupil response.
  - Reflexes.
- *Cognitive functions* (Box 14.1). It is important to determine whether the patient:
  - is orientated
  - can concentrate
  - has a memory problem
  - has any distortions of perception
  - has any aberration of thought content.

Box 14.1
Assessment of cognitive functions

This includes ascertaining the patient's:

- *Orientation.* Awareness of time, place, and personal data provide information on the patient's orientation. Confusion is disorientation regarding time, place, or person. It may result from organic disease, but may also be encountered in depression and psychosis
- *Attention and concentration.* Arithmetic tasks are usually used to check these dimensions. Disturbances can result from fatigue, affective change (e.g. excitement or depression), psychosis, or organic disorders. Disorganized attention is a key feature of delirium
- *Memory.* Accuracy of information provided, recall of recent events, and learning ability provide insight into memory function. Patients may be asked to name three items and then recall them 5–10 minutes later. The serial 7s test, which requires that the patient repeatedly subtract 7 from 100 (to give 93, 86, 79, etc.) may also be used. The key feature of dementia is impaired memory. Memory dysfunction may be:
  - Anterograde amnesia: post-traumatic amnesia occurs when new memories cannot be retained
  - Retrograde amnesia: this extends backwards in time and decreases as the patient recovers
- *Perception.* Disordered perceptions may present as:
  - Illusions: perceptual errors; sensory stimuli are falsely interpreted resulting in misperceptions
  - Hallucinations: involuntary false perceptions; are often auditory or visual
- *Thought content.* Careful questioning is required to recognize:
  - Delusion: illogical, false beliefs that are strongly held in the absence of any supporting evidence
  - Hypochondriacal ideas: extreme and inappropriate concern about health
  - Phobias: irrational and exaggerated fears are expressed
  - Obsessions: repetitive and intrusive thoughts are experienced; rituals may be performed
- *General intelligence and language function.* This includes understanding and verbal expression and is assessed by verbal fluency and an understanding of abstract concepts. Abstract reasoning may be checked by asking for an explanation of common proverbs or discussing the potential repercussions of current events. An attempt should be made to ascertain the patient's insight into their condition

- *Mood or affect.* This includes noting:
  - The quality of the prevailing mood. Mood may be depressed (depression) or elevated (euphoria). Extreme elation is encountered in mania.

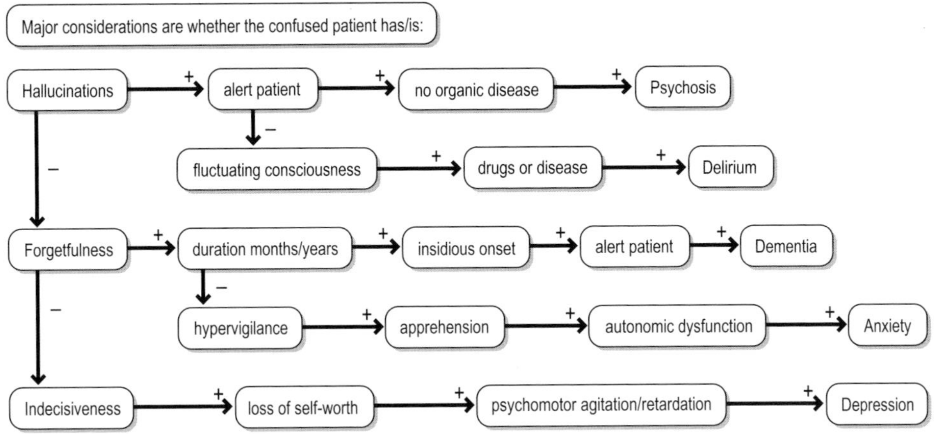

Figure 14.1 **Mental status examination.**

- Reaction to external influences. Inappropriate reactivity includes:
- Incongruity of affect given a particular situation. Examples include laughing on sad occasions or fear associated with normal everyday events (e.g. fear of shopping).
- Flattening or blunting of affect, as seen in schizophrenia where normal emotional responsiveness is reduced.
- Constancy. Patients with exaggerated changeability of mood in response to external influences are described as 'emotionally labile'.

The mental status examination provides some clues as to the nature of the patient's confused state (Fig. 14.1). A confused state may be encountered in:

- Organic mental disorders, such as:
  - Acute organic brain syndrome. Delirium is a relatively acute disorder in which orientation and attention are markedly impaired. Both perception and mood are affected.
  - Chronic organic brain syndrome. In dementia, the failure of higher mental functions is associated with impaired memory (particularly recent memory), understanding, and abstract reasoning. Dementia presents with progressively declining work performance, forgetting of appointments, difficulty with shopping, and getting lost, both geographically and in conversation. Patients are apathetic and disinterested without any lowering of consciousness. In dementia the predominant symptom is memory impairment.
- *Psychosis*. Features include:
  - Perceptual distortion with hallucinations and illusions. Perceptual problems can result in the patient being out of touch with reality.

  - Disorganized thinking with delusions.
  - Attention and concentration may be a problem.
- *Functional problems.* Persons under psychosocial stress may become forgetful or confused. Memory and mood can be affected by emotional and psychological stress or overload. Intense anxiety impairs thinking by blocking factual information and by reducing awareness of personal thoughts and feelings.

What is the cause of the patient's perceptual problem?

See Figure 14.2.

What is the cause of the patient's memory problem?

See Figure 14.3.

Does the patient need to be referred?

Referral is indicated for patients:

- With delirium.
- With a suspected psychiatric problem (e.g. evidence of psychosis).
- For specialized management of drug-related problems.
- With forgetfulness that affects their work or personal life, when:
  - specific treatment is required for the underlying problem
  - they may benefit from stress- or time-management counseling
  - investigations are indicated to exclude a treatable condition in a younger person.

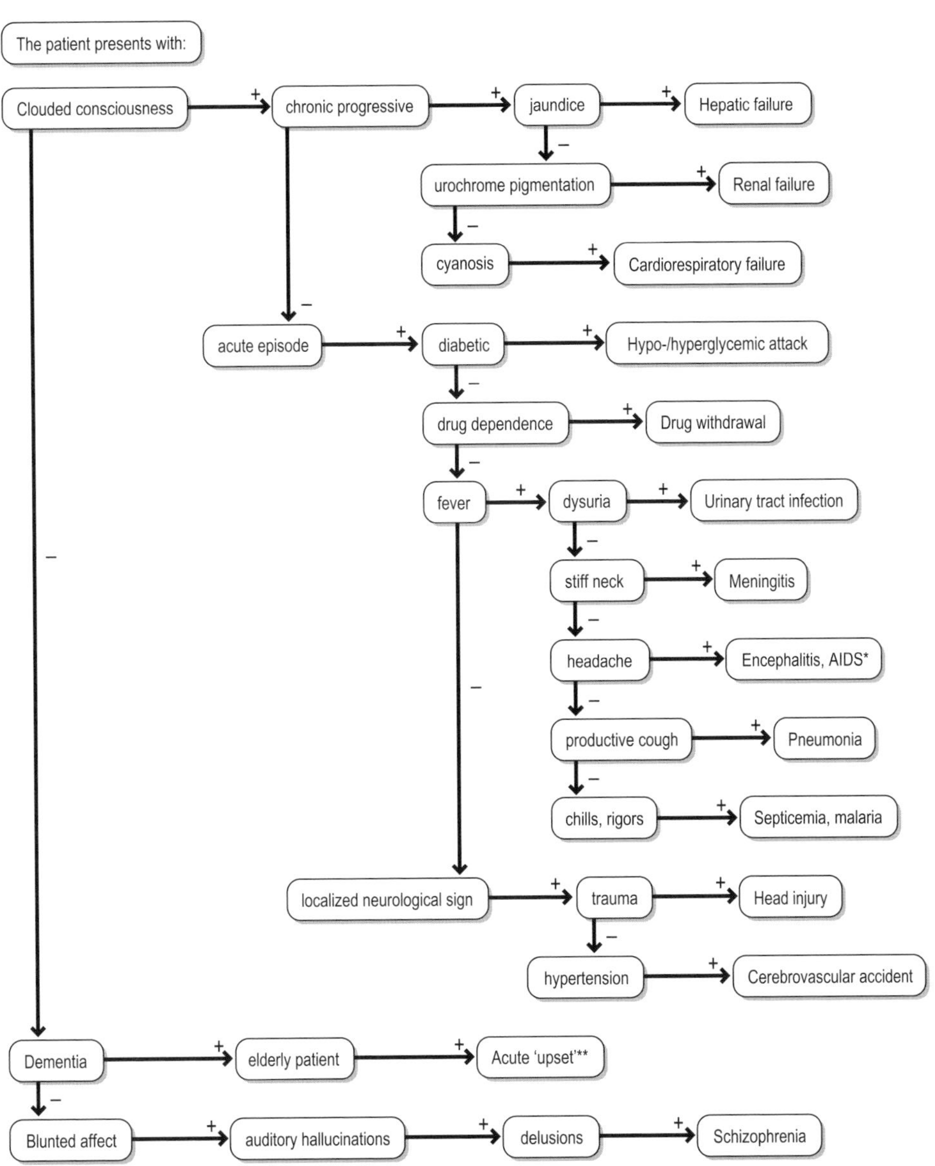

*AIDS: acquired immune deficiency syndrome
** Confusion may be precipitated by: pain, emotional upset, fecal impaction, urinary retention, or environmental change.

Figure 14.2 **Confusion.**

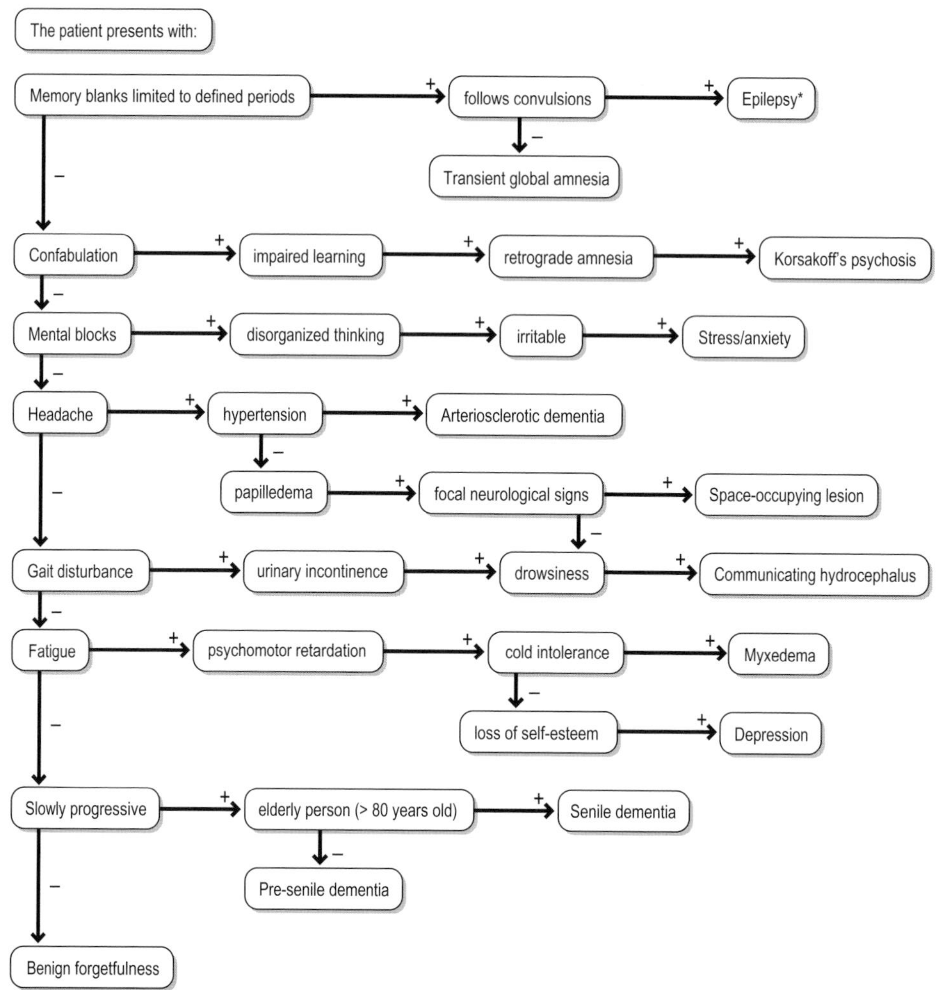

*Temporal lobe epilepsy may be associated with a period of confusion following an attack.

Figure 14.3 **Forgetfulness.**

FURTHER READING

Adelman A M, Daly M P 2005 Initial evaluation of the patient with suspected dementia. Am Fam Physician 71(9):1745–1750

Gleason O C 2003 Delirium. Am Fam Physician 67(5):1027–1034

PART TWO

CHAPTER 15

Constipation

CHAPTER CONTENTS

Does the patient have constipation?

Constipation may be functional due to poor dietary and/or bowel habits, or it may be attributable to bowel motility disorders and organic disease. Constipation is considered to be present when the patient:

- passes stools infrequently
- passes excessively hard stools
- cannot evacuate without prolonged straining.

What is the likely diagnosis?

See Figure 15.1.

Does the patient need to be referred?

Referral should be considered in patients with:

- an acute onset of severe constipation
- absent anal or perianal sensations (this suggests a neurological lesion which requires investigation)
- excessive perineal descent on straining (mechanical obstruction to defecation needs to be excluded)
- abdominal pain
- suspected colorectal disease:
  - weight loss
  - blood or mucus in the stool
- suspected anal lesions
- suspected appendicitis
- suspected endogenous depression
- suspected hypothyroidism, unless appropriate prescription therapy is available.

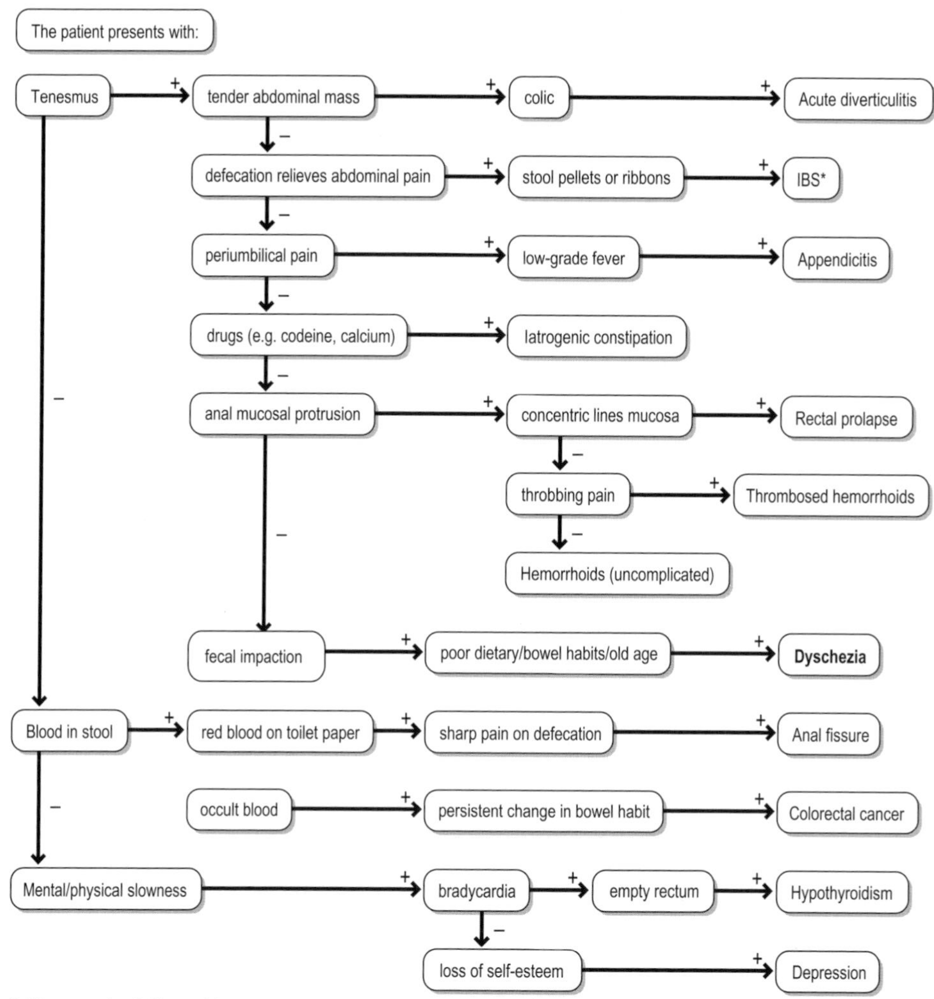

Figure 15.1 **Constipation.**

FURTHER READING

Arnaud M J 2003 Mild dehydration: a risk factor of constipation? Eur J Clin Nutr 57 Suppl 2:S88–95

Bosshard W, Dreher R, Schnegg J F, Bula C J 2004 The treatment of chronic constipation in elderly people: an update. Drugs Aging 2004;21(14):911–930

Muller-Lissner S A, Kamm M A, Scarpignato C, Wald A 2005 Myths and misconceptions about chronic constipation. Am J Gastroenterol 100(1):232–242

Prather C M 2004 Subtypes of constipation: sorting out the confusion. Rev Gastroenterol Disord 4 Suppl 2:S11–16

Wanitschke R, Goerg K J, Loew D 2003 Differential therapy of constipation – a review. Int J Clin Pharmacol Ther 41(1):14–21

CHAPTER 16

Cough

CHAPTER CONTENTS

What is the nature of the cough?

Coughing is attributable to enhanced sensitivity of the cough reflex or increased mucus production. It is important to ascertain whether a cough is:

- *Acute.* An acute cough lasts for days or weeks. In persons with an acute cough, bronchial irritation is temporary or self-limiting. When the cause persists or recurs, a chronic cough may develop.
- *Chronic.* Coughs which persist for more than 3 weeks are considered to be chronic. In patients with a chronic cough a chest radiograph may help discriminate between lung disease and sinus or gastroesophageal reflux problems.
- *Dry.* When coughing occurs in the absence of increased secretion production, a dry cough results. The underlying mechanism is an increase in the sensitivity of the cough reflex due to viral damage of the epithelium, bronchospasm, or drugs such as angiotensin-converting enzyme (ACE) inhibitors, which are used to treat hypertension and heart failure.
- *Productive.* A productive cough is one in which sputum is produced. Healthy people seldom cough, as ciliary action usually adequately clears the airways of mucus and other matter. When mucus production exceeds the capacity of the mucociliary transport system, material can be expelled from the airway by coughing. By narrowing the airways and increasing the velocity of airflow, coughing dislodges secretions from the respiratory mucosa.

What is the nature of the sputum?

See Figure 16.1.

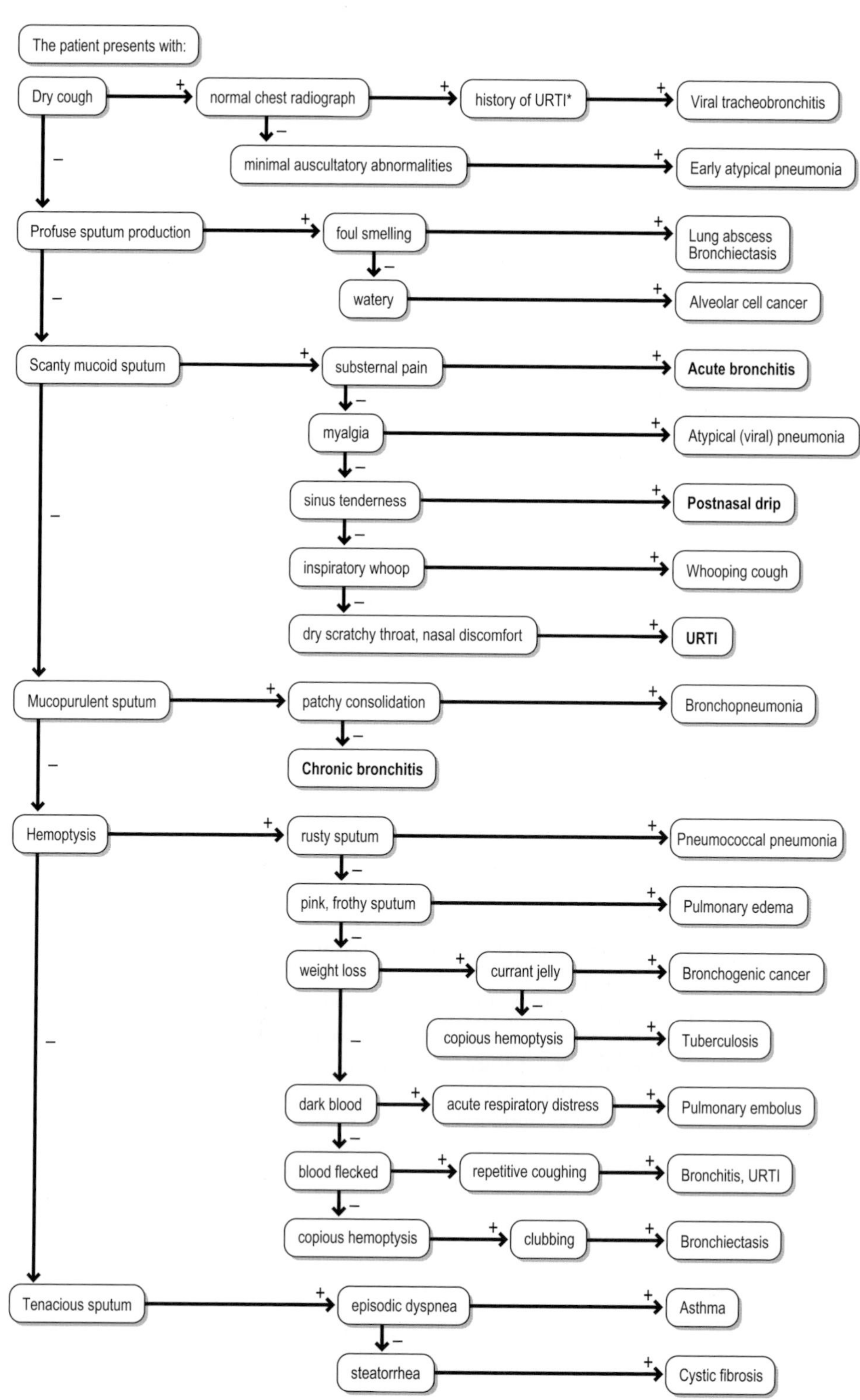

Figure 16.1 **Sputum.**

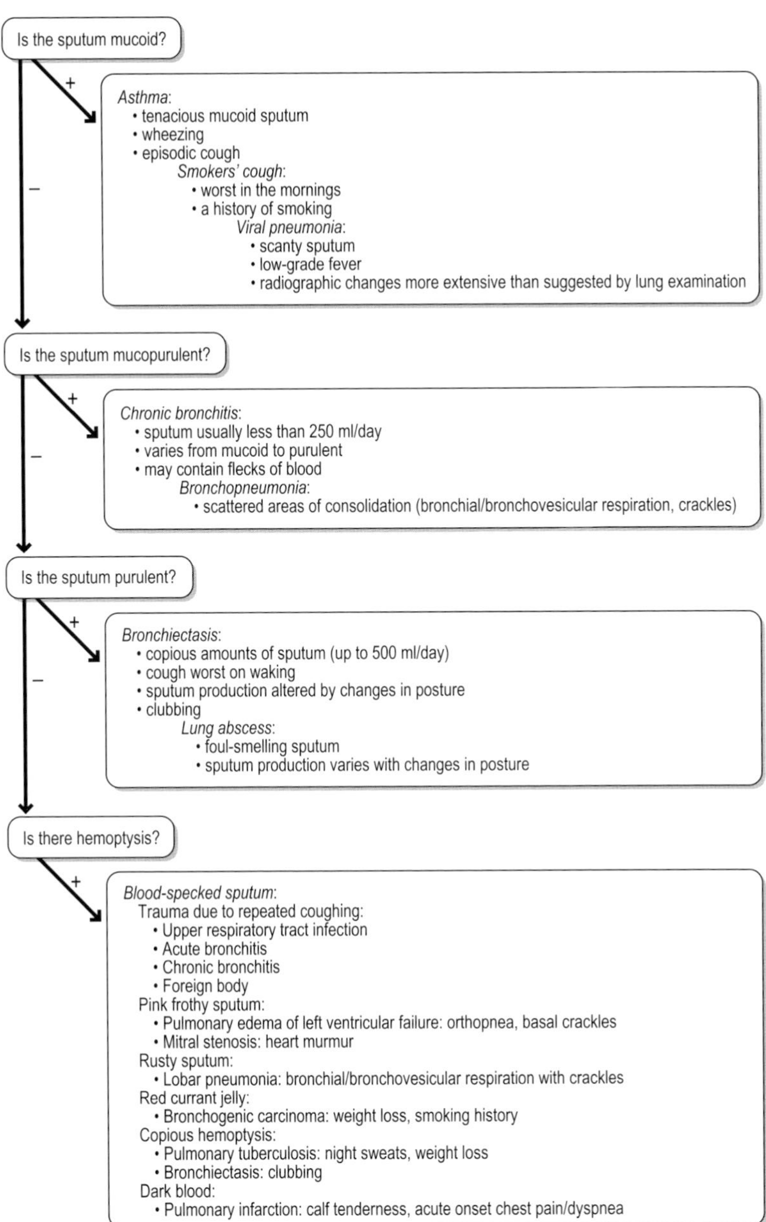

Figure 16.2 **A chronic productive cough: important questions to ask.**

What is the likely cause?

Figures 16.2 and 16.3 indicate some important questions involved in arriving at a diagnosis. In addition to sputum production, other clinical findings useful in the differential diagnosis of a cough include those shown in Figure 16.4.

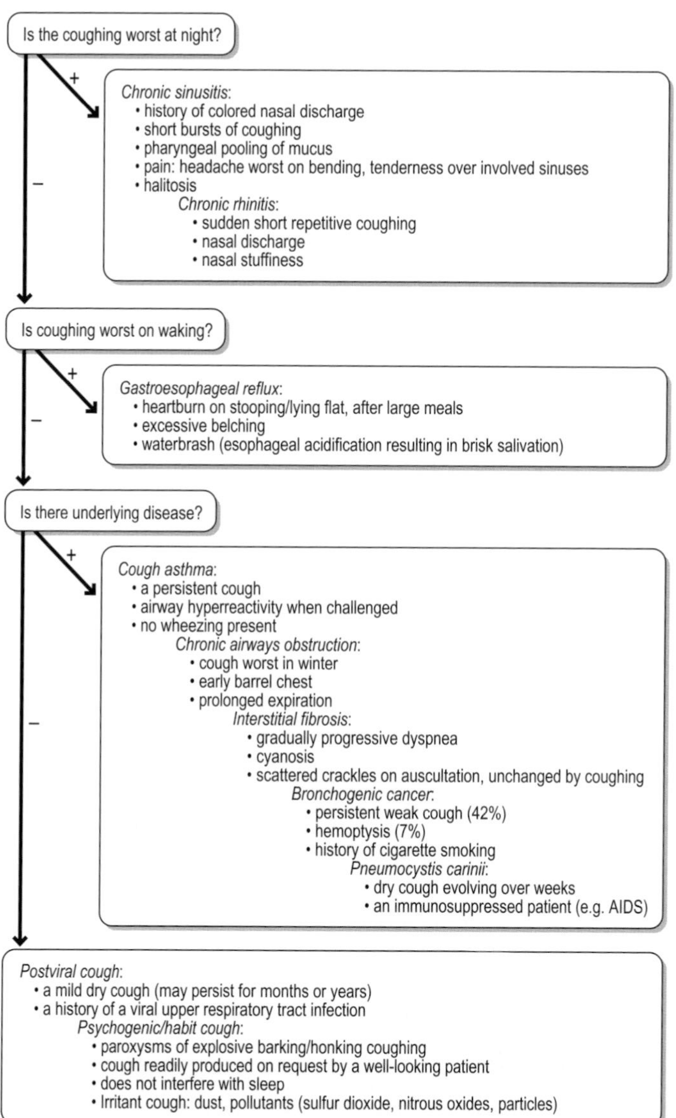

Figure 16.3 **A chronic dry or scanty cough: important questions to ask.**

Does the patient need to be referred?

In general medical practice less than one in 50 coughs is attributable to a serious cause. When the cough is bloodstained (hemoptysis), the likelihood of a serious cause is two to three times that of a trivial cause.

Patients should be referred if they fail to respond to treatment, especially if they have:

- hemoptysis
- a cough productive of purulent sputum
- a localized auscultatory abnormality

PART TWO

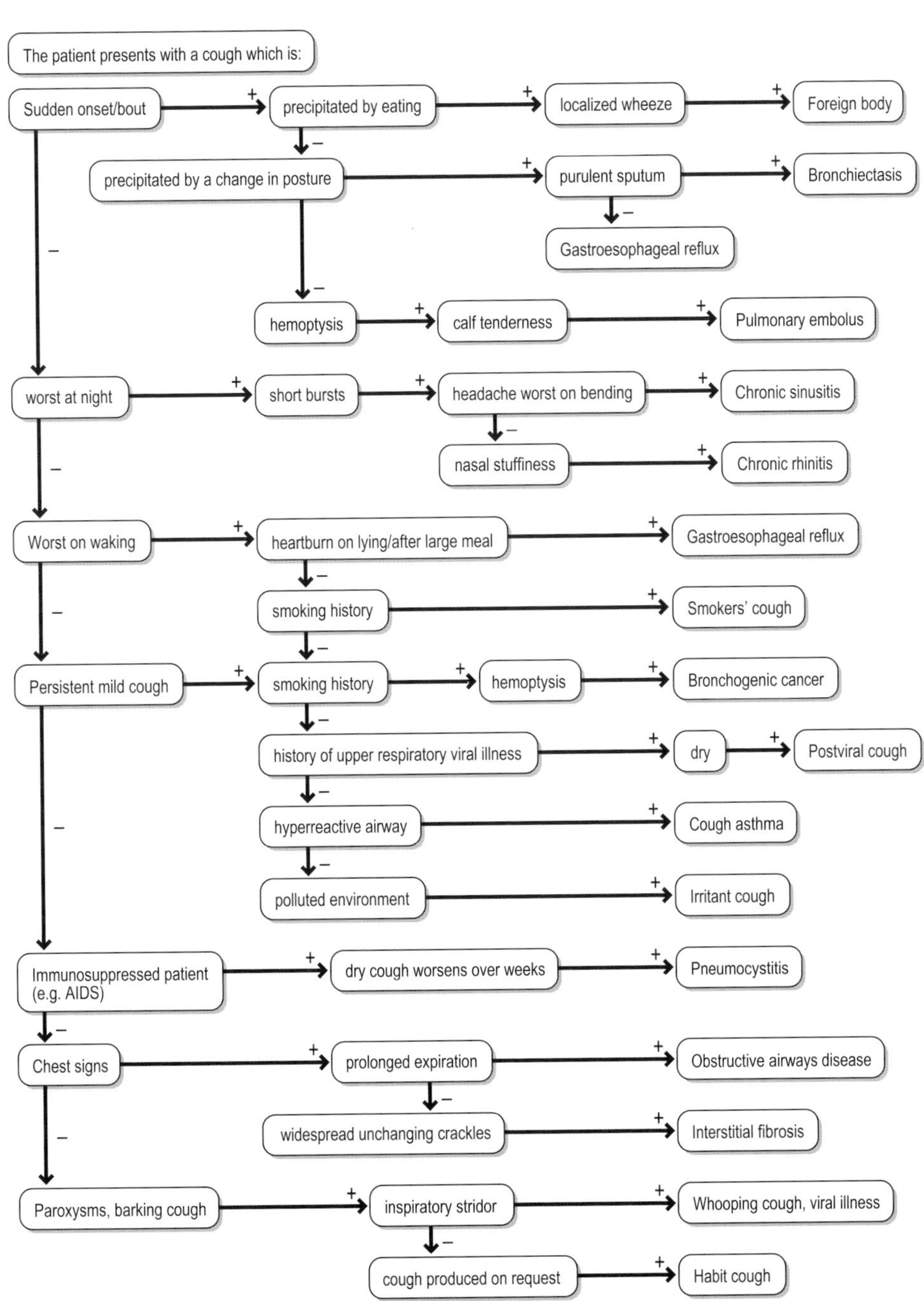

Figure 16.4 **Coughing.**

- a localized radiological abnormality
- a chronic cough.

Complications of coughing include:

- cough syncope
- rib fracture
- subconjunctival hemorrhage
- vomiting
- heart block
- urinary stress incontinence
- epistaxis
- pneumothorax
- uterine prolapse
- inguinal or femoral hernia
- postoperative wound dehiscence.

FURTHER READING

Chiu C Y, Wong K S, Lai S H, Hsia S H, Wu C T 2005 Factors predicting early diagnosis of foreign body aspiration in children. Pediatr Emerg Care 21(3):161–164

Fardy H J 2004 A coughing child: could it be asthma? Aust Fam Physician 33(5):312–315

Holmes R L, Fadden C T 2004 Evaluation of the patient with chronic cough. Am Fam Physician 69(9):2159–2166

Martinez F J, Standiford C, Gay S E 2005 Is it asthma or COPD? The answer determines proper therapy for chronic airflow obstruction. Postgrad Med 117(3):19–26

CHAPTER 17

Cyanosis

CHAPTER CONTENTS

Is the patient cyanosed?

Cyanosis is characterized by a dusty blue skin and mucosal discoloration. It is best detected by examination of mucous membranes and the nail beds. Cyanosis is attributable to an increase in the amount of deoxygenated (reduced) hemoglobin to above 5 g/100 ml. Cyanosis may be peripheral or central. The clinical causes and prognosis of central and peripheral cyanosis differ.

Does the patient have central or peripheral cyanosis?

Peripheral cyanosis is attributable to poor peripheral circulation. The clinical presentation of peripheral cyanosis is:

- blue discoloration limited to the extremities, such as the nail beds, the outer surface of the nose, the tips of the ears
- cold cyanosed extremities.

In peripheral cyanosis local vasospasm impairs perfusion, with resultant discoloration of the nail beds. Peripheral cyanosis is encountered on cold days or in persons with Raynaud's phenomenon. It is associated with normal arterial oxygen saturation and occurs when slowed circulation through peripheral capillary beds permits increased deoxygenation of hemoglobin. Other causes of peripheral cyanosis are venous obstruction and endarteritis.

Central cyanosis is due to low oxygen saturation, with a relative or absolute increase in deoxygenated hemoglobin. The clinical presentation of central cyanosis includes:

- discoloration of well-perfused areas, such as the lips, buccal mucosa, tongue, and conjunctiva, as well as the nail beds
- warm cyanosed areas.

Central cyanosis is usually indicative of cardiopulmonary disease. Causes of central cyanosis are right-to-left shunts within the heart, pulmonary arteriovenous fistulas, pneumonia, and chronic lung disease. In these, but not all, instances, cyanosis indicates hypoxia. Central cyanosis results from a generalized increase in reduced hemoglobin and is attributable to decreased oxygenation of available hemoglobin. Persons who have polycythemia have an increased mass of hemoglobin. They may thus achieve adequate tissue oxygenation even when the level of reduced hemoglobin is high enough to cause cyanosis. Likewise, the anemic patient, with their reduced mass of hemoglobin, may be hypoxic without being cyanosed. Cyanosis cannot appear when the hemoglobin level is less than 30%.

What is the cause of the patient's cyanosis?

See Figure 17.1.

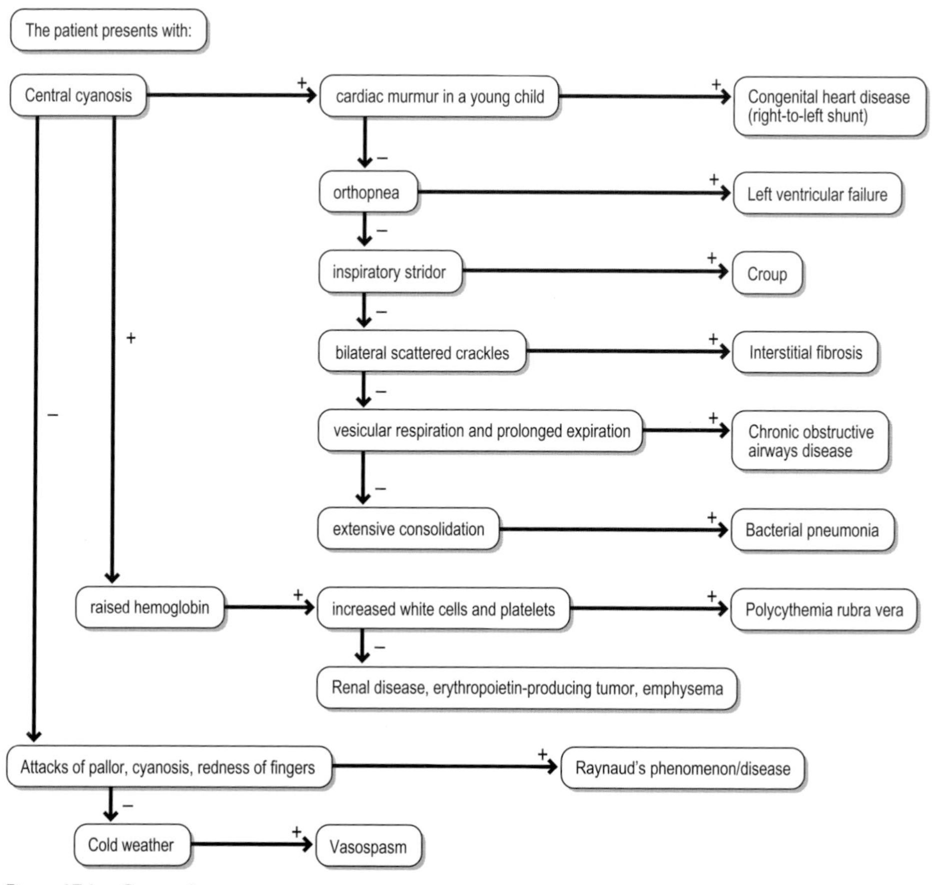

Figure 17.1 **Cyanosis.**

Does the patient need to be referred?

All patients without a definitive diagnosis should be referred. Cyanosis associated with cardiac or pulmonary disease in adults suggests that the underlying condition is advanced or extensive. Cyanosis associated with the following conditions requires further investigation and/or more vigorous treatment:

- left ventricular failure
- obstructive airways disease (cyanosis occurs late in chronic obstructive airways disease and is only present in severe attacks of asthma)
- pneumonia
- a child not under treatment for a congenital heart problem
- a myeloproliferative disorder
- suspected tumor
- uninvestigated:
  - renal disease
  - Raynaud's phenomenon.

FURTHER READING

Finesilver C 2003 Pulmonary assessment: what you need to know. Prog Cardiovasc Nurs 18(2):83–92

McDonnell J K 2002 Cardiac disease and the skin. Dermatol Clin 20(3):vii, 503–511

CHAPTER 18

Deafness and hearing impairment

CHAPTER CONTENTS

Is the patient's hearing impaired?

Holding a ticking clock to each ear is a useful clinical screening strategy to discern a hearing impairment. Confirmation and evaluation of the extent of deafness requires audiometry. Persons who fail to hear soft speech have lost approximately 20 dB of hearing and are mildly deaf. Persons who have difficulty hearing normal speech are moderately deaf, having lost around 40 dB. Severe hearing loss occurs when 60 dB have been lost and persons have difficulty hearing loud speech. Losses of over 60 dB result in profound deafness, and shouting is hard to hear.

Is it a conduction or sensorineural deafness?

Hearing loss may be attributed to nerve damage (sensorineural deafness) or to impaired transmission of sound (conduction deafness). Two tests, the Rinne and Weber tests, are routinely performed. Both tests require a 256 or 512 Hz tuning fork. The fork is struck, causing it to vibrate. Diagnostic findings are based on the duration or lateralization of the sound caused by the fork's vibration (Table 18.1).

Table 18.1
Testing for hearing loss

	Rinne test	**Weber test**
Health	AC better than BC	Midline sound
Conduction deafness	BC better than AC	Sound best heard in the 'deaf' ear
Sensorineural deafness	Both equally decreased	Sound best heard in the 'good' ear
Tuning fork position	Ear, then mastoid	Vertex (center) of forehead

AC, air conduction; BC, bone conduction.

Rinne's test is performed by placing a vibrating tuning fork over the mastoid bone. When the patient indicates that he or she no longer hears the sound, the vibrating end of the fork is held close to the external ear. In health, the sound will once again be detected, as air conduction is better than bone conduction. In patients with a conduction defect the sound is not detected (i.e. bone conduction is better than air conduction). In sensory or perceptive deafness, although both bone and air conduction are adversely affected, air conduction is better than bone conduction.

Weber's test is performed by placing the vibrating tuning fork on the vertex, or center, of the forehead. The patient is asked where he or she hears the sound. In health the sound is heard in the midline and equally well by both ears. In conduction deafness the sound is heard best in the affected ear. The affected ear has normal bone conduction but impaired air conduction, and therefore background noise in the room is masked. In sensorineural deafness the sound is loudest in the unaffected or good ear. The nerve is the final pathway for sound transmission and a problem at this level is unaffected by the mode in which sound is transmitted.

Conduction deafness is characterized by:

- paracusis (speech is heard better in a noisy environment)
- talking loudly or shouting increases speech intelligibility
- bone conduction is better than air conduction on the Rinne test
- sound lateralizes to or is louder in the deaf ear on the Weber test.

Disorders of the external and middle ear need to be investigated in conduction deafness. Impacted wax, otitis externa, and serous otitis media (glue ear) are the most common causes of conduction deafness.

Sensorineural deafness is characterized by:

- sensitivity to small increases in sound (people seem to be shouting)
- speech is often poorly understood, as high frequencies are lost early
- shouting may decrease intelligibility
- bone conduction lateralizes to the normal ear on the Weber test.

Lesions of the inner ear may cause sensorineural deafness, which should always be checked in patients complaining of tinnitus and/or vertigo.

What is the likely cause of the hearing loss?

See Figure 18.1.

PART TWO

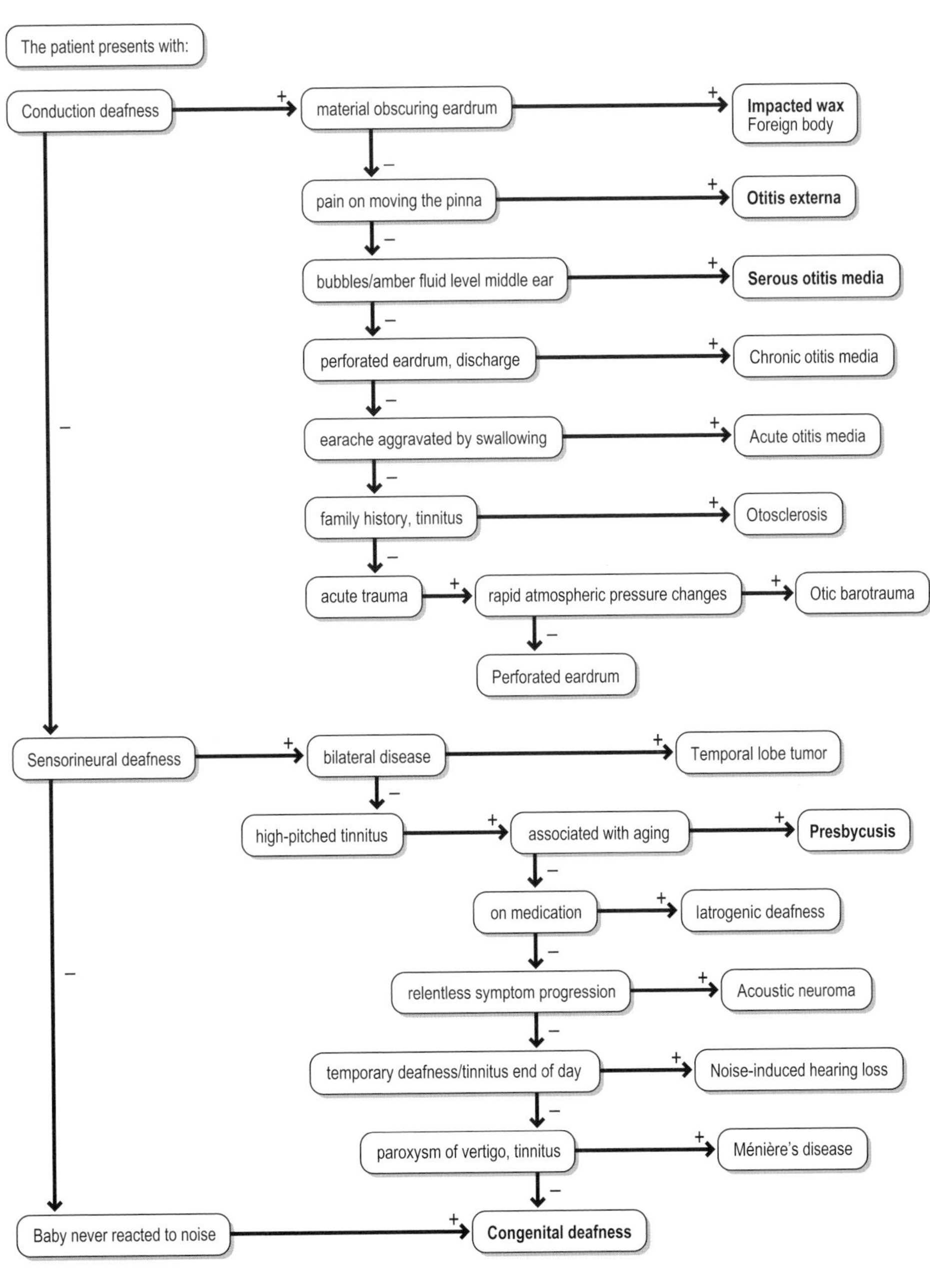

Figure 18.1 **Hearing impairment.**

Does the patient need to be referred?

Patients should be referred for evaluation and treatment, as necessary, for:

- recent sudden hearing loss
- an eardrum with:
  - a marginal perforation
  - an attic perforation
  - perforation and a purulent discharge
  - a large perforation with suspected skull fractures
  - a large perforation with significant hearing loss
- a discharge of:
  - pus draining through a ruptured eardrum
  - a clear fluid (cerebrospinal fluid) following trauma to the middle ear
  - a chronic discharge, especially if this is offensive
- nonresponsive bacterial infection
- acute mastoiditis with increasing deafness
- chronic otitis media with marked deafness
- previously undiagnosed sensorineural deafness
- a suspected central nervous system lesion.

FURTHER READING

Cohen S M, Labadie R F, Haynes D S 2005 Primary care approach to hearing loss: the hidden disability. Ear Nose Throat J 84(1):26, 29–31, 44

Isaacson J E, Vora N M 2003 Differential diagnosis and treatment of hearing loss. Am Fam Physician 68(6):1125–1132

Neff M J 2004 AAP, AAFP, AAO-HNS Release Guideline on diagnosis and management of otitis media with effusion. Am Fam Physician 69(12):2929–2931

Olajide T G, Olage F E, Alabi B S 2005 Management of impacted ear wax. Aust Fam Physician 34(5):395–396

Waddell A, Canter R 2004 Tinnitus. Am Fam Physician 69(3):591–592

CHAPTER 19

Depression

CHAPTER CONTENTS

PART TWO

Is the patient depressed?

Depression is diagnosed if two positive responses are offered to the following questions:

- Do you feel depressed?
- Has there been a change in your self-esteem?
- Are you more self-critical than usual?

Supportive findings may include:

- feeling helpless or hopeless
- a sense of giving up
- feeling guilty
- being pessimistic about the future.

Further diagnosis of depression involves exploring for:

- *Altered mood.* This is characterized by a loss of interest or pleasure in all usual activities, accompanied by feelings of sadness, hopelessness, and irritability. Mood disturbance is a prominent feature.
- *Changed vegetative symptoms.* Changes in appetite, sleep patterns, and psychomotor activity are encountered.
- *Cognitive symptoms.* These include feelings of worthlessness, excessive guilt, reduced concentration, slow thinking, indecisiveness, self-reproach, and thoughts of death and suicide.

Is the patient's depression physiological or clinical?

The duration of depression determines whether it should be considered a clinical problem. *Physiological depression*:

- is of less than 14 days' duration
- is not associated with loss of self-esteem

Table 19.1
Various types of depression

	Depression type			
Disturbance	**Physiological**	**Nonmelancholic**	**Endogenous**	**Neurotic**
Mood	–, or mild	Reactive	Diurnal change	Diurnal change
Psychomotor	–	–	+++	+
Psychosis	–	–	+	–
Self-esteem	Normal	Reduced	Reduced	Reduced
Duration	<14 days	>14 days	>14 days	>14 days

- has no diurnal mood variation
- has no or mild mood disturbance (the patient may express feelings of despair or rejection)
- carries no significant social impairment.

On the other hand, *clinical depression* is associated with significant mood disturbance or social impairment which has lasted longer than 14 days. Clinical depression falls into three major groups (Table 19.1):

- *Nonmelancholic depression* is diagnosed:
  - in the absence of observable psychomotor disturbance
  - when the mood is reactive, often improving during the consultation.
- *Psychotic melancholia* (endogenous depression) is diagnosed in cases of:
  - severe psychomotor disturbance (a poverty of movement, a paucity of ideas and agitation may be noted)
  - psychotic features, including delusions (false beliefs), hallucinations (erroneous sensory perceptions), and obsessive guilt
  - diurnal mood variation (depression is worst in the morning, and early morning waking is characteristic)
  - autonomic nervous system changes (e.g. constipation, anorexia)
  - psychosomatic complaints.
- *Nonpsychotic melancholia* (neurotic depression or reactive depression) is considered in cases with:
  - diurnal variation in mood (worst at night); the chronic mood disturbance involves sadness and loss of interest
  - chronic sleep disturbance, with difficulty getting off to sleep
  - a diurnal variation in and a lack of energy, but only a moderate psychomotor disturbance
  - no psychotic features.

In medically ill patients depressive disorders have been categorized as:

- a grief-like reaction
- an adjustive disorder with depressed mood
- a dysthymic disorder
- a major depressive episode
- an organic mood disorder.

Is there a risk of suicide?

Risk factors for suicide include persons who:

- are male, over 45 years of age, and white
- socially:
  - are separated, divorced, or widowed
  - live alone
- emotionally:
  - are depressed
  - experience feelings of hopelessness
- have psychotic symptoms
- have a general medical illness
- talk about suicide
- have a history of:
  - alcohol or drug abuse
  - a previous suicide attempt
  - previously attempted suicide by firearms, jumping, or drowning
- have a family history of:
  - substance abuse
  - suicide attempts.

The risk of suicide peaks during the period when the patient is beginning to improve from his or her depression and has more energy to carry out a suicide plan. This is the point when clinicians need to question the patient about suicide and make themselves readily available to patients, either personally or by telephone. There is no evidence that asking specific questions about suicide increases the likelihood of suicide or plants the idea in the patient's mind. If a significant risk for suicide exists, the idea is already there. Those who talk about suicide should be taken seriously. Some 80% of suicides give clear or subtle warning of their intentions.

Patients perceived to be at risk should be questioned with respect to:

- The specific method considered. It is important to ascertain whether the proposed strategy is:
  - practical and can be implemented
  - lethal (i.e. likely to be 'successful' if implemented).
- The strength of the suicidal ideation. Most suicide-risk patients seen by primary care practitioners have mild forms of suicidal ideation (i.e. weak intent and poorly formed plans).
- Any previous attempts.

Patients should also be asked whether they have thought about how the act would affect their family and friends.

A 'no suicide contract' to which the patient agrees until the next visit is a useful management strategy. In the contract, the physician outlines specific guidelines of how and when he or she can be contacted and the phone number and location of a psychiatric emergency room or other crisis service if suicide is contemplated in the interim. The patient is asked to sign the contract, and it is placed in the chart progress notes. If the patient is actively suicidal, he or she should be referred immediately for psychiatric evaluation.

Attempted suicide should be viewed as a cry for help.

What is the cause of the patient's clinical depression?

Depression may be psychological or physical.

Psychological depression is associated with loss. Bereavement, retirement, with its loss of role, status, and income and shrinking social network, loss of independence, or anxiety about the future may precipitate depression. It may be regarded as a normal response, provided it does not persist, in which case therapy is indicated.

Physical depression may result from aberrant cerebral metabolism or be associated with visceral disease. Infections, especially viral infections, and immune disorders are linked with depression. Excessive secretion of macrophage monokines is postulated to underlie the depression associated with rheumatoid arthritis, strokes, and ischemic heart disease, and is predictive of greater morbidity following cardiac surgery. Endocrine disorders of the thyroid, parathyroid, or adrenal glands and occult cancer, especially of the pancreas, and endocrine-secreting tumors, are all organic causes of depression.

Antihypertensive drugs, digitalis, steroids, levodopa, and nifedipine have also all been causally linked with depression. Recent evidence suggests that long-chain ω-3 fatty acids (especially docosahexenoic acid) may reduce the incidence of depression in alcoholism, multiple sclerosis, and postpartum depression.

Does the patient need to be referred?

Depressed patients should be referred if:

- underlying visceral disease requires investigation or specialist treatment
- moderate or marked depression is diagnosed
- specialist counseling is required
- a substantial suicide risk is detected
- the patient fails to respond to standard therapy.

PART TWO

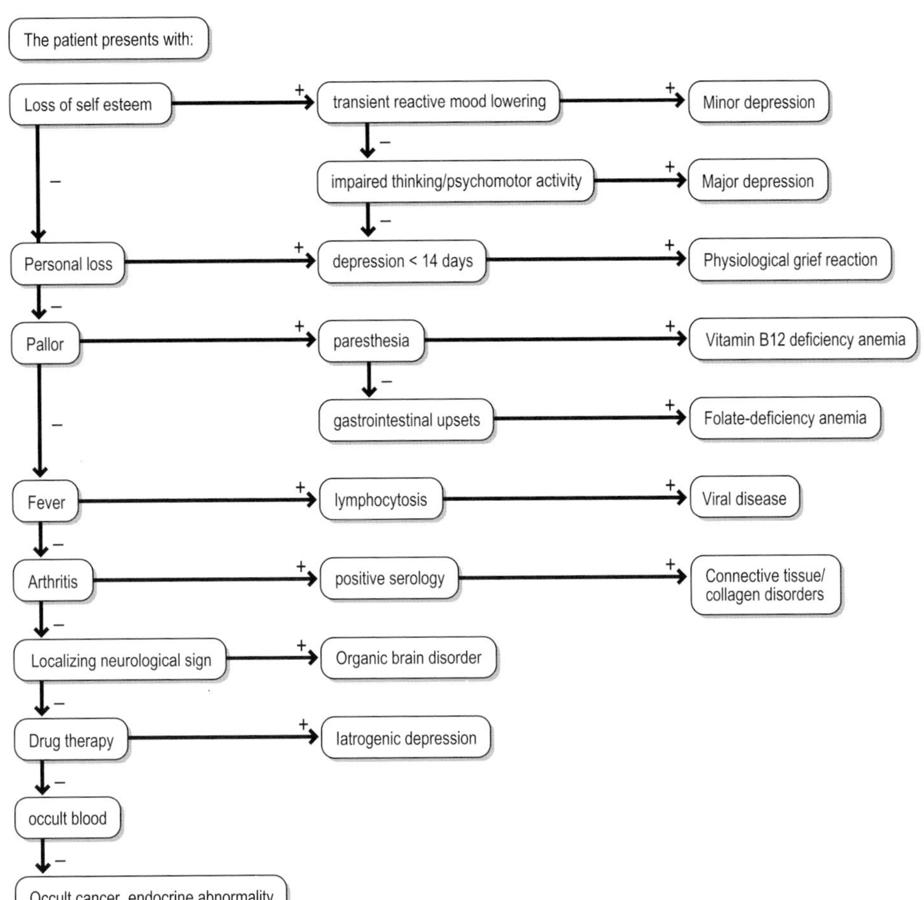

Figure 19.1 **Depression.**

FURTHER READING

Anisman H, Merali Z, Poulter M O, Hayley S 2005 Cytokines as a precipitant of depressive illness: animal and human studies. Curr Pharm Des 11(8):963–972

Birrer R B, Vemuri S P 2004 Depression in later life: a diagnostic and therapeutic challenge. Am Fam Physician 69(10):2375–2382

Deussing J M, Wurst W 2005 Dissecting the genetic effect of the CRH system on anxiety and stress-related behavior. C R Biol 328(2):199–212

Iverson G L, Thordarson D S 2005 Women with low activity are at increased risk for depression. Psychol Rep 96(1):133–140

Swann A C, Geller B, Post R M, Altshuler L, Chang K D, Delbello M P, Reist C, Juster I A 2005 Practical clues to early recognition of bipolar disorder: a primary care approach. Prim Care Companion J Clin Psychiatry 7(1):15–21

Thibault J M, Steiner R W 2004 Efficient identification of adults with depression and dementia. Am Fam Physician 70(6):1101–1110

Trigo M, Silva D, Rocha E 2005 Psychosocial risk factors in coronary heart disease: beyond type A behavior. Rev Port Cardiol 24(2):261–281

CHAPTER 20

Diarrhea

CHAPTER CONTENTS

PART TWO

Does the patient have diarrhea?

Diarrhea is the frequent passage of unformed stools. Stool size varies within cultures due to different eating habits. A patient has diarrhea if he or she passes:

- an increased number of stools (in western societies more than 200 g of stool each day for 30 days is considered diarrhea)
- stools that are increased in softness, fluidity, or volume.

Patients with diarrhea may complain of:

- urgency to defecate
- fear of incontinence (incontinence may actually occur in severe cases of diarrhea)
- abdominal cramping.

Does the patient require urgent attention?

It is important to establish the severity of the diarrhea and to examine the patient for signs of dehydration. The patient who is vomiting is at increased risk of fluid depletion and may need to be referred for intravenous fluids. Diarrhea may require urgent attention due to:

- *The severity of the underlying condition.* In chronic diarrhea, complications often result from the underlying condition. Chronic diarrhea is more likely to be complicated by malnutrition than dehydration. Patients with chronic diarrhea should be screened for evidence of:
  - weight loss
  - vitamin deficiencies.

- *Dehydration.* In acute diarrhea, the severity of the condition is determined by the total volume of fluid lost. Severe diarrhea combined with vomiting is a potent cause of dehydration. The risk of dehydration is greatest in children, particularly very young children. Adults with profuse diarrhea and uncontrolled vomiting also risk dehydration.

The dehydrated adult progressively experiences:

- a dry mouth
- thirst
- a reduced urinary output (oliguria); small volumes of dark urine are characteristic
- dizziness or light-headedness
- decreased skin turgor
- a low-volume pulse and/or low blood pressure.

In children, moderate dehydration can be recognized by:

- <10% loss of body weight
- restlessness, lethargy, irritability
- thirst and dry mucous membranes
- decreased tissue turgor
- cool extremities
- sunken eyes and fontanelles
- tachycardia and a normal blood pressure
- decreased urinary output.

Children with severe dehydration have/are:

- >10% loss of body weight
- stopped passing urine
- a rapid, feeble pulse
- a low blood pressure
- skin which retracts very slowly when pinched
- drowsy and apprehensive
- limp and cold.

It is important to prevent dehydration. Persons with diarrhea should be encouraged to maintain an adequate fluid intake by:

- sipping or drinking water and orange juice regularly to achieve urine which is pale in color
- drinking 200 ml fluid for each watery stool passed.

Oral rehydration therapy may be used for adults and non-dehydrated children to replace fluid and electrolytes. Ideally, 1 ℓ of replacement fluid should contain 90 mmol sodium, 20 mmol potassium, 80 mmol chloride, 10 mmol citrate, and 2% glucose. 'Oral rehydration' sachets, such as Gastrolyte, are available. Oral rehydration fluid may be made at home and should include water, electrolytes, and an energy source. Rehydration fluid should not be more salty than tears. As oral rehydration depends on the intestinal glucose-coupled sodium absorption mechanism, sugar-free cordial and low-calorie soft drinks are inappropriate. Oral rehydration therapy should not be used in dehydrated children, as it is ineffective and prolongs intestinal recovery.

Patients with acute diarrhea should rest and limit their diet to clear fluids such as water, tea, and thin soup. Once diarrhea and vomiting have stopped, a light bland diet should be eaten. Bran, fruit and vegetables, dairy products, and fatty and spicy foods should be avoided. It is often helpful to start with dry toast or plain biscuits, followed 12–24 hours later by mashed vegetables. Dairy products and meat should be delayed to the second or third day.

What is the nature of the diarrhea?

The underlying mechanism influences the clinical nature of diarrhea. Explanations for the frequent passage of an unformed stool include:

- Osmotically active substances being retained within the lumen. Osmotic diarrhea encountered in lactase deficiency, or mega-dosing with vitamin C or certain laxatives, leads to production of a watery stool.
- Disorders of intestinal secretion as a result of toxins (e.g. toxigenic *Escherichia coli* or cholera) or in response to local hormone secretion. An outpouring of fluid into the intestinal lumen causes an explosive watery diarrhea.
- Alterations in the absorptive capacity through mucosal changes (e.g. inflammation or villous atrophy in gluten sensitivity) or enzyme changes due to pancreatic insufficiency may cause a bulky stool.
- Alterations in transit time. Bowel motility may be disturbed due to increased bowel motility (e.g. thyrotoxicosis), autonomic neuropathy (e.g. diabetes), or intestinal stasis with altered bowel flora causing fecal breakdown in the intestine.

Diarrhea is described as:

- Acute, chronic, or intermittent. Acute diarrhea may persist and become chronic. The consequences and interventions in acute, chronic, and intermittent diarrhea are usually different.
- Functional or organic.
- Dysentery, if feces are bloodstained.
- Arising from the small or large bowel.

Acute diarrhea lasts for less than 2 weeks. Important causes of acute diarrhea are:

- food poisoning
- infective gastroenteritis
- drug-induced diarrhea
- dietary indiscretions (food consumed in the 24 hours prior to the onset of diarrhea is often implicated. In addition to asking

about the type of food eaten remember to inquire how food was prepared and who ate the suspect food)
- intense stress.

Chronic diarrhea persists for more than 3 weeks. Patients who have chronic or recurrent diarrhea or dysentery need to be investigated for:

- intestinal infections
- inflammatory bowel disease
- absorption defects (steatorrhea, which presents with a pale bulky offensive stool that is difficult to flush, suggests malabsorption, which may be due to pancreatic or mucosal defects)
- systemic disorders (evidence of an underlying systemic disorder should be suspected in patients with findings such as joint pain or backache, eye problems, polyuria, polyphagia, mouth ulcers, restlessness, or nervous tension)
- drug-induced diarrhea.

Intermittent diarrhea alternates with constipation. The patient notes a change in bowel habit. Intermittent diarrhea may be attributed to a trivial dysfunction or serious underlying pathology. A change in bowel habit may result either from a bowel abnormality or be secondary to another problem. Prevalent causes of fluctuating diarrhea with a vastly different natural history and prognosis include:

- Irritable bowel syndrome. This condition presents in young people and is postulated to be either a psychosomatic condition or to result from food intolerance. The presence of blood in the stool excludes irritable bowel syndrome.
- Bowel cancer. The prevalence of this cancer increases with age, and it is an important cancer in persons over 50 years of age. In colon cancer, pain is precipitated by eating, and a non-tender abdominal mass may be detected. In contrast, colorectal cancer causes a sensation of incomplete evacuation, and a mass may be detected on proctosigmoidoscopy.
- Diverticulitis (age of onset usually over 40 years). Diverticulitis causes cramps, and a tender mass, often in the left iliac fossa, may be detected.

Important considerations in differentiating between these three conditions are the patient's age, the presence of blood in the stool and the nature of any mass.

Both *psychosomatic and organic disorders* may cause diarrhea that is acute, intermittent, or chronic, yet they have a different prognosis and require diverse interventions. Before diagnosing functional diarrhea, organic causes must be excluded. Nervous diarrhea may be suspected in patients who present with:

- the frequent passage of a loose stool
- diarrhea that is most troublesome during periods of stress

- the absence of blood in the stool
- the absence of mucus in the stool.

Organic diarrhea should be diagnosed in the presence of:

- weight loss
- sleep disturbed due to diarrhea
- blood in the stool.

In organic diarrhea, the site of the intestinal lesion also influences the clinical presentation. In diarrhea due to a lesion of the upper gastrointestinal tract:

- the stools are:
  - copious
  - watery
  - pale yellow or green
  - offensive
  - fatty or float
  - contain undigested food
- borborygmi (loud rumbling) are characteristic
- defecation seldom relieves pain
- pain is experienced around the central umbilical area
- there is an increased risk of dehydration
- in cases of blood loss, the melena stool is dark.

In *colonic disease*, the stools:

- are small in volume and frequently passed
- vary in consistency
- are brown in color
- contain fresh blood or mucus.

Defecation may be associated with:

- Urgency.
- Tenesmus (straining at stool).
- Passing a stool on getting up in the morning.
- Relief of abdominal pain. Lower abdominal pain suggests colonic disorders. The left iliac fossa is a common site for pain arising from the colon.
- In cases of dysentery, blood is red and mucus is present. Red blood mixed with the stool suggests a colon lesion; blood limited to the surface of the stool suggests a rectal or anal lesion.

Stool microscopy and culture are indicated in cases of:

- food poisoning
- traveler's diarrhea
- dysentery
- diarrhea persisting for more than 7 days
- high fever (> 38.5°C)
- severe illness.

What is the likely cause of acute diarrhea?

Figure 20.1 lists important questions to ask if diarrhea is acute. Figure 20.2 illustrates an approach to the differential diagnosis of acute diarrhea.

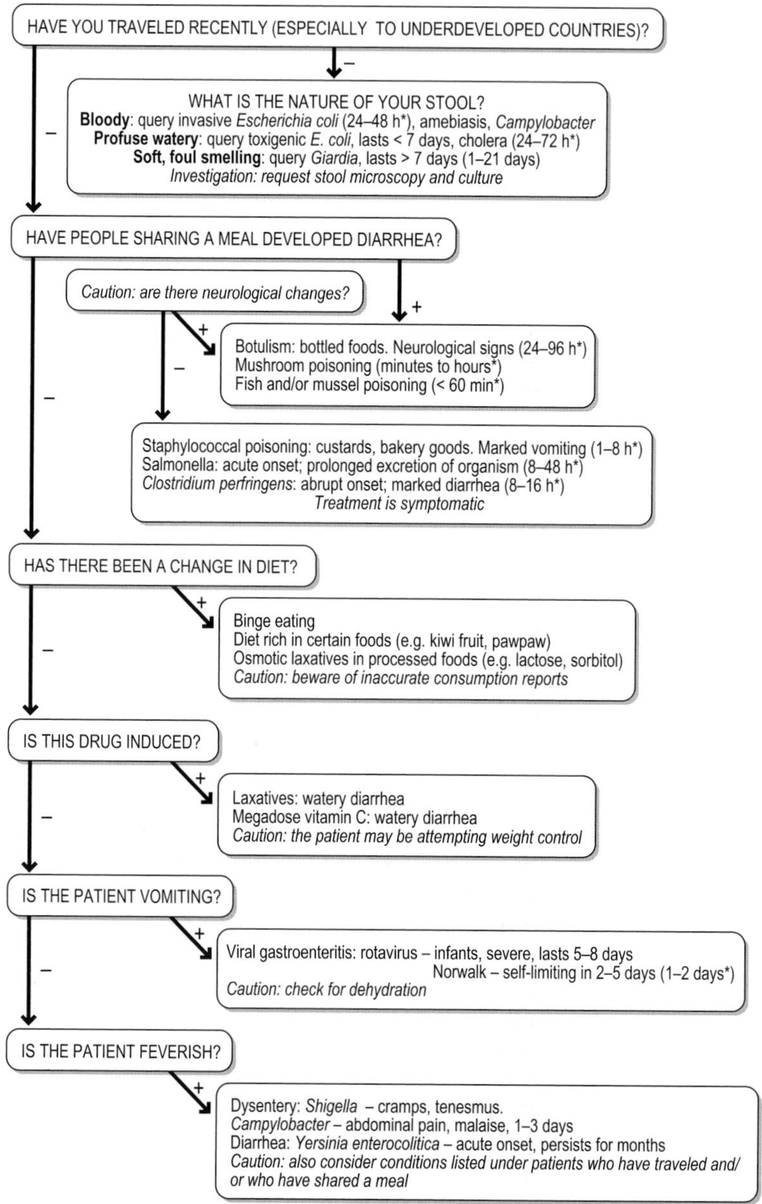

Figure 20.1 **Acute diarrhea: important questions to ask.**

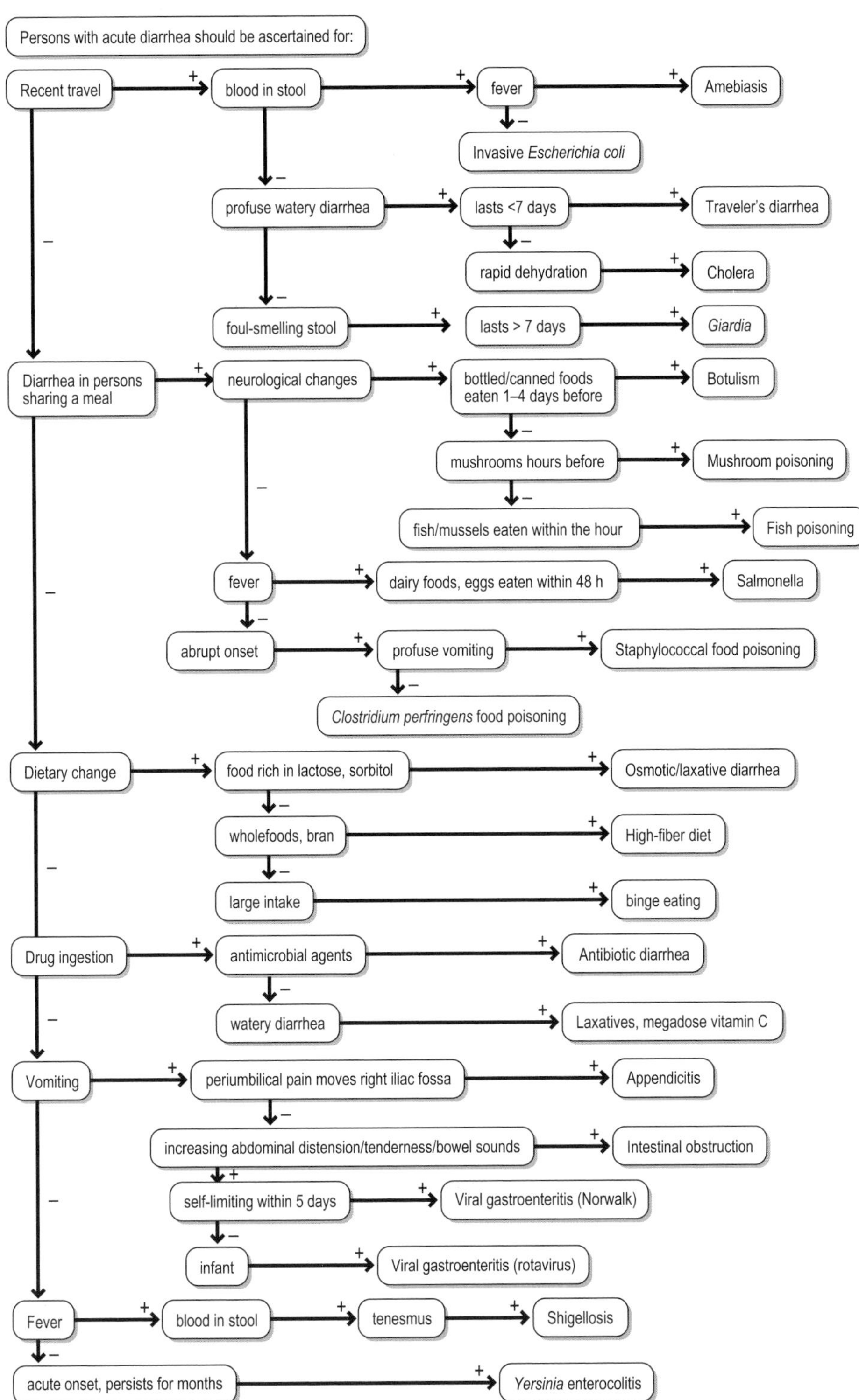

Figure 20.2 **The differential diagnosis of acute diarrhea.**

Does the patient with acute diarrhea need to be referred?

Acute diarrhea is usually self-limiting in 2–5 days. Persons with acute diarrhea should, however, be referred if:

- The patient is a neonate (< 28 days old).
- Moderate dehydration is noted in a child.
- Severe dehydration is present.
- The diagnosis is unlikely to be acute gastroenteritis (i.e. refer when one of the following is present):
  - diarrhea which persists for longer than 7 days
  - vomit is blood- or bile-stained
  - severe abdominal pain, anorexia, nausea, and vomiting in a young adult (appendicitis may be associated with diarrhea)
  - abdominal guarding, tenderness, distension
  - high fever (temperature > 39°C)
  - blood and mucus are present in the stool
  - pus or worms are noted in the stool
  - acute bloody diarrhea in an elderly patient who has experienced abdominal pain within the last 24 hours (acute ischemic colitis needs to be excluded).

What is the likely cause of chronic diarrhea?

Figures 20.3 and 20.4 list important questions to ask if diarrhea is chronic or intermittent. Figure 20.5 considers an approach to differential diagnosis of chronic diarrhea.

Does the patient with chronic diarrhea need to be referred?

Persons with chronic diarrhea may have underlying pathology which requires diagnosis and treatment. Clinical findings that suggest the need to refer include:

- Severe colic.
- Persistent nocturnal diarrhea.
- Dysentery (blood and mucus).
- Fever.
- Local abdominal tenderness and guarding.
- Abdominal distension and/or a succession splash. A splash may be produced by gently shaking the abdomen with your ear adjacent to the abdominal wall.
- An abdominal mass.
- An anal fistula.
- An elderly patient requiring treatment for fecal impaction.
- A significant change in symptoms in patients with a history of (cancer needs to be excluded):
  - irritable bowel syndrome
  - inflammatory bowel disease
  - diverticulitis.
- Diarrhea in long-term asymptomatic carriers of typhoid or paratyphoid fever.
- A suspected endocrine disorder.
- Failure to respond to treatment.
- Dehydration and/or persistent profuse watery diarrhea.

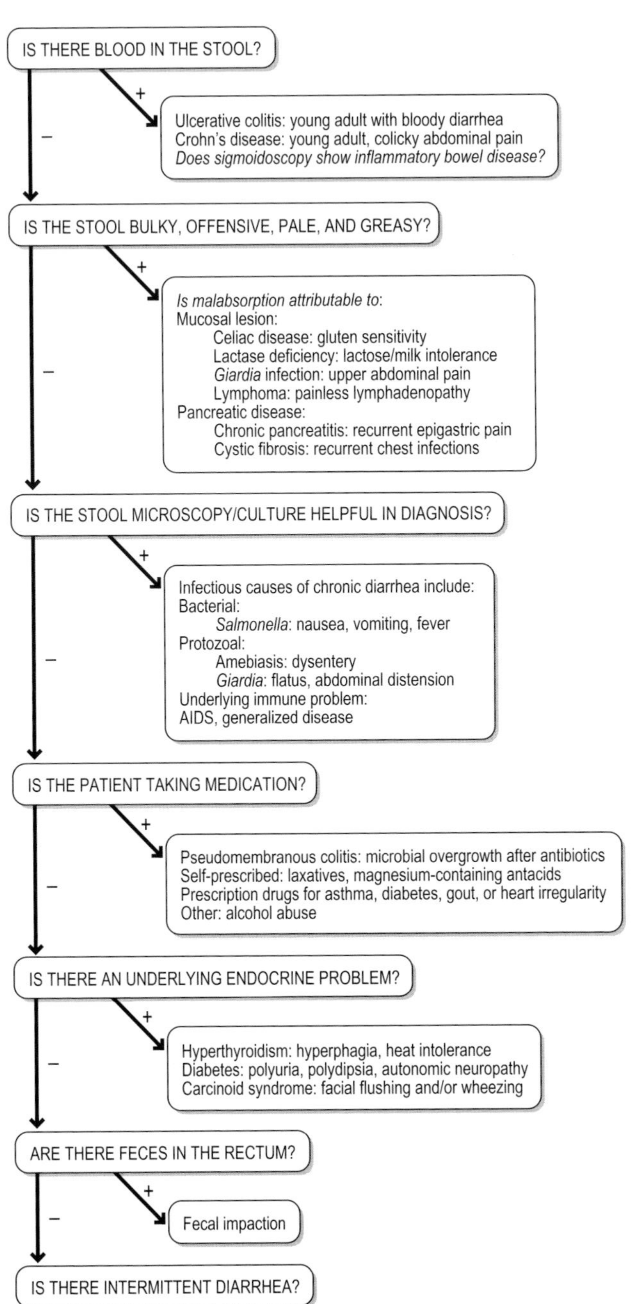

Figure 20.3 **Chronic diarrhea: important questions to ask.**

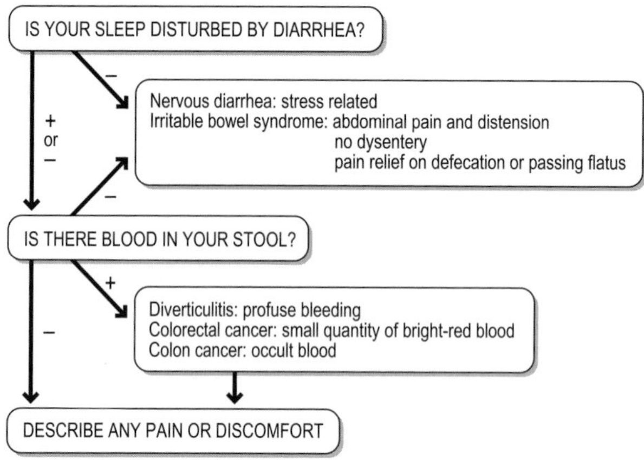

Figure 20.4 **Intermittent diarrhea: important questions to ask.**

- Complications of malabsorption, including:
  - edema secondary to hypoproteinemia
  - anemia due to malabsorption of iron, folic acid, or vitamin B_{12}
  - consequences of calcium malabsorption leading to paresthesia and tetany in the short term and osteoporosis in the long term
  - vitamin deficiencies leading to glossitis, angular stomatitis, dermatitis, peripheral neuropathy, and coagulation disturbances.
  - weight loss.

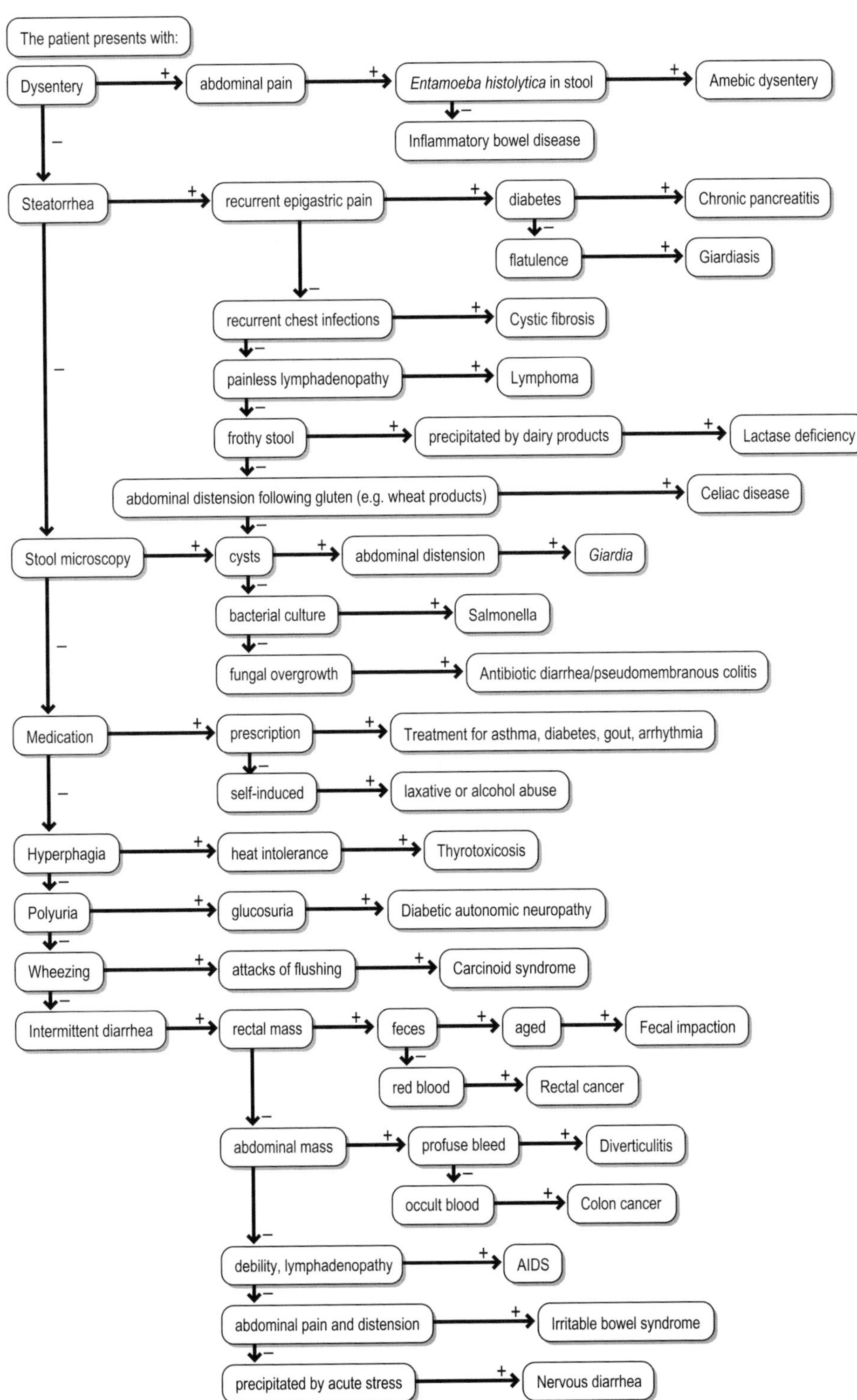

Figure 20.5 **Chronic diarrhea.**

FURTHER READING

Hunter P R 2003 Drinking water and diarrheal disease due to *Escherichia coli*. J Water Health 1(2):65–72

Kass B 2005 Traveller's diarrhea. Aust Fam Physician 34(4):243–247

Niyogi S K 2005 Shigellosis. J Microbiol 43(2):133–143

Widdowson M A, Bresee J S, Gentsch J R, Glass R I 2005 Rotavirus disease and its prevention. Curr Opin Gastroenterol 21(1):26–31

Dizziness

CHAPTER CONTENTS

What is the nature of the dizziness?

When patients complain of dizziness a distinction needs to be made between:

- *Vertigo*. Vertigo is a sensation of whirling or circular motion. It is usually episodic.
- *Giddiness*. Patients feel light-headed.
- *Presyncope*. In certain patients giddiness may progress and they may experience a sensation of impending loss of consciousness.

The severity, frequency, and duration of attacks should be documented.

Vertigo presents clinically with:

- a sensation of spinning
- a feeling of impulsion or being pulled to one side
- nausea and/or vomiting
- nystagmus (this may be absent)
- aggravation of symptoms by head movement.

Vertigo may arise from peripheral or central lesions. Vertigo of peripheral origin may result from a vestibular or VIIIth nerve lesion. Positional vertigo may be related to problems with the cervical spine. Findings suggestive of a peripheral cause of vertigo include:

- Tinnitus. This comprises a buzzing or ringing in the ears.
- Nystagmus. The patient is asked to look for more than 5 seconds at an object held in the midline. The object is moved up, down, medially, and laterally and held in each position. The patient is asked to fix his or her gaze on the stationary object in each position. Nystagmus is present when involuntary

rhythmical movements of the eye are detected. This is normal in extreme lateral gaze.

- Positional vertigo. Positional vertigo should be tested by rapidly taking the head, of a seated patient, down to 30° below the horizontal. This maneuver is repeated with the head: straight, rotated to the right, rotated to the left. In each position the head is held for 30 seconds and the patient is checked for vertigo and nystagmus. In positive cases there is a latent period of a few seconds before the onset of symptoms.
- Hearing loss. If this is present, the Weber and Rinne tests can be used to distinguish between sensory and conduction deafness (see Ch. 18).

Vertigo of central origin may be due to a cerebellar brainstem lesion. Suggestive associated findings include:

- dysarthria (difficulty in articulation)
- dysphagia (difficulty swallowing)
- diplopia (double vision)
- blurred vision
- paresis (muscle weakness)
- cranial nerve palsies.

Giddiness presents clinically as:

- light-headedness
- a symptom of presyncope.

Patients may experience giddiness due to psychogenic or physical causes. Psychogenic causes of giddiness may be mediated by hyperventilation. Patients can be screened by asking them to hyperventilate, by breathing 45 times within 2 minutes. Other causes of giddy light-headedness range from wax impinging on the eardrum to transient changes in cerebral perfusion which, unless rapidly corrected, may present as presyncope and progress to syncope.

Presyncope presents clinically with:

- a feeling of impending loss of consciousness
- giddiness, light-headedness, or faintness
- nausea
- fading hearing
- feeling hot or cold
- blurred vision
- symptoms are worst on standing and may be aborted by lying down.

When patients present with presyncope, examination must include taking the:

- blood pressure (blood pressure should be taken with the patient standing, seated, and lying down to check for postural hypotension)

PART TWO

- pulse rate and rhythm
- palpation of each carotid sinus.

Patients who complain of dizziness often experience a sensation of *disequilibrium*. Disequilibrium is, however, not always associated with dizziness. Patients who experience disequilibrium in the absence of any dizziness are ataxic (see Ch. 54). *Ataxia* presents clinically with:

- unsteadiness in the absence of any sensation of movement (cerebellar lesions cause unsteadiness, but true rotational vertigo is absent)
- disequilibrium without any fluctuation in consciousness
- an abnormal gait.

What is the likely cause?

See Figure 21.1.

Does the patient need to be referred?

Evidence suggesting a serious cause of the dizziness should be investigated. Danger signals include:

- cochlear signs:
  - hearing loss
  - tinnitus
- brainstem signs:
  - diplopia
  - dysarthria
  - paresis
- suspicion of cardiovascular causes:
  - cardiac arrhythmia
  - myocardial infarction.

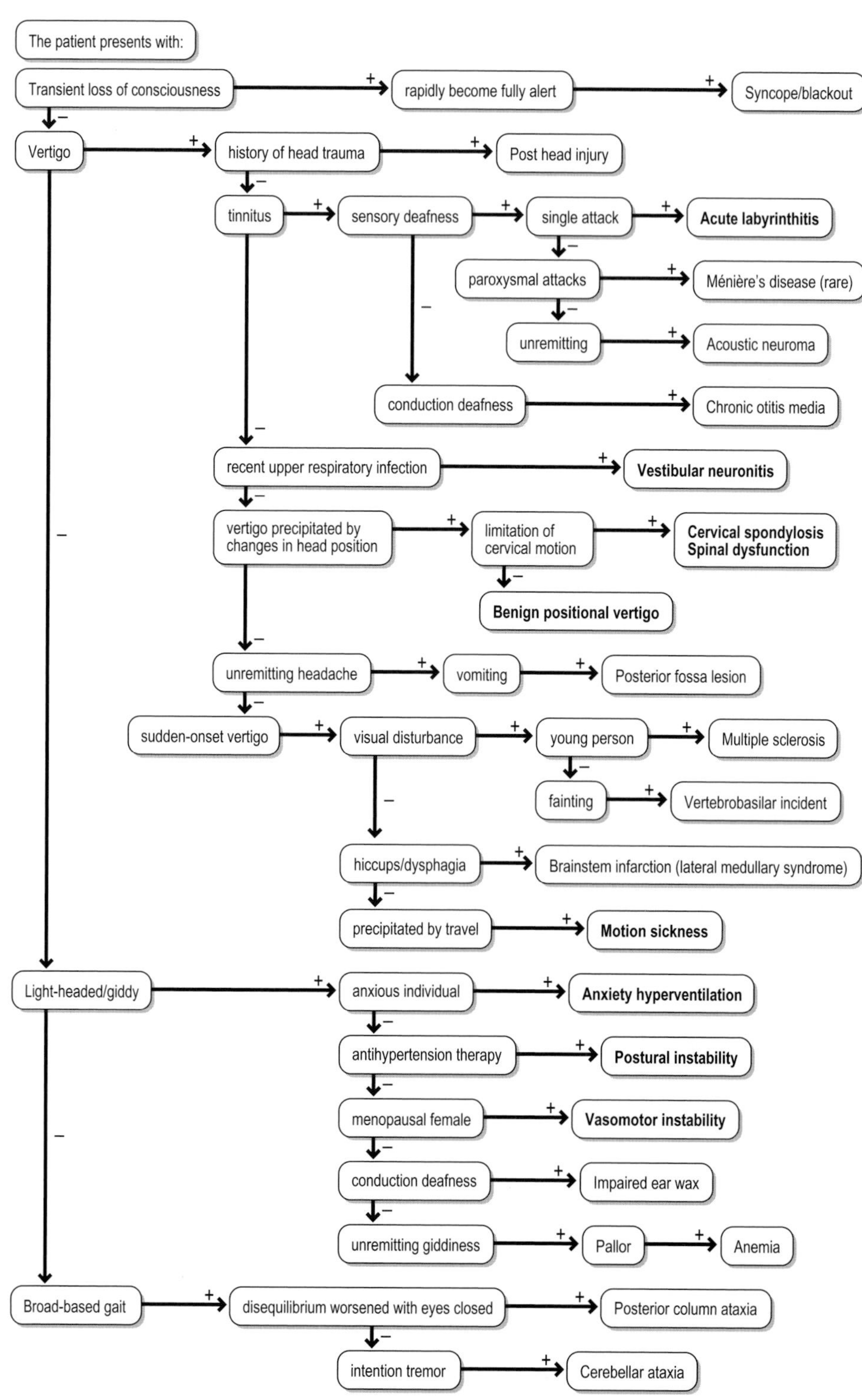

Figure 21.1 **Dizziness.**

FURTHER READING

Bradley J G, Davis K A 2003 Orthostatic hypotension. Am Fam Physician 68(12):2393–2398

Kwong E C, Pimlott N J 2005 Assessment of dizziness among older patients at a family practice clinic: a chart audit study. BMC Fam Pract 6(1):2

Salvinelli F, Firrisi L, Casale M, Trivelli M, D'Ascanio L, Lamanna F, Greco F, Costantino S 2004 Benign paroxysmal positional vertigo: diagnosis and treatment. Clin Ter 155(9):395–400

Swartz R, Longwell P 2005 Treatment of vertigo. Am Fam Physician 71(6):1115–1122

CHAPTER

22

Dysphagia

CHAPTER CONTENTS

Does the patient have dysphagia?

Dysphagia is difficulty in swallowing. The term used to describe painful swallowing is odynophagia. Patients with dysphagia may complain that food sticks, pauses, or does not pass into the stomach. About three out of every four cases of dysphagia in primary practice are attributable to trivial causes.

Is the dysphagia functional or organic?

Dysphagia may be functional or organic. Depending on the level of obstruction, dysphagia may be oropharyngeal or esophageal. Organic esophageal dysphagia may be associated with a lesion in the lumen, the wall, or outside the esophagus causing pressure on the esophageal wall. In cases of *esophageal dysphagia*, the patient reports that:

- the bolus catches in the cervical or retrosternal region
- there is a 15–30 second delay between swallowing and dysphagia.

Oropharyngeal dysphagia is characterized by a 'hold up' in the neck. The patient experiences a sensation of food sticking and has difficulty in initiating swallowing. Disordered bolus delivery to the esophagus is associated with:

- a dry mouth
- poor bolus control
- delayed swallowing initiation
- postnasal regurgitation
- coughing or choking during swallowing.

Oropharyngeal dysphagia is common and should be suspected in elderly patients with delirium, altered levels of consciousness, and a diminished cough. Underlying causes include: bulbar muscle dysfunction attributable to stroke, Parkinson's disease, motor neuron disease, myasthenia gravis, polymyositis, and thyrotoxic myopathy. Globus hystericus is a functional form of oropharyngeal dysphagia.

Functional dysphagia is associated with:

- a 'lump' in the throat
- subjective difficulty in swallowing, which is unrelated to eating or drinking
- no obstruction to food or fluid ingestion at meals
- a sensation of difficulty in swallowing saliva
- the absence of:
  - progressive dysphagia
  - reflux or regurgitation of esophageal contents

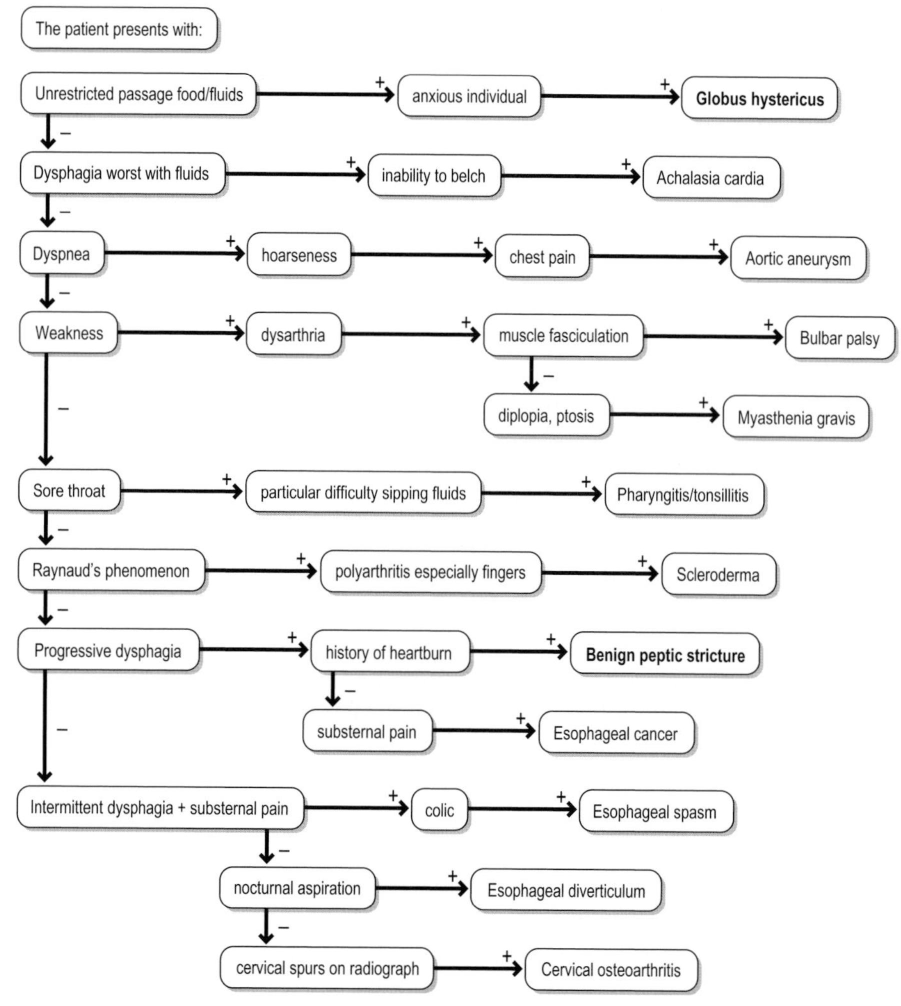

Bold type: most probable condition.

Figure 22.1 **Dysphagia.**

- substernal pain precipitated by eating or drinking
- weight loss.

What is the likely cause?

Any diagnostic protocol for dysphagia includes a statement on the character of dysphagia, the presence of associated symptoms and localization of the perceived obstruction (Fig. 22.1).

Does the patient need to be referred?

Referral may be considered for patients with:

- evidence of true dysphagia:
  - eating or drinking precipitates substernal pain
  - regurgitation manifest as the effortless spilling of gastric or esophageal contents into the mouth.
- weight loss
- progressive symptomatology.

FURTHER READING

Dusick A 2003 Investigation and management of dysphagia. Semin Pediatr Neurol 10(4):255–264

Lieu P K, Chong M S, Seshadri R 2001 The impact of swallowing disorders in the elderly. Ann Acad Med Singapore 30(2):148–154

Sitoh Y Y, Lee A, Phua S Y, Lieu P K, Chan S P 2000 Bedside assessment of swallowing: a useful screening tool for dysphagia in an acute geriatric ward. Singapore Med J 41(8):376–381

CHAPTER 23

Dysuria

CHAPTER CONTENTS

PART TWO

Is this dysuria?

Dysuria is uncomfortable or painful urination. Dysuria is often experienced as burning on micturition or the passage of 'hot' urine. It is usually the result of inflammation, often due to infection. Inflammation of the urinary tract may result from:

- Bladder infection (cystitis): pain is worst at the end of micturition.
- Urethral irritation (urethritis): pain is worst at the beginning of micturition.
- Vaginitis: discomfort occurs at the beginning and/or end of micturition and is experienced as an 'external' burning.

Associated findings are frequency and urgency. Strangury is severe pain on micturition followed by a persistent strong desire to void.

The discomfort of dysuria may be relieved by making the urine alkaline. In cases of urinary tract infection, citra soda masks the symptoms of dysuria without eliminating the organism. Alkalinization of the urine without simultaneously removing the organism may increase the risk of permanent renal damage.

What is the likely cause?

See Figure 23.1.

Does the patient need to be referred?

Dysuria is often an indication for prescription drugs or surgical correction. It is particularly important to note that:

- Patients with suspected urinary tract infection require antibiotics to minimize the risk of ascending infection and possible renal damage.

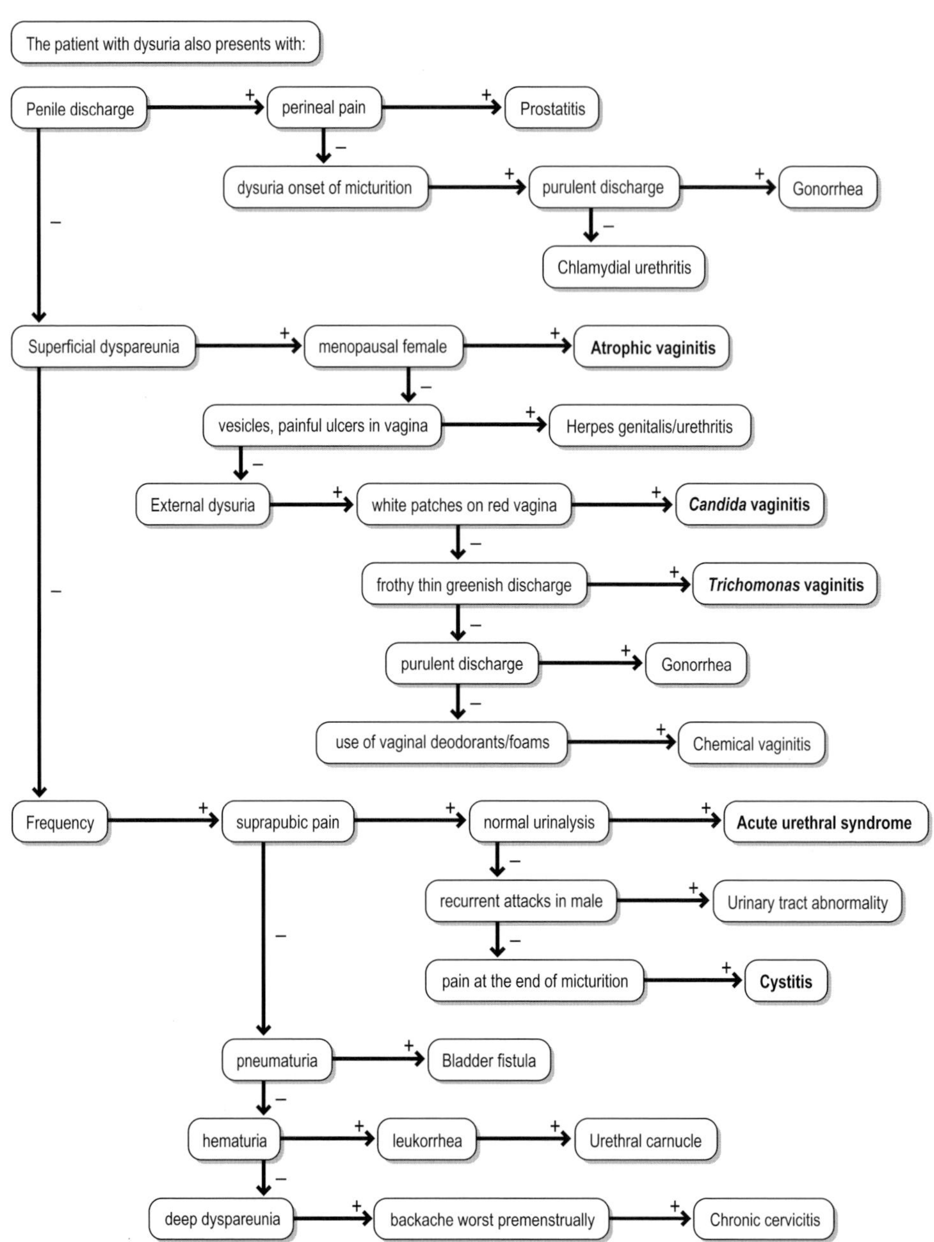

Figure 23.1 **Dysuria.**

- Both symptomatic patients and asymptomatic partners with sexually transmitted disease require treatment.
- Males with recurrent episodes of dysuria, frequency, and urgency require investigations to exclude abnormality of the urinary system. Unlike females, recurrent cystitis is unusual in males due to their long urethra.

FURTHER READING

Bent S, Nallamothu B K, Simel D L, Fihn S D, Saint S 2002 Does this woman have an acute uncomplicated urinary tract infection? JAMA 287(20):2701–2710

Bent S, Saint S 2003 The optimal use of diagnostic testing in women with acute uncomplicated cystitis. Dis Mon 49(2):83–98.

Bremnor J D, Sadovsky R 2002 Evaluation of dysuria in adults. Am Fam Physician 65(8):1589–1596

Simerville J A, Maxted W C, Pahira J J 2005 Urinalysis: a comprehensive review. Am Fam Physician 71(6):1153–1162

CHAPTER

24 Earache

CHAPTER CONTENTS

Does the patient have an aural problem?

Earache may be due to a local aural problem or may be referred from elsewhere. Analysis of associated findings provides an important clue to the origin of the pain. Patients with aural problems frequently present with any combination of:

- Hearing loss.
- Sound distortion (tinnitus).
- An abnormality of the tympanic membrane.
- A lesion of the external auditory canal.
- Earache. The character of the pain may be helpful in differentiating the underlying ear problems. In:
  - furunculosis, movement of the pinna causes extreme pain
  - occlusive otitis externa, pressure on the tragus causes pain
  - viral myringitis, pain occurs in cycles and is relieved when the bleb ruptures
  - acute otitis media, deep-seated throbbing earache is aggravated by swallowing
  - secretory otitis media, transient niggling pain is experienced
  - mastoiditis, persistent throbbing earache is associated with tenderness over the mastoid process.

Referred pain is likely when earache is experienced by a patient without any of these associated symptoms and/or a normal ear on clinical examination. Pain referred to the ear may arise from diverse structures and may be referred to anatomically discrete areas of the ear. Referred pain is frequently detected in one of three distinct areas depending on the source:

- Pain over the superior and anteromedial surface of the pinna and anterior surface of the eardrum may originate from:
  - Temporomandibular joint disease. Costen's syndrome (earache, tinnitus, and mild deafness (sometimes present)), may be attributable to abnormal stresses in the temporomandibular joint resulting from malocclusion. The pain is usually directly over the joint and may extend into the temporalis and other associated muscles. Joint tenderness may be noted. Patients may grind their teeth.
  - Dental problems/impacted molar.
  - Sphenoidal sinusitis (via the auriculotemporal nerve).
- Pain over the posterior junction of the pinna and scalp, the posterior portion of the eardrum, or the inner ear may be attributable to:
  - Glossopharyngeal (IX) or facial (VII) neuralgia. Lancinating ear and throat pain are found in glossopharyngeal neuralgia.
  - Carcinoma of the posterior third of the tongue.
  - Oropharyngeal lesion (e.g. tonsillitis, carcinoma). Earache and progressive dysphagia are suggestive of malignancy in the hypopharyngeal or laryngeal area.
- Pain over the posterior third, including the inferolateral surface of the pinna and the mastoid region, may result from:
  - cervical osteoarthritis
  - tense neck muscles
  - cervical soft tissue lesions (e.g. lymphadenopathy).

Once a possible source of the earache has been suggested by the area of pain, evidence of pathology in the source area should be sought.

PART TWO

What is the cause of the patient's earache?

See Figure 24.1.

Does the patient need to be referred?

Patients should be referred for further investigation, surgery, or prescription drugs in the presence of:

- earache that is:
  - severe, especially if sudden in onset
  - persistent
- pyrexia
- local changes such as:
  - a chronic purulent or foul-smelling aural discharge
  - a red, bulging eardrum with loss of light reflex/abnormal light reflex
  - a perforated drum with complications
  - edema and tenderness over the mastoid
  - facial palsy.

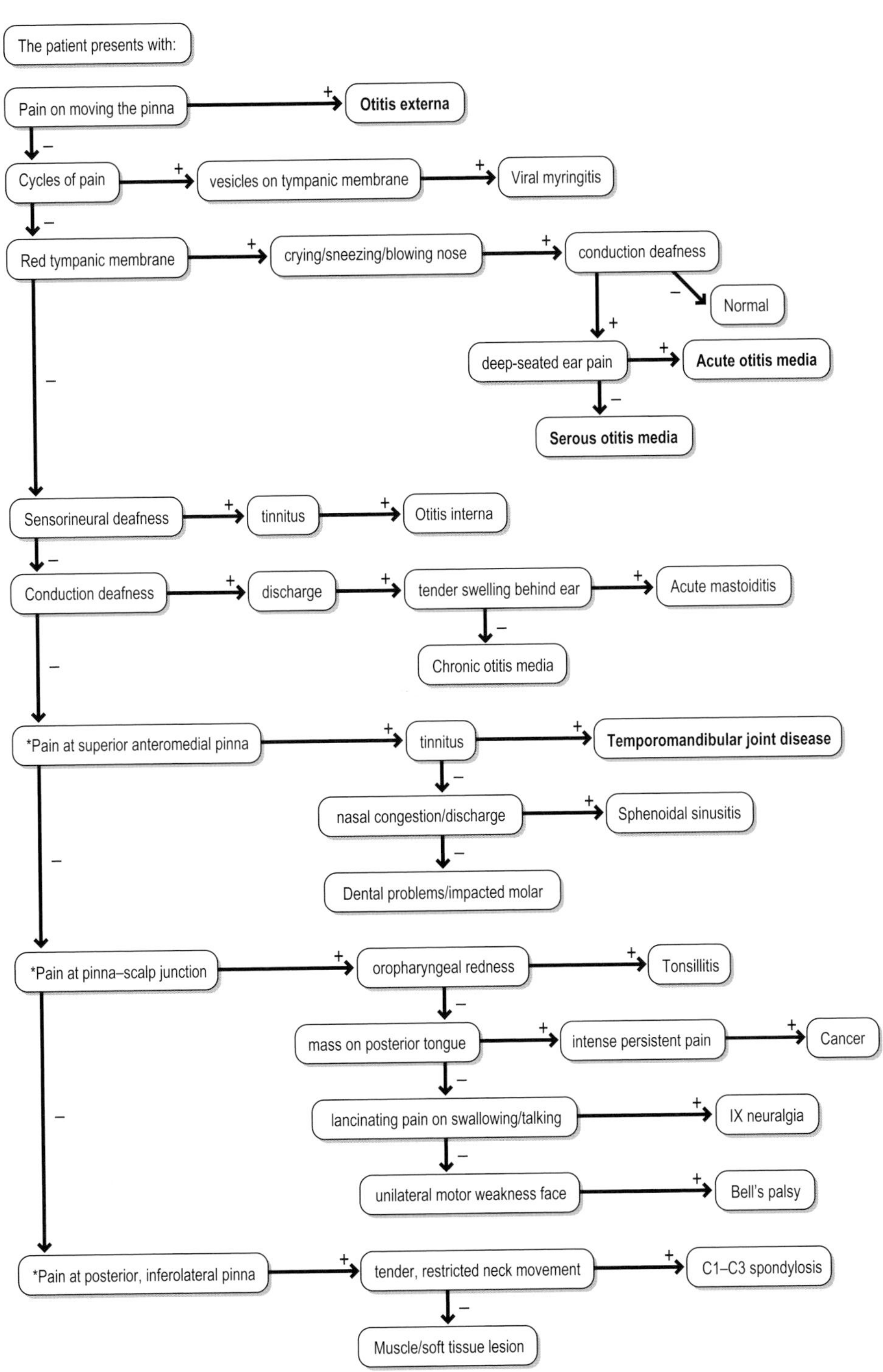

Bold face: most probable condition
*Referred pain

Figure 24.1 **Earache.**

FURTHER READING

Leung A K, Fong J H, Leong A G 2000 Otalgia in children. J Natl Med Assoc 92(5):254–260

Shah R K, Blevins N H 2003 Otalgia. Otolaryngol Clin North Am 36(6):1137–1151

CHAPTER 25

Facial pain

CHAPTER CONTENTS

PART TWO

Is the facial pain acute or chronic?

Facial pain may be local or referred. It can arise from any structure in the area of the face. Acute facial pain may result from:

- Acute infection. Acute sinusitis causes severe throbbing facial pain. When the maxillary or frontal sinuses are involved, marked facial tenderness is detected. A typical history is a cold and nasal discharge.
- An aneurysm. An aneurysm of the posterior communicating artery can cause pressure on the oculomotor nerve, leading to the rapid development of ptosis and an eye which is abducted and depressed due to impaired upward, downward, and medial movement. The pupil is dilated and nonreactive. Immediate surgical referral is indicated.
- Intracranial lesion. Patients may present with alterations of facial sensation. Areas of pain, paresthesia, or numbness may be indicative of intracranial disease.
- Eye disease. Patients with a red painful eye (see Ch. 48) should be checked for:
  - Acute glaucoma: raised intraocular pressure is diagnostic.
  - Acute uveitis/iritis: the patient complains of photophobia and decreased vision. The pupil is constricted and the direct light reflex is sluggish.
  - Corneal ulcer: the ulcer can be visualized using eyedrops containing fluorescein.

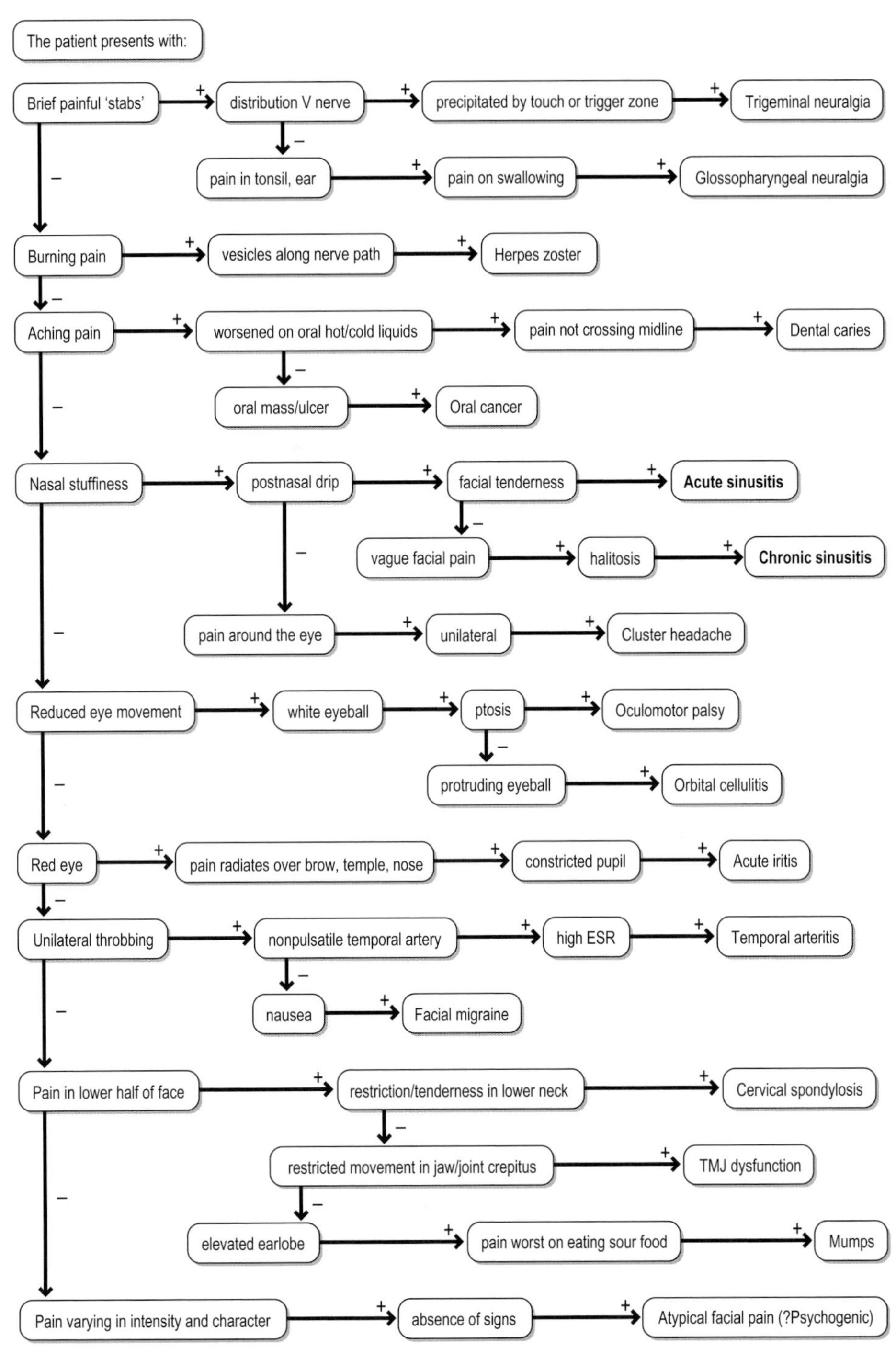

Figure 25.1 **Facial pain.**

Chronic or recurrent facial pain may arise from:

- Persistent infection of local structures:
  - chronic sinusitis
  - chronic dental disorders.
- Structural dysfunction:
  - temporomandibular joint (TMJ) disease.
  - cervical spinal dysfunction.
- Neuralgia attributable to:
  - no proven cause (idiopathic)
  - previous herpes infection.
- Vasospasm of cerebral arteries, causing migraine.

See Chapter 24, Earache.

What is the cause of the patient's facial pain?

See Figure 25.1.

Does the patient need to be referred?

Patients should be referred for further investigation and/or treatment when:

- acute facial pain is diagnosed and appropriate treatment is outside your scope of practice
- the patient is failing to respond to treatment
- there is a risk that a suspected infection will spread
- malignancy is suspected.

FURTHER READING

Horowitz M, Horowitz M, Ochs M, Carrau R, Kassam A 2005 Trigeminal neuralgia and glossopharyngeal neuralgia: two orofacial pain syndromes encountered by dentists. J Am Dent Assoc 2004 Oct;135(10):1427–1433

Zakrzewska J M 2002 Facial pain: neurological and non-neurological. J Neurol Neurosurg Psychiatry 72 Suppl 2:ii27–ii32.

Fatigue

CHAPTER CONTENTS

What is the nature of the patient's fatigue?

Fatigued patients present complaining of any combination of the following:

- lethargy, listlessness, a lack of energy
- tiredness, feeling worn-out
- weariness, exhaustion especially after prolonged exertion
- malaise, feeling unwell, or a feeling of depression
- feeling run down.

Fatigue may be categorized as:

- Acute or chronic: chronic fatigue is, by definition, fatigue that has lasted for more than 6 months.
- Mild, moderate, or severe: subjective evaluation by the patient of the intensity of their fatigue provides a helpful monitoring baseline.
- Functional or organic: Table 26.1 compares the characteristics of functional and organic fatigue.

Table 26.1 **Categorizing fatigue**

	Functional fatigue	Organic fatigue
Age	Young	Older
Onset	Gradual May follow an illness	Sudden Associated with signs (e.g. fever)
Duration	Months to years	Days to weeks
Progression	Fluctuating course	Gradually progressive
Sleep	No effect	Relieves fatigue
Circadian rhythm	Worst in the morning, improves as the day progresses	Best in the morning, worsens as the day progresses

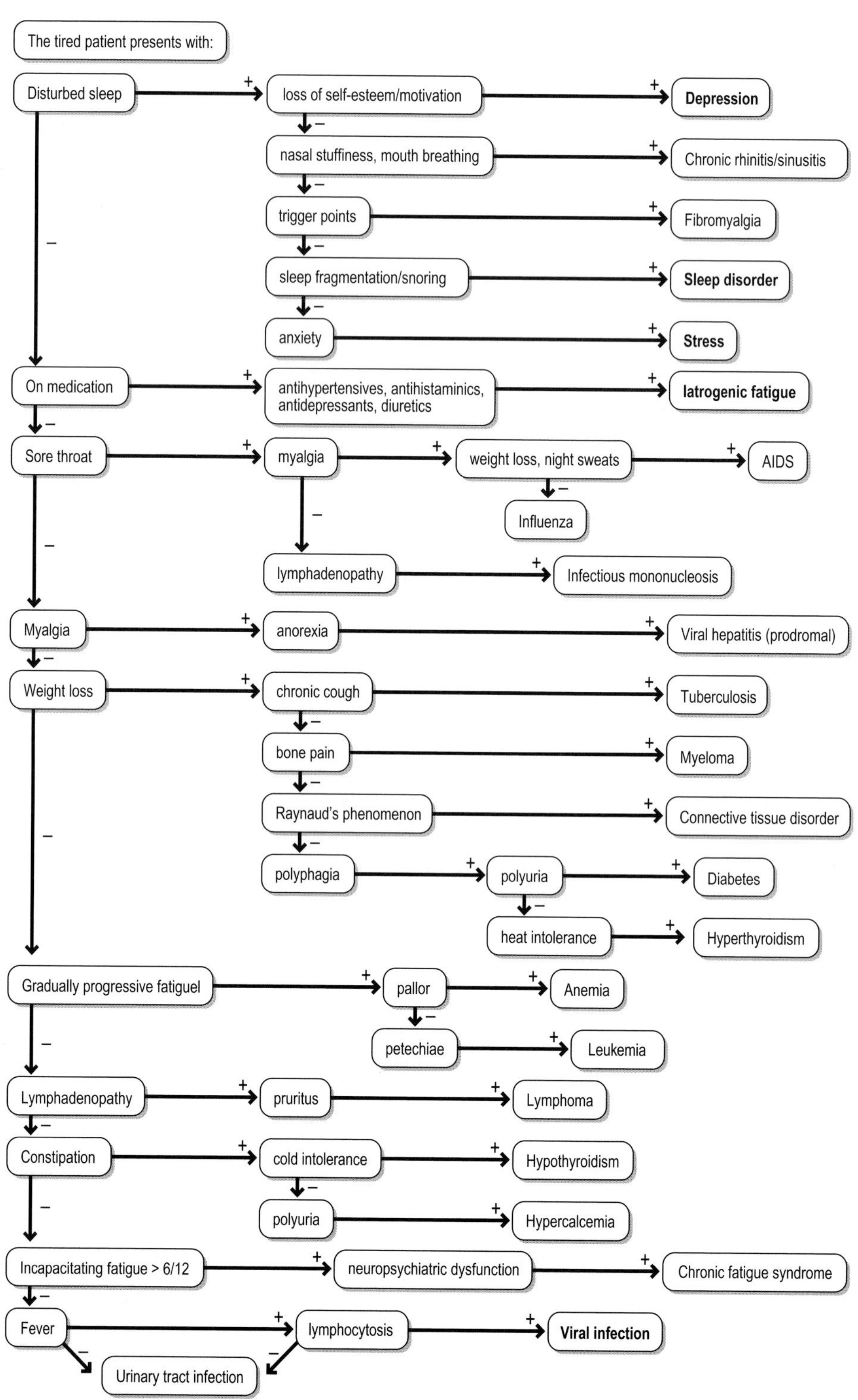

Bold face: common cause.

Figure 26.1 **Fatigue.**

What is the cause of the patient's fatigue?

See Figure 26.1.

Does the patient need to be referred?

Patients complaining of fatigue should be referred when:

- anemic
- underlying visceral disease is suspected
- bacterial infection is likely
- moderate or marked depression is diagnosed
- specialist counseling is required.

FURTHER READING

Andrea H, Kant I J, Beurskens A J, Metsemakers J F, Van Schayck C P 2003 Associations between fatigue attributions and fatigue, health, and psychosocial work characteristics: a study among employees visiting a physician with fatigue. Occup Environ Med 60 Suppl 1:i99–104

Darbishire L, Ridsdale L, Seed PT 2003 Distinguishing patients with chronic fatigue from those with chronic fatigue syndrome: a diagnostic study in UK primary care. Br J Gen Pract 53(491):441–445

Gerrity T R, Papanicolaou D A, Amsterdam J D, Bingham S, Grossman A, Hedrick T, Herberman R B, Krueger G, Levine S, Mohagheghpour N, Moore R C, Oleske J, Snell CR; CFIDS Association of America 2004 Immunologic aspects of chronic fatigue syndrome. Report on a Research Symposium convened by The CFIDS Association of America and co-sponsored by the US Centers for Disease Control and Prevention and the National Institutes of Health. Neuroimmunomodulation 11(6):351–357

Lerdal A, Wahl A, Rustoen T, Hanestad B R, Moum T 2005 Fatigue in the general population: a translation and test of the psychometric properties of the Norwegian version of the fatigue severity scale. Scand J Public Health 33(2):123–130

Meeuwesen L, Bensing J, van den Brink-Muinen A 2002 Communicating fatigue in general practice and the role of gender. Patient Educ Couns 48(3):233–242

Patarca R 2001 Cytokines and chronic fatigue syndrome. Ann N Y Acad Sci 933:185–200

CHAPTER 27

Fever (pyrexia)

CHAPTER CONTENTS

Does the patient have a fever?

A diurnal temperature fluctuation is normal, with the body temperature being lowest in the early hours of the morning and highest in late afternoon. The normal temperature range is 36.7–37.6°C. The temperature may be measured by placing a thermometer in the mouth, rectum, or axilla. The reading should only be taken after the thermometer has been in place for a number of minutes. To achieve an accurate reading, take the:

- oral temperature reading after 9 minutes or more have elapsed
- rectal temperature reading after 2 minutes
- axillary temperature reading after 11 minutes.

Failure to allow the recommended time lapse results in discrepant temperature readings between the three areas.

Fever, or pyrexia, is an elevation of temperature. In apyrexial patients a blood temperature in excess of 37.5°C stimulates the hypothalamus to trigger an autonomic nervous system shift towards vasodilatation and sweating. In pyrexia this homeostatic response fails. A fever progresses through a number of phases:

- In the early phases of pyrexia, heat production exceeds heat loss. Clinically, the patient presents with shivering or rigors.
- The temperature continues to rise then stabilizes once heat loss equals heat production. Clinically, patients are flushed and have a raised temperature.
- During defervescence, heat loss exceeds heat gain. Clinically, the patient's temperature drops and sweating is noted during the early phases.

Fevers are described as:

- *Continuous.* A continuous fever is a consistently elevated temperature, with only minor fluctuations in any 24-hour period. It may return to baseline. Streptococcal pharyngitis, meningitis, and typhoid are all associated with a continuous fever.
- *Intermittent.* In intermittent fevers the temperature is elevated then drops to normal or subnormal levels in any 24-hour period. The cycle is repeated. Gram-negative septicemia, malaria, and pyrogenic abscesses cause an intermittent fever.
- *Remittent.* In remittent fever an elevated temperature is sustained and, despite marked fluctuations, never returns to baseline. The fever associated with collagen or connective tissue disorders, such as rheumatoid arthritis, dermatomyositis, systemic lupus erythematosus (SLE), and necrotizing vasculitis is remittent.
- *Relapsing* or recurrent fever. The pattern of relapsing fever is several days of pyrexia followed by periods of normothermia. Lymphoma, poliomyelitis, brucellosis, and malaria all give rise to a relapsing fever.

Fever may be caused by release of endogenous pyrogens from polymorphs and other white cells as a result of inflammation. Fever is therefore extremely common in conditions in which the inflammatory process is pronounced, as in infections and immunological disorders. Other evidence of an inflammatory process includes a raised erythrocyte sedimentation rate (ESR) and C-reactive protein. Infections, in addition to general signs of inflammation, have white cell changes characteristic of the type of infection. Viral infections are associated with a lymphocytosis, bacterial infections with a leukocytosis, and parasitic infections with an eosinophilia. Conditions with a marked immune response may be diagnosed with the assistance of serological tests. The duration of the fever is a useful guide to diagnosis:

- *Fevers of less than 3 days.* The vast majority of patients will have self-limiting viral respiratory diseases. Localizing findings are useful diagnostic pointers (e.g. dysuria in urinary tract infection, spreading erythema in cellulitis).
- *Fevers of 4–14 days.* Most of the common viral diseases will have resolved after 4 days. Persons in this group require active investigation, including at least a full blood examination, blood culture, urinalysis, and chest radiograph.
- *Fevers of 14–21 days, with no diagnosis.* Pyrexia of unknown origin (PUO) is a fever that has persisted undiagnosed for 3 weeks. Some 40% of such cases are ultimately attributed to infection, 20% to neoplasms (lymphomas, solid tumors, metastatic disease), and 15% to collagen diseases (polymyalgia rheumatica, rheumatoid disease, polyarteritis nodosa, lupus erythematosus) and drug fevers. Some 10% are never diagnosed.

Is this an emergency?

A sustained rectal temperature in excess of 41°C is associated with permanent brain damage. Death from heat stroke may occur when the rectal temperature exceeds 43°C. Prevention of dangerously high temperature levels may usually be achieved by:

- A high intake of cool fluids.
- Tepid sponging.
- A cool fan.
- Antipyretic agents. Paracetamol and nonsteroidal anti-inflammatory drugs (NSAIDs) are important antipyretic drugs. They have a rapid, reversible effect. The antipyretic effect of NSAIDs is attributable to inhibition of prostaglandin E_2 synthesis in the anterior hypothalamus. The myalgia and muscle catabolism characteristic of a high fever is mediated via interleukin-1 acting via prostaglandin E_2. These drugs may also be used for their analgesic effect in certain viral infections, inflammatory disorders, and cancer.

What is the likely diagnosis?

See Figure 27.1.

Does the patient need to be referred?

Patients should be referred if:

- The cause of the fever cannot be identified (PUO).
- A serious underlying disease is suspected.
- The temperature cannot be adequately controlled.
- They appear ill and have no localizing signs.
- They fall into one of the following risk groups:
  - extremes of age (these patients may deteriorate rapidly)
  - immunocompromised (infections may become fulminant within hours)
  - overseas traveler or visitor (these patients may have highly contagious diseases that require early diagnosis and treatment).

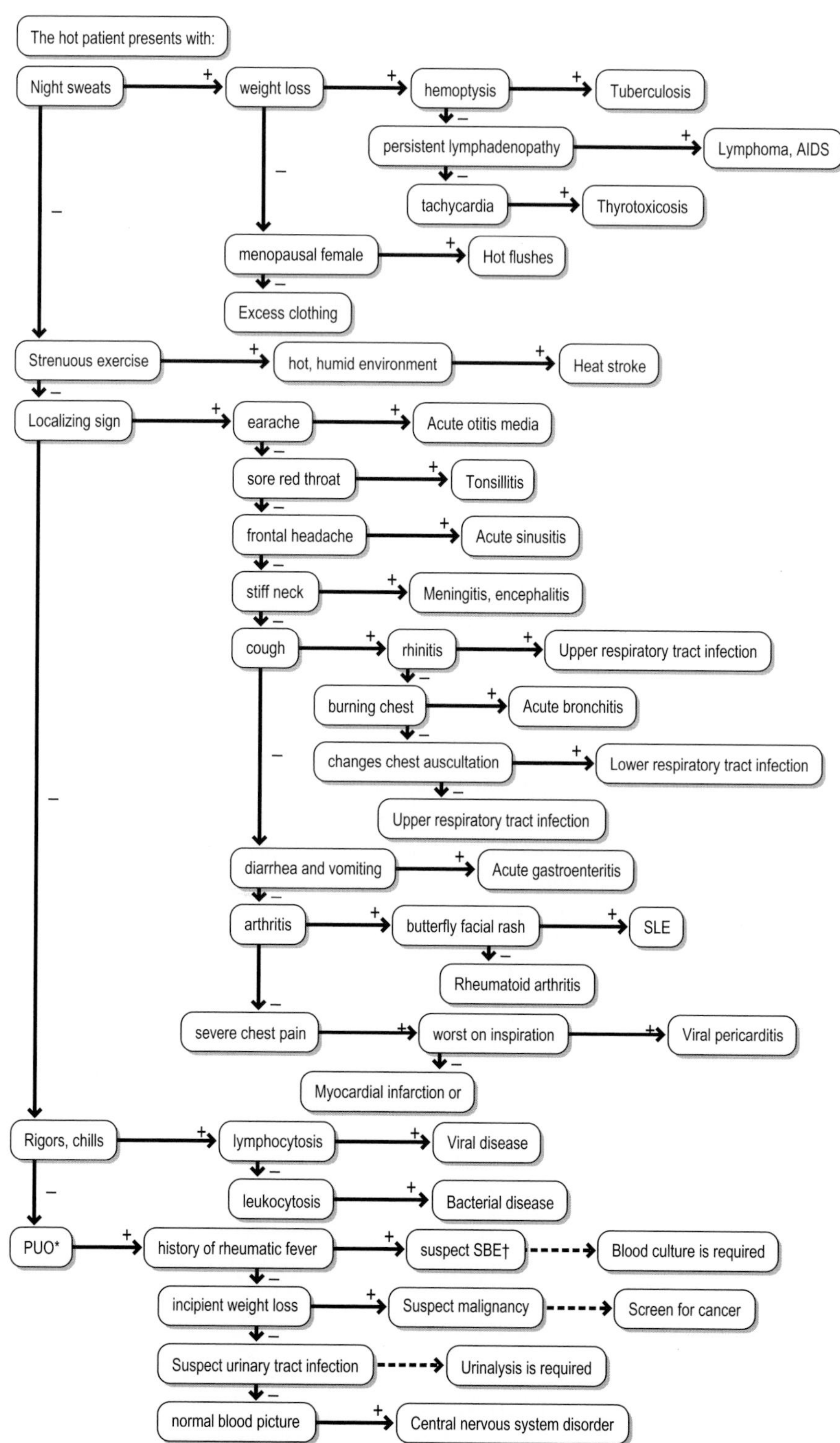

Figure 27.1 **Fever.**

FURTHER READING

Lo Re V 3rd, Gluckman S J 2003 Fever in the returned traveler. Am Fam Physician 68(7):1343–1350

Roth A R, Basello G M 2003 Approach to the adult patient with fever of unknown origin. Am Fam Physician 68(11):2223–2228

Woolery W A, Franco F R 2004 Fever of unknown origin: keys to determining the etiology in older patients. Geriatrics 59(10):41–45

CHAPTER 28

Flushing

CHAPTER CONTENTS

Does the patient show flushing?

Flushing is a temporary reddening of the face which may involve the ears, neck, and trunk. Active control of facial blood vessels is via vasodilatation rather than vasoconstriction. Blood to the skin is controlled by a combination of the autonomic nerve function, circulating vasoactive agents, and local release of vasoactive substances. Mediators involved in flushing include catecholamines, neuropeptides, kinins, histamine, leukotrienes, and prostaglandins. Bioflavonoids appear to restore endothelial structure and reduce hot flushes and vasodilatation. Peridin C, a tablet which contains hesperidin, a bioflavonoid, and vitamin C may provided some relief.

Flushing may result from:

- estrogen deprivation as in menopause (estrogen influences capillary tone and prevents excessive dilatation)
- hormonal secretion by tumors
- ingestion of certain foods or drugs
- emotion (psychological flushing, or blushing, is induced by emotion).

What is the likely cause?

See Figure 28.1.

Does the patient need to be referred?

Patients require referral if malignancy is suspected.

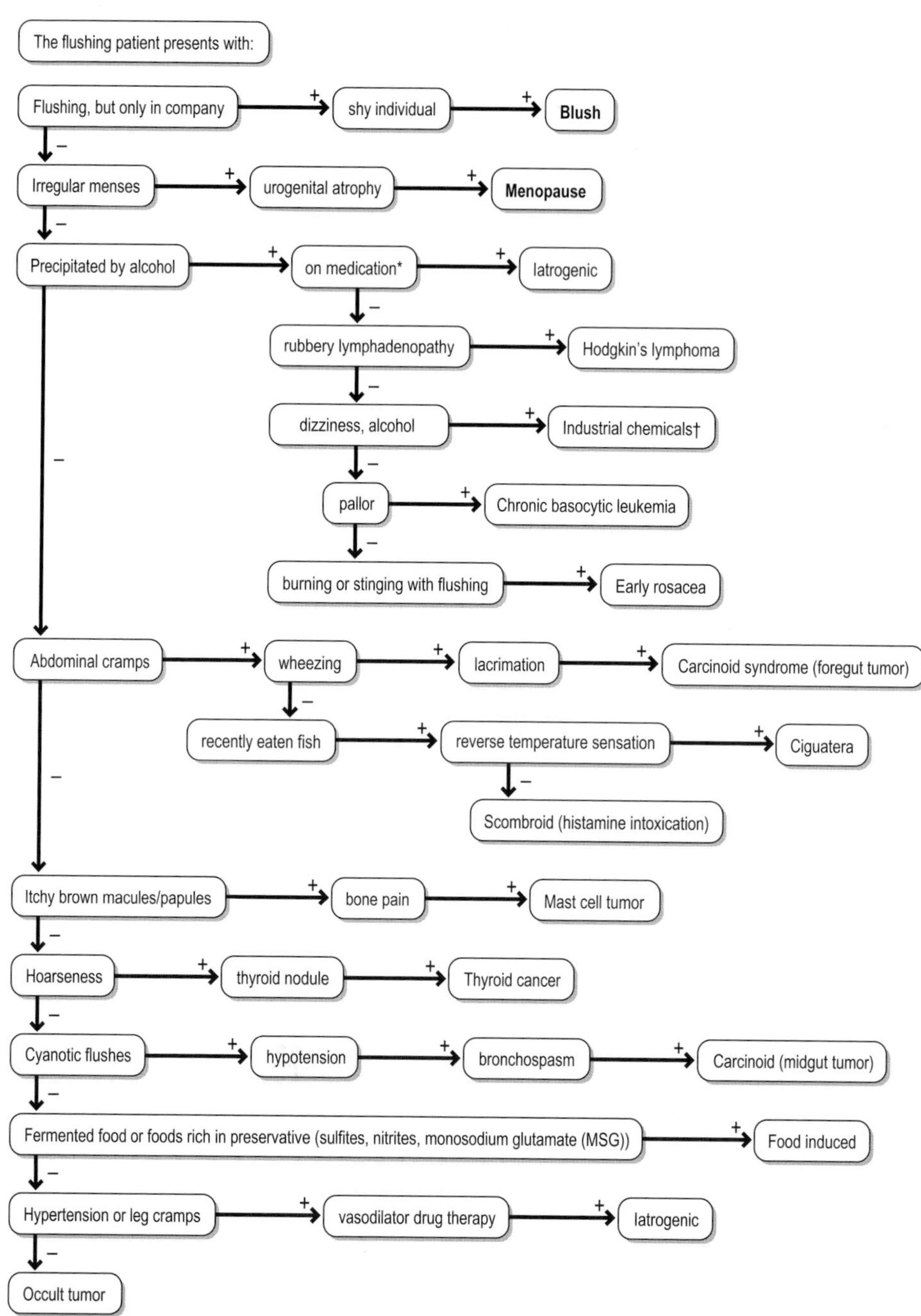

Bold face: most probable condition
*Alcohol-drug combinations associated with flushing include: disulfiram, chlorpropamine (antidiabetic), and various anti-microbial agents (metronidazole, griseofulvin).
† Alcohol-workplace chemical combination associated with flushing include: dimethylformealdehyde, trichloethylene, industrial solvents, and chemicals used in the rubber and printing industries.

Figure 28.1 **Flushing.**

FURTHER READING

Neff M J 2004 NAMS releases position statement on the treatment of vasomotor symptoms associated with menopause. Am Fam Physician 70(2):393–394, 396, 399

CHAPTER 29

Genital pain or discomfort

CHAPTER CONTENTS

Where is the pain?

In females genital discomfort is most often experienced during intercourse. Dyspareunia may be:

- *Superficial dyspareunia* is due to local lesions. Discomfort may:
  - be due to persistent local vulvovaginal irritation
  - result from psychogenic causes (vaginismus).
- *Deep dyspareunia* may result from lesions of the cervix, uterus, tubes, or ovaries. Vulval discomfort may be referred from the urinary tract.

Chronic pelvic pain in women is defined as continuous or episodic pain that has persisted for at least 6 months and is severe enough to affect the patient's daily functioning and relationships. Although primarily of gynecological origin, chronic pelvic pain may also be attributed to musculoskeletal, urinary, gastrointestinal, and psychological problems.

In males genital discomfort may be experienced in the scrotum, testis, or penis. Discomfort may be:

- Due to local lesions. Tenderness and swelling of any of these organs suggests a local lesion. Confirmation that the problem lies in the scrotum is obtained on finding:
  - scrotal tenderness
  - scrotal swelling
  - that the examiner's fingers can get above any mass in the scrotum.
- Referred. Scrotal discomfort may be referred from:
  - The urinary tract. In the absence of local tenderness or enlargement, pain is likely to have been referred. A urological problem is likely in patients whose scrotal pain is:
    Acute.

Associated with renal colic. Pain is referred to the scrotum when the lower end of the ureter on that side is distended. Pain may be referred to the testis when the ipsilateral upper ureter is distended.
Associated with urinary symptoms.
- The psyche. Psychogenic testing has shown marked similarities between patients with chronic orchalgia and low back pain. A high incidence of depressive disorders is also found in these patients.

Is the pain functional or organic?

Pain is likely to be organic if:

- A local lesion is detected.
- In the absence of a local lesion, evidence of dysfunction in another organ system suggests that pain is referred. For example, a spinal problem with nerve-root pressure is likely in patients who experience:
  - pain, paresthesia, or anesthesia in the dermatome supplied by L1
  - a dull mid–low backache
  - some limitation of movement in the region of the thora-columbar junction
  - pain in the genitalia is more pronounced than in the back.

Referred pain is likely to be functional:

- if it is nonspecific in nature
- if some degree of sexual dysfunction is present
- if it is chronic (pain is often found to have been present for some months).

Does the patient require urgent referral?

Gynecological conditions that require urgent referral are most likely to present as an acute abdomen. (See Figures 29.1 and 29.2 on pelvic or lower abdominal pain.)

Males with scrotal pain and swelling require urgent surgical referral if they have:

- Torsion of the testis. Twisting of the tunica vaginalis impairs testicular blood supply, and, unless perfusion is restored within 4 hours, permanent damage is likely to result.
- A strangulated indirect inguinal hernia. Obstruction to the blood supply of bowel which has descended into the scrotum along the inguinal canal can result in bowel necrosis and intestinal gangrene.

Patients should be referred if they:

- experience rapidly progressive severe constant pain
- are vomiting
- have an exquisitely tender testis which lies high and transverse in the scrotum
- a history of a hernia which has become irreducible
- paraphimosis.

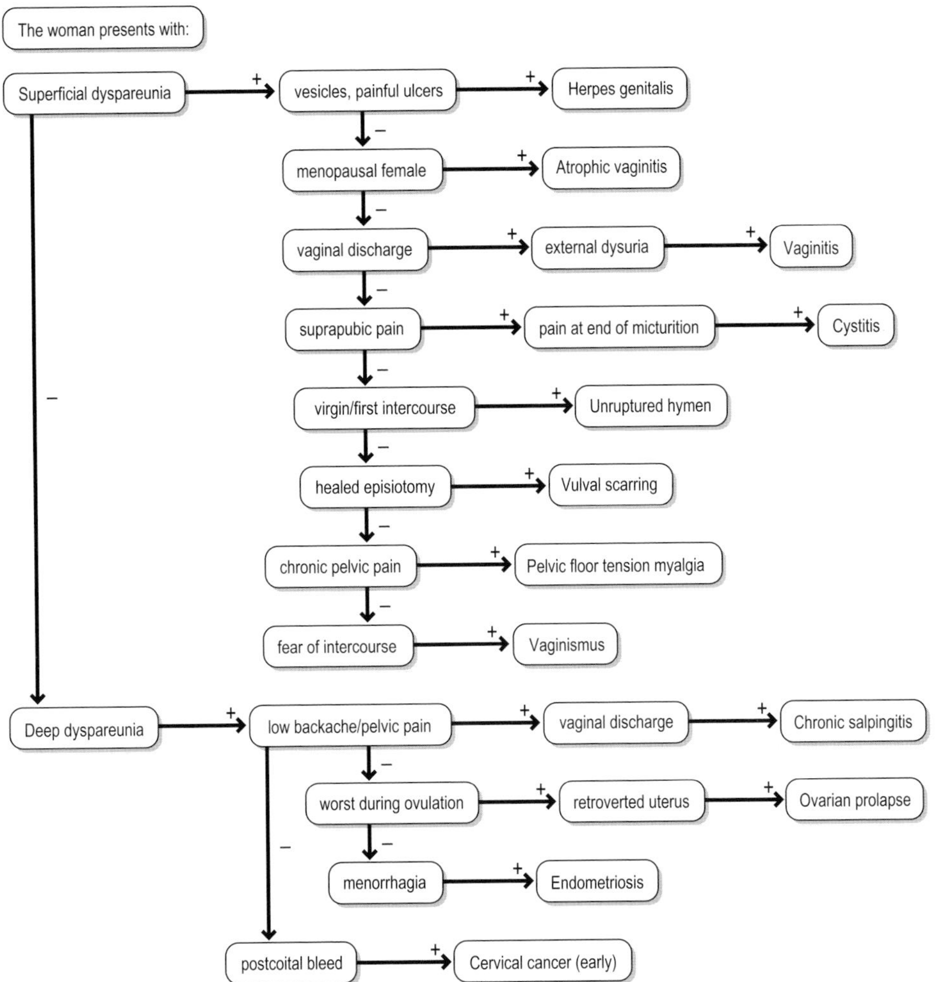

Figure 29.1 **Female genital pain (dyspareunia).**

What is the likely diagnosis?

See Figures 29.1 and 29.2.

Does the patient need to be referred?

Patients with genital pain should be referred if:

- a scrotal mass or testicular swelling is detected (malignancy must be excluded)
- vomiting persists despite primary attempts to achieve pain relief
- dysuria and frequency persist or recur
- intervention beyond the primary practitioner's scope of practice is indicated.

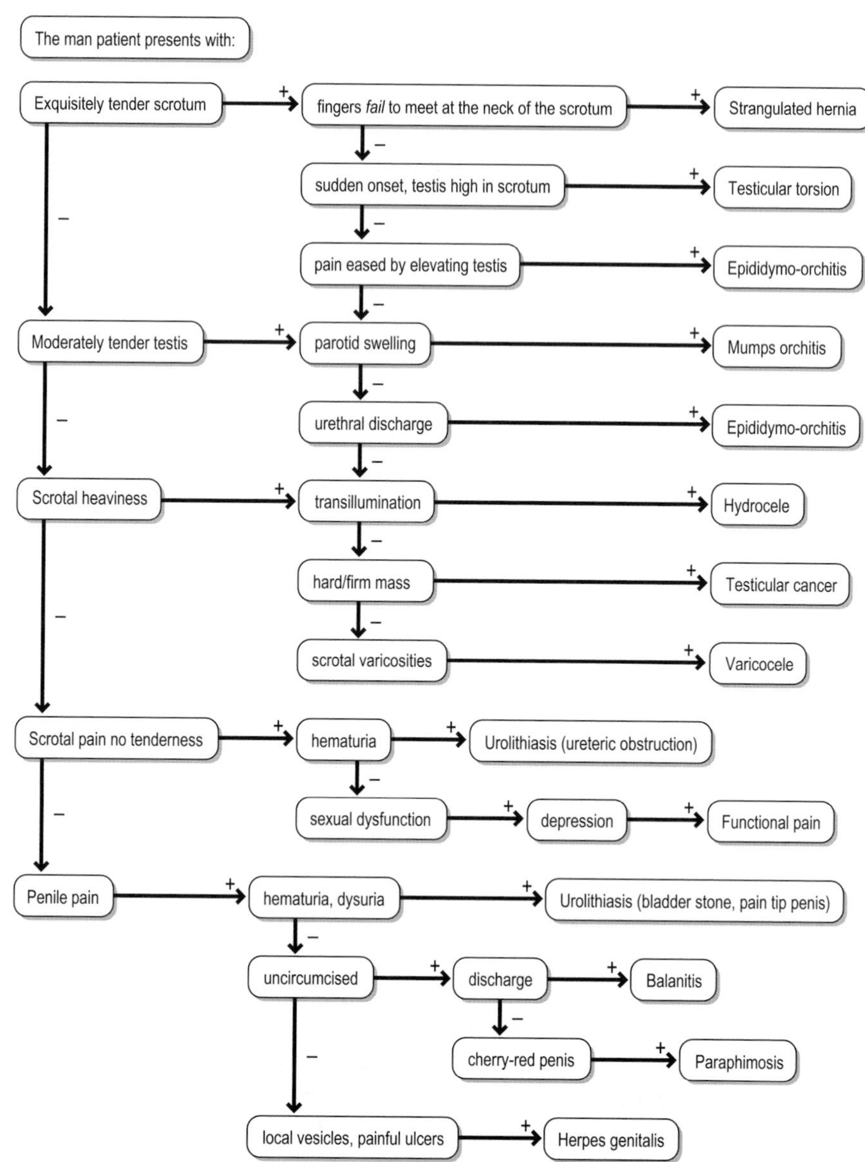

Figure 29.2 **Male genital pain.**

FURTHER READING

Banikarim C, Chacko M R 2004 Pelvic inflammatory disease in adolescents. Adolesc Med Clin 15(2):viii, 273–285

Luzzi G, Law L 2005 A guide to sexual pain in men. Practitioner 249(1667):73, 75, 77

Samraj G P, Curry R W Jr 2004 Acute pelvic pain: evaluation and management. Compr Ther 2004 Fall–Winter;30(3):173–184

PART TWO

CHAPTER 30

Halitosis

CHAPTER CONTENTS

PART TWO

What is the source of the halitosis?

Halitosis, or bad breath, may result from local or systemic disorders. Local sources include:

- nasal lesions (holding the nares closed while exhaling through the mouth helps to differentiate whether the source of the halitosis is nasal)
- oropharyngeal lesions
- impaired salivary flow
- poor oral hygiene and bacterial metabolism.

Infection and malodorous metabolic end-products are important systemic causes of halitosis. Systemic sources of halitosis include:

- the respiratory system
- the gastrointestinal tract
- metabolic disturbances.

Patients with serious disease seldom have halitosis as their presenting complaint. In such patients halitosis is more usually one of the signs characteristic of the underlying condition.

What is the likely diagnosis?

See Figure 30.1.

Does the patient need to be referred?

Patients with halitosis should be referred if:

- dental care is needed
- undiagnosed underlying disease is suspected
- intervention outside your scope of practice is required.

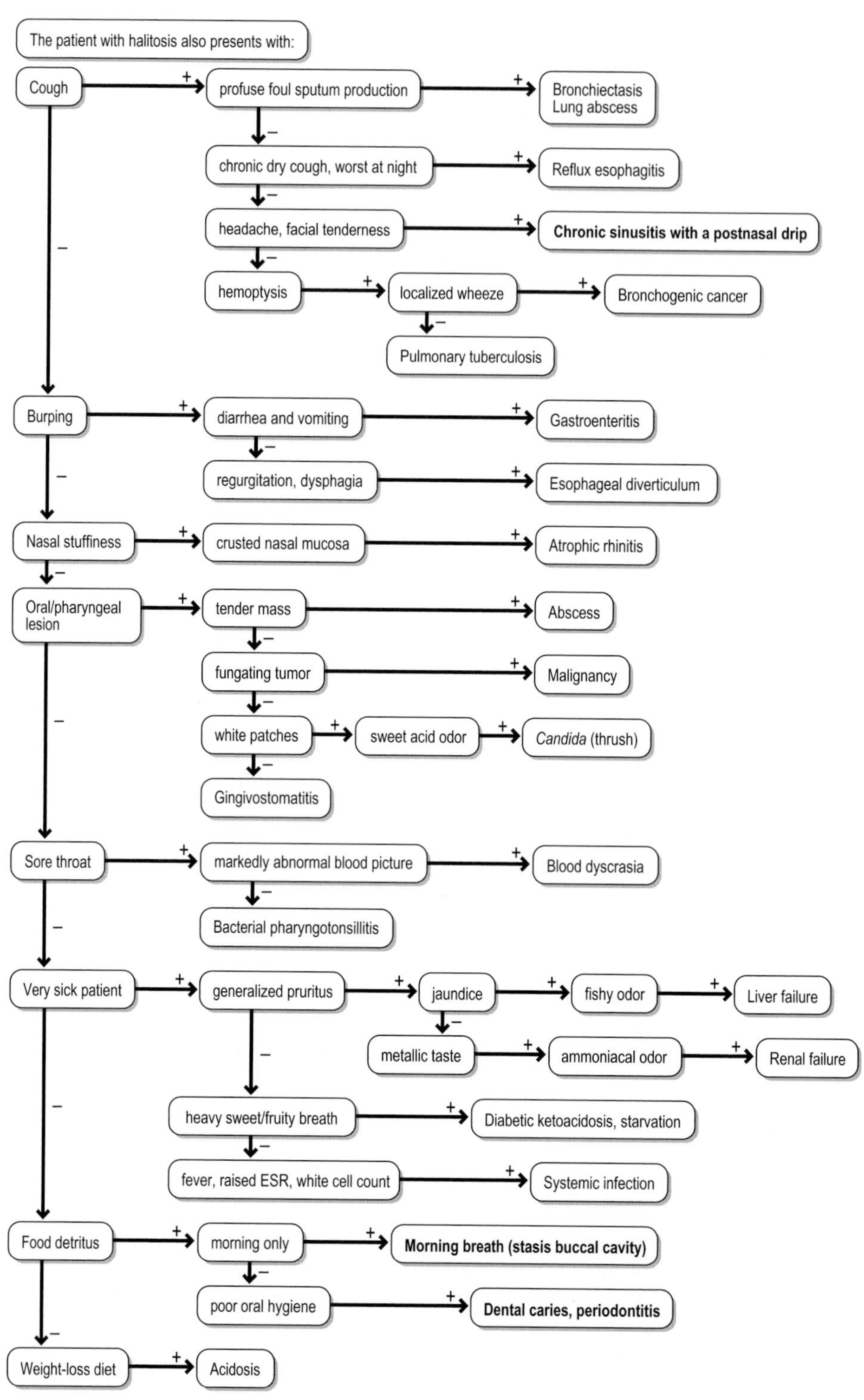

Bold face: most probable condition.
ESR, erythrocyte sedimentation rate.

Figure 30.1 **Halitosis.**

FURTHER READING

Feller L, Blignaut E 2005 Halitosis: a review. SADJ 60(1):17–19

Frydman A 2004 Oral malodor: a review. J West Soc Periodontol Periodontal Abstr 2004;52(1):5–10

CHAPTER 31

Headache

CHAPTER CONTENTS

PART TWO

What is the nature of the headache?

Headaches may be acute or chronic.

Potentially serious causes of *acute headaches or headaches of recent origin* which have been present for days or weeks include:

- *Meningitis.* Be wary of dismissing the patient with a fever and stiff neck.
- *Subarachnoid hemorrhage.* Suspect this in a patient with the sudden onset of headache and altered levels of consciousness.
- *Temporal arteritis.* Patients present with unilateral tenderness over the temple and a very high erythrocyte sedimentation rate (ESR).
- *Raised intracranial pressure.* A patient with papilledema and a headache which is worst on waking should be investigated for an intracranial lesion.

Important causes of *chronic or recurrent headaches* with a history over months and years include:

- *Muscle contraction headaches* due to tension headache and cervical spondylosis. Primary and secondary muscle contraction headaches are the most commonly encountered headaches.
- *Vascular headaches*, such as migraine and cluster headaches.
- *Post-traumatic headaches.* Some people who have had a moderate head injury may experience headaches for weeks or months after the injury. In some cases the headaches get worse and patients complain of lethargy, irritability, difficulty concentrating, and dizziness. Patients whose headache develops weeks after an often minor and forgotten head injury, and have fluctuating symptoms should have a subdural hematoma excluded. Alcoholics and patients on anticoagulants are at particular risk.

Is immediate referral indicated?

Meningeal irritation and structural intracranial disease are indications for immediate referral. Referral for special investigations can facilitate formulation of a definitive diagnosis and rapid initiation of appropriate treatment.

Structural intracranial disease is suspected in patients with:

- A recent substantial change in:
  - the frequency of headaches
  - the severity of headaches.
- Progressive worsening of headache despite appropriate therapy.
- Progressive development of focal neurological symptoms or signs.
- Evidence of raised intracranial pressure:
  - onset of headache with exertion, cough, or sexual activity
  - headache worst on waking
  - drowsiness
  - vomiting
  - bradycardia
  - papilledema.
- Onset of headache:
  - after the age of 40 years
  - and mental changes (e.g. dementia, personality change, apathy)
  - and epilepsy
  - and detection of an orbital bruit.

Patients with suspected structural intracranial disease should be referred for a computed tomography (CT) scan.

Meningeal irritation is present in patients with:

- Neck stiffness.
- A positive Brudzinski sign. Passive flexion of the neck in a supine patient with extended limbs causes involuntary muscle hip flexion.
- A positive Kernig sign. Attempts to extend the knee with the hip flexed results in pain in the hamstrings. This test is performed in the supine patient with the hip passively flexed to 90° and the knee flexed to 90°.

Patients with evidence of meningeal irritation should be referred for:

- Magnetic resonance imaging (MRI) when a posterior fossa lesion is suspected:
  - dull occipital or retro-orbital headache
  - papilledema
  - a recent onset of cough or exertional headache.
- Lumbar puncture when:
  - meningitis is suspected due to the sudden onset of an intense occipital headache, fever, or photophobia
  - subarachnoid hemorrhage is suspected due to focal neurologic defects or an altered level of consciousness.

What is the likely cause? See Figure 31.1.

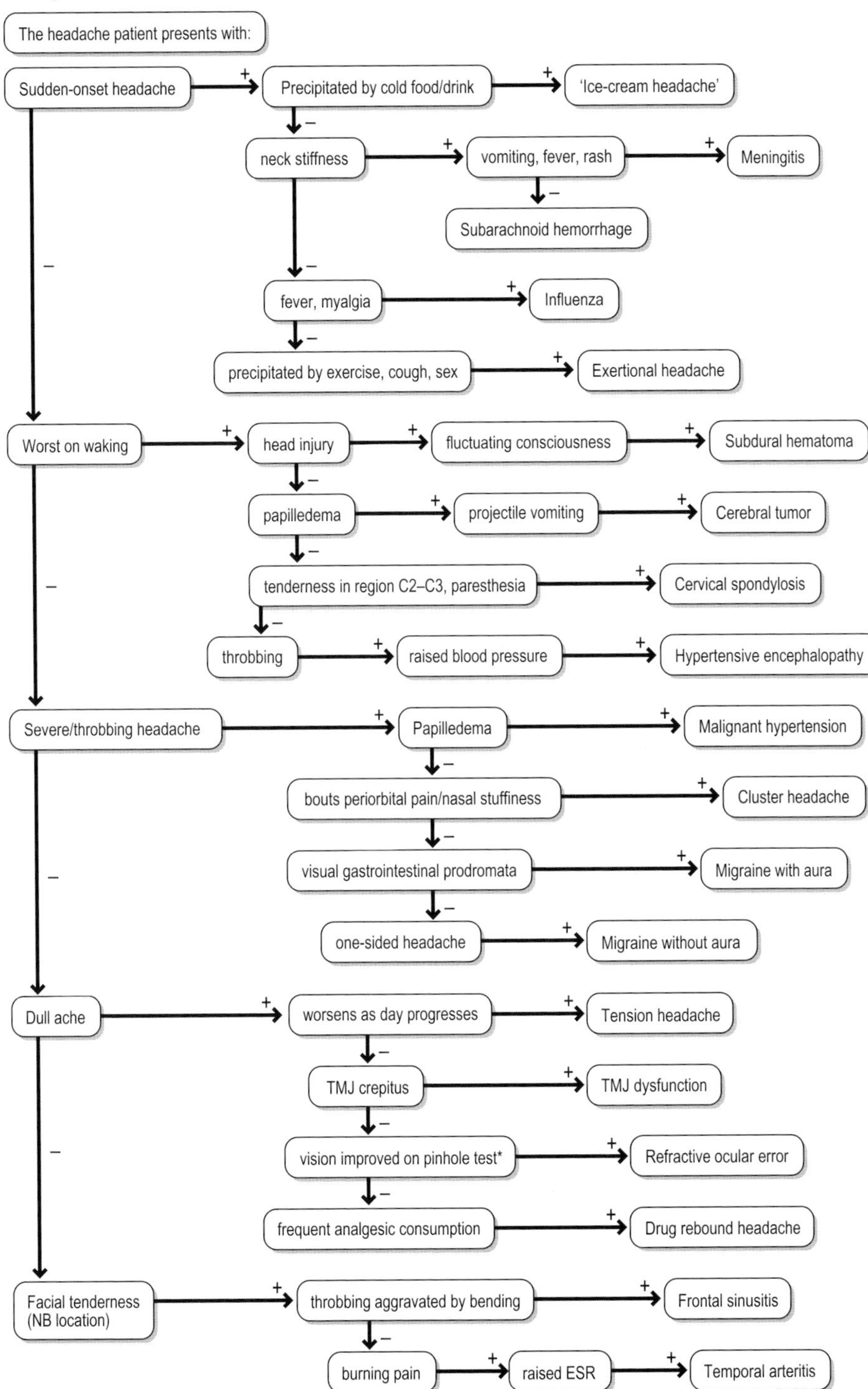

*This tests for refractive errors. Punch a 1 mm hole in a sheet of paper using a pen or large pin. Ask the patient to look at the Snellen chart through the pinhole. If their vision improves, they require glasses.
ESR, erythrocyte sedimentation rate; TMJ, temporomandibular joint.

Figure 31.1 **Headache.**

Does the patient need to be referred?

The prognosis of a headache is ultimately determined by the cause. Headaches suspected of having a serious prognosis should be referred. Clinical findings that suggest a serious prognosis include:

- Headaches of longer duration. All headaches that persist without respite for more than 24 hours are suspect, and the patient should be referred.
- A new headache in a headache-free patient.
- A sudden change in a chronic headache.
- A headache that is worst on waking, in the absence of cervical joint dysfunction.
- A persistent localized pain.
- A headache that worsens progressively.
- Pain aggravated by:
  - exertion
  - bending, stooping
  - coughing, sneezing, straining at stool.
- A headache associated with:
  - a progressive neurological deficit
  - a personality change
  - a memory disturbance
  - convulsions
  - projectile vomiting
  - papilledema
  - neck stiffness and fever
  - unequal pupil size
  - gradual rise in blood pressure and fall in pulse pressure
  - nystagmus
  - sudden deterioration in consciousness.

PART TWO

FURTHER READING

De Diego E V, Lanteri-Minet M 2005 Recognition and management of migraine in primary care: influence of functional impact measured by the headache impact test (HIT). Cephalalgia 25(3):184–190

Dowson A J, Bradford S, Lipscombe S, Rees T, Sender J, Watson D, Wells C 2004 Managing chronic headaches in the clinic. Int J Clin Pract 2004 Dec;58(12):1142–1151

Maizels M 2004 The patient with daily headaches. Am Fam Physician 70(12):2299–2306

Sadovsky R, Dodick D W 2005 Identifying migraine in primary care settings. Am J Med 118 Suppl 1:11S–17S

CHAPTER 32

Hematemesis

CHAPTER CONTENTS

Does the patient show a hematemesis?

Vomiting of blood is termed hematemesis. Vomited blood is:

- Frequently mixed with food particles.
- Dark in color due to acid degradation of hemoglobin.
- Associated with a history of:
  - dyspepsia
  - a dark-colored stool (melena)
  - brief episodes of hematemesis.

True hematemesis may result from lesions of the esophagus, stomach, or duodenum. False hematemesis may result from:

- A nosebleed. Blood can be swallowed and then vomited.
- A hemoptysis. Hematemesis needs to be differentiated from coughed blood (hemoptysis). In hemoptysis symptoms are different to and more persistent than those associated with a hematemesis.

What is the likely diagnosis?

See Figure 32.1.

Does the patient need to be referred?

All patients who vomit blood from a gastrointestinal source (a true hematemesis) should be referred for further investigation and treatment.

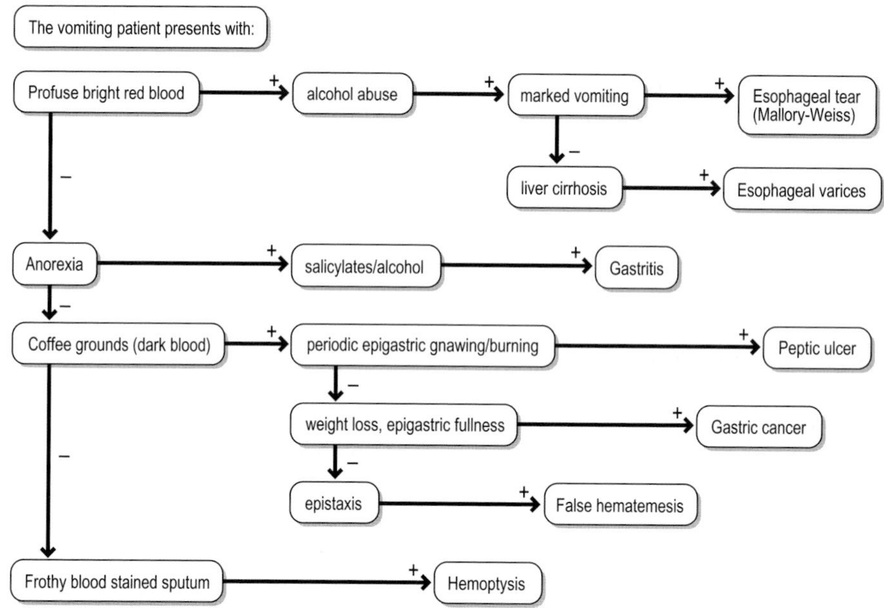

Figure 32.1 **Hematemesis.**

FURTHER READING

Arora N K, Ganguly S, Mathur P, Ahuja A, Patwari A 2002 Upper gastrointestinal bleeding: etiology and management. Indian J Pediatr 69(2):155–168

Barkun A, Fallone C A, Chiba N, Fishman M, Flook N, Martin J, Rostom A, Taylor A; Nonvariceal Upper GI Bleeding Consensus Conference Group 2004 A Canadian clinical practice algorithm for the management of patients with nonvariceal upper gastrointestinal bleeding. Can J Gastroenterol 18(10):605–609

Hematuria

CHAPTER CONTENTS

Is there blood in the urine?

Hematuria is blood in the urine. Hematuria may be macroscopic or microscopic.

Macroscopic hematuria. Hematuria is visible to the naked eye when blood reaches a concentration of 0.5 ml/500 ml of urine. Urine discoloration which may be confused with hematuria can result from:

- a diet rich in beetroot or berries (anthrocyanins)
- drugs such as phenolphthalein
- porphyrins
- red-colored sweets.

Microscopic hematuria. Hematuria may only be detectable by microscopy. Microscopic hematuria is significant when more than 10 red cells/mm^3 urine are detected. Microscopic hematuria can also be detected on chemical testing with a dipstick. A dipstick becomes positive in the presence of 0.15 g/l free hemoglobin. False-positive results for hematuria may be obtained on dipstick testing when:

- Microbial peroxidase is present. Peroxidase action of bacteria is most likely to occur in urine that is left standing at room temperature.
- A sample is contaminated with povidone iodine.
- Residues of oxidizing cleaning agents are left in the collection container.
- Hemoglobinuria or myoglobinuria is present.

False-negative results on dipstick testing may occur in urine:

- With a high specific gravity (SG).

- Rich in ascorbic acid. The rate of false-negative results on dipstick testing is 70% for people on vitamin C and 10% for those not taking vitamin C. Doses of at least 250–500 mg vitamin C are required before false-negative dipstick readings are induced. This applies for both blood and glucose tests.

Does the blood arise from the kidney or the urinary tract?

The source of blood in the urine is an important diagnostic consideration. Blood in the urine which is unrelated to the kidneys or urinary system may arise from:

- menstruation
- perineal inflammation
- a urethral caruncle
- a prepucal lesion.

The presence of dysmorphic red cells or red cell casts on examination of the urinary sediment suggests renal rather than urinary tract involvement.

In persons over the age of 50 years a tumor is responsible for over half of the cases of macroscopic hematuria. In the absence of clot colic, tumors are responsible for painless hematuria, while the passage of stones is associated with painful hematuria. Menstrual blood must always be excluded as a cause of macroscopic hematuria in females.

Microscopic hematuria is found in systemic conditions such as subacute bacterial endocarditis and various renal conditions, including papillary necrosis. Microscopic hematuria may be the only sign of certain serious disorders such as renal cell carcinoma and proliferative glomerulonephritis. A smoky rather than overtly macroscopic hematuria is characteristic of acute glomerulonephritis. A high proportion of cases of asymptomatic microscopic hematuria are due to thin membrane disease, a nephropathy in which the basement membrane in the glomerulus is thinner than normal and allows red cells to leak into the urine. In general, the prognosis in cases of isolated microscopic hematuria is good, as long as blood pressure and renal function are normal.

Investigation of patients with hematuria includes evaluation of renal function and visualization of the urinary tract.

What is the likely diagnosis?

See Figure 33.1.

Does the patient need to be referred?

If referring a case for investigation of the kidney and urinary system on the basis of a dipstick result, first exclude possible causes of a false-positive test result. Positive microscopy resolves dipstick errors.

All patients with hematuria should be referred, except for:

- men who have fallen astride and had minor local trauma
- women who have false hematuria due to menstruation.

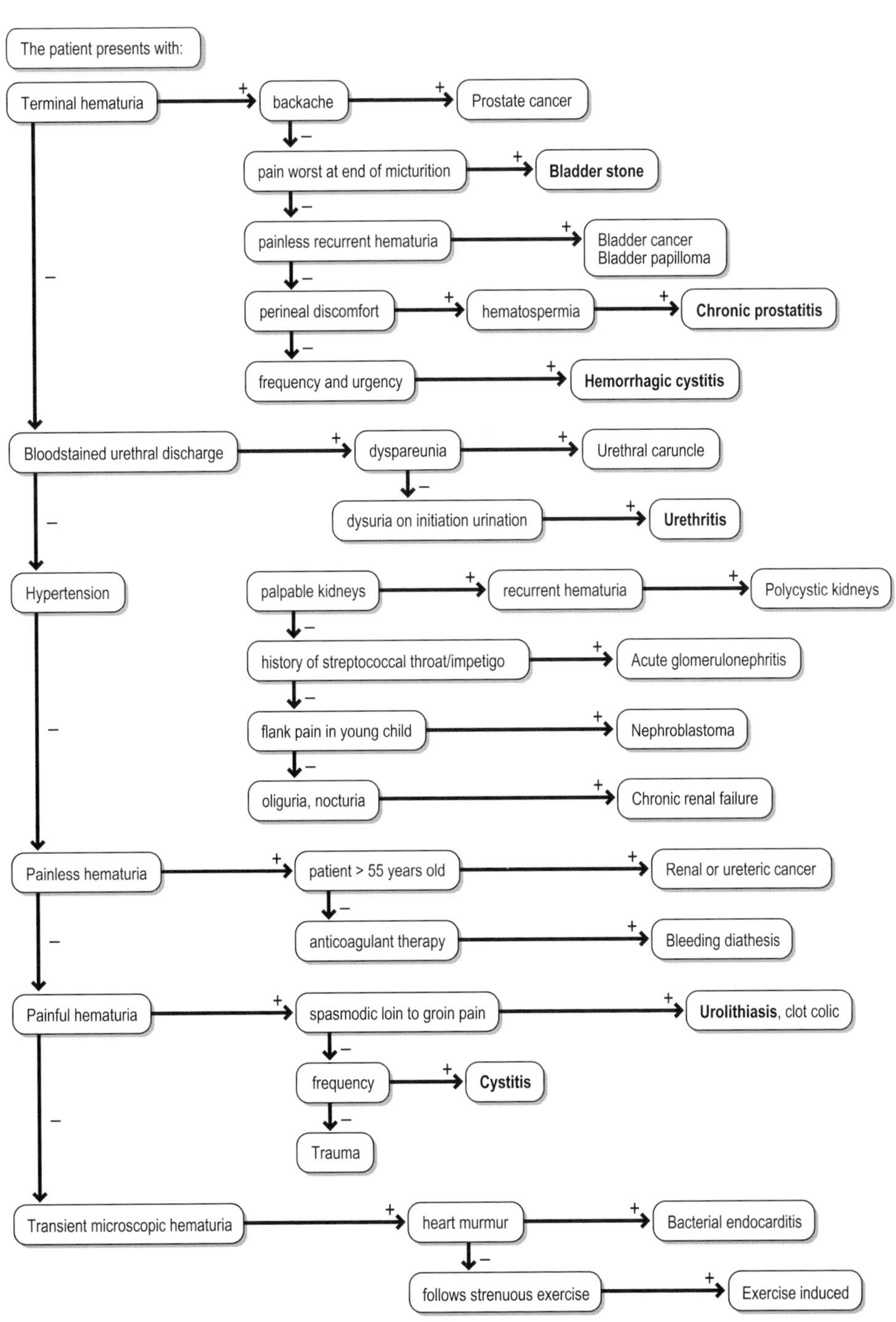

Figure 33.1 **Hematuria.**

Patients with hematuria and any one of the following should be referred for further evaluation or specialist management:

- old age (all elderly patients with hematuria should be referred)
- renal failure
- hematuria after trauma
- suspected malignancy
- suspected infection
- suspected impaired renal function:
  - oliguria
  - edema
  - hypertension
- unexplained microscopic hematuria
- more than a trace (> 200 mg/l) of proteinuria on dipstick testing.

FURTHER READING

Dooley R E, Pietrow P K 2004 Ureteroscopy for benign hematuria. Urol Clin North Am 31(1):137–143

Francis R S, Tomson C R 2004 A GP guide to glomerulonephritis. Practitioner 248(1664):848–855

Huussen J, Koene R A, Hilbrands L B 2004 The (fixed) urinary sediment, a simple and useful diagnostic tool in patients with hematuria. Neth J Med 62(1):4–9

Packham D K, Perkovic V, Savige J, Broome M R 2005 Hematuria in thin basement membrane nephropathy. Semin Nephrol 25(3):146–148

CHAPTER 34 Hirsutism

CHAPTER CONTENTS

Does the patient show physiological or pathological hirsutism?

Hirsutism is the appearance of coarse terminal hair in women in areas normally found in post-pubertal men. Hypertrichosis is the appearance of excess, usually fine, hair in non-androgen-dependent areas.

Hirsutism may be associated with:

- acne
- diffuse thinning of scalp hair (androgenetic alopecia)
- hyperkeratosis of hair follicles (keratosis pilaris); spiky follicular lesions are especially distributed on the upper arm and legs
- intractable infection of apocrine sweat glands in the groin and axilla (hidradenitis suppurativa).

In most cases hirsutism is physiological and constitutes nothing more than a cosmetic problem. It may, however, also be a sign of organic disease. Virilization due to ovarian and adrenal pathology needs to be excluded.

What is the likely cause?

See Figure 34.1.

Should the patient be referred?

Findings that suggest underlying organic disease, and should prompt the clinician to refer patients for special investigations and therapy, include:

- The recent and rapid development of hirsutes in an adult.
- Severe hirsutism that warrants medical rather than cosmetic intervention.
- Hirsutism associated with one or more of:
  - amenorrhea (except in menopausal females)
  - virilization: deepening of the voice, frontal baldness, enlargement of the clitoris.

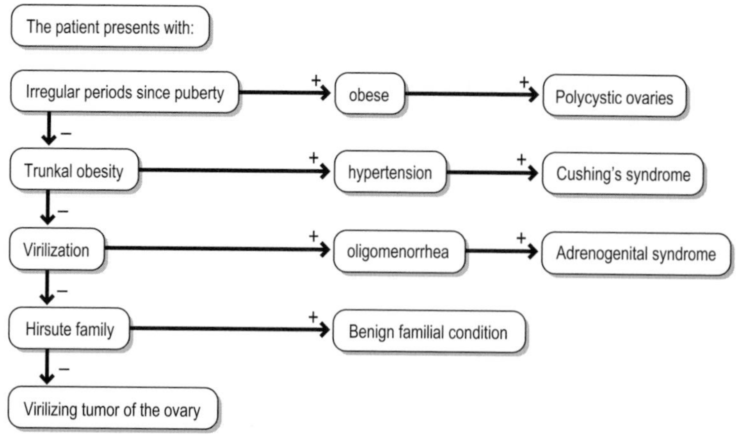

Figure 34.1 **Hirsutism.**

FURTHER READING

Ali I, Dawber R 2004 Hirsutism: diagnosis and management. Hosp Med 65(5):293–297

Chang R J 2004 A practical approach to the diagnosis of polycystic ovary syndrome. Am J Obstet Gynecol 191(3):713–717

Impotence

CHAPTER CONTENTS

Does the patient show impotence?

Impotence is the inability of a male to achieve an erection of sufficient quality to achieve satisfactory sexual intercourse. Erectile dysfunction may be confused with premature ejaculation by the patient. Impotence affects 1 in 10 males. Patients with *psychogenic causes* of impotence usually:

- Have normal erections in the following circumstances:
  - early morning
  - nocturnally
  - on masturbation.
- Have an erection:
  - of good quality
  - they are unable to maintain.
- Experience the sudden onset of impotence.
- Have an underlying performance anxiety or relationship problems.
- Experienced impotence with only one partner.

Medical causes of impotence which must be considered are:

- *Vascular disorders.* Both arterial insufficiency and venous disease need to be considered.
- *Diabetes.* The neuropathy of diabetes is a particular risk in patients with poorly controlled blood sugar levels.
- *Trauma.*
- *Endocrine problems.* Reduced testosterone levels need to be excluded.
- *Drugs.* At worst, thiazides may affect up to 32% of patients with impotence, spironolactone 80%, beta blockers 43%, antipsychotics 54%, and monoamine oxidase inhibitors (MAOIs)

31%. Antihypertensives, psychotropics, digoxin, high-dose steroids, and hypolipidemic agents may all impair sexual function.

What is the likely diagnosis?

See Figure 35.1.

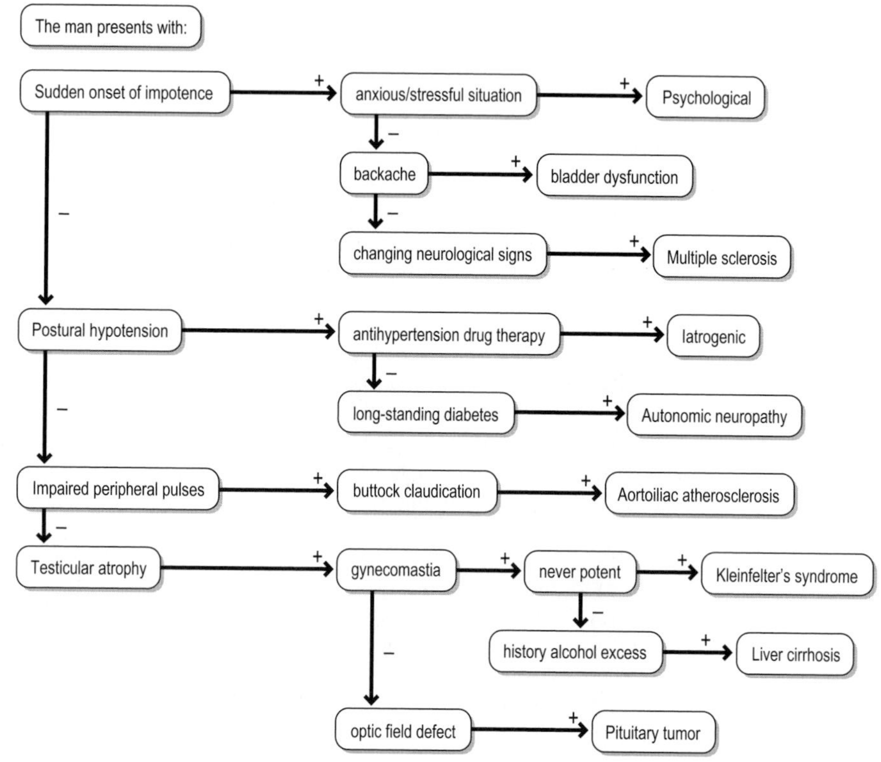

Figure 35.1 **Impotence.**

Does the patient need to be referred?

Refer all patients who are concerned by their impotence. Specialist referral may also be required to manage the underlying problem, whether this be medical or psychological.

FURTHER READING

Tomlinson J 2005 The patient with erectile dysfunction. Practitioner 249(1667):104, 106, 108

PART TWO

CHAPTER 36

Indigestion

CHAPTER CONTENTS

PART TWO

Does the patient have functional or organic dyspepsia?

Indigestion or dyspepsia is discomfort related to meals. It encompasses heartburn, epigastric discomfort or fullness, abdominal distension, belching or flatulence, nausea, or regurgitation. Dyspepsia may result from organic obstruction at or near the pylorus, dysmotility of the stomach, or be attributable to emotion. The prevalence of functional compared to organic dyspepsia is 6:1.

Functional dyspepsia may present as:

- ulcer-like dyspepsia
- reflux-like dyspepsia
- dysmotility-like dyspepsia.

Ulcer-like dyspepsia is diagnosed when two or more of the following are present:

- pain relieved by food on >25% of occasions
- pain often relieved by antacids
- pain often experienced before meals or when hungry
- periodic pain (pain-free intervals of weeks)
- night-time pain (disturbs sleep).

Reflux-like dyspepsia is diagnosed when the following are present:

- Retrosternal and/or upper abdominal discomfort especially:
  - on stooping
  - after large meals
  - on lying flat.
- One or more of:
  - heartburn experienced more than once every fortnight
  - acid regurgitation experienced more than once every week
  - nonspecific nausea or excessive belching

- waterbrash (esophageal acidification may cause sudden brisk salivation).

Dysmotility-like dyspepsia is diagnosed when three or more of the following are present:

- nausea or vomiting, experienced more than once every second month
- hunger followed by early satiety
- postprandial discomfort
- epigastric heaviness aggravated by food or milk (fatty foods are a particular problem)
- discomfort often relieved by belching
- abdominal fullness, bloatedness, and distension
- diffuse, often severe, pain that does not disturb sleep
- variable and multiple food intolerances
- symptoms tend to be continuous.

Acute stress can slow stomach emptying.

Over half the patients with functional dyspepsia have delayed gastric emptying and show no evidence of gastric hypersecretion. Delayed gastric emptying, which is associated with decreased gastric motility and chronic stasis of gastric contents, produces the sensations of early satiety and bloating. In a percentage of patients with gallstones dyspepsia, removal of the gallstones does not affect the dyspepsia.

What is the cause of the patient's dyspepsia?

See Figure 36.1.

The major causes of dyspepsia, in order of prevalence, are:

- functional (nonulcer) dyspepsia
- peptic ulceration
- reflux esophagitis
- rare causes include gastric cancer, pancreatitis, pancreatic cancer, giardiasis, diabetes, scleroderma, lupus, and intestinal angina.

Does the patient need to be referred?

Patients with organic dyspepsia may require referral. As organic dyspepsia has a significant morbidity, further investigation is indicated in all patients with suspected organic dyspepsia. Organic dyspepsia is most likely to be present when:

- An individual over 45 years of age presents with dyspepsia.
- There is a loss of periodicity, with the development of daily pain or symptoms.
- Evidence of reflux disease is complicated by:
  - dysphagia
  - odynophagia
  - nocturnal coughing
  - choking
  - hematemesis.

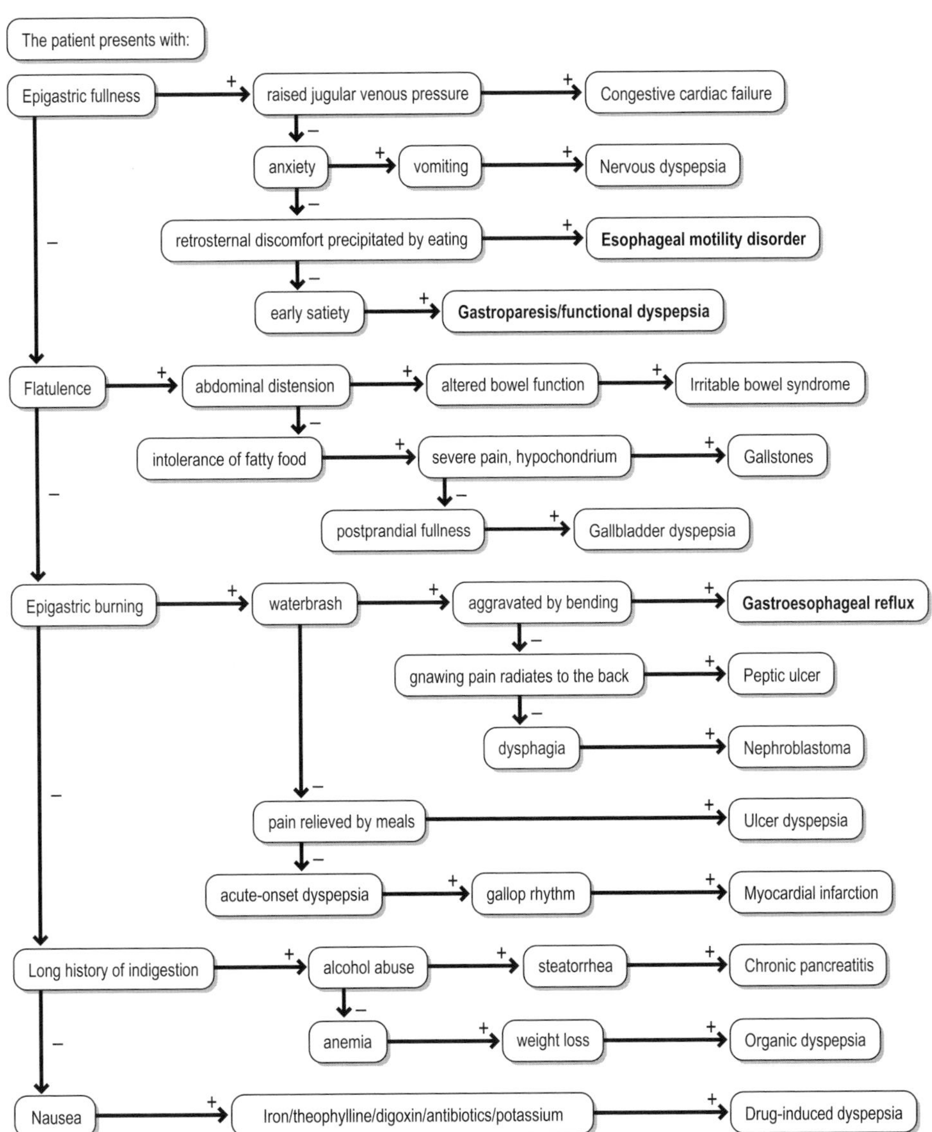

Figure 36.1 **Dyspepsia.**

- Evidence of ulcer dyspepsia is complicated by:
  - a previous personal or family history of ulcer dyspepsia
  - heavy cigarette or alcohol use
  - regular use of nonsteroidal anti-inflammatory drugs (NSAIDs), including high doses of aspirin (the risk is particularly great in patients on prolonged, high-dose and/or multiple NSAID therapy)
  - a family history of gastric cancer

  - failure to respond to symptomatic treatment
  - rapid recurrence of symptoms.
- There is clinical evidence of organic disease:
  - bleeding
  - anemia
  - weight loss
  - recurrent vomiting
  - dysphagia
  - pain radiating to the back
  - jaundice
  - abdominal mass.

FURTHER READING

Dickerson L M, King D E 2004 Evaluation and management of nonulcer dyspepsia. Am Fam Physician 70(1):107–114

Greenwald D A 2004 Aging, the gastrointestinal tract, and risk of acid-related disease. Am J Med 117 Suppl 5A:8S–13S

Layke JC, Lopez PP 2004 Gastric cancer: diagnosis and treatment options. Am Fam Physician 69(5):1133–1140

Schroeder B M 2003 Evaluation of epigastric discomfort and management of dyspepsia and GERD. Am Fam Physician 68(6):1215–1216, 1219–1220

CHAPTER 37

Itch

CHAPTER CONTENTS

What is the nature of the itch?

Pruritus is defined as the desire to scratch. Pain and pruritus, or itching, although different sensations, are conducted along the same pathways. An itch can:

- If severe, disturb sleep and cause marked irritability
- Be subdued by counter-irritation. A sign of severe pruritus is excoriation. In addition to scratching, cold, heat, and vibration may serve as counterirritants. Pruritus is often relieved by cooling the skin. Patients complaining of itchiness should soak the area in water and apply wet cloths.
- Be relieved by analgesics and anti-inflammatories. If scratching is irresistible, antihistamines and/or steroids may be required. If infection is present the patient may require an antibiotic or antifungal agent.
- Be referred.

Itching may result from infections, infestations, allergies, metabolic disturbances or local lesions.

Pruritus may be local or generalized.

Local pruritus. Pruritus may be localized to a region as a result of:

- The behavior of the infesting or infecting organism:
  - the location of *Tinea* depends on the particular species of dermatophyte involved
  - itching that is worst at night and associated with a skin rash suggests an infestation (e.g. lice or scabies).
- Local conditions in the area favoring pruritus:
  - limited skin exposure results in isolated patches of pruritus as in contact dermatitis

  - impaired venous drainage predisposes to pruritus in patients with a postphlebitic leg
  - the relative warmth and dampness of flexures and the anogenital region favors a particular group of skin rashes.

Generalized pruritus. The presence or absence of a skin rash provides useful information.

- Generalized pruritus associated with a skin rash may indicate:
  - systemic disease (e.g. atopic dermatitis (eczema))
  - dry skin; pruritus in the elderly is often the result of dry skin, although, more rarely, it may be a manifestation of underlying disease.
- Generalized pruritus without a skin rash. The presence of normal skin, albeit marred by scratch marks, suggests a:
  - psychogenic cause (constitutional symptoms are absent)
  - systemic cause; malignancy should be suspected if pruritus is precipitated by consuming alcohol or taking a hot shower.

It is useful to consider the likely causes of widespread and local pruritus.

What is the likely cause of widespread pruritus?

See Figure 37.1.

What is the likely cause of localized pruritus?

See Figure 37.2.

Should the patient be referred?

Referral is indicated when:

- underlying untreated systemic disease is suspected
- specific antimicrobial therapy is indicated and is outside your scope of practice.

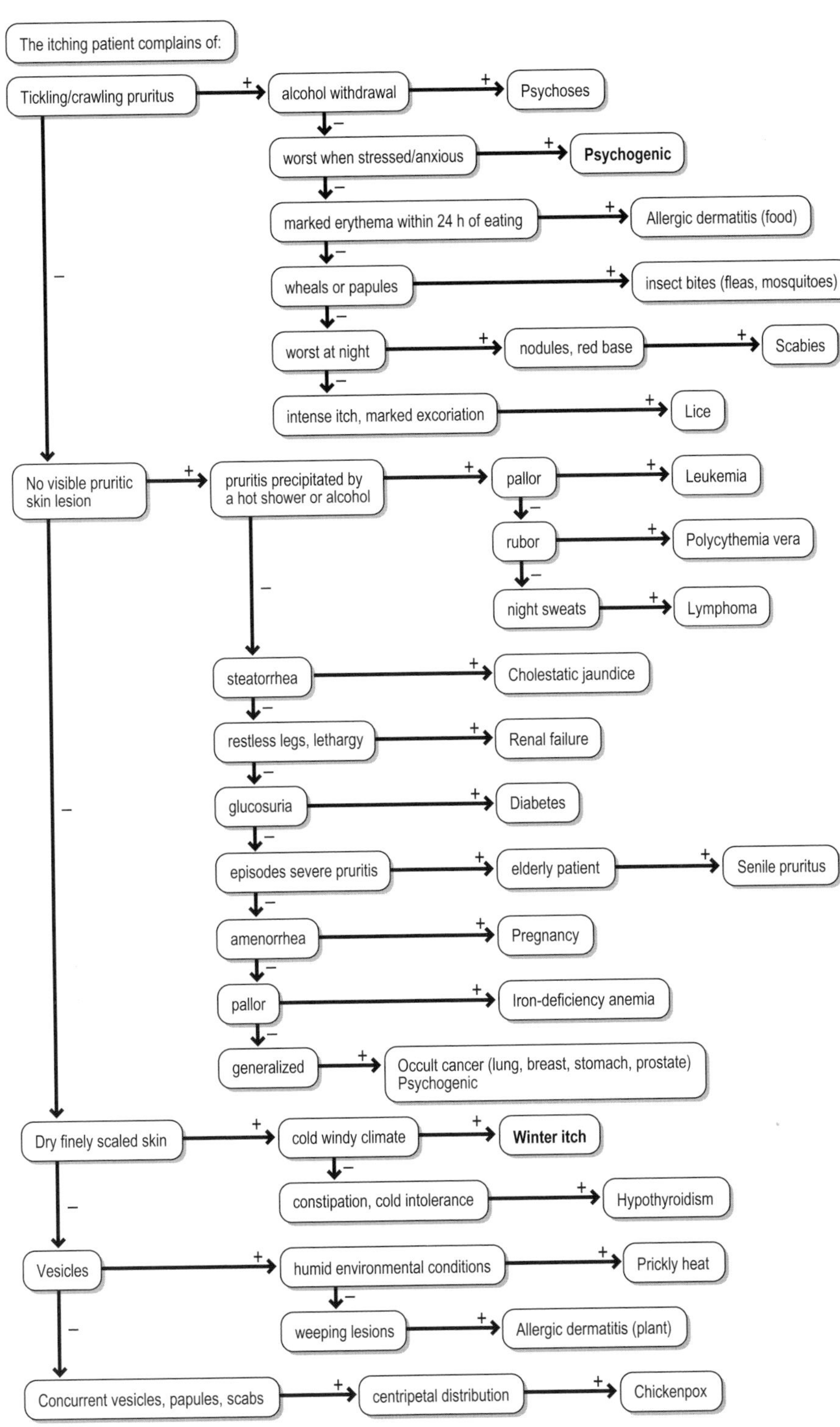

Bold face: most probable condition.

Figure 37.1 **Generalized pruritus.**

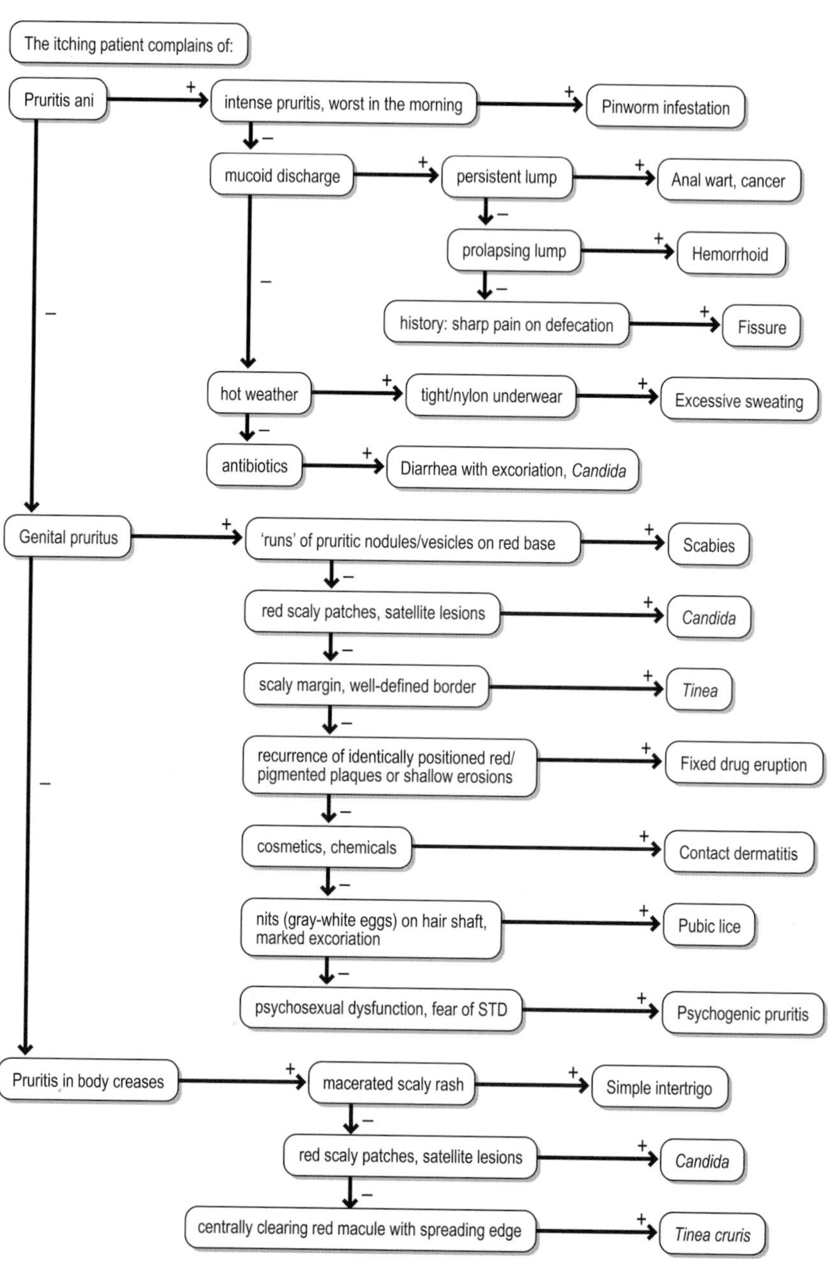

STD, sexually transmitted disease.

Figure 37.2 **Localized pruritus.**

FURTHER READING

Flinders D C, De Schweinitz P 2004 Pediculosis and scabies. Am Fam Physician 69(2):341–348

Moses S 2003 Pruritus. Am Fam Physician 68(6):1135–1142

Muller B A 2004 Urticaria and angiedema: a practical approach. Am Fam Physician 69(5):1123–1128

CHAPTER 38

Jaundice

CHAPTER CONTENTS

Is the patient jaundiced?

Jaundice presents as a yellow discoloration of the skin and mucous membranes. The yellow discoloration is caused by high levels of bilirubin. Bilirubin is a breakdown product of hemoglobin, myoglobin, and cytochromes. The porphyrin of these compounds is excreted as bilirubin.

Red cells are the major source of bilirubin. Removal of iron and globin from hemoglobin produces unconjugated bilirubin. This is transported to the liver attached to albumin. The liver converts water-insoluble unconjugated bilirubin into water-soluble conjugated bilirubin, which is excreted in the bile. Intestinal organisms act upon biliary conjugated bilirubin, converting it into stercobilinogen. Stercobilinogen gives fecal material its brown color. Some of the stercobilinogen is absorbed and re-excreted in the bile. A percentage of the resorbed stercobilinogen is excreted in the urine as urobilinogen.

Jaundice is detected by:

- *Yellow discoloration of the sclera.* Such yellowing is detectable when serum bilirubin exceeds 50 µmol/l. If lighting is poor, jaundice may be difficult to detect at serum levels below 85 µmol/l. The sclera should be inspected using natural light.
- *Yellow skin discoloration.* This is usually detected later than discoloration of the sclera. Jaundice should not be confused with carotinemia, which also causes a yellow skin discoloration. Carotinemia does not cause yellowing of the sclera. Carotinemia is a benign condition in which skin yellowing occurs due to excess ingestion of carotene-rich foods such as carrots, pumpkins, and pawpaw.

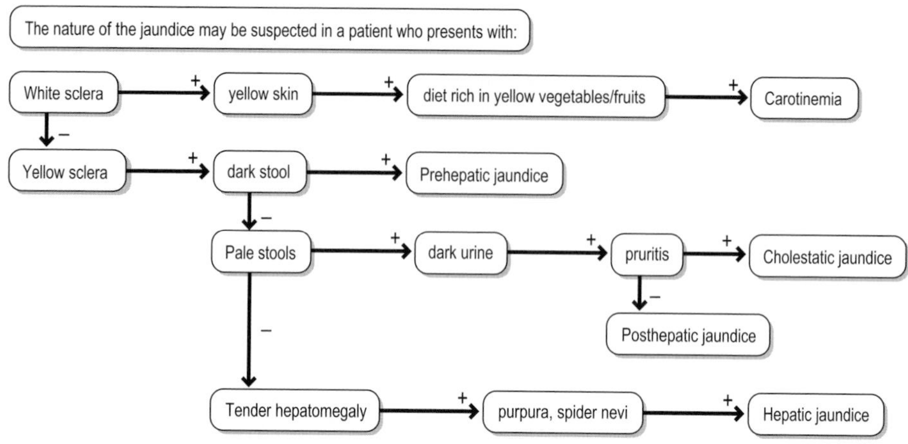

Figure 38.1 **A classification of jaundice.**

- *Laboratory investigations.* The exact biochemical picture depends on the cause of the jaundice. Diagnostic findings include:
  - raised serum bilirubin levels (conjugated bilirubin levels are negligible in the plasma of healthy people)
  - increased levels of urobilinogen
  - urinary bilirubin.
- Additional findings such as:
  - very dark or pale feces
  - dark urine.

What sort of jaundice is present?

Depending on the site of the lesion, jaundice may be prehepatic, hepatic, or posthepatic (Fig. 38.1).

Prehepatic jaundice is associated with excessive destruction of red cells, resulting in increased work for a normal liver. The homeostatic response to red-cell destruction is reticulocytosis. Hemolytic anemia, septicemia, malaria, and leukemia may all give rise to prehepatic jaundice. Prehepatic jaundice is characterized by:

- light yellow jaundice
- a dark stool
- increased urinary urobilinogen
- bilirubinemia (predominantly unconjugated)
- a normal or slightly enlarged liver
- a low hemoglobin
- reticulocytosis.

Hepatic (hepatocellular) jaundice occurs when the primary problem resides in the liver. Liver inflammation (hepatitis) due to infection, drugs, or alcohol, primary liver cancer (hepatoma), cirrhosis, or congestive cardiac failure may all cause hepatic jaundice. Hepatic jaundice is characterized by:

- Jaundice.
- Tender hepatomegaly.
- Altered bilirubin metabolism:
  - markedly raised urinary urobilinogen
  - bilirubinuria
  - raised serum conjugated and unconjugated bilirubin.
- Raised liver enzymes:
  - gammaglutamyl transferase/transpeptidase
  - transaminases.
- Impaired liver function, which may manifest as:
  - Edema. Edema attributable to hypoalbuminemia due to reduced albumin synthesis by the liver is aggravated by impaired hepatic inactivation of aldosterone.
  - A prolonged prothrombin time. Reduced levels of clotting factors produced in the liver result in purpura, epistaxis, melena, and menorrhagia.
  - Elevated estrogen levels. Possible clinical manifestations include:
    spider nevi, telangiectasia, palmar erythema, clubbing
    Dupuytren's contracture (palmar fibrothickening)
    gynecomastia and testicular atrophy in males.
  - Impaired detoxification of nitrogenous products resulting in:
    fetor hepaticus
    a flapping tremor
    mental changes.

Posthepatic jaundice may be found in intra- or extrahepatic obstruction to bile flow. Posthepatic jaundice is characterized by:

- A pale stool. The flow of bilirubin to the intestine is impaired, less intestinal production of stercobilin occurs, and the stool is a light color.
- A dark urine. Conjugated bilirubin regurgitated into the blood is excreted in the urine, giving it a dark shade.
- Raised liver enzymes. Alkaline phosphatase and 5′-nucleotidase are substantially raised in posthepatic jaundice.
- Findings in extrahepatic obstruction that reflect the underlying cause:
  - in gallstone jaundice a positive Murphy's sign is detected
  - in cancer of the head of the pancreas the gallbladder is enlarged and is palpable
  - in hepatic metastasis a hard, irregular liver is palpated.
- Cholestasis. Cholestasis is the term used to describe biliary obstruction. Extrahepatic cholestasis may occur late in posthepatic jaundice attributable to gallstones or cancer of the head of the pancreas or bile ducts, or pancreatitis. Intrahepatic cholestasis is encountered in pregnancy, oral contraceptive usage, autoimmune biliary cirrhosis, alcoholic cirrhosis, viral hepatitis, and drug use. Findings attributable to cholestasis include those attributable to:

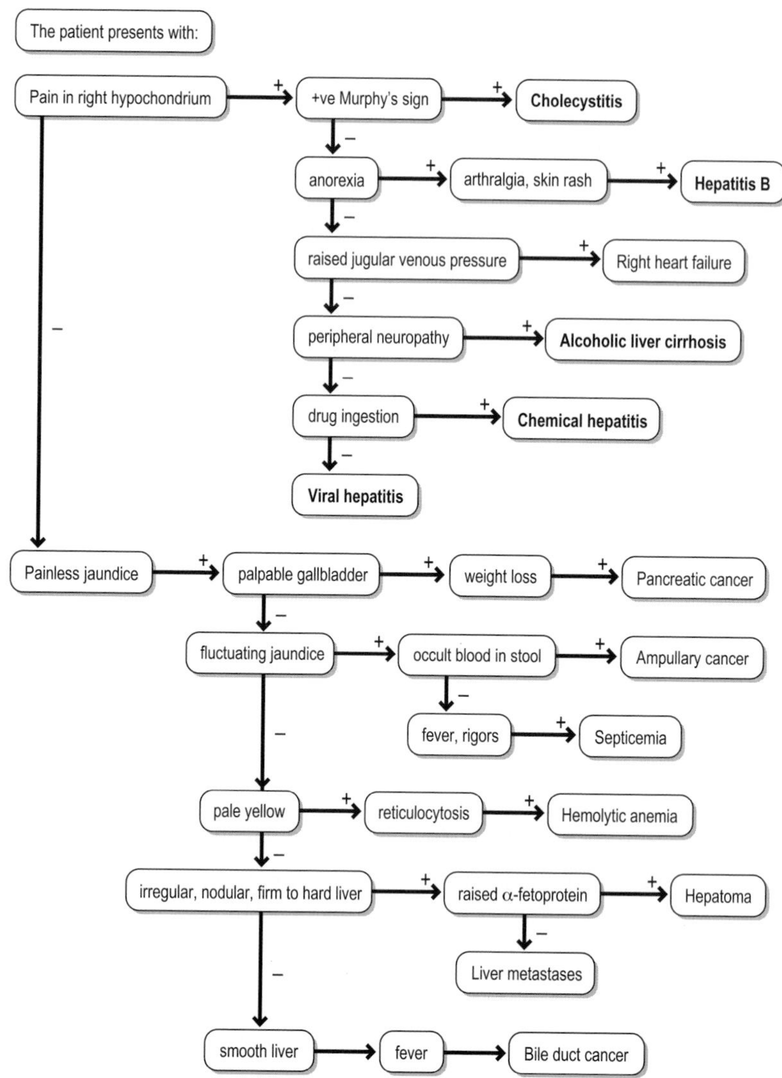

Bold face: most common condition.
*Many drugs are hepatotoxic. Alcohol aggravates drug hepatotoxicity. Classes of prescription drugs associated with hepatotoxicity include: nonsteroidal anti-inflammatory (NSAIDs) and slow-acting antirheumatic drugs (SAARDs), antimicrobials, anticonvulsants, psychotropics, cardiovascular agents, and steroids such as estrogens and androgens. Paracetemol in overdose can cause fulminant liver failure in 24–72h. Vitamin A in overdose is potentially lethal.

Figure 38.2 **Jaundice.**

- impaired excretion of:
  bile salts, leading to pruritus
  cholesterol, resulting in hypercholesterolemia and xanthomatosis
- impaired fat absorption presenting as:
  steatorrhea
  prolonged prothrombin time
  malabsorption of vitamins A, D, and K.

What is the likely diagnosis?

See Figure 38.2.

Does the patient need to be referred?

Patients should be referred for investigation to make a definitive causal diagnosis of jaundice. Painless jaundice may be a clinical manifestation of malignant disease.

FURTHER READING

Roche S P, Kobos R 2004 Jaundice in the adult patient. Am Fam Physician 69(2):299–304

Yazbeck M F 2004 Clarifications on patients presenting with jaundice. Am Fam Physician 271(3):425–426

No authors listed 2005 Advising patients with hepatitis C in primary care. Drug Ther Bull 43(3):22–24

CHAPTER 39

Joint pain

CHAPTER CONTENTS

PART TWO

Is this an arthritis or arthralgia?

Arthritis is inflammation of one or more joints. In arthritis the joint is tender on examination. Laboratory investigations are helpful in diagnosing arthritis due to the underlying inflammatory process. They are of little use in diagnosing arthralgia. Arthralgia means joint pain. The pain in arthralgia may be due to mechanical joint dysfunction or be referred.

Orthopedic tests are used to differentiate between mechanical and referred arthralgia. As pain from deep-lying structures is referred, palpation used alone may deceive. Orthopedic tests are mechanical procedures designed to reproduce or aggravate the patient's symptoms. By positioning or moving the area involved, the practitioner can reproduce the patient's pain or elicit a sign. By manually applying selective tension, orthopedic tests exert controlled stresses on anatomical structures to reproduce or aggravate the presenting complaint. Structures are challenged with isometric contraction and end-range stretch. As orthopedic tests are designed to reproduce a patient's complaint and/or to demonstrate impaired function, they provide vital information about whether the problem is local or referred.

Orthopedic testing explores joint function by:

- Stretching ligaments and the joint capsule.
- Stretching and/or contracting muscles and tendons.
- Palpating and compressing bone.
- Stretching and compressing nerves. Nerves are also tested indirectly with contraction.

Joints are tested using passive and resisted movements. Function is assessed by assuming various joint positions that stretch, compress, and/or contract soft tissue.

Mechanical arthralgia presents with:

- Pain and stiffness that worsens with use and is improved by rest.
- Local pain.
- Effusion may be present.
- Upon orthopedic testing, two or more of the following:
  - impaired joint motion
  - tenderness in the vicinity of the joint margin
  - pain on weight bearing or physical stressing of the joint
  - pain experienced in the joint (periarticular pain is felt adjacent to the joint).

Referred arthralgia presents with:

- Dull heaviness uninfluenced by movement.
- Little diurnal 'pain' variation.
- Poorly localized and diffuse pain.
- The absence of signs of joint disease in the vicinity of the pain.
- Mechanical sensitivity of skin and deep tissues.

Arthritis is characterized by:

- Prolonged stiffness, which tends to ease with use and responds to rest.
- Pain at night.
- Local pain with some spread.
- Localized joint swelling, effusion, and warmth.
- Associated systemic findings (malaise, fever).
- General signs of inflammation (raised erythrocyte sedimentation rate (ESR), C-reactive protein).
- Signs of the inflammatory process characteristic of the disease:
  - immunological evidence (rheumatoid factor, antinuclear antibodies, HLA B27 antigen, lupus erythematosus cells)
  - infection (leukocytosis, positive blood culture)
  - metabolic disorder (raised uric acid).

What is the likely diagnosis?

See Figure 39.1.

Does the patient need to be referred?

Referral criteria for a patient presenting with polyarthritis are:

- weight loss
- fever
- lymphadenopathy
- extensive rash
- symptoms in more than one system
- vasculitis
- heart murmurs
- severe pain/disability
- extreme fatigue
- increasing severe/intractable joint pain.

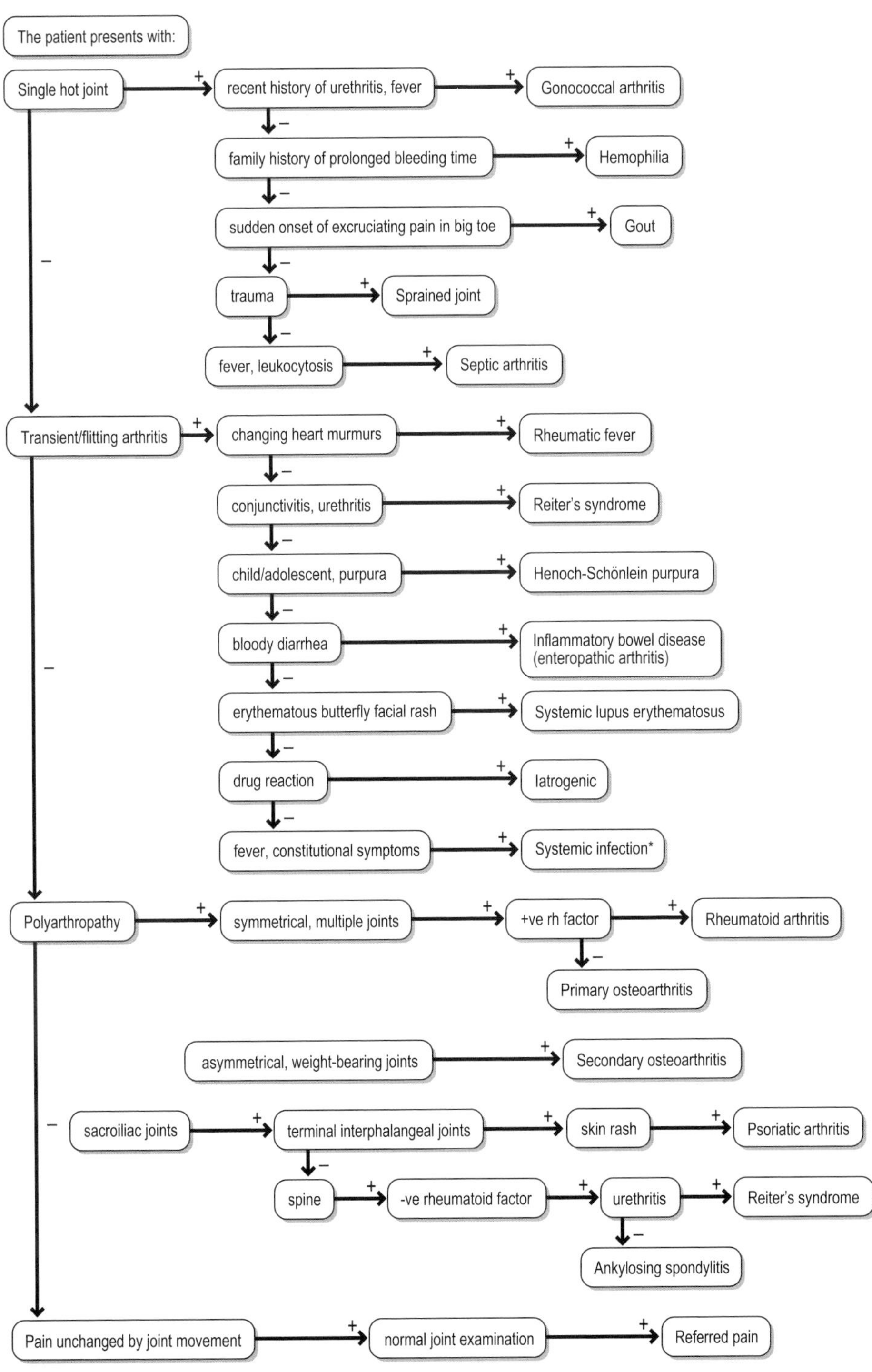

*Gonococcal/meningococcal septicemia, bacterial endocarditis, rubella, infectious mononucleosis, infective hepatitis, mycoplasma pneumonia.

Figure 39.1 **Joint pain.**

FURTHER READING

Calmbach W L, Hutchens M 2003 Evaluation of patients presenting with knee pain: Part I. History, physical examination, radiographs, and laboratory tests. Am Fam Physician 68(5):907–912

Calmbach W L, Hutchens M 2003 Evaluation of patients presenting with knee pain: Part II. Differential diagnosis. Am Fam Physician 68(5):917–922

Kataria R K, Brent L H 2004 Spondyloarthropathies. Am Fam Physician 69(12):2853–2860

Mies Richie A, Francis M L 2003 Diagnostic approach to polyarticular joint pain. Am Fam Physician 68(6):1151–1160

Siva C, Velazquez C, Mody A, Brasington R 2003 Diagnosing acute monoarthritis in adults: a practical approach for the family physician. Am Fam Physician 68(1):83–90

CHAPTER 40

Limb pain

CHAPTER CONTENTS

Is the pain locally produced or referred?

Limb pain may be produced by local structures or referred. Locally produced limb pain is often:

- Associated with local pathology or dysfunction. In the absence of any associated local lesion or functional disruption, a referred source of pain should always be carefully explored.
- Precisely delineated. Widespread hyperalgesia is nonetheless regularly found in musculoskeletal disorders such as fibromyalgia or diffuse cervicobrachial pain.

Limb pain may arise from a local lesion of the bone, joint, peri-articular tissues, muscle, nerve, or vessels. The nature of the pain experience may also help to identify the tissue involved:

- Bone pain is nagging and worst at night.
- Muscle pain is experienced as tender points over the muscle belly.
- Nerve pain is described as burning, shooting, itching, or pins and needles.
- Vascular pain is severe and throbbing.

When no local lesion can be detected in the limb, the source of the pain must be sought elsewhere. In the case of upper limb pain possible sources are the heart and pleura, diaphragm, and lower cervical or upper thoracic vertebrae. Limb pain may arise in the chest, abdomen, or spine. The level of the spinal lesion determines if pain is referred to the upper or lower limb. Referred pain frequently:

- Is an aching pain or deep discomfort.
- Has a general, diffuse, or patchy distribution. Pain from central nervous system lesions, carcinomatosis, and psychogenic pain 'cannot be localized'.

Is there a local soft tissue lesion?

In order to accurately attribute pain to its source, special testing is required. Just as radiological investigations are used to detect osseous lesions, so are orthopedic tests used to determine soft tissue lesions.

Determining local lesions using orthopedic testing requires:

- *An understanding of local anatomy.* Pain at the outer elbow referred down the back of the forearm suggests lateral tennis elbow (epicondylitis), while a similar ache on the inner side of the elbow suggests medial epicondylitis. Pressure on the median nerve causes carpal tunnel syndrome, while pressure on the posterior tibial nerve causes tarsal tunnel syndrome.
- *A search for pathology.* Osseous lesions may present as a fracture; soft tissue lesions may present as tendonitis, sprain of a ligament, strain or trigger points in a muscle, neural lesions as entrapment with compression of the nerve trunk, or radiculopathy with pressure on the nerve root. In each instance, further information is gathered to create a clinical picture. Fractures are, for example, aggravated by activity, relieved by rest, and have marked restriction of movement, muscle spasm, and deformity.
- *Consideration of the underlying process.* A history of injury with an emphasis on the mechanism whereby the lesion developed is important. Asymmetric pain is often associated with trauma, while symmetrical pain, especially when the patient complains of fatigue, malaise, and weight loss, may result from underlying systemic disease, including malignancy, collagen disease, or chronic infection.

Specific orthopedic tests have been developed to assess particular dysfunctions. However, certain generalizations are possible. Passive movements are used to assess problems associated with joint capsules, ligaments, fasciae, bursae, dura mater, or the dural sheaths to nerve roots. A limitation of passive movement is indicative of a problem in one of these inert tissues. The extent of limitation of passive movement, partial or full range, has diagnostic significance. Inert structures are put under tension by stretching; contractile structures are tested using resistance.

Joints are tested using passive and resisted movements. Function is assessed by assuming various joint positions that stretch, compress, and/or contract soft tissue. Two of the following are suggestive of joint disease:

- impaired joint motion
- tenderness in the region of the joint margin
- pain on weight bearing.

Stability testing of each joint is undertaken by stabilizing one side of a joint while moving the other. *Extra-articular lesions* rarely limit passive joint movement. In such cases the amount of limitation in one joint is dictated by the position of another. Disproportionate limitation with gross restriction in one direction and full painless range in all others may also be found.

Diagnosis of a *capsular lesion* is made on detection of a capsular pattern of pain or movement limitation characteristic of that joint. In instances of internal derangement, joint movement is restricted to 1–4 movements. At the extreme of each passive movement of the joint 'a springy block-end feel' sensation is transmitted to the examiner's hands. A sprain is a complete or partial ligamentous injury and usually occurs following trauma or twisting injuries. Sprains are graded:

Grade I	Pain and tenderness over the joint is not associated with lax ligaments.
Grade II	The joint is intact, but there are lax ligaments and bruising over the joint.
Grade III	In addition to tenderness, swelling, and bruising, no end-point is felt on stressing the joint. In cases of ligamentous sprain, pain is limited to one passive movement. Usually pain is felt at the extreme range when movement is in the contralateral direction (e.g. a lesion of the ulnar collateral ligament causes pain on extreme radial deviation).

In *bursitis* a lack of organic resistance creates a sensation of 'empty end feel'. This sensation may also be encountered in abscesses or neoplasms. Other findings that help in the diagnosis of patients with bursitis are:

- Complaints of joint pain, despite a full range of motion being present on examination.
- Pain is experienced above and below the joint during physical examination. Direct pressure in the region of the 'joint' results in discomfort. Flexion aggravates the lesion.
- There is exquisite tenderness when the examiner exerts slight pressure on a particular area in the vicinity of the joint. In 'knee' pain this trigger point is found on the medial side of the tibia about 2–3 in. below the joint margin over the insertion of the pes anserinus. In 'hip' pain the tender point lies over the

greater trochanter. In 'shoulder' pain, pressure applied laterally just under the acromion precipitates severe pain.
- Pain peaks with use.
- Night pain.
- Focal, brief morning stiffness.

In contrast to inert structures, contractile structures are tested using resisted movement. The lesion is identified by detecting a pattern of congruous positive and negative findings. When a resisted movement causes pain, a muscle, tendon, or bony attachment is the source. Passive movements are full range and pain free. Except for partial muscle rupture, scar tissue, or adhesion, a contractile structure does not produce limitation on passive movement. Pain to all resisted movements suggests either a gross capsular lesion or psychogenic problems.

The testing procedure for resisted movements requires that:

- The joint must be held in midrange to avoid stretching inert structures.
- No movement should take place at the joint.
- Muscles other than those being tested must not be included.
- The patient exerts himself or herself.
- Focus on appropriate relative positioning of the examiner and patient.
- Accurate assessment of muscle weakness requires bilateral comparison.

Findings are interpreted as follows:

- Strong and painless movement implies no lesion of a contractile structure.
- Strong and painful movement suggests a minor lesion.
- Weak and painful movement suggests a serious problem such as a fracture or metastases. Radiological investigations are helpful.
- Weak and painless movement implies impaired neural innervation, unless complete rupture of muscle or tendon has occurred.

A *strain* is complete or partial disruption of a muscle or tendon, and is frequently associated with overuse. Pain, tenderness, and weakness are localized.

Inflammation of a tendon, usually at the site of bony insertion or the point of muscle origin, causes tendonitis. *Tendonitis* presents clinically with:

- Pain and tenderness over the affected tendon
- Focal, brief morning stiffness
- Mild heat and erythema of the overlying skin
- Pain aggravated by active movement
- Locking or instability is unusual, except for a rotator cuff tear or trigger finger.

Neural lesions frequently accompany musculoskeletal problems. The nature and distribution of pain are also helpful in locating the site of neural compression:

- Discomfort attributable to spinal cord compression tends to be bilateral, disregards body segmentation, and presents as paresthesia rather than pain.
- Nerve root compression produces pain in the relevant dermatome. Paresthesia and/or numbness may also be encountered. Weakness to resisted movements may be detected.
- Nerve trunk compression leads to weakness and paresthesia rather than pain.
- Small-nerve compression does not cause weakness, but numbness with a well-defined edge is detected. Pain is referred distally.

What is the likely cause of buttock pain?

See Figure 40.1.

What is the likely cause of hip pain?

See Figure 40.2.

What is the likely cause of knee pain?

See Figure 40.3.

What is the likely cause of thigh or leg pain?

See Figure 40.4.

What is the likely local cause of ankle or foot pain?

See Figure 40.5.
For referred pain, see Nerve root and entrapment.

What is the likely local cause of shoulder pain?

See Figure 40.6.
Pain restricted to above the elbow suggests a shoulder lesion.

What is the likely cause of referred shoulder pain?

See Figure 40.7.

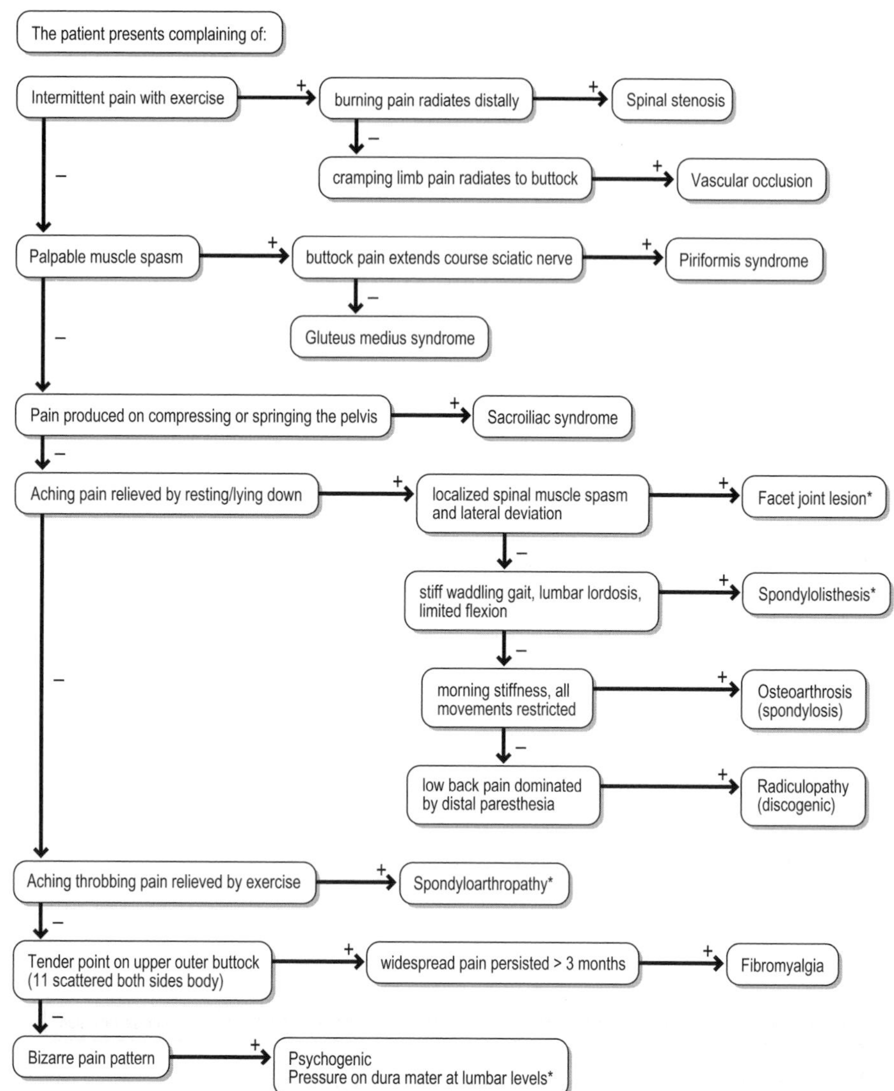

The dominant complaint in a patient with buttock pain may be back pain.
*Bilateral or unilateral pain, which may extend from the lower thorax posteriorly over the buttocks and groin and go down to the ankles.

Figure 40.1 **Buttock pain.**

What is the likely cause of arm and hand pain?

See Figure 40.8.

Arm and hand pain requires consideration of the various types of arthritis, overuse strain syndromes, tendonitis, and neural pain, both from nerve-root pressure arising in the spine and nerve entrapment.

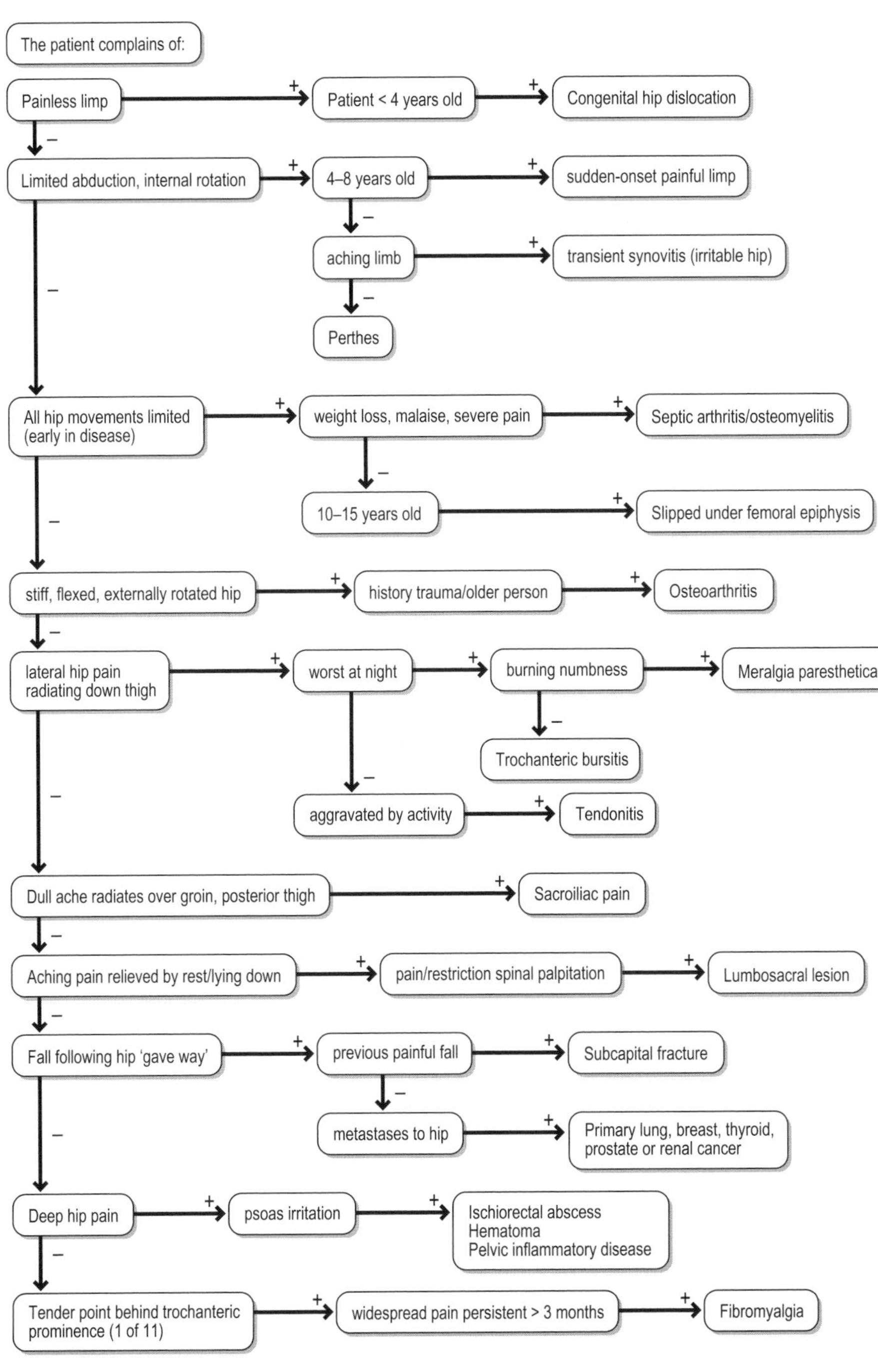

Figure 40.2 **Hip pain.**

PART TWO

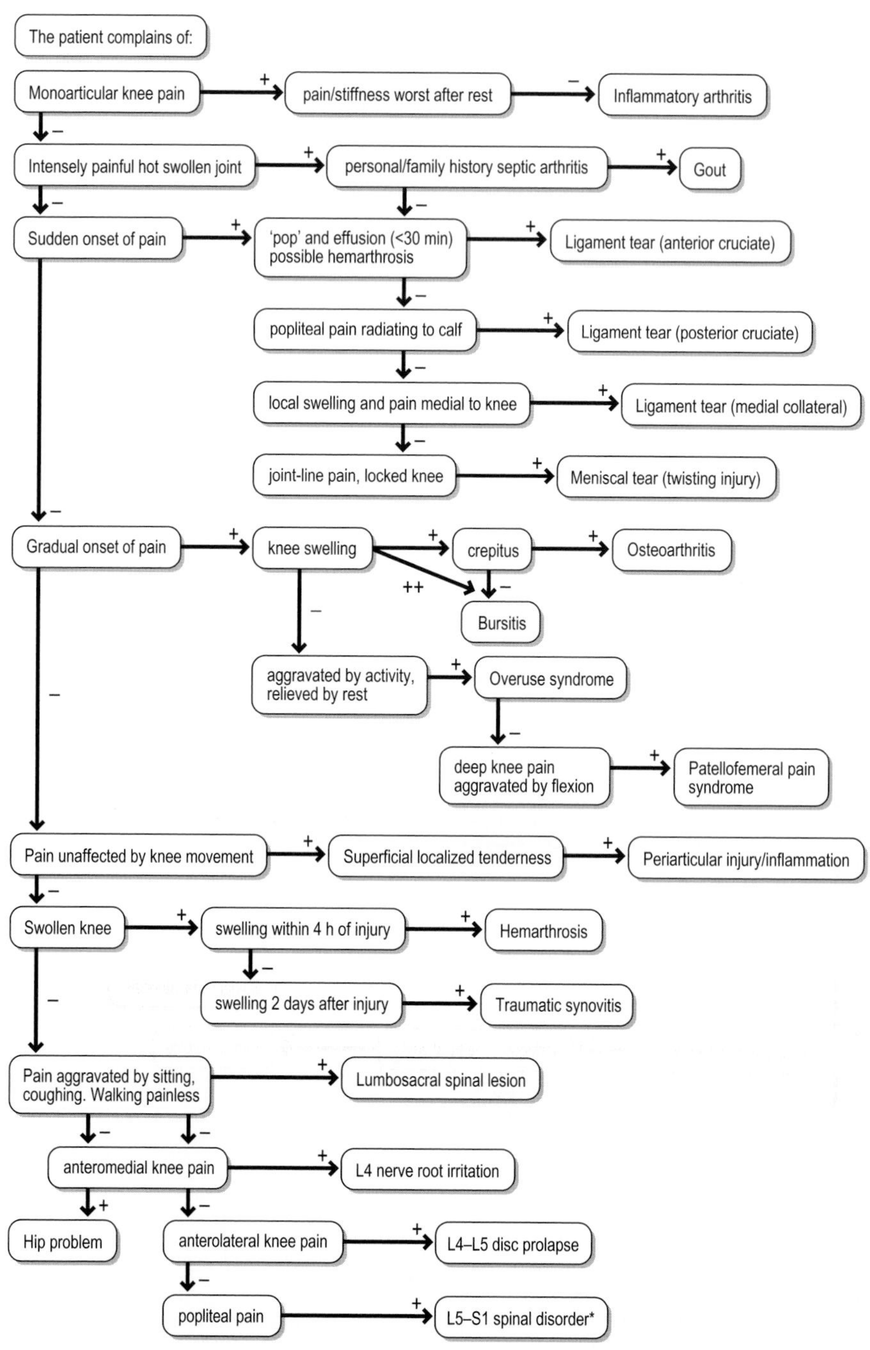

*Medial knee pain may be referred from hip osteoarthritis, osteomyelitis, Paget's, or metastases.

Figure 40.3 **Knee pain.**

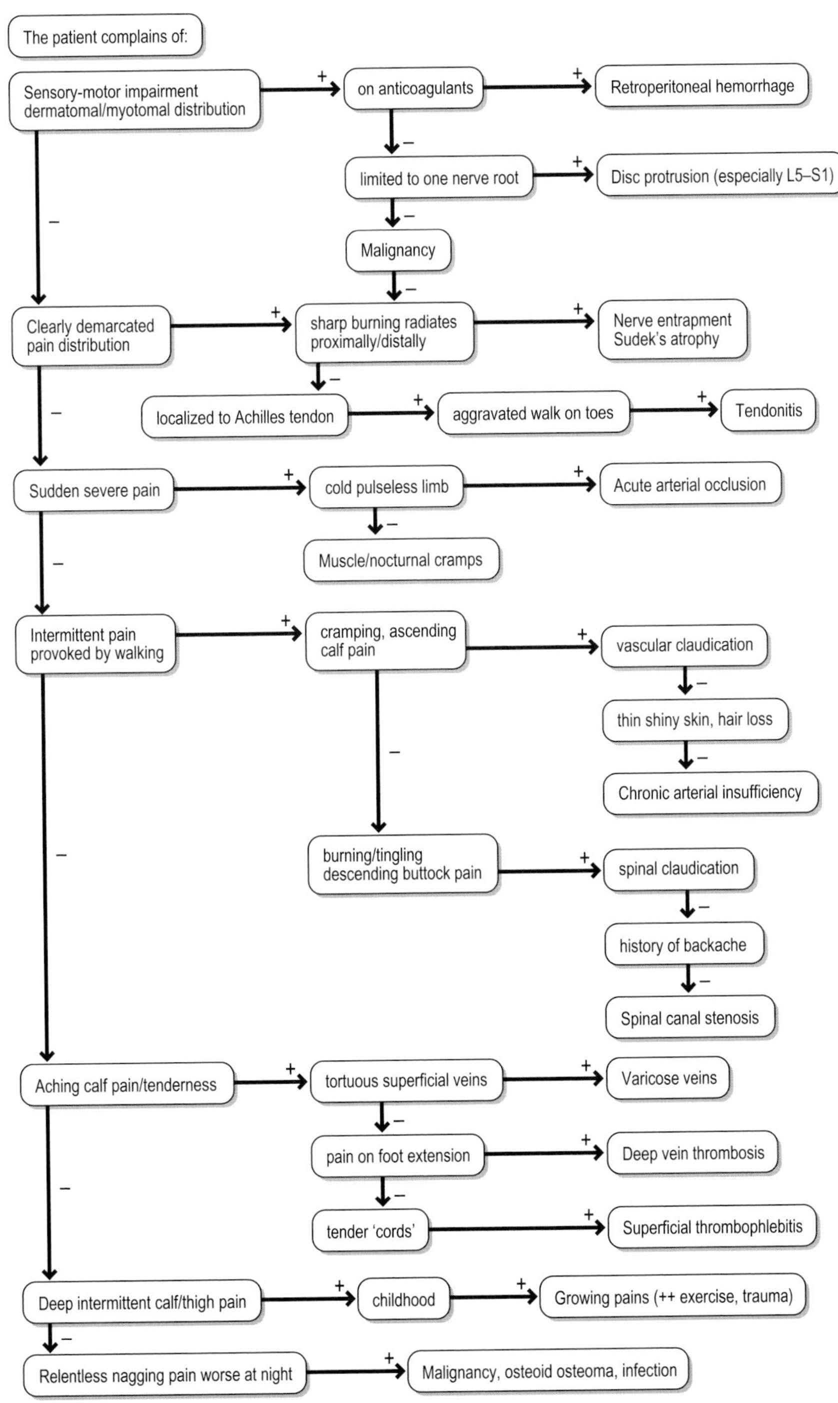

Figure 40.4 **Thigh and leg pain.**

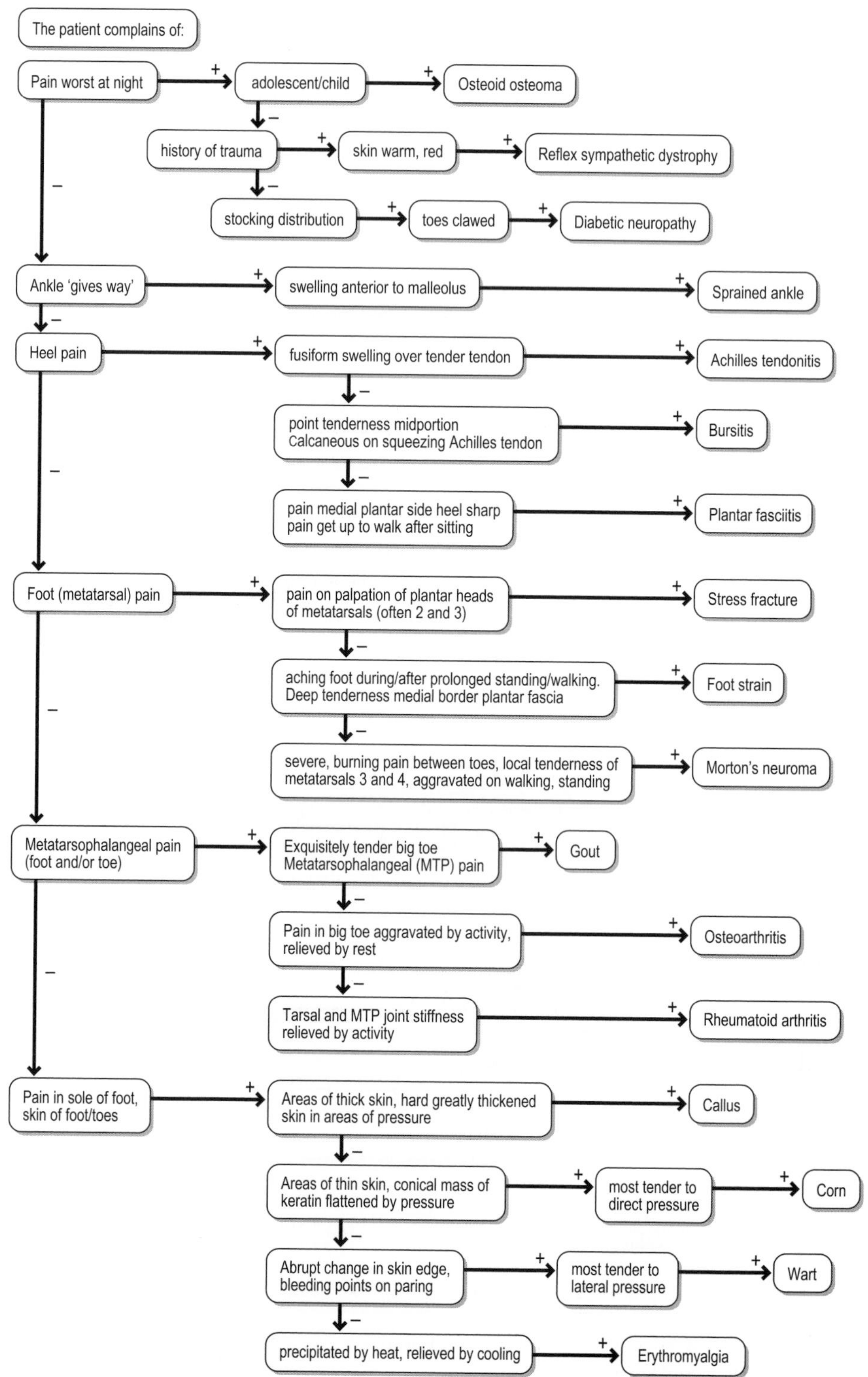

Figure 40.5 **Ankle and foot pain.**

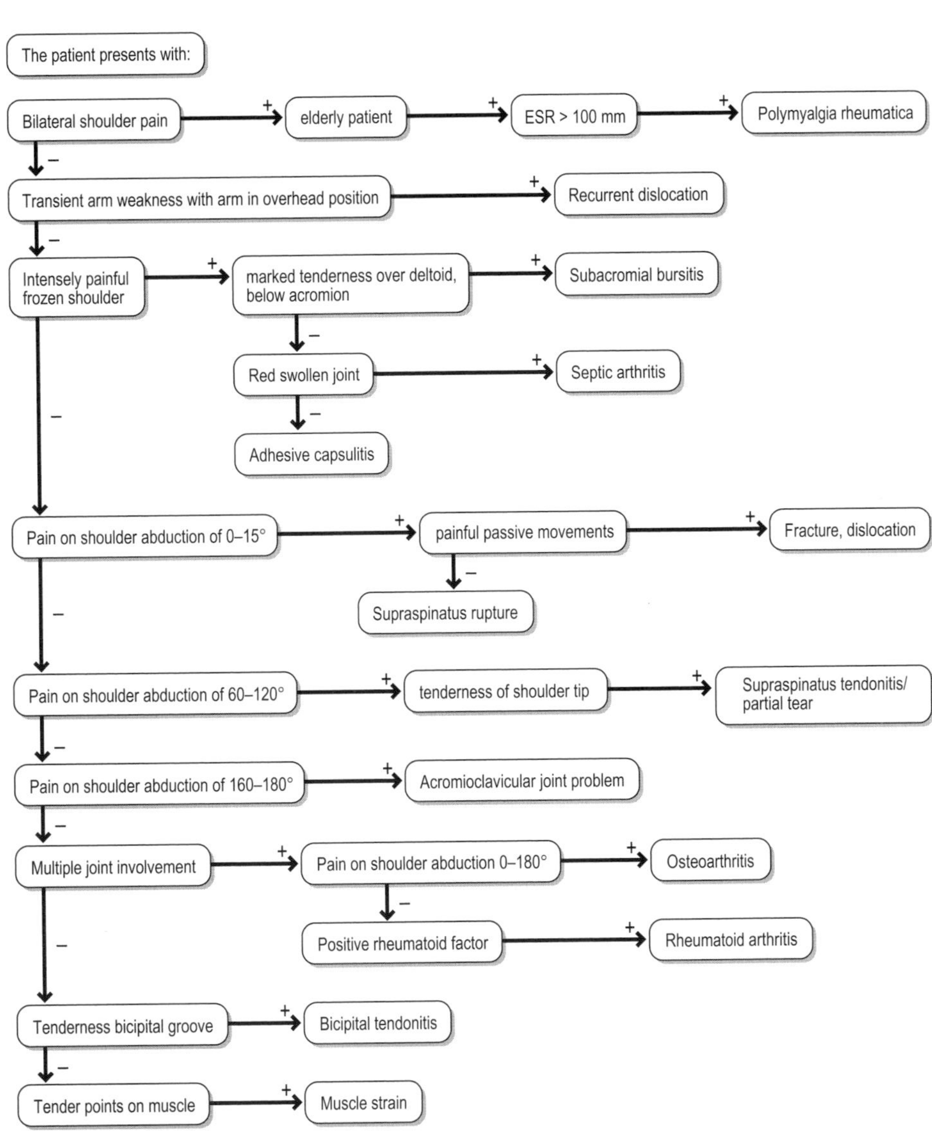

ESR, erythrocyte sedimentation rate.

Figure 40.6 **Shoulder pain.**

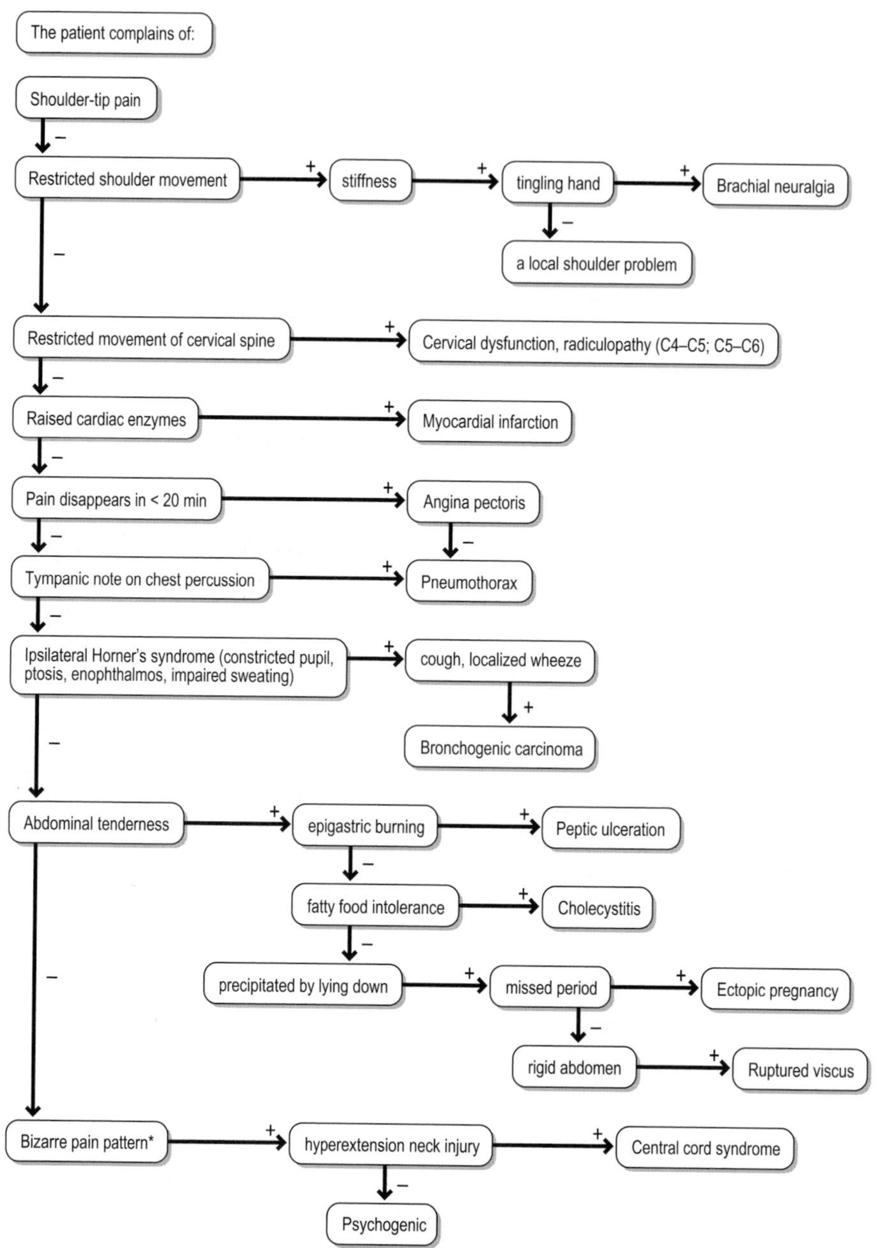

*Pain from pressure on the dura mater at cervical levels may be experienced from the head to midthorax; pressure at thoracic levels may cause pain from the base of the neck to the trunk, front and back.

Figure 40.7 **Pain referred to the shoulder.**

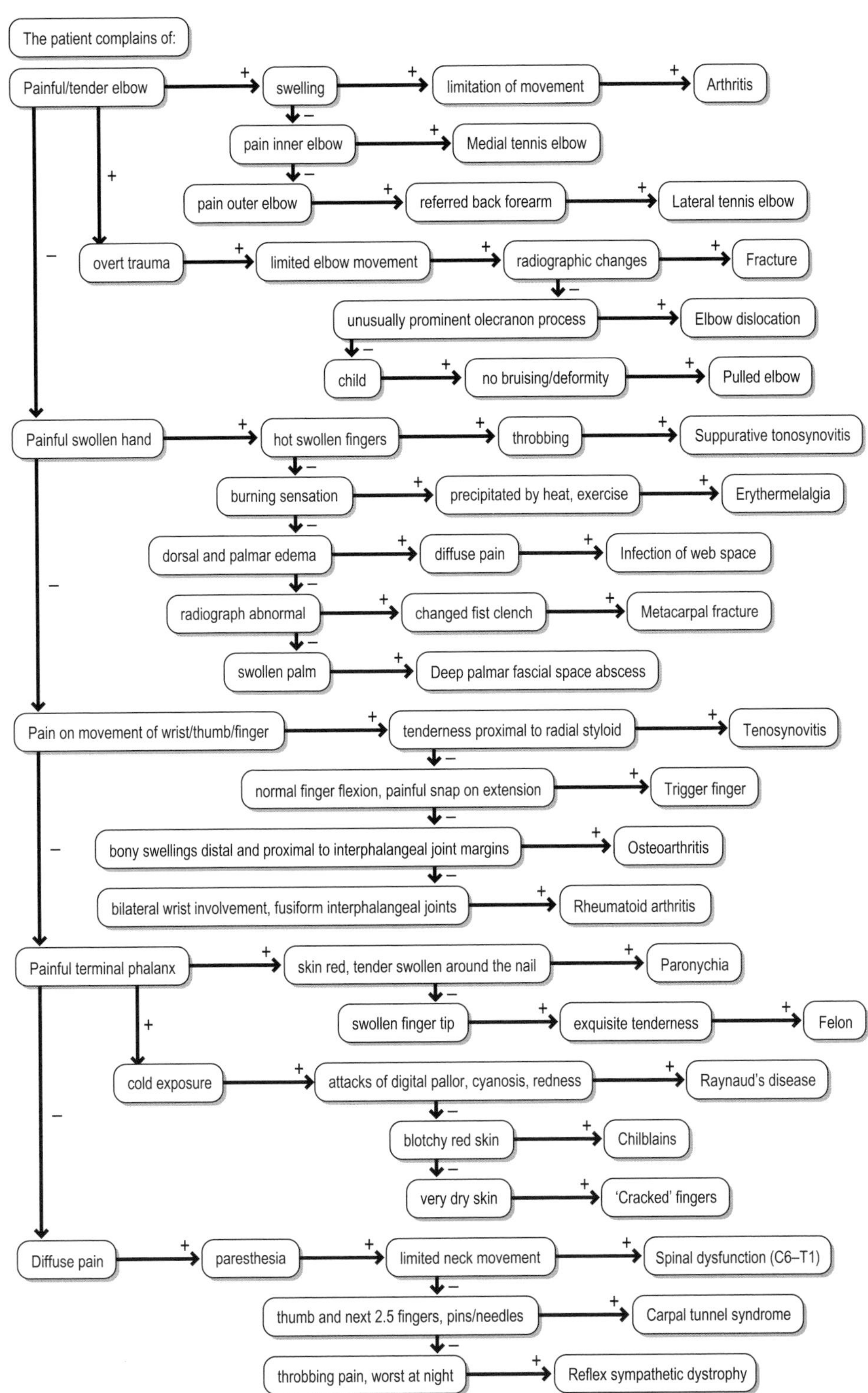

Figure 40.8 **Arm and hand pain.**

Does the patient need to be referred?

Conditions in which referral for special investigations, surgery, or drug therapy are indicated include:

- Suspected fracture:
  - history of trauma
  - pain aggravated by activity relieved by rest
  - marked restriction of movement
  - deformity
  - muscle spasm.
- Polyarthritis associated with:
  - weight loss
  - fever
  - lymphadenopathy
  - extensive rash
  - symptoms in more than one system
  - vasculitis
  - heart murmurs
  - severe pain/disability
  - extreme fatigue
  - increasing severe/intractable joint pain.
- Suspected vascular disorder:
  - acute arterial occlusion (sudden onset of pain, pulselessness, limb weakness, and coldness)
  - worsening chronic arterial occlusion (rest pain, worsening intermittent claudication)
  - popliteal aneurysm
  - suspected deep venous thrombosis (calf pain and swelling)
  - superficial thrombophlebitis of the thigh.
- Spinal dysfunction suggestive of:
  - disc protrusion (patients present with unilateral signs)
  - spinal cord compression (emergency referral is required).
- Suspected joint dislocation, subluxation, or instability.
- Persistence of symptoms such as night pain, stiffness, or restriction of movement.

FURTHER READING

Aldridge T 2004 Diagnosing heel pain in adults. Am Fam Physician 70(2):332–338

Gey D C, Lesho E P, Manngold J 2004 Management of peripheral arterial disease. Am Fam Physician 69(3):525–532

Koester M C, George M S, Kuhn J E 2005 Shoulder impingement syndrome. Am J Med 118(5):452–455

Oudega R, Moons K G, Hoes A W 2005 Limited value of patient history and physical examination in diagnosing deep vein thrombosis in primary care. Fam Pract 22(1):86–91

Stansby G 2005 The patient with intermittent claudication. Practitioner 249(1670):318, 320–321, 323–324

Lump

CHAPTER CONTENTS

Is the lump a benign or malignant tumor?

As the prognosis of benign and malignant lumps is vastly different, it is important to determine the nature of a mass. Masses are more likely to be malignant if they have the following properties:

- *Hard*. Although malignant tumors are often stony hard, they may sometimes be:
  - soft
  - firm
  - fluctuant (the central necrosis of a malignant tumor that has outgrown its blood supply can produce a lesion that resembles a cyst or abscess).
- *Irregular surface*. Fast-growing malignancies may, however, have a smooth surface.
- *Ill-defined edge*. An exception is a rapidly growing tumor that compresses surrounding tissue to form a false capsule. Benign tumors, in addition to having a well-defined margin, are usually mobile.
- *Fixed*, due to local invasion of surrounding tissue. Malignancy may be confused with inflammatory masses, which may also be difficult to separate from the surrounding tissue.
- *Nontender*. Inflammatory masses are tender.
- *Nonpulsatile*. Pulsatile masses suggest a vascular source and should be checked for bruits.
- *Evidence of spread*:
  - stony hard fixed regional lymphadenopathy suggests lymph node spread
  - skin edema may result from lymphatic obstruction.

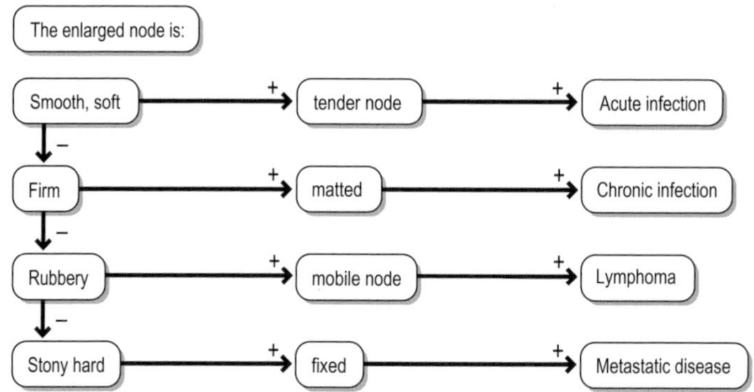

Figure 41.1 **Lymphadenopathy.**

- Associated with unexplained systemic findings such as:
  - weight loss
  - fever
  - migratory thrombosis
  - pruritus
  - endocrine anomalies.

Particular findings that suggest that a lump in the breast is malignant include:

- A nontender, fixed and hard mass.
- a deformity or alteration to the shape of the breast:
  - nipple/breast elevation
  - nipple retraction
  - dimpling of skin (peau d'orange)
  - localized skin rash.

Is the lump an enlarged lymph node?

Enlarged lymph nodes may result from acute or chronic infection, lymphoma (primary malignancy) or metastases. In all instances it is important to:

- Determine the character of the node.
- Examine the drainage area. The cause of the lymphadenopathy may be apparent (e.g. an infected lesion). The consequences of prolonged lymph node obstruction may also be detected as brawny nonpitting edema of the drainage area.
- Determine whether the lymphadenopathy is localized or generalized.

The major production and 'residential' sites for red cells, leukocytes, and platelets are the bone marrow and blood; the major sites for lymphocytes are the spleen, lymph nodes, and blood. In any disorder of white cells, always examine the lymph nodes, the spleen, the bone marrow, the blood and, in the event of extramedullary hematopoiesis, the liver. The character of the node is helpful in differential diagnosis (Fig. 41.1).

What could the patient's lump be?

The anatomical site of the lump is helpful in making the diagnosis (Fig. 41.2).

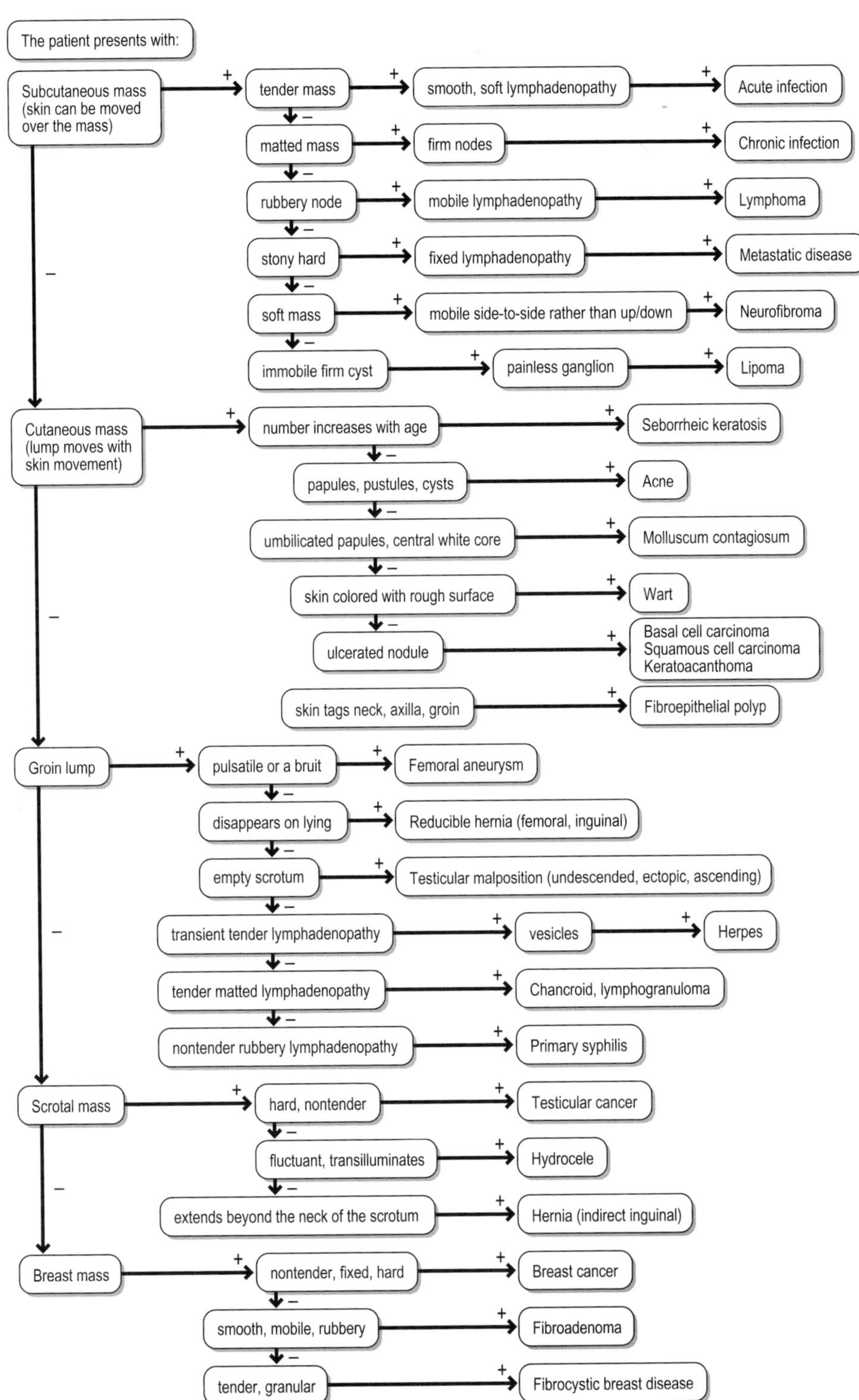

Figure 41.2 **A mass.**

Does the patient need to be referred?

Patients with a lump need to be referred for investigation and definitive diagnosis if there is:

- Diagnostic or therapeutic uncertainty.
- Suspected malignancy, including:
  - tumors over 1 cm
  - recurrent tumors
  - overlying ulceration which fails to heal.
- Unexplained:
  - localized lymphadenopathy
  - generalized lymphadenopathy
  - fever, night sweats, cachexia.

FURTHER READING

Dumitrescu R G, Cotarla I 2005 Understanding breast cancer risk – where do we stand in 2005? J Cell Mol Med 9(1):208–221

Franco E L, Harper D M 2005 Vaccination against human papillomavirus infection: a new paradigm in cervical cancer control. 1: Vaccine 23(17–18):2388–2394

Freak J 2005 Identification of skin cancers 1: benign and premalignant lesions. Br J Community Nurs 10(1):8–12

Freak J 2005 Identification of skin cancers 2: malignant lesions. Br J Community Nurs 10(2):58–64

Klein S 2005 Evaluation of palpable breast masses. Am Fam Physician 71(9):1731–1738

CHAPTER 42

Menstrual problems

CHAPTER CONTENTS

Is the genital blood loss abnormal?

Genital bleeding is normal in women of reproductive age. Genital blood loss is abnormal:

- Before puberty.
- After menopause.
- Between periods.
- If menstruation has:
  - a cycle of less than 21 days' duration
  - a flow of longer than 8 days' duration
  - a flow intensity that causes clotting and pain
  - a heavy–light–heavy flow sequence.
- In a woman with a hemoglobin of less than 9 g/dl without any other source of blood loss.

What is the nature of the bleed?

Abnormal genital bleeding may present as:

- *Metrorrhagia.* Metrorrhagia is excessive acyclic or intermenstrual bleeding. A patient who has genital bleeds between periods has metrorrhagia.
- *Menorrhagia.* Menorrhagia is excessive menstrual blood loss as a result of an increased volume of blood lost during a cycle of normal duration. A patient with heavy periods is menorrhagic.
- *Menometrorrhagia.* Menometrorrhagia implies excessive random uterine bleeding. Menometrorrhagia may result from any of the causes of metrorrhagia or from a complication of pregnancy.
- *Metrostaxis.* Metrostaxis describes continuous bleeding and/or premenstrual staining (spotting) less than 8 days prior to menstruation.

- *Polymenorrhea.* Polymenorrhea describes a frequent, often profuse, menstrual cycle of less than 21 days. A patient with short cycles, often with heavy periods, has polymenorrhea. Polymenorrhea is found in anovulatory cycles or patients with abnormal estrogen due to liver cirrhosis.

What is the cause of the patient's abnormal genital blood loss?

See Figure 42.1.

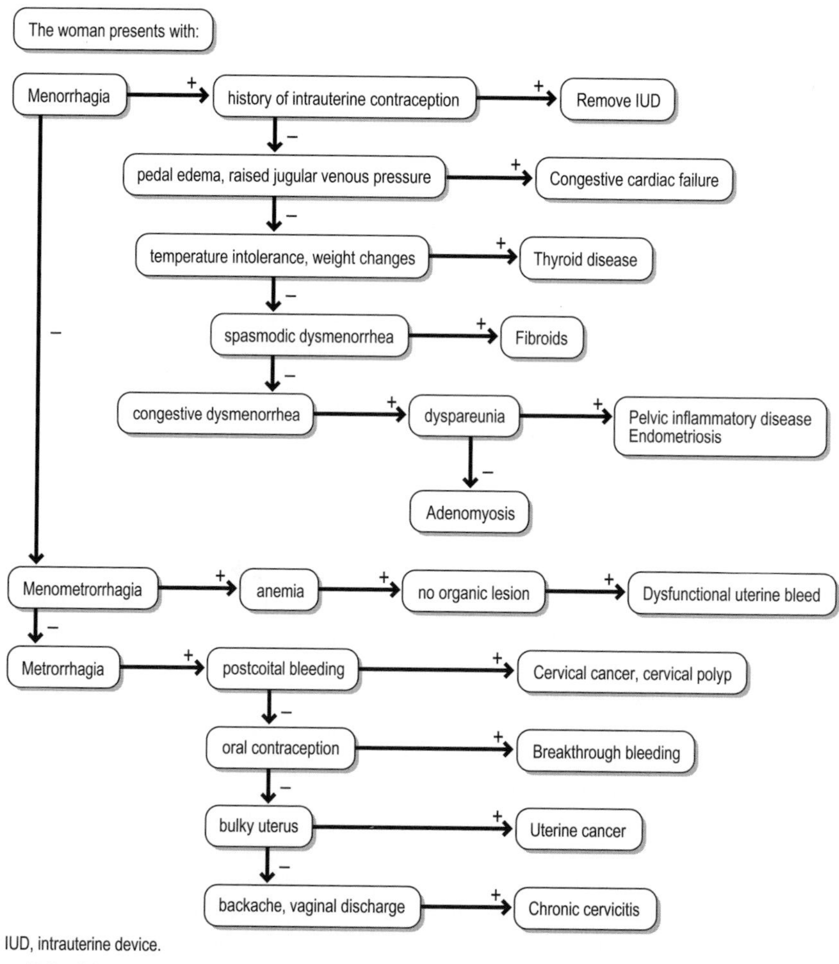

IUD, intrauterine device.

Figure 42.1 **Menstrual disorders.**

Does the patient need to be referred?

Patients with any of the following should be referred for investigation and causal diagnosis:

- metrorrhagia
- anemia
- suspected thyroid disease
- cardiac failure
- suspected infection.

FURTHER READING

Albers J R, Hull S K, Wesley R M 2004 Abnormal uterine bleeding. Am Fam Physician 69(8):1915–1926

Eliakim A, Beyth Y 2003 Exercise training, menstrual irregularities and bone development in children and adolescents. J Pediatr Adolesc Gynecol 16(4):201–206

Farrell E 2004 Dysfunctional uterine bleeding. Aust Fam Physician 33(11):906–908

Kouides P A 2002 Menorrhagia from a hematologist's point of view. Part I: initial evaluation. Hemophilia 8(3):330–338

Mitan L A 2004 Menstrual dysfunction in anorexia nervosa. J Pediatr Adolesc Gynecol 17(2):81–85

Moodley M, Roberts C 2004 Clinical pathway for the evaluation of postmenopausal bleeding with an emphasis on endometrial cancer detection. J Obstet Gynecol 24(7):736–741

Warren M P, Goodman L R 2003 Exercise-induced endocrine pathologies. J Endocrinol Invest 26(9):873–878

Pallor

CHAPTER CONTENTS

Why is the patient pale?

Pallor implies a lack of oxyhemoglobin. This may be due to reduced perfusion or anemia.

Reduced perfusion. Pallor limited to the extremities (fingernails) suggests local vasospasm, often in response to cold. In an acute hemorrhage any pallor detected is due to generalized vasoconstriction. It takes some 48–72 hours for the circulating volume to be restored and anemia to develop after an acute hemorrhage. Blood loss or oligemic (hypovolemic) shock and not pallor is the presenting complaint in cases of overt hemorrhage.

Reduced hemoglobin, or anemia. Pallor of the conjunctiva and lips suggest a low hemoglobin. Patients with pallor attributable to anemia may also experience:

- lethargy, easy fatiguability
- tachypnea on exertion
- palpitations
- dizziness
- faintness, blackouts
- confusion
- claudication and/or angina.

Anemia is confirmed on laboratory testing. A full blood count includes:

- A low hemoglobin: a value of less than 13 gm/dl in men or 12 gm/dl in women.
- A reduced red cell count: a count of less than 4.5×10^{12}/l in men or less than 3.8×10^{12}/l in women.
- A packed cell volume of less than 40% in men and 37% in women.

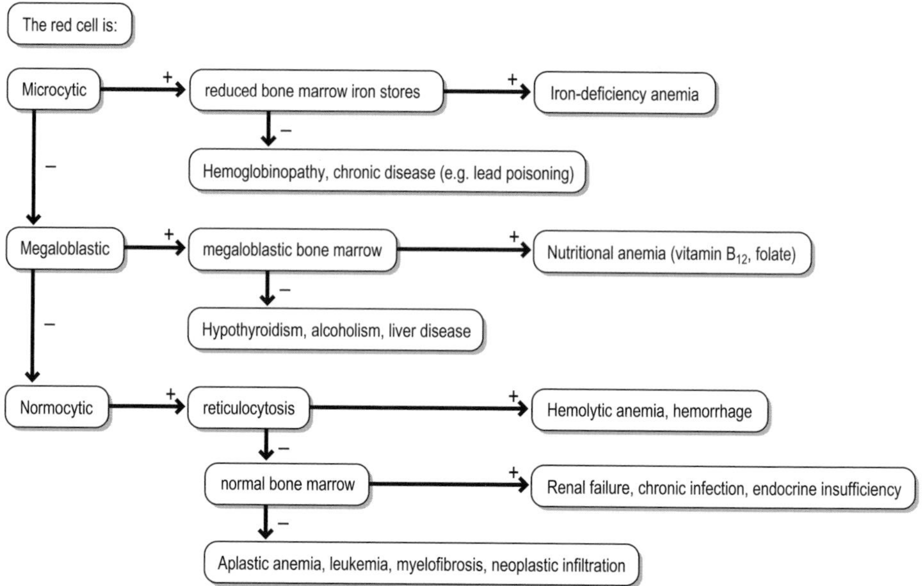

Figure 43.1 **Erythrocyte morphology.**

- A mean cell volume, which may demonstrate microcytic, normocytic, or macrocytic cells. Red-cell morphology provides useful diagnostic information.

The appearance of the red cell may aid diagnosis (Figure 43.1).

Anemia may result from an imbalance in red-cell production and destruction (loss). Deficiencies in red-cell production (dyshemopoiesis) may be attributable to:

- Defective heme production. Erythropoiesis may be suppressed by toxins (e.g. uremia, alcoholism) and chronic diseases.
- Defective globin production, as in thalassemia.
- Defective DNA production due to vitamin B_{12} or folic acid deficiency.
- Marrow hypoplasia due to bone marrow suppression by drugs or irradiation.
- Marrow replacement by malignant cell or fibrous tissue (myelofibrosis).

Increased loss of red cells may be due to:

- Bleeding. Anemia is one of the earliest signs of chronic blood loss. While iron-deficiency anemia may be the presenting sign in occult blood loss, it is not a sign in acute hemorrhage.
- Destruction (hemolysis) of fragile erythrocytes. A healthy bone marrow responds by increasing red-cell production and the laboratory finds an increased reticulocyte count. Increased hemoglobin catabolism also results in enhanced bilirubin production, and jaundice may be noted.

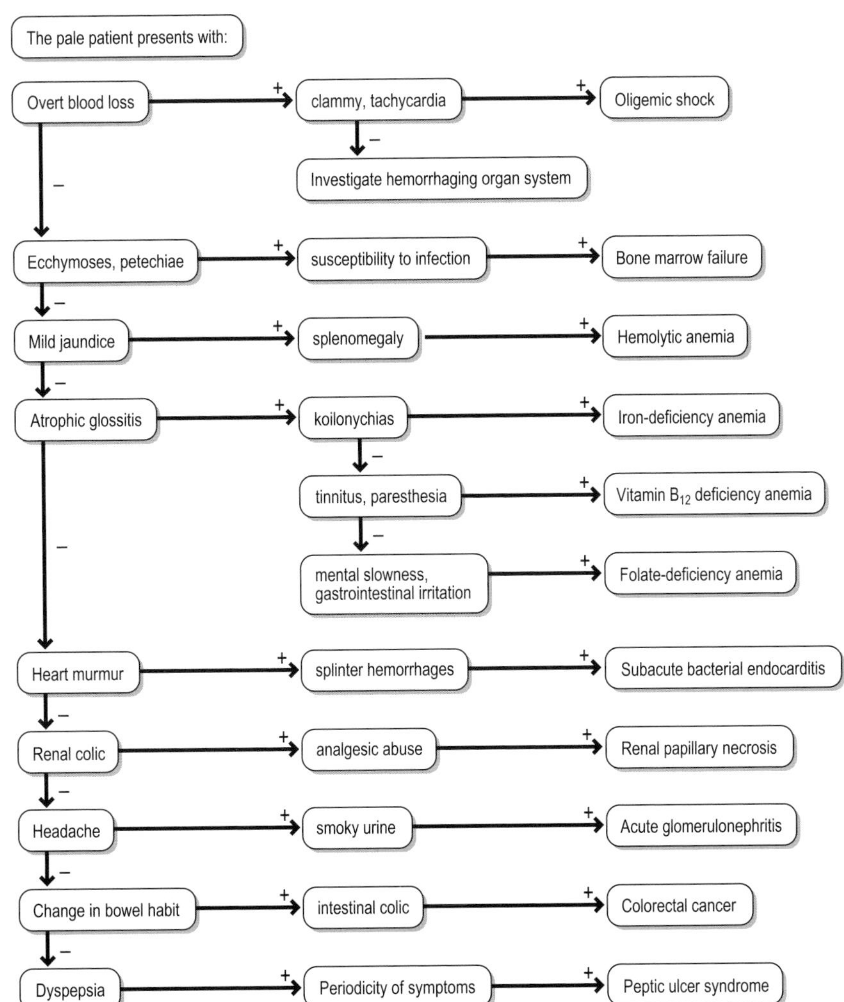

Figure 43.2 **Pallor.**

What is the likely diagnosis?

See Figure 43.2.

Does the patient need to be referred?

Refer pale patients for investigation in cases of:

- Unexplained anemia. Exclusion of microscopic hematuria and occult blood in the stool is an integral component of any such investigation. The morphology of the red cells is also helpful in formulating a working diagnosis.
- Easy bruising.
- Unexplained bleeding into the skin and mucous membranes.

FURTHER READING

Bizzarro M J, Colson E, Ehrenkranz RA 2004 Differential diagnosis and management of anemia in the newborn. Pediatr Clin North Am 51(4):xi, 1087–1107

Chowdhury M E, Chongsuvivatwong V, Geater A F, Akhter H H, Winn T 2002 Taking a medical history and using a color scale during clinical examination of pallor improves detection of anemia. Trop Med Int Health 7(2):133–139

Palpitations

CHAPTER CONTENTS

Does the patient have a cardiac arrhythmia?

Palpitations are an unpleasant awareness of the heartbeat and are usually related to a variation in the rate, regularity, or force of cardiac contraction. Arrhythmias are usually described as awareness that the heartbeat is pounding, skipping, stopping, or racing. People vary greatly in their awareness of an arrhythmia.

Normal rhythm is regular, with impulses originating at the sinoatrial node (nodal rhythm). Normal sinus rhythm is a regular pulse of 65–95 beats/min. A heart rate outside these limits is defined as:

- tachycardia, when the heart rate exceeds 100 beats/min
- bradycardia, when the heart rate is less than 60 beats/min.

Irregular rhythms may present as regular or irregular irregularities. Extrasystoles or ectopic beats leading to premature contraction may cause a regular irregularity. On exercise the rate increases and the irregularity disappears. Irregular irregularity may be caused by random transmission of atrial stimuli through the atrioventricular node. Patients commonly describe ectopic beats as a skipped beat followed by a stronger beat. A ventricular ectopic (symptomatic premature ventricular beat) is a common arrhythmia encountered in primary practice.

Palpitations may have a cardiac or noncardiac origin. Palpitations are most likely to have a cardiac cause if they are:

- associated with:
  - syncope
  - dizziness.

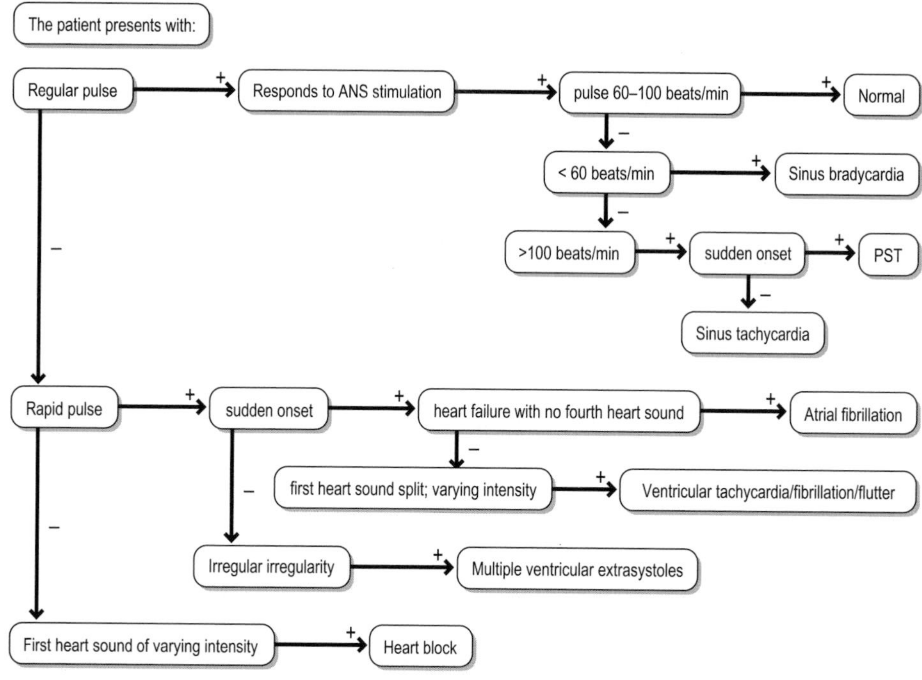

ANS, autonomic nervous system; PST, paroxysmal supraventricular (atrial) tachycardia.

Figure 44.1 **Classification of cardiac arrhythmias.**

- the following precipitating factors are absent:
  - emotion
  - fever
  - exercise.

Figure 44.1 considers how cardiac arrhythmias may be classified.

Is the arrhythmia pathologic?

Arrhythmias may be pathological or nonpathological. Nonpathological arrhythmias:

- respond to autonomic nervous system (ANS) stimulation:
  - Sympathetic stimulation increases heart rate in bradycardia. This may be achieved by exercise.
  - Vagal (parasympathetic) stimulation slows a tachycardia. This may be achieved by:
  - carotid sinus massage (carotid sinus massage is contraindicated in persons over 75 years of age, and in those with a carotid bruit, with hemodynamic instability, or with possible digitalis toxicity)
  - pressure on the eyeballs
  - retching, gagging, or self-induced vomiting
  - breath-holding
  - applying ice or cold water to the face.

- Have a regular pulse (sinus arrhythmia). Conduction passes through the atrioventricular (AV) node and, therefore, the beat is regular.
- May be fast or slow:
  - sinus tachycardia, with a rate of 100–150 beats/min
  - sinus bradycardia, with a rate around 40 beats/min.

Should the patient be urgently referred?

Urgent referral should be considered for potentially life-threatening arrhythmias such as:

- Ventricular tachycardia:
  - a rapid pulse of up to 200 beats/min
  - a first heart sound of varying intensity and often split
  - unresponsive to vagal stimulation.
- Complete heart block:
  - no increase in heart rate with exercise
  - syncope
  - ventricular asystole (asystole of more than 3 minutes is usually fatal).
- Sick sinus syndrome:
  - atrial fibrillation
  - dizziness or syncope
  - bradycardia–tachycardia made worse by digoxin.
- Silent myocardial infarction presenting as an arrhythmia:
  - Raised cardiac enzymes: after infarction, measure creatine kinase in the first 48 hours (creatine kinase MB isomer is not affected by intramuscular injections), aspartate transferase in the next 24–72 hours, and lactic dehydrogenase in the next 3–14 days.
  - Electrocardiogram (ECG) changes: transient inversion of the T wave, elevation of the ST segment, and development of broad, deep Q waves.

What is the likely diagnosis?

See Figure 44.2.

Does the patient need to be referred?

In general it may be prudent to refer patients for further investigation or treatment if they have any one of the following:

- A bradycardia of:
  - less than 50 beats/min
  - 50 beats/min in patients on beta blockers
  - less than 60 beats/min in a patient on digoxin.
- A tachycardia at rest of 120 beats/min.
- An irregularity that is new and has not been investigated previously.
- Syncope or dizziness associated with an arrhythmia.
- Systolic blood pressure of 90 mmHg or less.
- Paroxysmal arrhythmia.

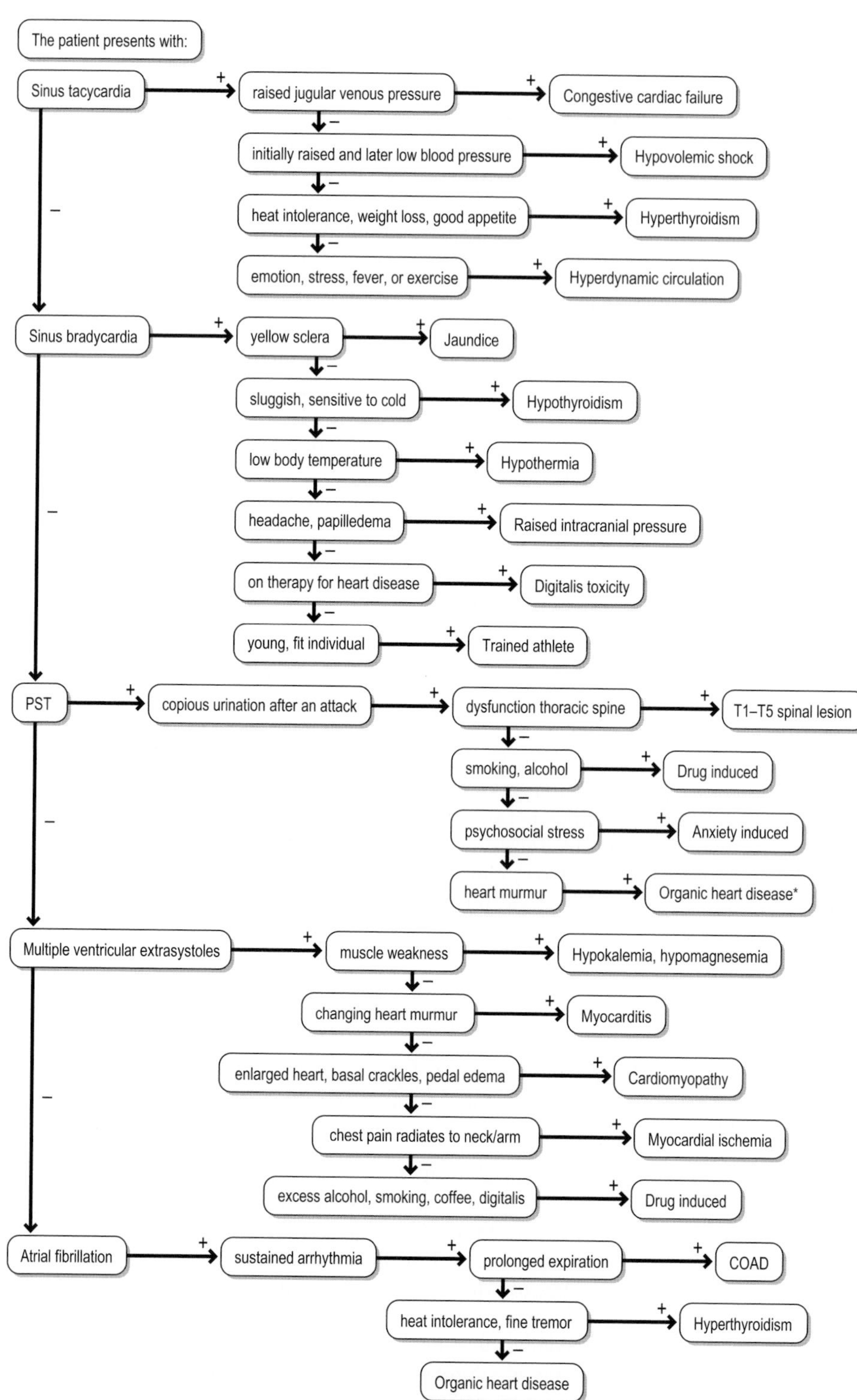

*Includes consideration of rheumatic fever resulting in valvular lesions, especially mitral stenosis, myocarditis, atherosclerotic heart disease, cardiomyopathy, and hypertension.
COAD, chronic obstructive airways disease; PST, paroxysmal supraventricular tachycardia.

Figure 44.2 **Arrhythmia.**

- Chronic or sustained atrial fibrillation if the patient is not on anticoagulant therapy.
- Symptomatic patients with:
  - Pulsus paradoxus. When blood-pressure fluctuation between inspiration and expiration exceeds 15 mmHg, pulsus paradoxus is diagnosed. The physiological arterial pressure fluctuation associated with respiration between expiration (higher) and inspiration (lower) is usually 5–15 mmHg. Pulsus paradoxus is encountered when cardiac flow into the left side of the heart is impeded (e.g. chronic obstructive airways disease (COAD), constrictive pericarditis, pericardial effusion).
  - Pulsus alternans. Pulsus alternans refers to a changing stroke volume that results in an arterial pulse of varying amplitude. Pulsus alternans is found in left ventricular failure.
  - Pulse deficit. A discrepancy between the heart rate and the pulse rate is called a pulse deficit. Cardiac irregularity may result in a variable stroke volume. When the stroke volume decreases to a level insufficient to elicit a palpable arterial pulse, a pulse deficit is diagnosed.

FURTHER READING

Abbott A V 2005 Diagnostic approach to palpitations. Am Fam Physician 71(4):743–750

Beery T T 2005 The genetics of cardiac arrhythmias. Biol Res Nurs 6(4):249–261

Ressel G W 2004 AAFP and ACP release practice guideline on management of newly detected atrial fibrillation. Am Fam Physician 2004 69(10):2474–2475

Period pains

CHAPTER CONTENTS

Does the patient have spasmodic or congestive dysmenorrhea?

Pain with menstruation is termed dysmenorrhea. Patients complaining of period pain may have either spasmodic or congestive dysmenorrhea.

Spasmodic dysmenorrhea occurs in young nulliparas. It is thought to be associated with overproduction of prostaglandins. Spasmodic dysmenorrhea presents clinically with pain which:

- is cramp-like and begins within 12 hours of the onset of menses
- is relieved some 24–48 hours after the onset of the period
- presents as low midline abdominal pain and radiates to the thighs and lower back
- may be associated with nausea or vomiting.

In *congestive dysmenorrhea* the normal congestion of the pelvic organs associated with the increasing levels of estrogen and progesterone prior to menstruation may be aggravated by pelvic infection and/or endometriosis. Congestive dysmenorrhea is characterized by:

- pain which starts up to 7 days prior to the onset of menses
- a feeling of heaviness and/or a dull pain in the lower abdomen which worsens until the onset of menstruation
- an increased risk of dyspareunia and/or infertility.

What is the likely cause?

See Figure 45.1.

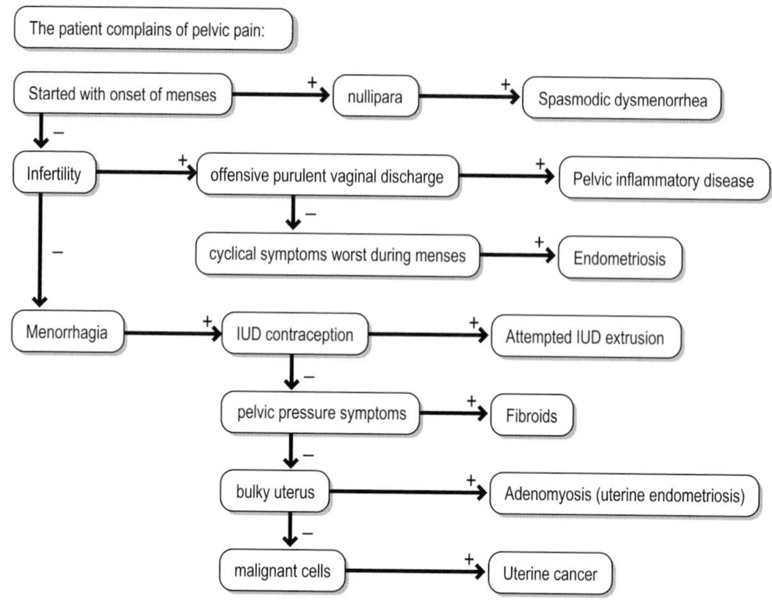

Figure 45.1 **Dysmenorrhea.**

Does the patient need to be referred?

Unless the primary practitioner has access to appropriate therapy it may be necessary to refer patients whose:

- Dysmenorrhea:
  - started with the first menses
  - began after the age of 25 years
  - is associated with anovulatory cycles.
- Pain is:
  - increasing or changing
  - unrelieved by treatment
  - interfering with her duties.
- History suggests pelvic inflammatory disease.
- Personal or family history includes a problem with endometriosis.
- Desire is to become pregnant.

FURTHER READING

Dick M L 2004 Chronic pelvic pain in women: assessment and management. Aust Fam Physician 33(12):971–976

French L 2005 Dysmenorrhea. Am Fam Physician 71(2):285–291

Marjoribanks J, Proctor M L, Farquhar C 2003 Nonsteroidal anti-inflammatory drugs for primary dysmenorrhea. Cochrane Database Syst Rev (4):CD001751

Wilson M L, Murphy P A 2001 Herbal and dietary therapies for primary and secondary dysmenorrhea. Cochrane Database Syst Rev (3):CD002124

Pins and needles

CHAPTER CONTENTS

Does the patient show paresthesia?

Patients with paresthesia experience abnormal sensation including:

- pins and needles
- tingling
- burning
- itching.

Other alterations in sensation include:

- anesthesia (the absence of touch sensation)
- hypoesthesia (reduced sensitivity to touch)
- hyperesthesia (heightened sensitivity to touch).

Paresthesia may result from:

- Prolonged pressure on:
  - A peripheral nerve: tingling is experienced in the area supplied by the nerve.
  - A nerve root: tingling is experienced in the distribution of the dermatome.
  - The spinal cord in the region of the spinothalamic tract: the patient experiences a sensation of 'water running over the skin'.
- Vasospasm of cerebral vessels. Migraine patients may describe transitory tingling in one limb that spreads to the face.
- Aberrant electrical activity resulting from:
  - Localized cerebral hyperactivity: focal seizures may be associated with a short episode of local paresthesia.
  - Metabolic aberration: electrolyte and acid–base disturbances may produce unilateral or bilateral paresthesia.

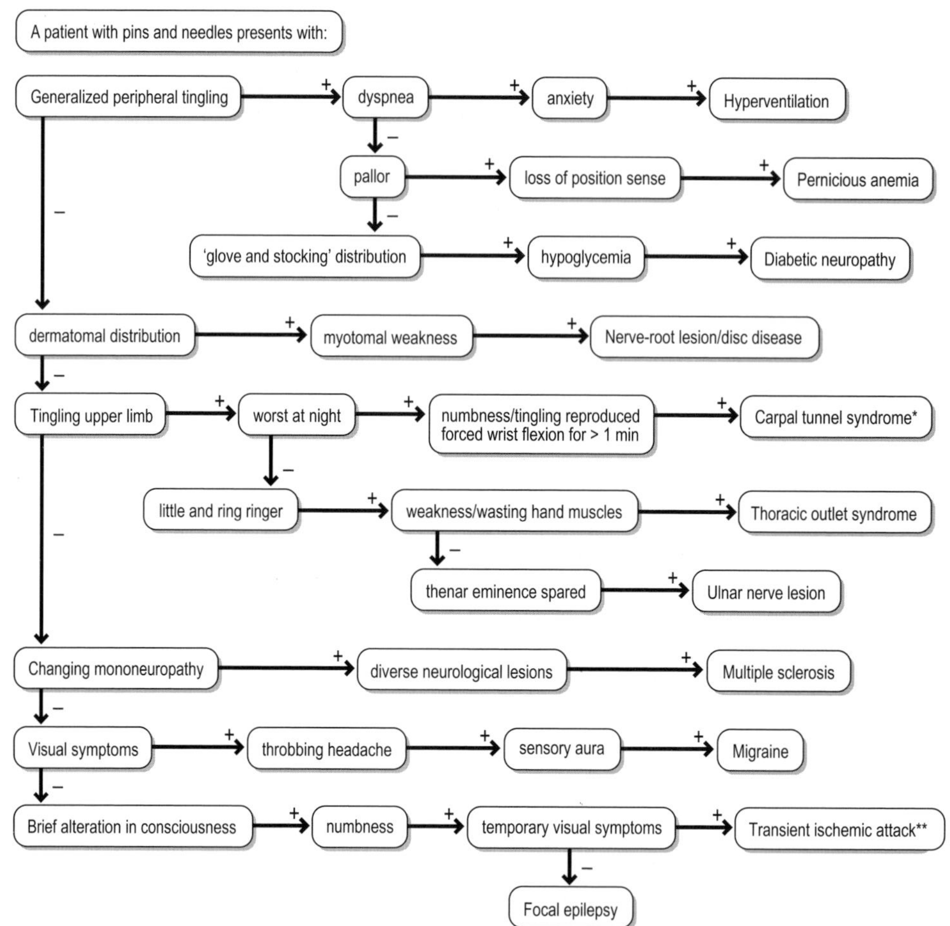

*Median nerve entrapment.
**Cardiovascular accident, sensory cortex; brainstem, numbness of hand.

Figure 46.1 **Paresthesia.**

What is the likely diagnosis?

See Figure 46.1.

Does the patient need to be referred?

Referral for definitive therapy may be required for patients requiring:

- release of pressure on nerves
- control of cerebral hyperactivity
- correction of metabolic imbalances
- anticoagulant therapy.

FURTHER READING

Alexandre A, Coro L, Azuelos A, Pellone M 2005 Thoracic outlet syndrome due to hyperextension–hyperflexion cervical injury. Acta Neurochir Suppl 92:21–24

Duby J J, Campbell R K, Setter S M, White J R, Rasmussen K A 2004 Diabetic neuropathy: an intensive review. Am J Health Syst Pharm 61(2):160–173

CHAPTER 47

Rash

CHAPTER CONTENTS

What does the rash look like?

The appearance provides helpful clinical information. It also forms the basis of the terminology used for referring dermatological patients (Table 47.1). Combinations of the features listed in Table 47.1 are also common.

Three major descriptions of a maculopapular rash are:

- *scarlatiniform*, when the rash is diffusely erythematous
- *morbilliform*, when the rash is blotchy
- *rubelliform*, when the rash is fine and discrete.

What is the likely cause based on its morphology?

Lynch and Edminster have taken this notion further and produced an algorithm, based on morphology (appearance), to assist in the classification of skin lesions (Fig. 47.1).

Maculopapular rashes are frequently associated with fever. Causes of maculopapular rashes and fever include:

- Viral infections: measles, rubella, infectious mononucleosis, Ross river, Dengue fever, acute human immunodeficiency virus (HIV) infection.
- Bacterial infections: meningococcemia, streptococcal scarlet fever, and staphylococcal diseases such as toxic shock syndrome.
- Rickettsial infections: typhus.
- Drugs.
- Immunological/collagen-type disorders: systemic lupus erythematosus, erythema multiforme, and juvenile rheumatoid arthritis.

Table 47.1
Dermatological terminology

Appearance of the skin	Nomenclature
Redness	Erythema
Dilated small cutaneous blood vessels	Telangiectasia
A transient red raised area, pale in the center	Wheal
Bleeding into the skin	Purpura Petechiae (purpura < 2 mm) Ecchymosis (large purpura)
A flat discolored area	Macule (< 1.5 cm diameter) Patch (> 1.5 cm diameter)
A palpable mass	Papule (< 1.5 cm diameter) Nodule (> 1.5 cm diameter; spherical) Plaque (> 1.5 cm diameter; flat topped)
Fluid-filled papule	Vesicle (< 1.5 cm diameter) Bullous (> 1.5 cm diameter) Pustule vesicle with neutrophils (pus)
Collection of pus	Pustule (< 1 cm) Abscess (> 1 cm)
An infected hair follicle	Folliculitis (small, pulsatile) Furuncle: boil (large) Carbuncle (collection of boils)
A keratin or sebum plug in a dilated sebaceous gland	Comedo: Open comedo (blackhead) Closed comedo (whitehead)
Accumulation of dried exudate on the skin	Crust
Scratch marks/superficial skin abrasions	Excoriation
Diffuse thickening and scaling due to chronic rubbing	Lichenification
Deep epithelial defect	Ulcer
Dry or greasy dead epidermal cells being shed	Scales

Scaliness may also be a useful consideration when diagnosing a rash (Fig. 47.2).

What is the likely cause based on its distribution?

Certain skin lesions are particularly prevalent in particular areas of the body. When a lesion is detected in these regions the particular condition should be considered; when the lesion is absent from the anatomical site, the condition is not automatically excluded. Figure 47.3 provides some clues as to the common rashes that should be considered if a lesion is encountered in various anatomical areas.

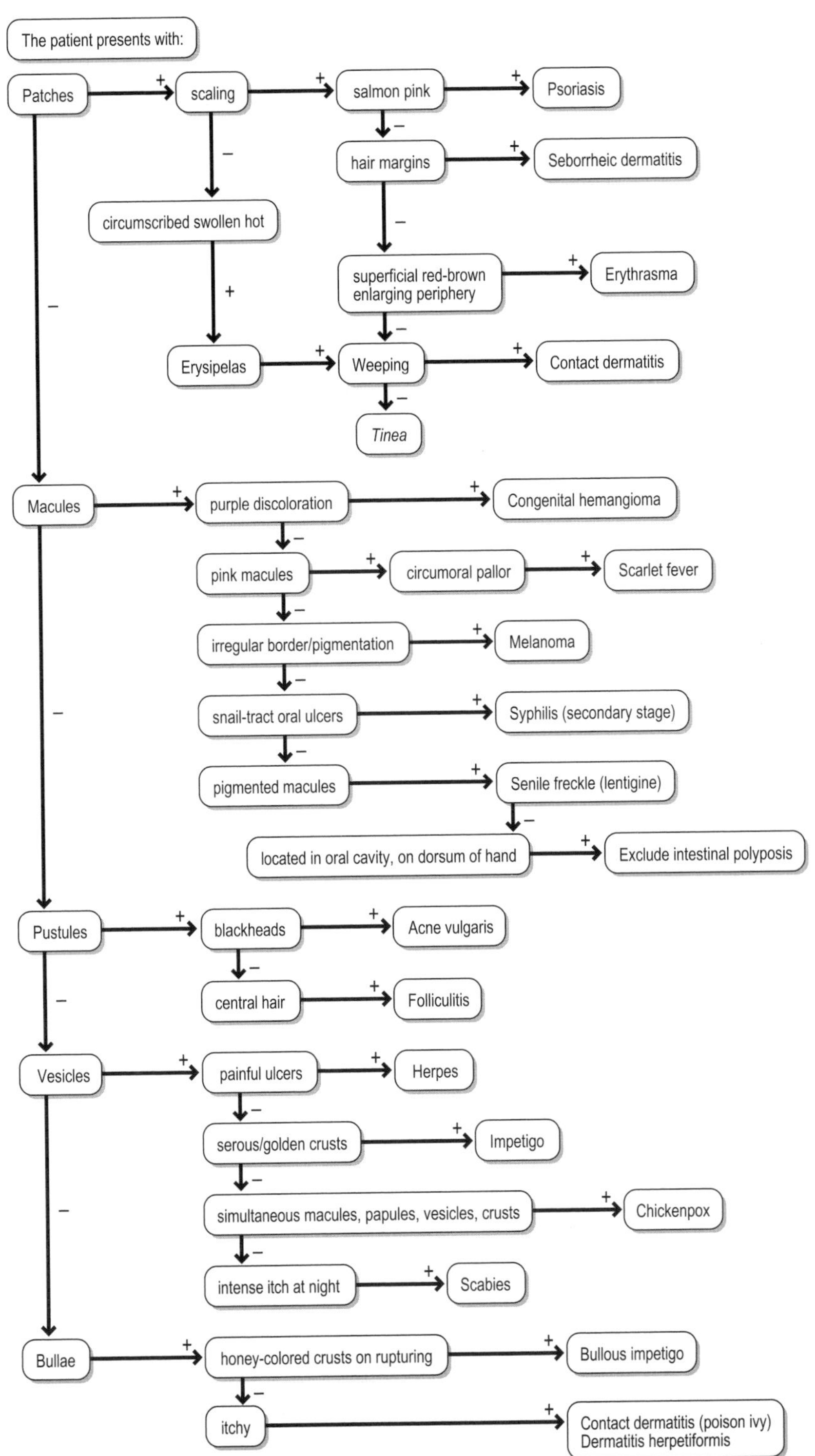

Figure 47.1 **Skin rash – by morphology.**

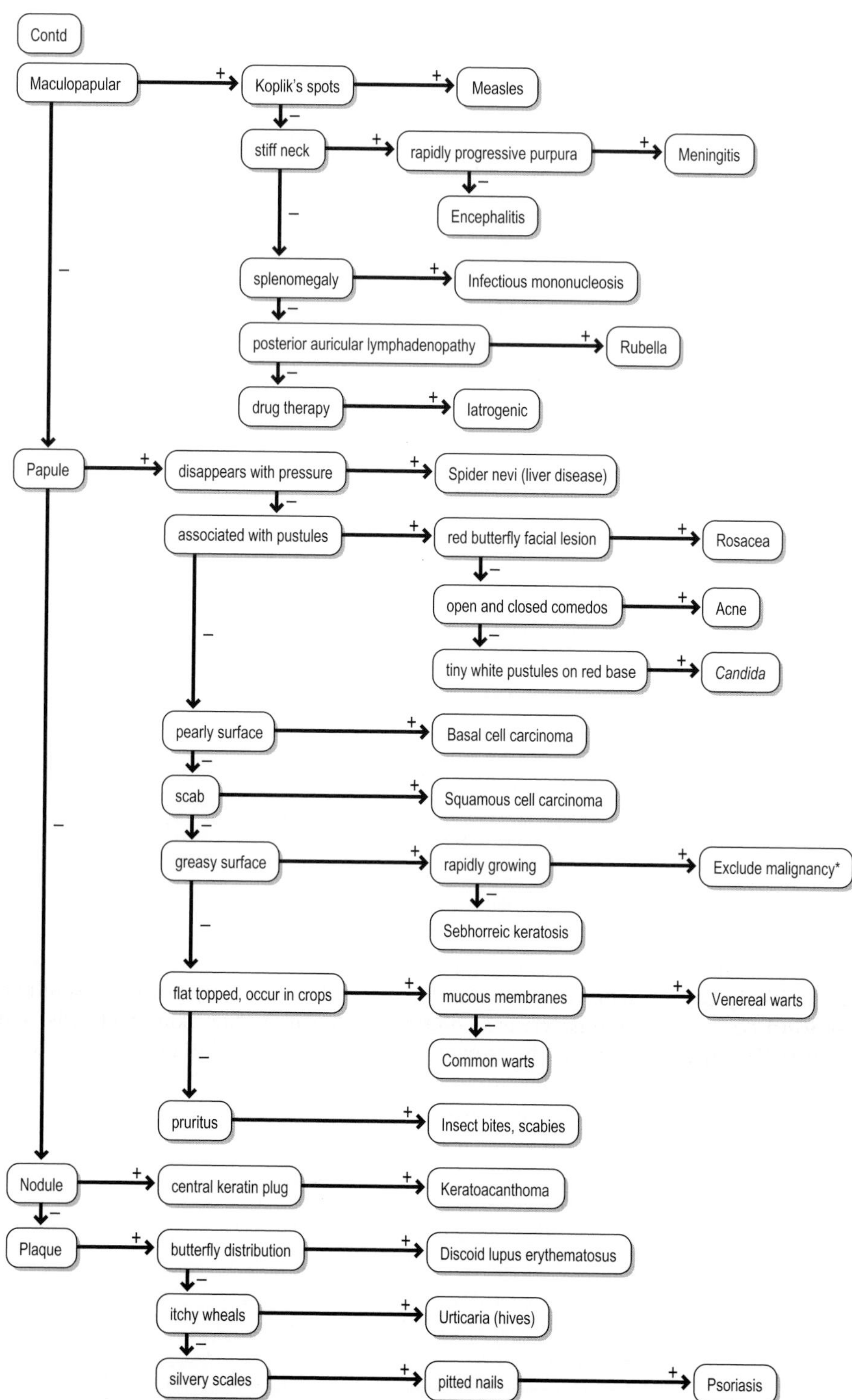

*Rapidly growing seborrheic keratosis may be a skin manifestation of metaplasia, lymphoproliferative disorders, or adenocarcinoma of the gastrointestinal tract.

Skin rash – by morphology contd.

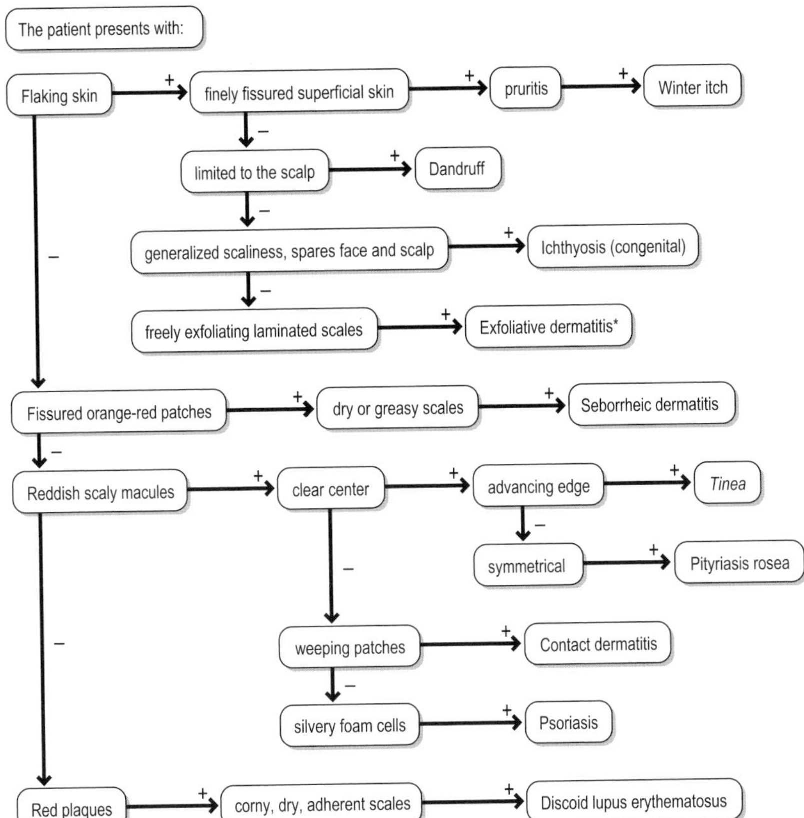

*This is a descriptive term for a skin condition the cause of which may be unknown or be the result of medication, leukemia, lymphoma, or dermatitis.

Figure 47.2 **Scaly skin rash.**

Which rashes are unlikely to respond to topical therapy?

Topical therapy for skin lesions is usually determined by the local skin response. Treatments include dusting powders, soothing lotions, creams, ointments to soften the skin, and gels and solutions to promote drying of weeping inflamed areas. Acute skin lesions are usually treated with water-based mixtures, and chronic lesions with oils and greases. Important causes of skin lesions that may require therapy beyond dermatological relief are those attributable to malignancy, infection, or systemic disease. It is therefore important to actively consider these possibilities.

Findings suggestive of a *dermatological malignancy* include:

- Asymmetrical lesions with an irregular border and variable color, of more than 5 mm in diameter.
- Scaly erythematous patches with a sandpaper texture.
- Flesh-colored nodules with everted or pearly edges.
- Nodules with central ulceration or overlying telangiectatic vessels.

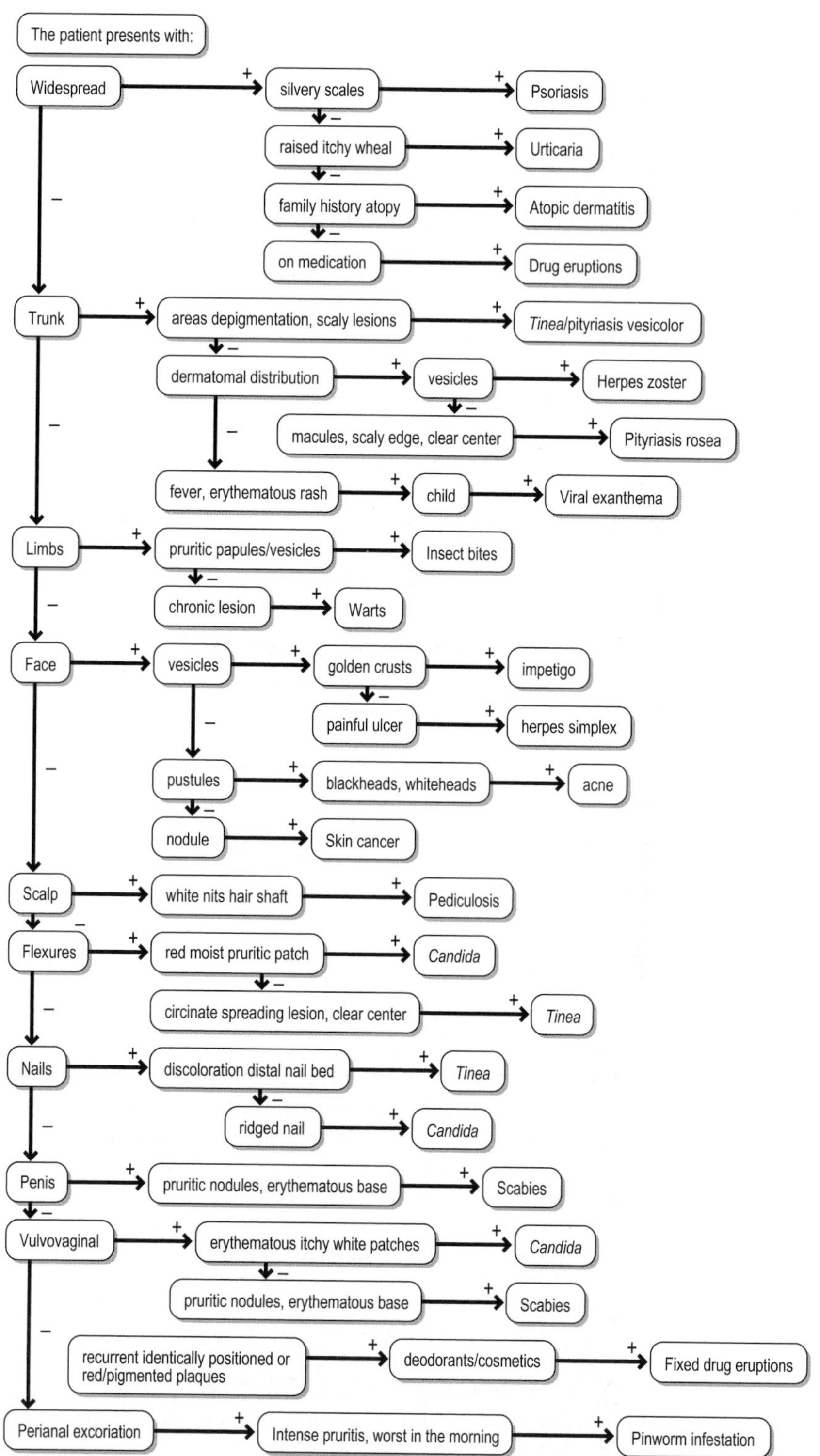

Figure 47.3 **Skin rash – by distribution.**

Although a skin lesion may itself be benign, a rash may be a marker for malignancy elsewhere. Benign skin lesions that herald malignancy elsewhere include:

- Generalized pruritus in the absence of a rash.
- Acanthosis nigricans: a velvety hyperpigmented nodule. When detected in the axilla, neck, or groin this nodule may be indicative of adenocarcinoma of the stomach, pancreas, liver, or gallbladder.
- Ichthyosis: thickening of the palm and soles with dry scaly skin may be associated with Hodgkin's disease.
- Seborrheic keratosis: greasy verrucous lesions may be associated with malignancy, especially of the lymphoid tissue or gastrointestinal tract.
- Lentigines: these pigmented macules are associated with intestinal polyposis in the Peutz–Jeghers syndrome. Persons with this syndrome are at increased risk of bowel cancer.

Skin rashes may also be associated with *systemic disease*. General findings suggestive of systemic disease include:

- malaise, weight loss
- fever
- abnormalities on hematological and/or blood chemistry investigation.

Specific lesions that are associated with systemic disorders include:

- Tan macules (café-au-lait spots). When five or more tan macules over 1 cm in size are present the patient should be investigated for neurofibromatosis (von Recklinghausen's disease). If the macules are jagged and limited to one side of the body, Albright's syndrome of premature puberty, fibrous dysplasia, and cystic bone lesions seen on radiography should be investigated.
- Recurrent symmetric red skin lesions, target lesions with clear centers, and any combination of macules, papules, bullae, and purpura are encountered in erythema marginatum. Erythema marginatum, a primary skin disorder, can also be a manifestation of underlying systemic disease, including ulcerative colitis, rheumatoid arthritis, and lupus erythematosus.
- Painful red nodules on the leg, erythema nodosum, is found in patients with drug sensitivity, syphilis, rheumatic fever, or fungal infection.

All chronic skin lesions need to have both malignancy and systemic disease included in the differential diagnosis.

Infection is an important cause of an acute skin lesion. The infection may be local or systemic. The infectious diseases of childhood result from droplet spread and present with a confluent maculopapular rash that desquamates in the case of measles, a discrete pink macular rash in rubella, and a centripetal rash with macules, papules, and vesicles in chickenpox. The presentation of local infections may be determined by the organism and the site of infection. Infection of a hair follicle by *Staphylococcus aureus* can result in: folliculitis, a pustule of the hair follicle; furunculosis, a boil, or abscess around the hair follicle; or carbuncles in which cysts involve a number a hair follicles and discharge through a number of orifices. Other variables also influence the nature of the skin rash. In the case of *Streptococcus pyogenes*, cellulitis, an area of well-defined erythema and erysipelas, an intense raised erythematous area with a defined border, arise from direct infection; scarlet fever results from toxin production, and erythema nodosum and erythema marginatum from a hypersensitivity response. Both these organisms can also give rise to impetigo, with its vesicles and golden-yellow crusts.

As many infections and infestations require specific antimicrobial therapy, it is important to consider an infection in patients with:

- a scaly pruritic lesion
- a purulent exudate
- an altered white cell count (an eosinophilia is suggestive of a parasitic disorder)
- positive microscopy or culture on examination of scrapings from the lesion (organisms, ova, or parasites may be visualized or illuminated).

See Figure 47.4 for conditions that need to be considered when lesions persist despite topical therapy.

Does the patient need to be referred?

Skin rashes are common and difficult to diagnose. For the primary practitioner it is important to ascertain the discomfort associated with the lesion and its prognostic implications.

Skin lesions that may require referral in an effort to modify the natural history of the condition include those that are:

- malignant
- a manifestation of an undiagnosed systemic condition
- infected or caused by a parasite or microorganism
- a reaction to a prescription drug
- a manifestation of a severe allergic reaction
- characterized by an intense local reaction (steroids may be indicated).

Skin lesions that may be amenable to intervention at the primary level include self-limiting conditions and those attributable to local irritants.

In general, it is wise to refer patients with skin lesions if:

- diagnosis is uncertain
- a serious cause is suspected
- the problem recurs

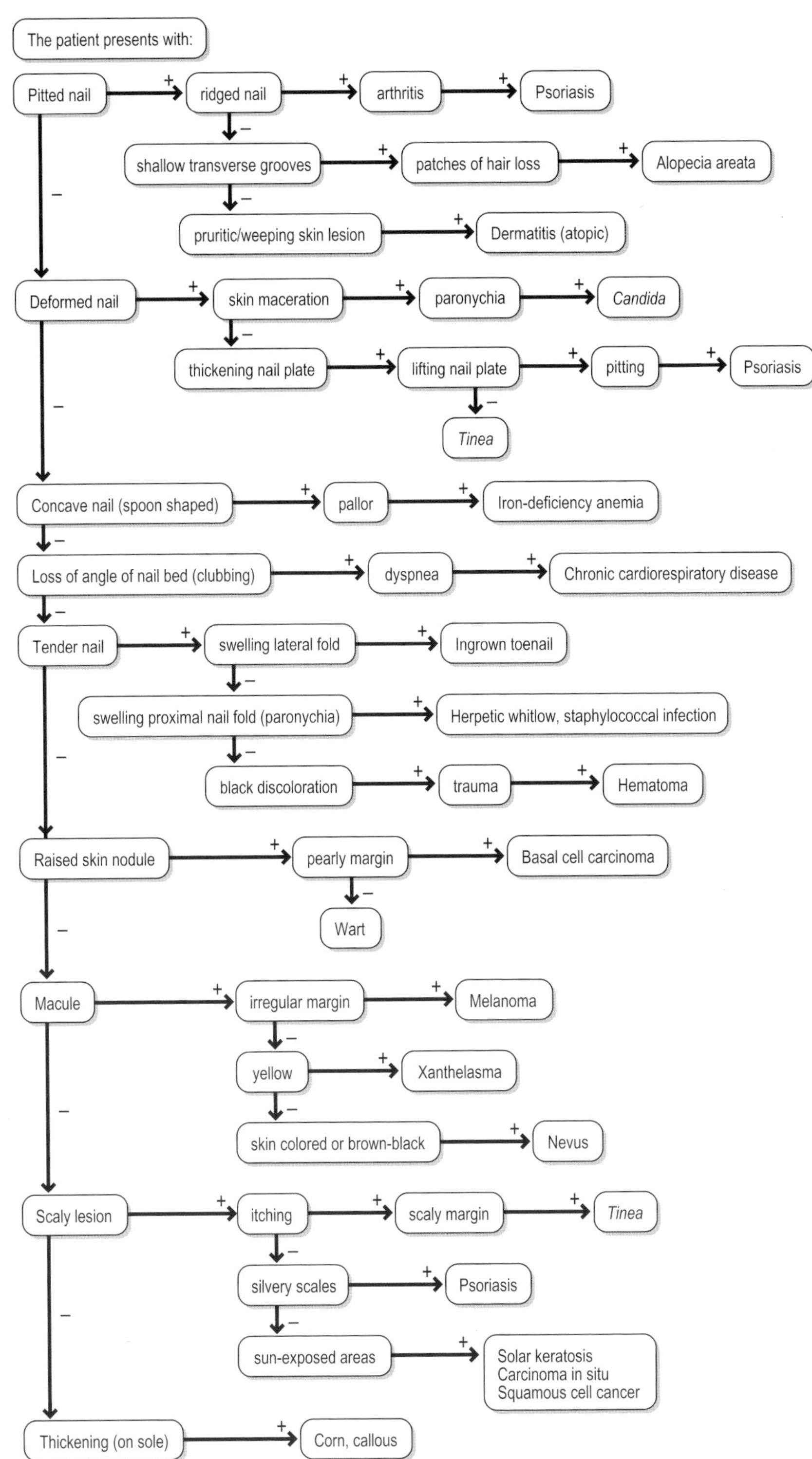

Figure 47.4 **Persistent lesions.**

- the condition is chronic and not responding to treatment
- systemic signs or symptoms are noted
- the rash is worsening
- the rash is generalized (particularly if it is peeling, weeping, or bullous).

FURTHER READING

Cahill J, Sinclair R 2005 Cutaneous manifestations of systemic disease. Aust Fam Physician 34(5):335–340

Chuh A A, Wong W C, Wong S Y, Lee A 2005 Procedures in primary care dermatology. Aust Fam Physician 34(5):347–351

Fawcett R S, Linford S, Stulberg D L 2004 Nail abnormalities: clues to systemic disease. Am Fam Physician 69(6):1417–1424

Feldman S, Careccia R E, Barham K L, Hancox J 2004 Diagnosis and treatment of acne. Am Fam Physician 69(9):2123–2130

Jones J R, Parman C L 2004 Cutaneous manifestation of a systemic disease. Am Fam Physician 69(1):145–146

Stulberg D L, Clark N, Tovey D 2003 Common hyperpigmentation disorders in adults: Part I. Diagnostic approach, café au lait macules, diffuse hyperpigmentation, sun exposure, and phototoxic reactions. Am Fam Physician 68(10):1955–1960

Stulberg D L, Clark N, Tovey D 2003 Common hyperpigmentation disorders in adults: Part II. Melanoma, seborrheic keratoses, acanthosis nigricans, melasma, diabetic dermopathy, tinea versicolor, and postinflammatory hyperpigmentation. Am Fam Physician 68(10):1963–1968

CHAPTER 48

Red eye

CHAPTER CONTENTS

Does the patient have a sore red eye?

Red eyes are often painful. Pain varies in patients with a red eye from a deep pain in cases with a more serious prognosis, to mild discomfort in cases with conjunctivitis, to being absent in a patient with a subconjunctival hemorrhage. The nature and intensity of pain provides diagnostic clues:

- chronic itching/burning may result from local irritation such as atmospheric pollution or be an indication of systemic disease (e.g. rheumatoid arthritis)
- mild burning suggests conjunctivitis
- unilateral pain, especially if gritty, exacerbated by blinking or lid movement suggests corneal damage or a foreign body
- a dull ache and photophobia may result from spasm of the pupillary sphincter in iritis, or from irritation of nerve ending in keratitis
- deep pain may be encountered in conditions of the orbit or sclera (check intraocular pressure).

As a general rule, the more severe or deep-seated the pain the more serious the prognosis.

Is the redness ocular or extraocular?

Redness may involve the eye or the tissue around the eye.

Extraocular redness may involve:

- Both lids. Orbital cellulitis is a serious condition which requires urgent referral.
- One lid. A stye may cause localized redness of one lid.

Table 48.1
The differential diagnosis of a red eye

Disorder	Lid swelling	Discharge	Redness	Pain	Photo-phobia	Pupil	Effects on vision
Subconjunctival hemorrhage*	–	–	Focal	Absent	Absent	Normal	None
Bacterial conjunctivitis	Variable	Purulent, profuse	Generalized	Slight/ irritation	Minimal	Normal	Minimal
Viral conjunctivitis†	Variable	Profuse, watery	Generalized	Slight/gritty	Slight	Normal	Minimal
Herpetic keratitis	–	Reflex lacrimation	Circumcorneal	Severe	Severe	Normal	Variable depending on site
Chlamydial conjunctivitis	Scarring	Serous	Generalized	Slight	Slight	Normal	Variable
Allergic conjunctivitis‡	Present	Mucoid, stringy	Generalized	Minimal/ itch	Slight	Normal	Variable
Foreign body (corneal)	–	Reflex lacrimation	Circumcorneal	Often severe/ gritty	Often severe	Normal	Variable depending on site
Anterior uveitis	–	Reflex lacrimation	Circumcorneal	Moderate/ severe	Moderate	Small	Decreased
Acute glaucoma	–	Reflex lacrimation	Circumcorneal/ generalized	Severe	Severe	Large	Decreased
Scleritis	–	Reflex lacrimation	Focal to diffuse	Severe	Variable, severe	Normal	Minimal/variable

*Often spontaneous. Associated with venous congestion (e.g. whooping cough). Found in persons with arteriosclerosis.
†Occasional tender preauricular lymph nodes.
‡Chronic recurrent condition, may be associated with hay fever.

PART TWO

Ocular redness may be:

- Unilateral or bilateral. A unilateral red eye often indicates a more serious problem than bilateral generalized redness.
- Focal redness. Focal redness may result from episcleritis, a benign inflammatory condition of the deep conjunctiva, or scleritis, a necrotizing vasculitis of the sclera. Patients with scleritis have an underlying autoimmune condition (e.g. rheumatoid arthritis), and are at risk of eye perforation.
- Diffuse. Generalized redness, when bilateral, is usually associated with conditions that do not threaten vision (e.g. conjunctivitis). When unilateral, a foreign body needs to be considered.
- Circumcorneal. A ciliary flush is generally associated with more serious conditions such as acute glaucoma, iridocyclitis (anterior uveitis), or keratitis. A red eye associated with impaired vision suggests serious ocular disease.

The differential diagnosis of a red eye is considered in Table 48.1.

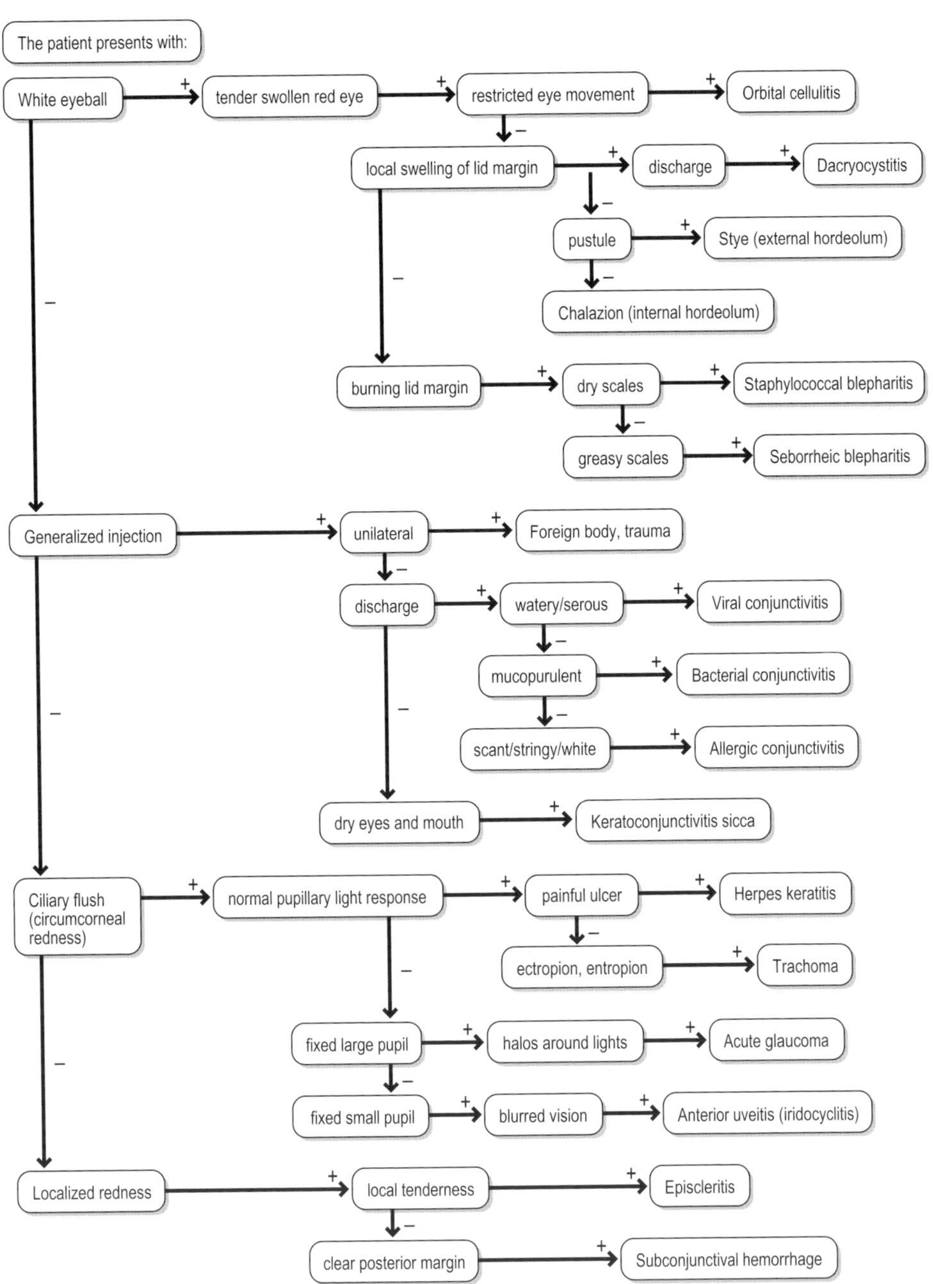

Figure 48.1 **Red eye.**

PART TWO

What is the likely diagnosis? See Figure 48.1.

Does the patient need to be referred?

Referral is indicated in the event of:

- Ocular pain.
- Unilateral redness.
- A ciliary flush.
- Visual disturbance.
- A suspected infection:
  - orbital cellulitis
  - a purulent discharge (unless antibiotics can be prescribed).
- A red eye associated with:
  - trichiasis (eyelashes rubbing the cornea)
  - entropion (eyelids bent into the eye)
  - ectropion (eyelids everted).

FURTHER READING

Cunha-Vaz J, Bernardes R 2005 Nonproliferative retinopathy in diabetes type 2. Initial stages and characterization of phenotypes. Prog Retin Eye Res 24(3):355–377

Hajj-Ali R A, Lowder C, Mandell B F 2005 Uveitis in the internist's office: are a patient's eye symptoms serious? Cleve Clin J Med 72(4):329–339

Lee A G, Beaver H A, Brazis P W 2004 Painful ophthalmologic disorders and eye pain for the neurologist. Neurol Clin 22(1):75–97

Lee A G, Brazis P W 2003 The evaluation of eye pain with a normal ocular exam. Semin Ophthalmol 18(4):190–199

Runny nose

CHAPTER CONTENTS

What is the nature of the rhinorrhea?

Rhinorrhea, or nasal catarrh, are terms used to describe a runny nose. A nasal discharge is a sign of rhinitis, due to acute irritation or chronic inflammation of the nasal mucosa. Rhinitis is one of the six most common chronic disorders encountered in primary practice.

Rhinorrhea may be:

- Unilateral or bilateral. Local lesions must be excluded in unilateral rhinorrhea and systemic causes should be investigated in bilateral rhinorrhea.
- Acute or chronic.

Acute rhinorrhea may be:

- unilateral when caused by a foreign body
- bilateral when caused by coryza or irritant inhalation.

Chronic or recurrent rhinitis may be associated with:

- structural changes which are unilateral (e.g. a foreign body, nasal polyps, tumors, deviated septum)
- mucosal changes which are bilateral (e.g. allergy, vasomotor activity, atrophy, or drugs).

The discharge may be:

- watery or mucoid, suggesting irritation or viral infection
- purulent, suggesting bacterial infection
- bloodstained, suggesting trauma (epistaxis) or neoplasia and the need to investigate.

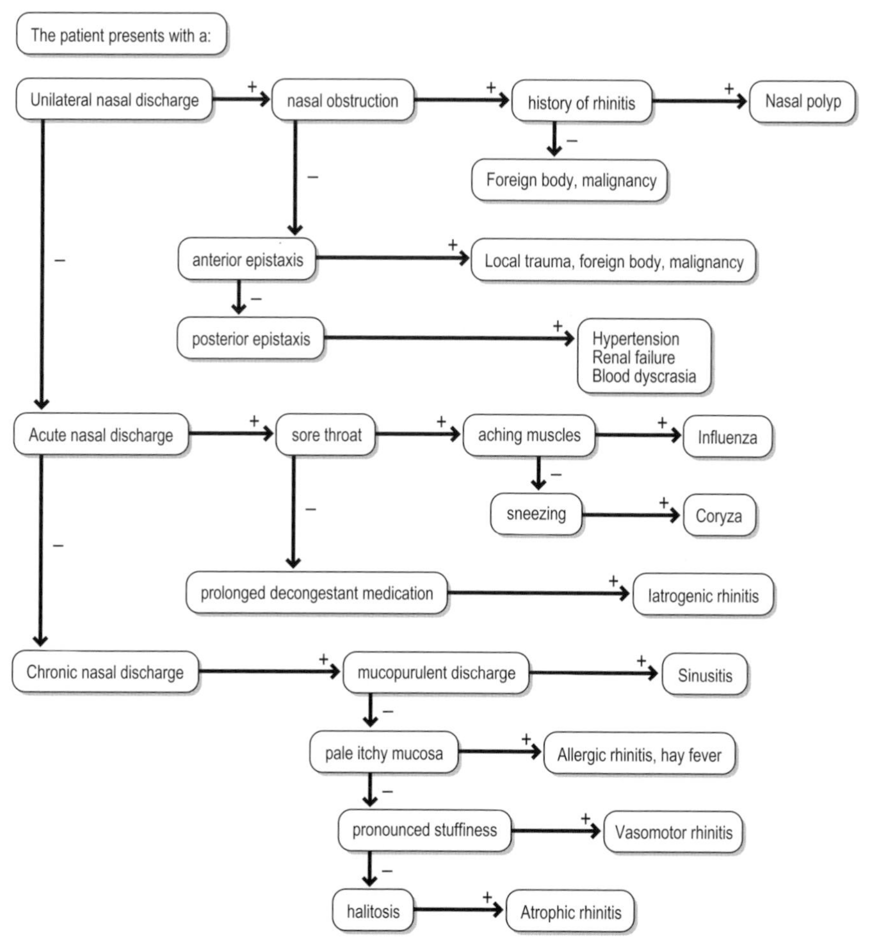

Figure 49.1 **Rhinorrhea.**

What is the likely cause of the patient's rhinorrhea?

See Figure 49.1.

Does the patient need to be referred?

Indications for referral for definitive diagnosis and treatment are a:

- unilateral rhinorrhea
- purulent discharge
- bloodstained discharge.

FURTHER READING

Fendrick A M 2003 Viral respiratory infections due to rhinoviruses: current knowledge, new developments. Am J Ther 10(3):193–202

Greenberg S B 2003 Respiratory consequences of rhinovirus infection. Arch Intern Med 163(3):278–284

Mallikarjun P, Oyebode F 2005 Understanding seasonal affective disorder. Practitioner 249(1667):116–119

Staevska M, Baraniuk J N 2005 Persistent nonallergic rhinosinusitis. Curr Allergy Asthma Rep 5(3):233–242

CHAPTER 50 Sore throat

CHAPTER CONTENTS

What is the cause of the sore throat?

A sore throat is a common complaint in primary practice. Patients with a sore throat complain of difficulty with swallowing. It is usually more painful for a patient with a very sore throat to sip than to fill their mouth with fluid and then swallow.

A throat may be sore due to:

- Local inflammation. The patient should be examined for:
  - Oropharyngeal redness. However, healthy throats may be red, and therefore this is an unreliable sign.
  - An exudate. Pharyngeal and tonsillar exudates suggest infection. In general exudative tonsillitis is more likely to result from bacterial tonsillitis than viral pharyngitis. Furthermore, the exudate of a streptococcal and viral throat is removable, unlike that of diphtheria, infectious mononucleosis, and candida which resists wiping.
  - Petechiae on the soft palate.
  - Cervical lymphadenopathy.
- Irritation:
  - Smoking or air pollution.
  - Acid reflux. A patient with a chronic mildly sore throat, especially if associated with nocturnal coughing, should be investigated for gastroesophageal reflux.
- Immune deficiency. Recurrent sore and infected throats may be indicative of immunological inadequacy.
- Referred pain. A patient who presents complaining of a severely sore throat, without any significant local signs, should be investigated for angina or myocardial infarction.

Table 50.1 **Differentiating a viral and streptococcal throat**

	Streptococcal throat	Viral throat
Pyrexia	> 37.7°C	< 37.7°C
Dry cough, hoarseness	Uncommon	Common
Conjunctivitis	Rare	Common
Rhinorrhea	Seldom present, mucopurulent	Common, watery
Throat	Marked erythema. Petechiae on posterior pharynx	Varies with virus involved
Lymphadenopathy	Anterior, more tender	Posterior, less tender

Does the patient require penicillin?

Over 50%, and possibly 70%, of sore throats are caused by viruses. Antibiotics are not required. About 30% are caused by bacteria, invariably *Streptococcus pyogenes*. It is important to differentiate between these causes of a sore throat, as streptococcal pharyngotonsillitis requires treatment to avoid the potentially serious disease rheumatic fever. Immunologically susceptible patients who react to a streptococcal throat by producing cardiac antibodies can be protected against rheumatic fever and rheumatic heart disease with penicillin. Penicillin prevention is, however, only effective if given early, before the immune system has produced antibodies. Early diagnosis and treatment is therefore essential. Table 50.1 identifies potential differences between a viral and streptococcal throat. In practice, however, it is often difficult to discriminate between the two. Although the child with a streptococcal throat is usually sicker, overlaps between the extremes of these conditions make it difficult to make a definitive diagnosis clinically. A throat swab sent for microscopy, culture, and sensitivity is often the only definitive means of differentiation.

What is the likely diagnosis?

See Figure 50.1.

Does the patient need to be referred?

Patients with a sore throat should be referred in cases of:

- Suspected bacterial tonsillitis. Recurrent streptococcal sore throats are cause for concern, as these may predispose the patient to rheumatic fever and, less commonly, acute glomerulonephritis.
- Suspected underlying systemic disease.
- Suspected complications.
- Difficulty with swallowing saliva (drooling).
- Recurrent severe tonsillitis (> 6 attacks in 12 months).
- Grossly enlarged tonsils, causing sleep apnea.
- A history of peritonsillar abscess.
- Persistence of symptoms after 4 weeks of therapy.

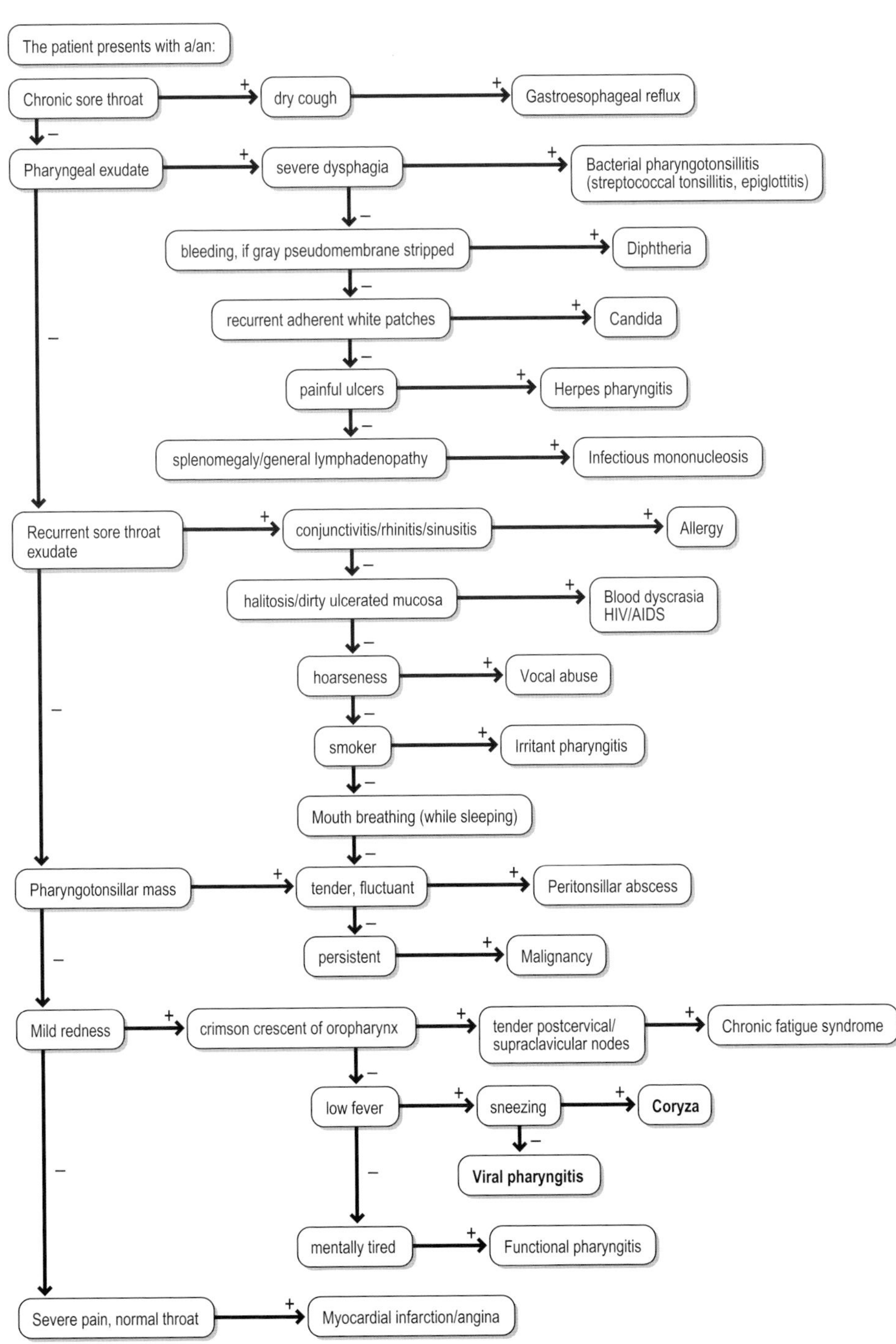

Figure 50.1 **Sore throat.**

FURTHER READING

Schroeder B M 2003 Diagnosis and management of group A streptococcal pharyngitis. Am Fam Physician 67(4):880, 883–884

Vincent M T, Celestin N, Hussain A N 2004 Pharyngitis. Am Fam Physician 69(6):1465–1570

Swollen ankles

CHAPTER CONTENTS

Is there ankle swelling?

Ankle swelling may be detected by:

- Checking for pitting edema. In patients with swollen ankles, exerting thumb pressure over the tibia causes the skin to become depressed (pitted) as fluid is displaced from the underlying tissue. The depression is temporary and the tissue gradually regains its normal contour.
- Noting puffiness in or loss of the depression between the Achilles tendon and the medial and lateral malleolus on each side of the ankle.

Ankle swelling is an indication of edema. Patients with edema may also present complaining of:

- swollen hands (rings become tight)
- sudden weight gain or weight fluctuations in the absence of dietary change
- fluid retention.

Body fluid is distributed as intracellular and extracellular fluid. Extracellular fluid is distributed as intravascular and interstitial fluid. Edema is the accumulation of excess interstitial fluid. The relationship between intravascular and interstitial fluid is determined by:

- The permeability of the vascular system.
- The hydrostatic pressure in the vessel. The total circulating fluid volume and the contractility of the heart influence hydrostatic pressure. The hydrostatic pressure is high (around 32 mmHg) on the arterial side and low (around 12 mmHg) on the venous side of the capillary bed. Fluid tends to move out of the blood vessel at the arterial end of the capillary bed.

- The osmotic pressure of the intravascular fluid. Compared with the interstitial fluid, plasma is rich in protein, particularly albumin. Plasma proteins exert a force of around 25 mmHg and draw fluid back into the vasculature. The osmotic pressure draws fluid back into the vasculature on the venous side of the capillary bed, where the hydrostatic pressure is relatively low.
- Lymphatic drainage of interstitial fluid.

Fluid that accumulates in the interstitial fluid may be:

- An exudate. Exudates are accumulations of protein-rich fluid with a high specific gravity and a tendency to clot (due to fibrinogen). Exudates occur when there is increased vascular permeability.
- A transudate. Transudates are accumulations of fluid of low specific gravity and low protein content. Transudates develop as a result of a hydrostatic imbalance between the intravascular and interstitial compartment.

Edema may be generalized or localized. Bilateral ankle swelling is associated with *generalized edema*. Generalized edema is usually linked to excess sodium retention. Considerable fluid retention may be necessary before ankle swelling is detected. Mild edema is just detectable when there is a 15% (2–3 liters) increase of extracellular fluid. Pitting ankle edema becomes apparent when patients have retained enough fluid to demonstrate a weight gain of 4.5 kg. In severe generalized edema, extracellular fluid can double. Generalized edema may result from:

- Reduced plasma volume due to decreased serum albumin. This is the mechanism in nutritional edema.
- Increased plasma volume following retention of sodium and water. This is the mechanism underlying the edema of renal disease and cardiac failure. The gravity-determined distribution of dependency or pedal edema in ambulatory cardiac patients is enhanced by the increased hydrostatic pressure in the venous system due to an incompetent pump. Lying down causes redistribution of fluid.

Unilateral ankle swelling suggests *local edema*. Obstruction to venous and/or lymph drainage may result from ankle trauma and venous thrombosis. Local edema is associated with:

- Inflammation. Increased permeability of the vasculature permits fluid to accumulate in the interstitial fluid. A fluid exudate is common.
- Venous obstruction or incompetent veins. The hydrostatic pressure on the venous side of the capillary bed is raised, and the normal differential between the osmotic and hydrostatic pressures is impaired.
- Lymphatic obstruction. Obstruction to lymphatic drainage causes interstitial accumulation of a transudate rich in protein.

Persistence of this protein-rich transudate stimulates fibrosis. A brawny edema which, in time, resists pitting on thumb pressure is the result. Malignant obstruction of lymphatics gives rise to the coarse orange peel (peau d'orange) appearance of the skin, best described in breast cancer.

Congenital lymphedema may also be bilateral and present with gross ankle and leg swelling.

What is the likely diagnosis?

See Figure 51.1.

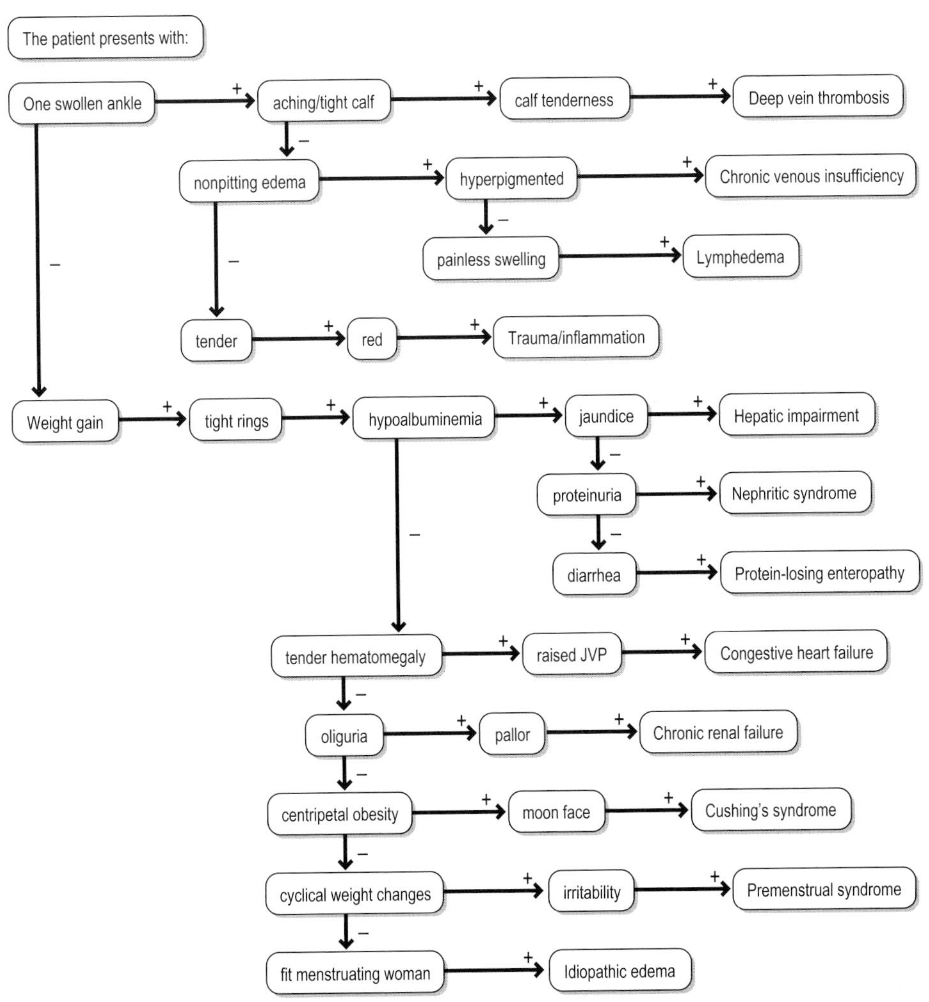

JVP, jugular venous pressure.

Figure 51.1 **Ankle edema.**

Does the patient need to be referred?

Patients should be referred when:

- The cause of edema:
  - has not been diagnosed
  - requires specialist or medical intervention
  - worsening renal failure (potassium level exceeds 6.5 mmol/l, pH < 7.2)
  - worsening heart failure (pulmonary edema is not responding to treatment).
- Underlying malignancy is suspected in lymphatic edema.

FURTHER READING

Leslie S J, Imray E A 2005 Chronic heart failure: a review. Practitioner 249(1669):262, 264–266, 268

Skaner Y, Backlund L, Montgomery H, Bring J, Strender L E 2005 General practitioners' reasoning when considering the diagnosis heart failure: a think-aloud study. BMC Fam Pract 6(1):4

Tremor

CHAPTER CONTENTS

PART TWO

What is the nature of the tremor?

A tremor is rhythmic shaking, usually of the hands or arms. Tremors may be physiological or pathological.

Physiological tremors are more likely to be noted by the clinician than complained of by the patient. Physiological tremors:

- Occur at a rate of 8–12 cycles/s.
- Can be induced in most people by having them hold out their hands for a period.
- Become pronounced in stressful situations, alcoholism, thyrotoxicosis, and metabolic disorders.

Pathological tremors may be classified as:

- *Resting.* A resting tremor is present at rest and decreases with active movement. Distraction of the patient evokes the tremor.
- *Postural.* A postural or action tremor is present throughout movement and is enhanced by voluntary contraction. Patients are best examined with outstretched arms and with the fingers splayed.
- *Intention.* An intention tremor is a coarse oscillating tremor that is absent at rest and exacerbated by movement. It is tested by running the heel down the shin of the opposite leg or by finger–nose–finger touching. Past pointing is a feature.
- *Flapping.* A flapping or metabolic tremor involves slow coarse jerky movements of the wrist. It is best tested with the arms extended and the wrists hyperextended.

What is the likely diagnosis?

See Figure 52.1.

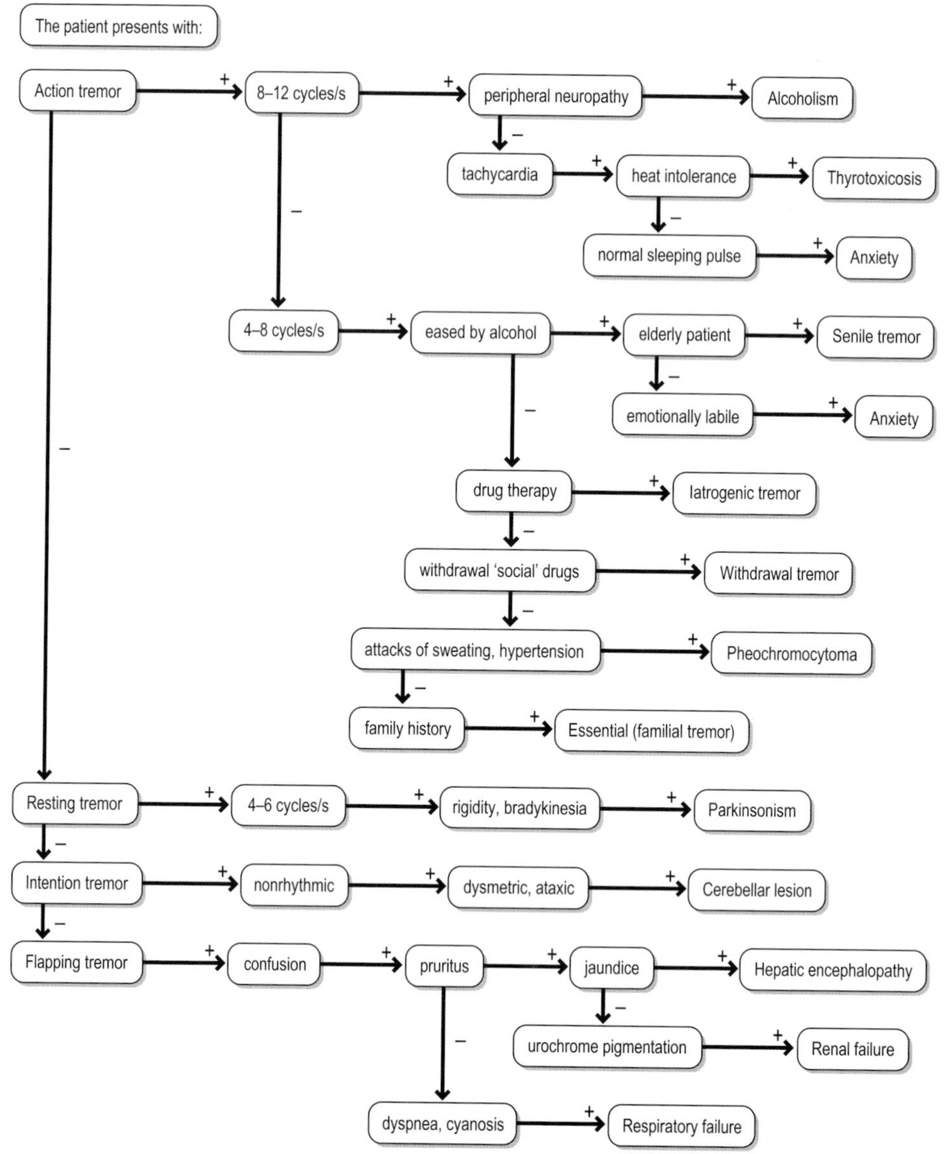

Figure 52.1 **Tremor.**

Does the patient need to be referred?

Referral may be indicated for therapy of the underlying condition.

FURTHER READING

Smaga S 2003 Tremor. Am Fam Physician 68(8):1545–1552

Klein C 2005 Movement disorders: Classifications. J Inherit Metab Dis 28(3):425–439

Ulcer

CHAPTER CONTENTS

PART TWO

What is an ulcer?

An ulcer is a raw area which results when the epithelial layer of the skin or mucous membrane is disrupted. Ulcers may result from:

- Mechanical trauma. Persons particularly susceptible to traumatic ulcers are those with neuropathy, loss of sensation, and those with 'friable' skin due to nutritional deficiencies or hormonal imbalance.
- Impaired arterial perfusion.
- Impaired venous drainage.

Any abnormality of the skin or mucosa, such as a tumor, increases the propensity for skin to ulcerate.

What is the likely cause?

The appearance and location of an ulcer are helpful in diagnostic decision-making (Fig. 53.1). In instances in which the diagnosis indicates a lesion in another system (e.g. arterial, venous, or neurotrophic ulcers), the underlying problem needs to be treated. The site of the ulcer may suggest diagnostic possibilities (Fig. 53.2).

Does the patient need to be referred?

Patients with ulcers that fail to heal should be referred:

- for a definite diagnosis
- for treatment of the underlying cause.

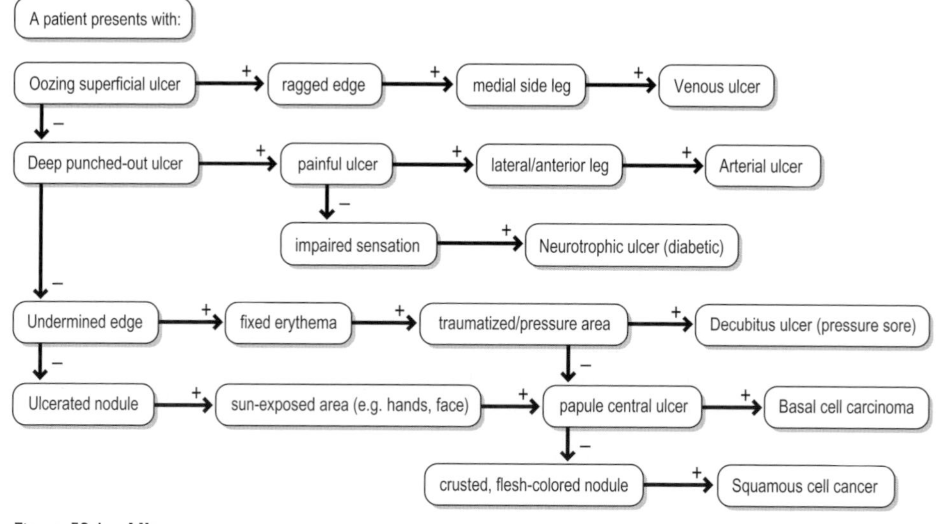

Figure 53.1 **Ulcer.**

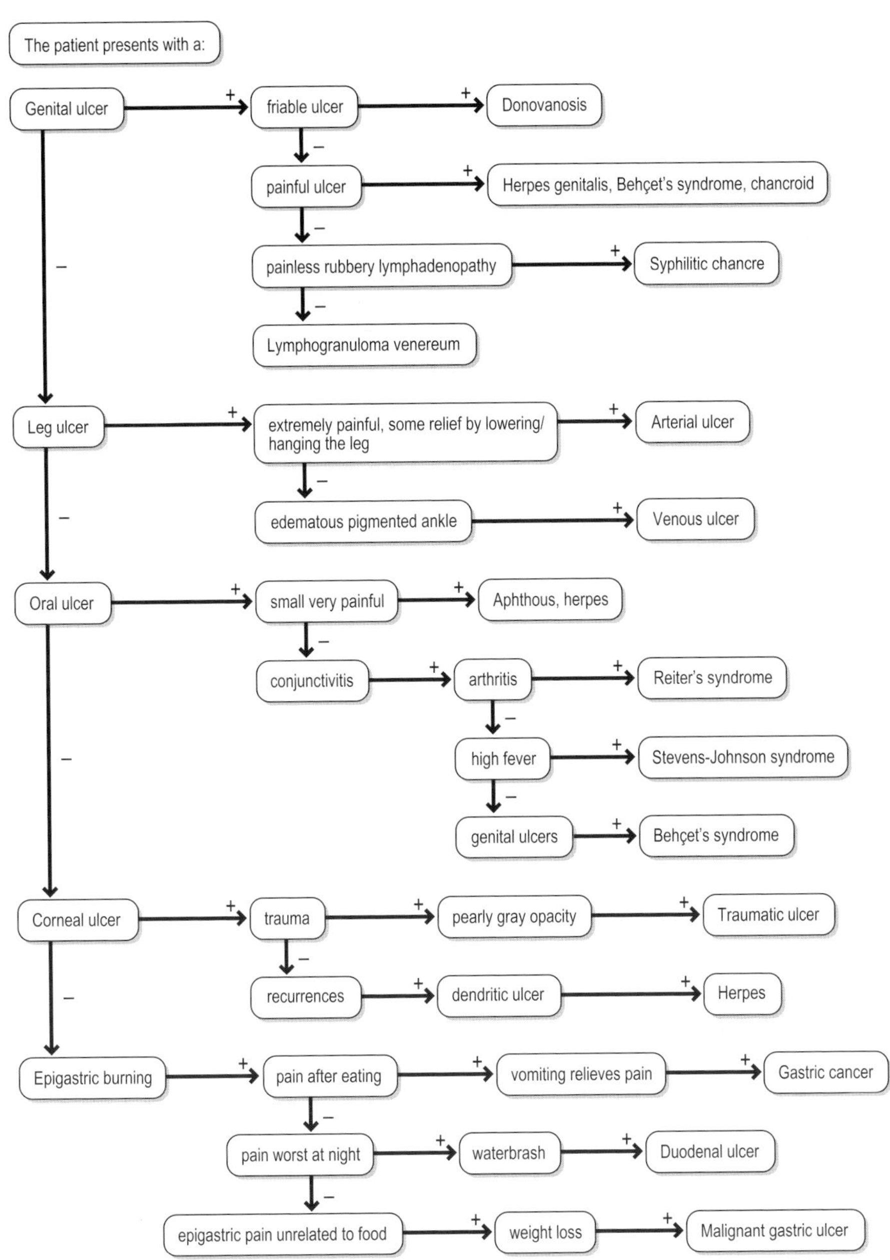

Figure 53.2 **Regional ulcer.**

FURTHER READING

McMullen M 2004 The relationship between pain and leg ulcers: a critical review. Br J Nurs 13(19):S30–36

Singh N, Armstrong D G, Lipsky B A 2005 Preventing foot ulcers in patients with diabetes. JAMA 293(2):217–228

CHAPTER 54

Unsteadiness

CHAPTER CONTENTS

What is the nature of the unsteadiness?

Unsteadiness may be due to:

- Dizziness (see Ch. 21).
- Ataxia. Lack or loss of muscular coordination may be attributable to:
  - neurological imbalances or lesions in the brain, spinal cord, nerve roots, or peripheral nerves
  - muscular disorders (myopathy due to muscle disorders needs to be differentiated from myopathy due to deficiencies with innervation).
- Local disorders. Leg or foot pain arising from local tissue lesions or vascular insufficiency may cause difficulty with walking.

What is the patient's gait?

The patient's gait is an important source of information. Disturbances of gait have been specifically associated with diverse conditions.

- A *limp* may be found in patients with a local lesion of the foot, a musculoskeletal problem, or vascular claudication.
- A *festinating gait* occurs in patients with an extrapyramidal lesion. The patient starts with a small step shuffle, leans forward, seeming to lose balance, and quickly takes small steps in an attempt to compensate. Associated findings that suggest a lesion of the basal ganglion/extrapyramidal system include:
  - slowness of movement (bradykinesia)
  - paucity of movement (the arm does not swing when walking, the face is expressionless)
  - altered tone (smooth persistent 'lead pipe' or intermittent 'cog-wheel' rigidity may be found on passive movement)

- involuntary movements:
  tremor, worst at rest
  choreiform movements presenting as quasipurposive, nonrepetitive, jerky movements of the face, tongue, and limbs
  athetoid movements, which present as slow writhing of the face and limbs
  dystonia, which affects the proximal part of the limb and trunk, causing rotation and prolonged abnormal posture.

- A *reeling gait*, with a tendency to lurch from side to side, is encountered in cerebellar lesions. Associated findings that confirm a cerebellar problem include:
  - muscle hypotonia (muscles are flaccid on palpation)
  - reduced or pendular reflexes
  - horizontal nystagmus
  - poor coordination resulting in:
    dysmetria: movements are not accurately adjusted and past pointing occurs
    dyssynergia: movements involving more than one joint, instead of being smoothly integrated, are broken up into their component parts
    intention tremor: dysmetria and dyssynergia combine to cause finger zigzagging when reaching to touch a target
    dysdiadochokinesia: rapidly alternating movements are jerky and clumsy
    slurred, explosive, or scanning speech.

Cerebellar ataxia may be found in: multiple sclerosis, alcoholic cerebellar degeneration, spinocerebellar degeneration, or space-occupying lesions.

- A *sensory ataxic* gait is broad based with a high step. Associated findings supporting a lesion involving the posterior column include:
  - ataxia, made worse in darkness
  - an inability to recognize limb position
  - loss of two-point discrimination (patients fail to identify that two objects are present when they are placed (or touched) 75 mm apart in the thigh or upper arm, or 40 mm apart on the chest or upper arm, or 8 mm apart on the fingertip)
  - loss of vibratory sensation
  - a positive Romberg sign (patients are unable to stand with their eyes closed and their feet together for 5 seconds without swaying; disequilibrium is worsened by closing the eyes)
  - astereognosis (the patient lacks the ability to identify familiar objects or distinguish their form by touch, e.g. coins placed in the hand are not recognized).

Sensory ataxia may be encountered in Guillain–Barré syndrome and vitamin B_{12} deficiency.

- A *waddling gait*. Patients with muscle girdle (proximal muscle) weakness as in muscular dystrophy have a wide-based gait and throw their thighs forward by twisting their pelvis. Steps are regular but uncertain. Bilateral hip dislocation causes a similar gait. Proximal muscle weakness may also result from Guillain–Barré syndrome, myopathy, or motor neuron disease.
- A *slapping or high-stepping gait* is found in patients with foot drop. Patients with weakness of dorsiflexion walk with their feet wide apart and lift their foot/feet high. In cases due to a lower motor neuron lesion, associated findings include:
  - muscle weakness or paralysis
  - loss of muscle tone (flaccidity)
  - muscle atrophy (wasting is detected within 14–21 days of the lesion developing, in time muscle contractures may develop)
  - loss of reflexes.
- A *foot-dragging or hemiplegic gait*. On the affected side, the arm is flexed and stationary, the hip and knee are poorly flexed, and the leg is swung out, with toes laterally, while walking. Patients with a cerebral lesion tend to walk by dragging the foot in a semicircle on the affected side. Signs of an upper motor lesion are confined to one side of the body.
- A *spastic gait*. The leg is held stiffly and walking is jerky with short steps. The whole foot is dragged over the floor.
- A *scissor gait*. Spasticity of the lower limbs with adductor spasm tends to cause the legs to cross. Legs are held close together and the feet are further apart. Scissor gait is found in spastic paraplegia and cerebral palsy.

An upper motor neuron lesion may present with:

- Muscle weakness
- Increased muscle tone (spasticity). 'Clasp-knife' rigidity is demonstrated by increased resistance to passive movements, which is maximal at the beginning of the movement, smoothly sustained, and then suddenly released.
- Hyperreflexia.
- A Babinski reflex (extensor planter response).
- Absence of muscle atrophy.
- A hemiplegic, spastic, or scissor gait, depending on the nature of the upper motor neuron lesion.

What is the likely diagnosis?

See Figure 54.1.

Does the patient need to be referred?

Referral is recommended for:

- children with an undiagnosed limp
- specialist intervention, where indicated.

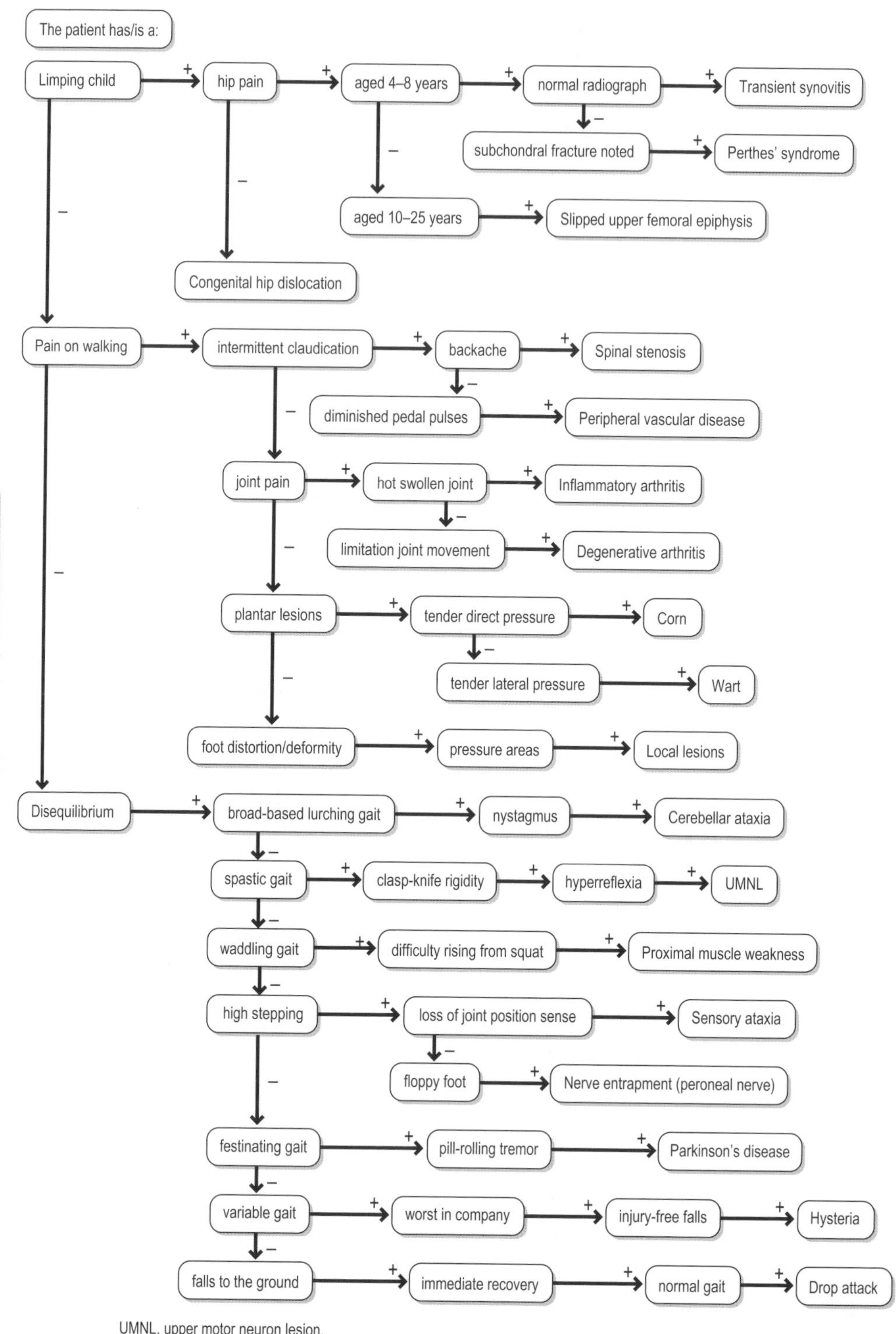

Figure 54.1 **Unsteadiness.**

FURTHER READING

Perlman S L 2004 Symptomatic and disease-modifying therapy for the progressive ataxias. Neurologist 10(5):275–289

Urinary frequency

CHAPTER CONTENTS

PART TWO

Is there urinary frequency?

In this text, urinary frequency is the subjective assessment of a patient who feels they are passing urine more often than usual. The patient may be aware of urinary frequency due to their sleep being disturbed by nocturia (passing urine at night). They may be aware of a full bladder and needing to pass large volumes of urine, or of frequently passing small volumes of urine, either because of associated burning or due to uncontrolled leakage. In establishing the nature of urinary frequency it is important to determine the volume of urine passed on each occasion. Urine may be passed with increased frequency if:

- Small volumes of urine are passed with increased frequency. This may be attributable to:
  - Irritation of the urinary tract mucosa. Associated findings are urgency and dysuria. Pain is worst:
    at the end of micturition in patients with cystitis or bladder infections
    at the beginning of micturition in patients with urethritis
    either at the beginning or the end of micturition accompanied by an 'external' discomfort in vaginal infections.
  - Stress incontinence. Increased intra-abdominal pressure may result in the uncontrolled leakage of small volumes of urine from a full bladder due to urethral sphincter incompetence. Patients 'leak' small volumes of urine when sneezing or coughing.
- An increased volume of urine is passed. Although polyuria, the passage of more than 2500 ml of urine in 24 hours, merely implies increased urinary volume, the passage of this increased volume may result in increased frequency. Oliguria is the

passage of less than 400 ml of urine in 24 hours, and anuria is the passage of less than 100 ml in 24 hours. Polyuria may result from:
  - An increased intake of fluids. Patients complain of thirst, and polydipsia (increased drinking) is noted. A number of endocrine disorders may cause polyuria and polydipsia.
  - An inability of the kidneys to concentrate urine. A light-colored urine of fixed specific gravity (isosthenuria) is passed regardless of the volume of fluid consumed. Renal disease should be suspected in patients with nocturia and isosthenuria. A lack of antidiuretic hormone (ADH) secretion by the pituitary has a similar clinical outcome (diabetes insipidus).
  - An increased solute concentration resulting in an osmotic diuresis. This is encountered in diabetes and certain stages of renal failure.

Associated findings help to establish whether the likely cause of urinary frequency resides in the urinary tract or elsewhere.

What is the likely cause?

See Figure 55.1.

Does the patient need to be referred?

Referral for definitive assessment or prescription drugs should be considered in patients with:

- Suspected urinary tract infection:
  - frequency, urgency, dysuria
  - dipstick test positive for nitrites
  - leukocytes without apparent bacteriuria.
- Relapsing infections.
- Sexually transmitted disease.
- Suspected urolithiasis:
  - persistent pain
  - recurrent pain
  - worsening obstruction.
- Suspected endocrine disorders.
- Persistent enuresis.
- Surgically responsive incontinence.

Urgent surgical referral is indicated in cases with:

- stone obstruction in a patient with a solitary functioning kidney
- bilateral calculus obstruction.

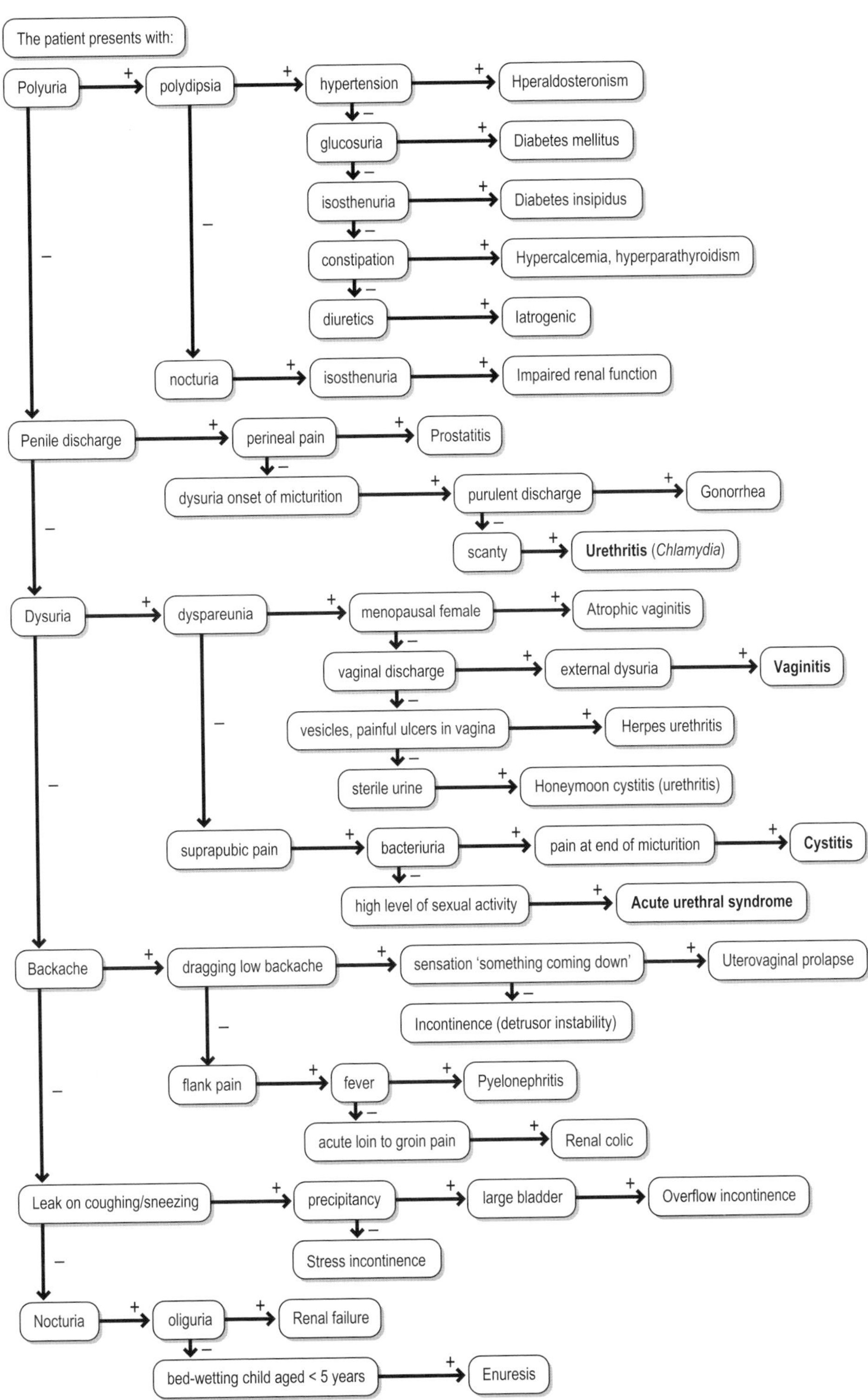

Figure 55.1 **Urinary frequency.**

FURTHER READING

Bent S, Saint S 2003 The optimal use of diagnostic testing in women with acute uncomplicated cystitis. Dis Mon 49(2):83–98

Bo K 2004 Urinary incontinence, pelvic floor dysfunction, exercise and sport. Sports Med 34(7):451–464

Finer G, Landau D 2004 Pathogenesis of urinary tract infections with normal female anatomy. Lancer Infect Dis 4:631–635

Rosenberg M T, Dmochowski R R 2005 Overactive bladder: evaluation and management in primary care. Cleve Clin J Med 72(2):149–156

Vaginal discharge

CHAPTER CONTENTS

Is the vaginal discharge abnormal?

The vaginal discharge varies depending on the stage of the cycle. A normal vaginal discharge falls within the following limits:

- a thin whitish transudate from the vaginal wall.
- a mucoid cervical discharge, which becomes particularly thick and sticky at ovulation
- a translucent thinner cervical discharge before and after ovulation
- a volume that varies from 60 ml to a peak of 700 ml at ovulation and premenstrually.

Some women are unaware of normal variations in the volume and consistency of a physiological vaginal discharge, and present complaining of a discharge and odor.

Physiological or psychosexual vaginitis is diagnosed:

- when clinical findings are normal
- when laboratory findings are normal
- in anxious, introverted, fastidious women
- in women who are ignorant in sexual matters.

Abnormal vaginal discharges are more likely to be encountered in women who:

- are sexually active
- have or have had many sexual partners
- do not use condoms.

Vaginal discharges are abnormal if they are:

- bloodstained
- malodorous

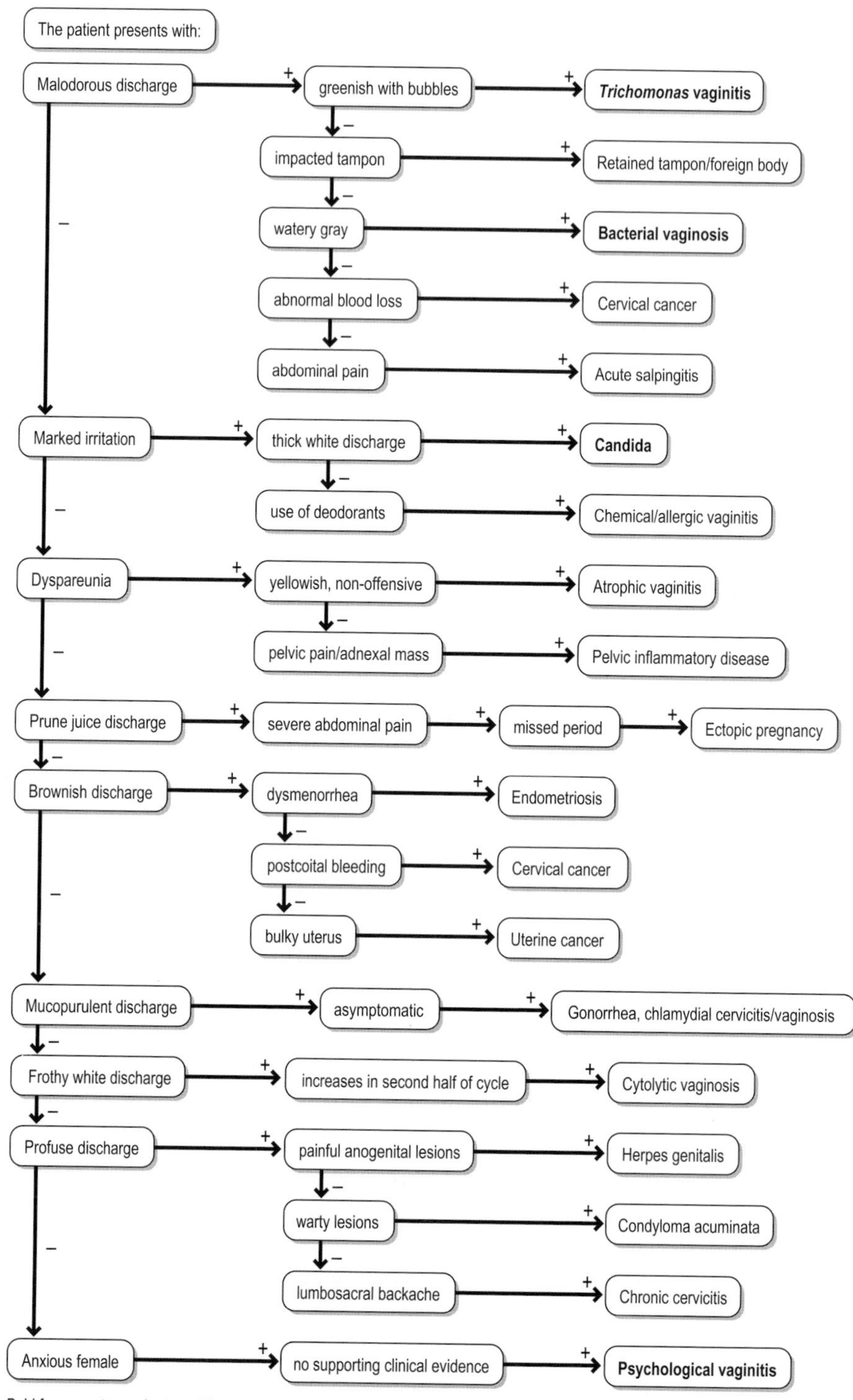

Figure 56.1 **Vaginal discharge.**

- irritating
- discolored.

What is the likely cause?

An abnormal vaginal discharge may be associated with infection, chemical irritants or neoplasia (Fig. 56.1).

Does the patient need to be referred?

Patients with a vaginal discharge who should be referred include those:

- lacking a definitive diagnosis
- suspected of genital cancer
- requiring antimicrobial therapy, if you do not have prescription rights.

FURTHER READING

Anderson M R, Klink K, Cohrssen A 2004 Evaluation of vaginal complaints. JAMA 291(11):1368–1379

French L, Horton J, Matousek M 2004 Abnormal vaginal discharge: using office diagnostic testing more effectively. J Fam Pract 53(10):805–814

Mitchell H 2004 Vaginal discharge – causes, diagnosis, and treatment. BMJ 328(7451):1306–1308

Sheeley A 2004 Sorting out common causes of abnormal vaginal discharge. JAAPA 17(10):15–16, 18–20, 22

CHAPTER 57

Visual impairment

CHAPTER CONTENTS

PART TWO

Does the patient have visual impairment?

When screening for visual impairment, any aberrations in vision, such as flashes, halos, blurring, and double vision, as well as loss of vision, should be noted. When checking for visual impairment in primary practice, it is usual to ascertain:

- visual acuity
- visual fields
- diplopia
- nystagmus.

Visual acuity may be impaired by lesions of the macula or by interruptions to the passage of light to the retina. Loss of the red reflex suggests an opacity between the cornea and the retina.

- The *Snellen chart* checks visual acuity. The Snellen, or E, charts provide information on macular vision. The test procedure requires that:
  - The patient is seated 6 meters away from the Snellen chart. In children, an E chart may be used. Daylight or normal room lighting are required. Patients who wear spectacles keep them on for the test.
  - Each eye is tested separately. The eye not being tested is covered with a card.
  - Visual acuity is scored as a fraction. The distance the patient is seated away from the chart, usually 6 meters, is expressed relative to the size of the letter the patient can read. Normal visual acuity is 6/6.

  - If the patient is unable to see any letters on the chart, rather than recording 0/6, it is more helpful to record the ability to count fingers, see movements, or perceive light.

  The test interpretation is:
  - 6/6 indicates normal macular vision.
  - Less than 6/12 is an indication for referral. Patients who are unable to read the 6/12 line are not granted a driver's licence.
  - 6/60 is legal blindness. These patients cannot read the largest letter when standing at 6 meters from the chart.
- The *pinhole test* checks light convergence and is useful in the evaluation of blurred vision. Patients who normally wear glasses should keep their glasses on unless their prescription is for long-distance vision. The test procedure requires that:
  - A 1-mm hole is punched in a sheet of paper (use a pen or large pin).
  - The patient looks at the Snellen chart through the pinhole. The test is interpreted as follows:

    If vision improves, suspect a refractive error due to difficulty in focusing. A refractive cause is more likely if the problem is bilateral and/or either near or far vision, but not both, are affected.

    If vision is unchanged or deteriorates, consider vitreous or retinal disease.

Visual fields are tested using the confrontation test. A more accurate assessment can be made if the patient is referred for a perimetry test. The *confrontation test* procedure requires that:

- Each quadrant of the visual field is tested by comparing the patient's visual field with that of the clinician. The visual field of both eyes and each eye is tested. Care is taken to check both the perimeter of the visual fields and to explore the inside of the 'circle' for blind spots.
- The clinician introduces an object into his visual field at a point equidistant from himself and the patient.
- A finger, or a white or red target is used.
- The test is reported as:
  - Normal, if vision is present in all quadrants.
  - An altitudinal visual defect, if blindness is detected above or below a horizontal line. A retinal problem is likely.
  - Hemianopia, if blindness is detected in the temporal or nasal half of the field. A cortical problem is likely.
  - Quadrantanopia, if blindness is confined to one quadrant.
  - Tunnel vision, if concentric diminution of the outer border of the visual field is present.
  - A scotoma, if an area of blindness is detected within any one of the quadrants.

Diplopia is double vision. Patients with double vision may have extraocular or ocular lesions. If the images overlap an ocular lesion is likely, including:

- A refractive error. This is corrected by the pin-hole test.
- A cataract. The red reflex is absent.

If the images are separate, ocular malalignment from impaired extraorbital musculature is more likely. Tests used to ascertain double vision due to an extraocular source are:

- The *cover test* screens for a latent squint. The test procedure is to ask the patient to focus on an object with the one eye covered, and then remove the cover. If the covered eye moves on removing the cover, a latent squint has been exposed.
- The *H-test*: checks eye movement by activating the extraocular muscles. The test procedure is to test each of the extraocular muscles by asking the patient to gaze in the direction that muscle moves the eyeball. The test interpretation is as follows:
  - Failure of the eye tested to swivel inferomedially suggests a lesion of the superior oblique muscle or the trochlear nerve.
  - Failure of the eye tested to swivel laterally suggests a lesion of the lateral rectus muscle or the abducent nerve.
  - Failure of the eye tested to move in all directions suggests a neural lesion or a problem with one of the muscles innervated by the oculomotor nerve.

Nystagmus is a series of rhythmic oscillations of the eye. The direction of nystagmus is defined by the direction of the fast component. Nystagmus may be present in:

- Normal people. A fine nystagmus is present when the eyes are voluntarily fully deviating.
- In persons with severely impaired vision. It is described as:
  - Pendular: oscillations are equal in speed and amplitude in both directions.
  - Jerking: oscillations are unequal.
  - Rotatory: oscillations occur as a series of rotations around a central axis.

Major causes of nystagmus are:

- Ocular lesions impairing vision. Pedular or jerking nystagmus may result from an inability to fix gaze.
- Vestibular lesions. Jerking nystagmus affects both eyes when there is an imbalance of labyrinthine stimuli.

Is there an indication for emergency referral?

Referral is always indicated when vision is threatened (Table 57.1). Three fundamental criteria suggesting the necessity for immediate referral in ocular cases are:

- a change in visual acuity
- pain
- redness, particularly in one eye.

Table 57.1
Threatened vision

Characteristic	Threatened vision	No threat to vision
Visual acuity	Impaired	Normal
Visual field	Altered	Normal
Redness	Absent or circumcorneal	Diffuse, focal
Photophobia	++	–
Pain	Deep ache	Itch, burn
Topical anesthesia	No effect on pain	Pain sometimes decreased

Indications for urgent referral include:

- Flashing lights. Flashes that last seconds rather than minutes suggest ocular rather than cortical problems.
- Transient unilateral blindness. Blindness lasting seconds or minutes may be indicative of carotid occlusive disease.
- Rapid loss of vision. Retinal detachment, intraocular infection, or a serious neurovascular lesion may all cause rapid loss of vision.

Is the loss of vision painful or painless?

Loss of vision may be painful or painless. The nature and intensity of pain may provide diagnostic clues:

- Unilateral pain, especially if gritty, exacerbated by blinking/lid movement suggests corneal damage or a foreign body.
- A dull ache and photophobia may result from spasm of the pupillary sphincter in iritis, or from irritation of nerve endings in keratitis.
- Deep pain may be encountered in conditions of the orbit or sclera. Check the intraocular pressure.
- Deep pain on moving the eye suggests retrobulbar optic neuritis.
- Mild headaches may be due to refractive errors, ocular muscle imbalance, or sinusitis, among other causes.

Table 57.2 compares four important causes of visual impairment in a painful red eye. Table 57.3 provides an overview of conditions in which loss of vision is painless.

What is the likely diagnosis?

See Figure 57.1.

The information used to make a working diagnosis is based on the results of the three diagnostic procedures: the red reflex, the pupillary light reflex, and ophthalmoscopy.

The red reflex. The red reflex is the result of the retina shining through the pupil. The test procedure is to:

- Stand 60 cm away from the patient. Ask the patient to look past your head.

Table 57.2
Impaired vision in a patient with a painful red eye

	Conjunctivitis	Keratitis	Iritis	Acute glaucoma
Involvement				
Uni/bilateral	+/+	++/+	++/–	++/–
Anatomy	Conjunctiva	Cornea	Inflammation iris and ciliary body	Shallow anterior chamber
Pain intensity	+ (gritty)	3+ (sharp)	2+ (aching)	4+ (nausea/vomiting)
Eyeball	–	–	Tender	Hard, tender
Discharge	Purulent	Clear/pus	Reflex tearing	Reflex tearing
Vision				
Blurring	Intermittent	Slightly	Slightly	Marked
Photophobia	–	– or +	++	++
Redness	Diffuse	Local	Circumcorneal	Global
Cornea	Clear	Hazy/ulcer	Clear	Cloudy
Pupil				
Size	*n*	*n*	< *n*	> *n* (fixed)
Light reflex	*n*	*n*	Slow	Fixed
Diagnostic aid	MCS discharge	Fine white precipitates	–	Tonometry (raised intraocular pressure)

MCS – microscopy, culture, and sensitivity.

Table 57.3
Painless loss of vision

Disorder	Onset	Pupil response	Red reflex	Retinal examination
Chronic glaucoma	Insidious	Normal	Normal	Cupping of the optic disc
Diabetic retinopathy	Insidious	Normal	Normal	Dot and blot hemorrhages, exudates
Macular degeneration	Insidious	Normal	Normal	Mottling and pigment changes in macular area
Optic atrophy	Insidious	Absent (direct)	Normal	Pale optic disc
Optic neuritis*	Sudden	Absent (direct)	Normal	Optic disc normal, swollen, possibly pale
Central retinal artery occlusion	Sudden	Absent (direct)	Normal	Cherry-red macula, pale fundus with thread-like vessels
Central retinal vein occlusion	Sudden	Normal/–	Normal	Tortuous vessels, congestion, hemorrhages
Vitreous hemorrhage	Sudden	Variable	Variable	Obscured by blood in vitreous humor
Retinal detachment	Sudden	Normal/–	Normal	Balooning of retina

*Pain on moving the eye.

PART TWO

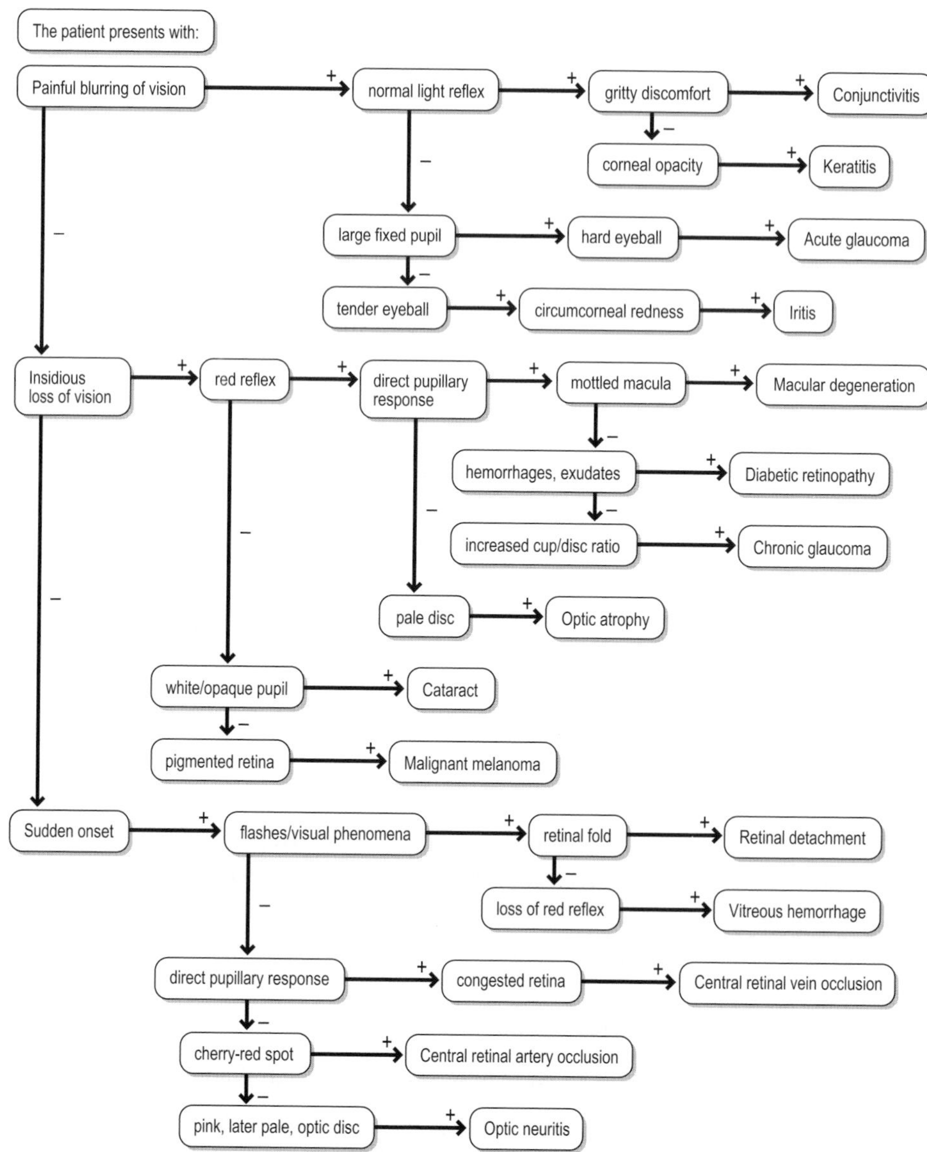

Figure 57.1 **Impaired vision.**

- With the ophthalmoscope at zero, focus the light beam on the pupillary area of the cornea.

In health, a red/pink color is detected. Light has passed from the external light source to shine uninterrupted on a well-perfused retina. If, instead of a red reflex, a white or dark color is evident, then a lesion of the retina, vitreous, or lens is present.

The pupillary light reflex. The test procedure is to shine a bright light into the pupil:

- In the eye tested the pupil constricts briskly and remains constricted while exposed to light. This is a normal direct light reflex.
- In the opposite eye, the pupil also constricts. This is a normal consensual light reflex.

Reflexes are absent in cases of severe optic nerve damage, and sluggish or absent on the affected side in inflammation of the iris.

Ophthalmoscopy. The test procedure is to examine:

- The cornea and anterior chamber by slanting the light beam. Abrasions of the cornea, keratic precipitates (cloudiness), and a narrow anterior chamber may all be visualized.
- The retina. By focusing on the retina, the optic disc, general background, vessels, and macula are examined in sequence.

Does the patient need to be referred?

Clinical findings that suggest a risk to vision and should be considered for referral include:

- Recent uni- or bilateral proptosis (protruding eye).
- A squint of recent onset, or reduced ocular movements.
- A unilateral red eye.
- Corneal ulceration or opacification, irregular corneal light reflex.
- Pupil abnormalities (e.g. a pupil that is irregular or non-reactive to direct light).
- A shallow anterior chamber.
- Raised intraocular pressure.
- Sudden loss or blurring of vision in one or both eyes.
- Trauma with any complication including:
  - a hyphema (bleeding occurs into the anterior chamber)
  - a hypopyon (pus is found in the anterior chamber)
  - corneal or scleral laceration
  - impairment of vision
  - a penetrating injury (do not attempt to remove the foreign body if this is still present!).

Conditions that require emergency referral are:

- Central retinal artery occlusion. First aid is to immediately attempt to reduce intraocular pressure by massaging the eye. The procedure is to repeat the following cycle 20 times:
  - 5 seconds of pressure
  - 5 seconds during which the pressure is released.
- Acute angle-closure glaucoma. Immediately instil pilocarpine or equivalent, if possible.
- Ischemic optic atrophy. Immediately start prednisone, if possible.
- Keratitis.
- Retinal detachment.
- Infections:
  - in the eye (ophthalmitis)
  - around the eye (orbital cellulitis).

Conditions that require referral within 48 hours are:

- Retinal or vitreous hemorrhage.
- Acute maculopathy.
- Retinal vein occlusion.
- Optic neuritis.
- Visual cortex/occipital infarction.

Leisurely referral is recommended for:

- Gradual loss of vision.
- Chronic glaucoma:
  - increased optic cup to disc ratio
  - raised eyeball tension.
- Cataracts. The red reflex is lost.
- Disorders of refraction. The pinhole test improves vision.

Referral for management of an underlying condition should be considered in:

- Hyperthyroidism with eye signs, including:
  - exophthalmos or ocular proptosis
  - myopathy of the extraocular muscles, especially the inferior rectus
  - palpebral edema
  - conjunctival swelling with blurring of vision
  - diplopia
  - retraction of the upper eyelid with lid lag.

Eye signs may progress despite adequate control of thyroid hormone levels.

- Diabetes mellitus with:
  - ophthalmoplegia resulting in diplopia (diabetes, unlike other causes of third nerve palsy, does not cause a dilated pupil)
  - decreased visual acuity, whether by cataracts or transient changes in intraocular pressure
  - diabetic retinopathy with macula edema.
- Increased intracranial pressure detected by papilledema, whether at the stage of:
  - congested retinal veins
  - increased redness
  - blurred margins most marked on the nasal side
  - filling of the physiological cup
  - elevation of the optic disc
  - hemorrhage in and around the optic disc.

Visual acuity is relatively well preserved, although some peripheral constriction of visual fields and an enlarged blind spot may be found.

FURTHER READING

Gariano R F, Kim C H 2004 Evaluation and management of suspected retinal detachment. Am Fam Physician 69(7):1691–1698

Ressel G W; American Academy of Pediatrics Section on Ophthalmology; American Association for Pediatric Ophthalmology and Strabismus; American Academy of Ophthalmology 2003 AAP releases policy statement on eye examinations. Am Fam Physician 68(8):1664, 1666

Schoenleber D B 2005 Preventing vision loss from glaucoma: putting data from clinical trials into practice. Mo Med 2005 102(1):51–54

Vomiting

CHAPTER CONTENTS

Is the patient vomiting?

Vomiting is the forceful expulsion of gastric contents. It may result from local disorders of the gastrointestinal tract or from central stimulation of the emetic center. Stimulation of the emetic center in the medulla causes simultaneous relaxation of the gastroesophageal sphincter and integrated contraction of the diaphragm, stomach, and abdominal muscles.

Vomiting needs to be differentiated from:

- Regurgitation. This is the effortless passage of contents through an incompetent gastroesophageal sphincter. Waterbrash is a particular example of regurgitation encountered in persons with duodenal ulcers.
- Retching. This is characterized by the simultaneous contraction of abdominal muscles and abortive, spasmodic respiratory movements against a closed glottis.

Vomiting may be associated with:

- retching
- anorexia (the diminution or loss of appetite)
- nausea (the desire to vomit).

The nature of the vomiting provides useful information:

- Projectile vomiting is found in pyloric stenosis and raised intracranial pressure. The absence of nausea suggests raised intracranial pressure rather than a gastrointestinal problem.
- Acute, short-lasting, self-limiting vomiting is characteristic of gastroenteritis.
- Early morning vomiting is a feature of pregnancy and excess alcohol intake.

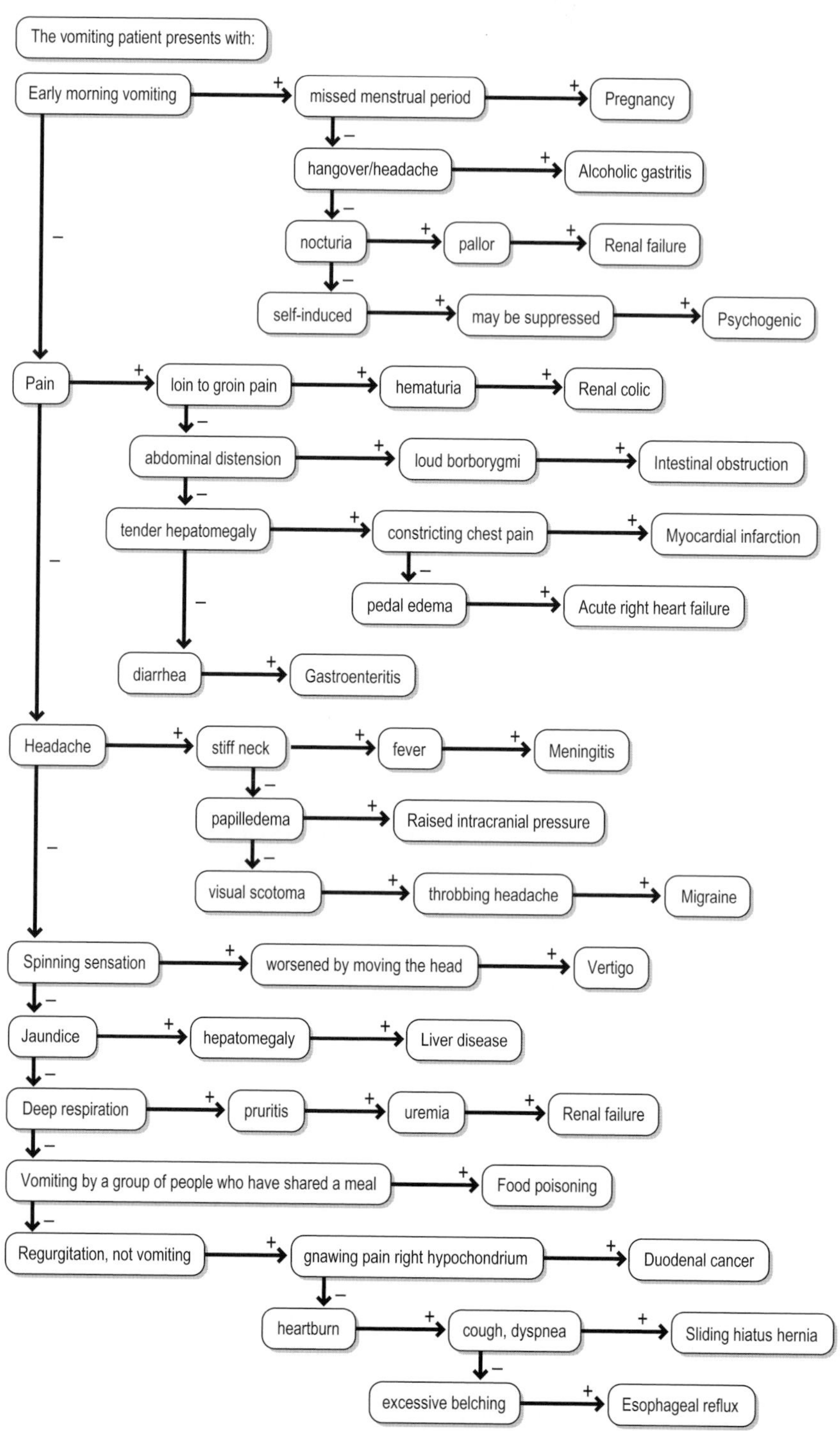

Figure 58.1 **Vomiting.**

- Vomiting that persists for more than 1 hour after eating suggests:
  - an obstruction to gastric outflow
  - impaired gastric motility.

The nature of the vomitus also provides useful information:

- Undigested food. This is encountered in regurgitation from a pharyngeal pouch, esophageal stricture, or achalasia.
- Blood or 'coffee ground' is found when there is bleeding in the upper gastrointestinal tract. Hematemesis must be differentiated from hemoptysis. Hematemesis, the vomiting of blood, is associated with:
  - dyspepsia
  - the production of dark blood mixed with food
  - blood passed in the stool as melena.

Hemoptysis, the coughing of blood, is associated with underlying respiratory disease and the production of bright red blood mixed with sputum.

- Old food. Vomiting yesterday's meal suggests an obstruction to gastric outflow such as pyloric stenosis.
- Bile implies a small intestine obstruction distal to the ampulla of Vater.
- Feculent vomit implies a large-intestine obstruction or a gastrocolic fistula.
- Large volumes of vomit are produced in intestinal obstruction.

What is the likely diagnosis?

See Figure 58.1.

Does the patient need to be referred?

Patients may need to be referred:

- if there is a risk of dehydration
- for specialist management of the underlying condition.

FURTHER READING

Spiller R C 2004 Inflammation as a basis for functional GI disorders. Best Pract Res Clin Gastroenterol 18(4):641–661

Weakness

CHAPTER CONTENTS

What is the nature of the weakness?

The patient's complaint of weakness needs to be explored to establish if they:

- Feel tired. A lack of energy is associated with a general lack of drive rather than the inability to perform specific functions. Questioning finds the patient is capable of doing most things but lacks the will to do so.
- Experiences poor muscle strength. Patients complain of difficulty in carrying out certain tasks. Patients may present with:
  - Proximal generalized weakness. Proximal upper limb weakness causes difficulties when working above shoulder height (e.g. hanging out washing, brushing hair). Proximal lower limb weakness may be experienced when getting out of a chair or taking a high step into a vehicle.
  - Distal generalized weakness. Difficulty may be experienced doing tasks that require fine finger movements. Tripping due to dropping of the foot and dragging of the toes may result in falls.
  - Specific patterns of weakness, as in hemiplegia, paraplegia, and nerve palsies.

What is the likely diagnosis?

See Figure 59.1.

Does the patient need to be referred?

Patients may need to be referred:

- for a definitive diagnosis
- therapy outside your scope of practice.

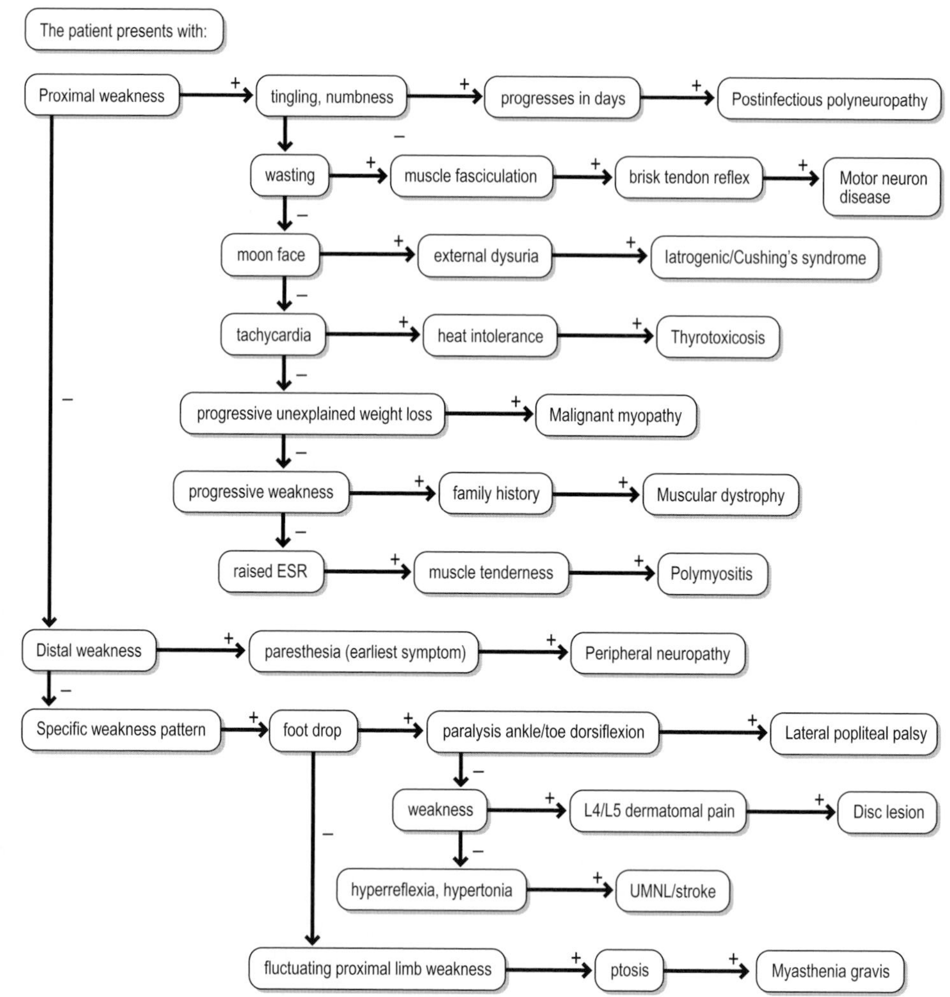

ESR, erythrocyte sedimentation rate; UMNL, upper motor neuron lesion.

Figure 59.1 **Weakness.**

FURTHER READING

Meriggioli M N, Sanders D B 2004 Myasthenia gravis: diagnosis. Semin Neurol 24(1):31–39

Saguil A 2005 Evaluation of the patient with muscle weakness. Am Fam Physician 71(7):1327–1336

Solenski N J 2004 Transient ischemic attacks: Part I. Diagnosis and evaluation. Am Fam Physician 69(7):1665–1674

Younger D S 2005 The myopathies. Med Clin North Am 87(4):ix, 899–907

Weight problems

CHAPTER CONTENTS

What is the weight problem?

Identify the nature of the complaint by determining if the problem is one of:

- A change in weight. Determine whether the patient's complaint of an involuntary change of weight is clinically significant by ascertaining:
  - The rapidity with which the change in weight has occurred. Sudden weight gain and weight fluctuations are more usually attributable to fluid retention than fat. The initial steep weight-loss curve in an individual who goes on a weight-loss diet is largely due to changes in fluid balance. During their menstrual cycle, women may experience fluid retention and weight fluctuations due to changes in their sex hormone levels. Gradual changes in weight, without any associated change in eating or exercise habits, implies underlying disease, which needs to be investigated.
  - The patient's body mass index (BMI = weight (kg)/height (m^2)). A BMI between 20 and 25 is within acceptable limits.
- A change in abdominal girth. Tightness or looseness of a waistband may have led the patient to conclude they have gained or lost weight.

Does the patient show weight gain or abdominal distension?

Weight gain may be attributed to (Fig. 60.1):

- Increased energy consumption. This may be due to eating more energy-dense foods or due to increasing the amount of food eaten.
- Reduced energy utilization. This may be due to a reduced requirement for energy due to a reduction of:

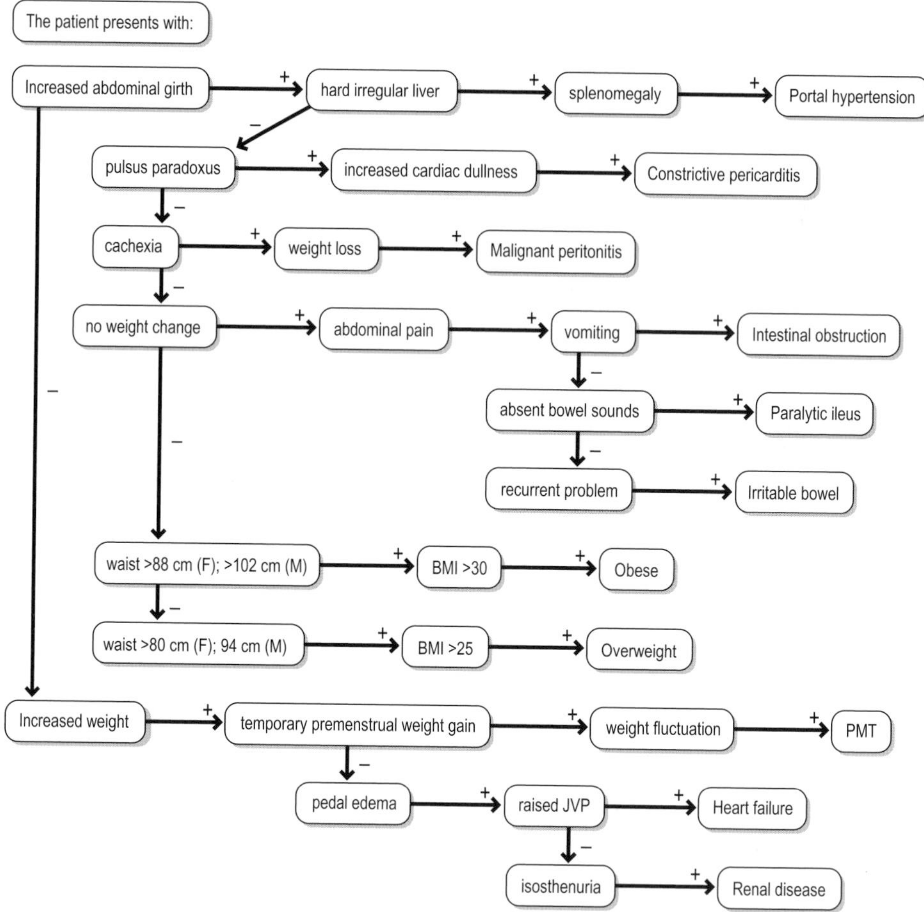

Weight, body mass index; JVP, jugular venous pressure; PMT, premenstrual tension.

Figure 60.1 **Weight gain.**

  - exercise or activity levels
  - the basal metabolic rate, which may result from endocrine disorders (such as hypothyroidism) or loss of lean body mass due to yoyo dieting.
- Fluid retention. Check for complaints of tight rings or swollen ankles (see Ch. 51).

An increased abdominal girth may be attributed to (Fig. 60.1):

- Fat deposition. An abdominal girth in excess of 94 cm in males and 80 cm in females correlates with being overweight. A large abdominal girth is associated with an increased risk of ischemic heart disease. Fat deposition results in a gradual increase in abdominal girth.
- Ascites. Fluid may accumulate in the abdominal cavity. A transudate is found in patients with renal, cardiac, or liver disease. An exudate is found in patients as a result of irritation

to the peritoneal cavity. A large amount of fluid in the peritoneal cavity may result in a relatively sudden increase in abdominal girth.

- Gas. Bowel distension may be associated with an increase in abdominal girth.

Does the patient show voluntary or involuntary weight loss?

Voluntary weight loss implies a deliberate attempt to reduce energy intake with the aim of decreasing total body mass. In order to achieve and maintain a reduced body weight the individual is advised to:

- Reduce their energy intake.
- Eat a low fat, high complex carbohydrate diet.
- Lose no more than 0.5–1 kg/week.
- Exercise regularly to protect lean body mass and increase basal metabolic rate.
- Adapt a lifestyle change rather than go on a temporary 'diet'.

Voluntary weight loss is consistent with improved health.

Involuntary weight loss implies some underlying pathology that requires investigation, diagnosis, and treatment. *Sudden weight loss* suggests a change in fluid balance. This may be associated with a diuresis or diarrhea. Patients with sudden weight loss should be checked for dehydration. *Gradual involuntary weight loss* may be attributed to diverse mechanisms:

- Cancer, humeral substances such as bombesin, and somatostatin play a role in satiety and anorexia. Weight loss may be noted long before other signs of malignancy are detectable.
- Infection, cytokines, such as interleukin-1, and tumor necrosis factor cause cachexia. Cachectin, a product of activated blood monocytes, macrophages, and fibroblasts, causes anorexia. Tuberculosis, brucellosis, subacute bacterial endocarditis, and protozoal infections are significant causes of weight loss.
- Hyperthyroidism. The increased basal metabolic rate, motor activity, and decreased bowel transit time all contribute to weight loss.
- Diabetes mellitus. Early weight loss is due to fluid loss associated with an osmotic diuresis. As the condition progresses, calorie losses due to glucosuria, insulin deficiency, and glucagon excess impair protein synthesis, accelerate proteolysis, and lipolysis. Loss of weight may be an early indication of metabolic dysfunction in more severe cases.
- Medications are an important cause of involuntary weight loss. They may cause anorexia, nausea, and diarrhea and inhibit gastric emptying.
- Bowel motility disorders associated with delayed gastric emptying and/or constipation may impair the appetite. Dyspepsia is associated with weight loss because patients change their diet to alleviate discomfort.

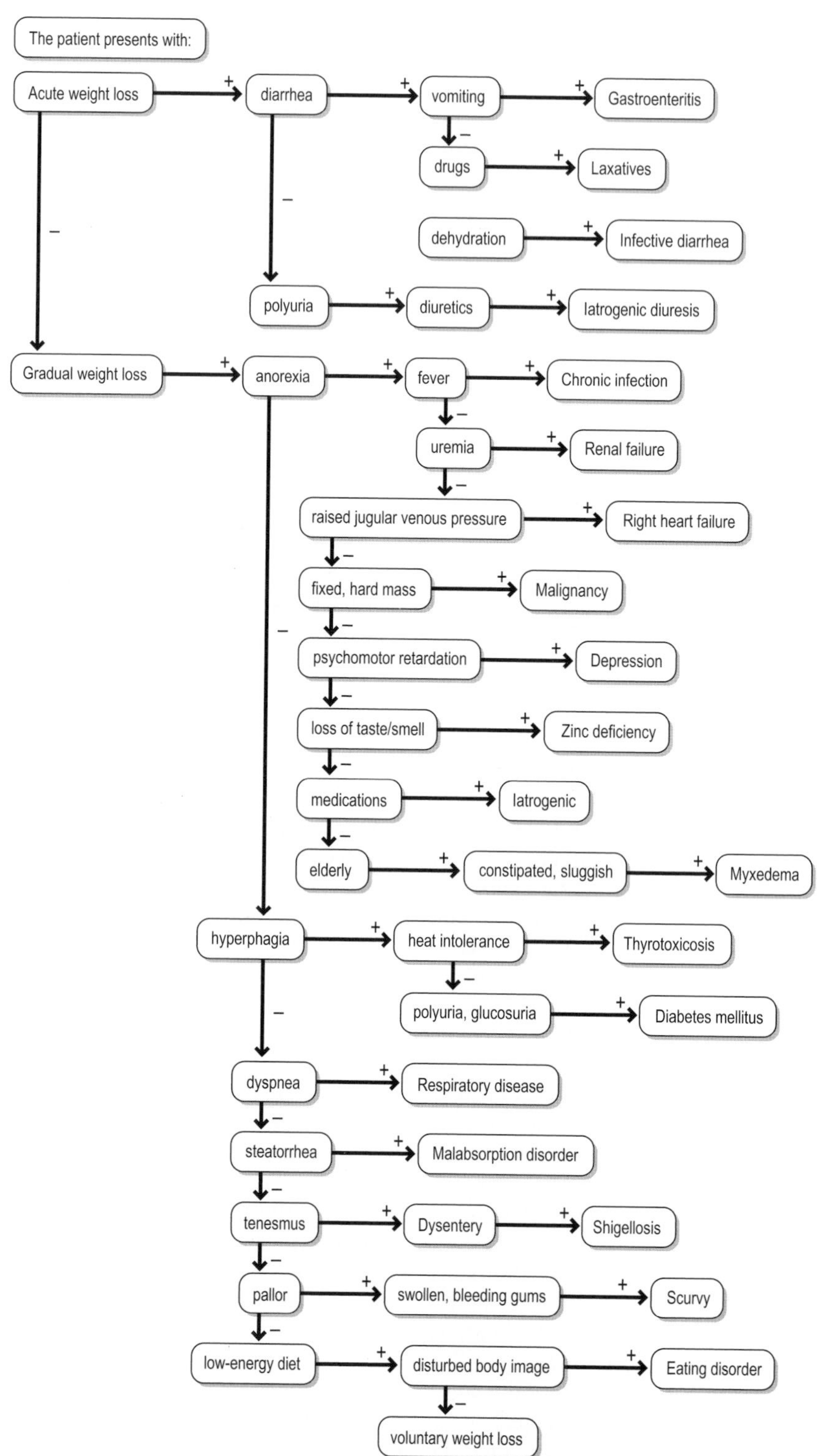

Figure 60.2 **Weight loss.**

- Cardiac disorders increase metabolic demands and cause anorexia.
- Respiratory problems may cause weight loss both due to dyspnea impairing eating and swallowing of expectorate may lead to anorexia. Weight loss along with night sweats are prominent symptoms in pulmonary tuberculosis.
- Old age. Weight loss in the elderly may be due to anorexia attributable to zinc deficiency, a cholecystokinin exaggerated satiety effect, or reduced responsiveness of the opioid system of food regulation.
- Uremia, connective tissue disorders, and depression are also associated with involuntary weight loss.

What is the likely cause?

See Figure 60.2.

Does the patient need to be referred?

Patients who may require referral are those with:

- acute weight loss who require rehydration
- gradual involuntary weight loss of unknown origin
- weight loss attributable to a psychogenic cause.

Chronic infections associated with weight loss include:

- tuberculosis
- subacute bacterial endocarditis
- brucellosis
- protozoan infections.

FURTHER READING

Rohrer J E, Rohland B M, Denison A, Way A 2005 Frequency of alcohol use and obesity in community medicine patients. BMC Fam Pract 22;6(1):17

Diaz V A, Mainous A G 3rd, Koopman R J, Geesey M E 2004 Undiagnosed obesity: implications for undiagnosed hypertension, diabetes, and hypercholesterolemia. Fam Med 36(9):639–644

Hagarty M A, Schmidt C, Bernaix L, Clement J M. 2004 Adolescent obesity: current trends in identification and management. J Am Acad Nurse Pract 16(11):481–489

Pritts S D, Susman J 2003 Diagnosis of eating disorders in primary care. Am Fam Physician 67(2):297–304

Ressel G W; American Academy of Pediatrics 2003 AAP releases policy statement on identifying and treating eating disorders. Am Fam Physician 67(10):2224, 2226

Saper R B, Eisenberg D M, Phillips R S 2004 Common dietary supplements for weight loss. Am Fam Physician 70(9):1731–1738

Wheeze

CHAPTER CONTENTS

What is the character of the wheeze?

A wheeze is a high-pitched musical note that occurs when air is forced past an obstruction. As wheezing results from partial obstruction to airflow, wheezing is frequently heard in association with vesicular respiration with prolonged expiration. Narrowing of the bronchial tree may be attributable to:

- Bronchospasm. Exaggerated smooth muscle reactivity may narrow the airway.
- Excessive mucus production. Mucous gland hypertrophy may lead to increased mucus production.
- Edema of bronchial mucosa. Inflammation and/or venous back-pressure may cause narrowing of the airway.
- Tumor growth.

  Wheezes are described with respect to their:
- Distribution:
  - A localized wheeze is suggestive of limited obstruction. It may be caused by a bronchogenic carcinoma or a foreign body.
  - Generalized wheezing with little daily variation is suggestive of chronic bronchitis, emphysema, or chronic obstructive airways disease.
- Periodicity
  - Inspiratory and expiratory wheezing in a child of 3–36 months suffering marked respiratory distress suggests bronchiolitis.
  - Intermittent, nocturnal, or early morning expiratory wheezing suggests asthma.
  - Wheezing which occurs after lying down suggests pulmonary edema or aspiration.

  - The sudden onset of localized wheezing suggests pulmonary embolism or a foreign body.
- Associated findings. As wheezing is a sign of airflow obstruction, it is invariably associated with dyspnea. Wheezing, although more usually encountered in pulmonary disease, can also be caused by cardiac problems. Wheezes in cardiac disease are associated with dyspnea which is:
  - largely inspiratory
  - develops rapidly
  - mainly experienced on exertion.

Wheezing in pulmonary disease is not aggravated by lying down. The severity of the underlying pulmonary disease is best gauged by the variability of peak flow and the minimum peak flow rate. The maximum peak flow rate is an index of best lung function.

Is the patient acutely distressed?

Severe bronchospasm is suggested by:

- Severe dyspnea. This presents as:
  - breathlessness when sitting
  - speaking using words (breathlessness prevents the use of phrases or sentences)
  - increasing chest tightness.
- A notably reduced air entry. This is detected as:
  - a silent chest
  - a peak flowmeter reading of <50 l/min in children or <200 l/min in adults, or <40% of predicted normal.
- A loud wheeze or a wheeze that becomes quiet.
- Cyanosis.
- Use of accessory muscles of respiration.
- Sternal retraction in young children.
- Confusion/altered consciousness.
- Pulsus paradoxus. A fluctuation of arterial pressure of more than 15 mmHg during the respiratory cycle indicates impaired outflow of blood from the lungs into the left ventricle.
- Signs of hypoxia:
  - restlessness
  - tachypnea
  - a pulse rate of >140/min in children or >110/min in adults.

During an acute attack of bronchospasm, before specific therapy takes effect, the patient should be assisted to resist the gulping inspiration and forced expiration, which enhances air trapping, by instructing the patient to:

- Lean forward on their forearms (not hands).
- Flex at the hips to facilitate diaphragmatic movement by relaxing the abdominal wall.
- Avoid coughing.
- Huff (i.e. giving hard sharp wheezy expirations to clear the bronchial tree).

PART TWO

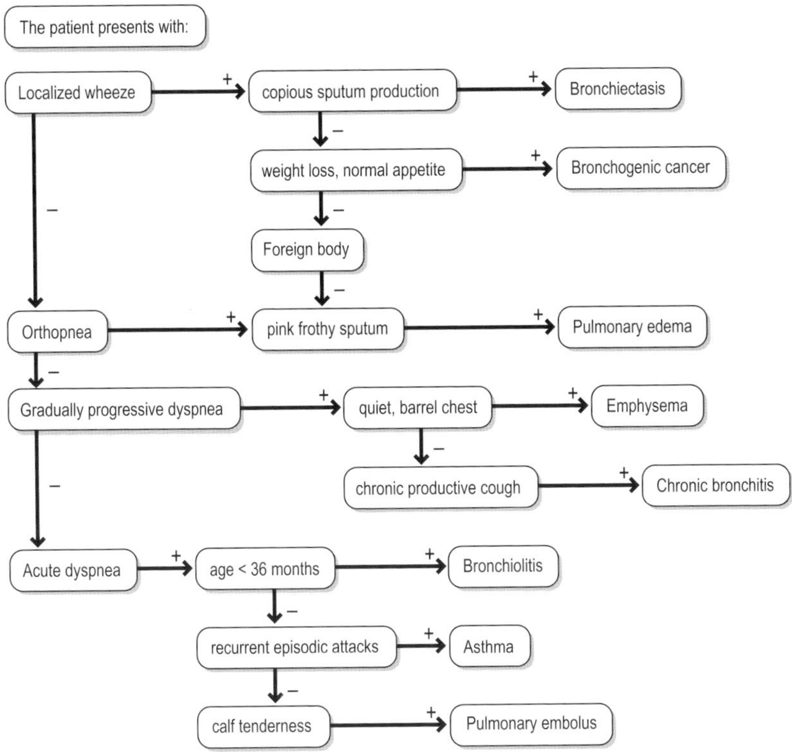

Figure 61.1 **Wheeze.**

- Breathe abdominally. With the chest relaxed and the abdomen flat, stand with the head up, the chin, shoulder, and chest relaxed downwards, the buttocks tucked slightly in, and the weight of the body tilted slightly forward.
- Alternate between huffing and abdominal breathing.

Check that any bronchodilator is being correctly inhaled. Common errors in use of metered-dose inhalers include:

- failure to synchronize the inhaler release with a steady, deep inhalation
- attempting more than one puff in a single breath
- omission of the necessary 10-second breathhold after inhaling.

What is the likely cause?

See Figure 61.1.

Does the patient need to be referred?

Patients should be referred for definitive diagnosis when they have a:

- persistent localized wheeze
- wheeze associated with:
  - hemoptysis
  - unexplained dyspnea
  - respiratory distress.

PART TWO

FURTHER READING

Hewitt J, Smeeth L, Bulpitt C J, Tulloch A J, Fletcher A E 2005 Respiratory symptoms in older people and their association with mortality. Thorax 60(4):331–334

Lilly C M 2005 Diversity of asthma: evolving concepts of pathophysiology and lessons from genetics. J Allergy Clin Immunol 115(4 Suppl): S526–531

Schonberger H, van Schayck O, Muris J, Bor H, van den Hoogen H, Knottnerus A, van Weel C 2004 Towards improving the accuracy of diagnosing asthma in early childhood. Eur J Gen Pract 10(4):138–145, 151

Tan W C 2005 Viruses in asthma exacerbations. Curr Opin Pulm Med 11(1):21–26

PART

3

Clinical conditions

PART THREE

ABORTION

Abortion should be investigated in a woman who presents with:

- central lower abdominal cramps
- a recently missed period followed by a heavy 'period'
- bright red vaginal bleeding.

ACHALASIA CARDIA

Achalasia cardia presents with:

- dysphagia which:
  - has a very gradual onset
  - is for liquids and solids
  - is most pronounced for liquids
  - fluctuates
  - progresses over years
- an inability to belch
- regurgitation
- substernal pain.

Definitive diagnosis can be made by:

- asking the patient to swallow a bolus of water (>10 ml) while lying down.
- auscultating the stomach and noting the time taken between swallowing and the 'squelch' as the liquid bolus enters the stomach.

If the bolus takes 30 seconds or more to enter the stomach, achalasia is diagnosed. This test for achalasia is 100% sensitive and 88% specific.

ACNE

- Acne vulgaris is a common condition caused by inflammation of the sebaceous glands. It is usually worst around adolescence when androgen levels increase. The lesions of acne progress through a number of phases:
  - *Comedos*. Excessive sebum production is trapped under a plug of keratin in the duct of the gland, resulting in the formation of papules. Open comedos are called *blackheads*, closed comedos are termed *whiteheads*.
  - *Pustules or pimples*. Lipases break down the sebum and release free fatty acids, which act as irritants and provoke an inflammatory reaction.
  - *Cysts*. Breakdown of the sebum results in cyst formation.
- Lesions resolve slowly, often leaving scars.

Lesions occur mainly over the face, neck, upper chest, back, and shoulders.

ACOUSTIC NEUROMA

Patients present with:

- early sensorineural hearing loss
- early vertigo
- dizziness and unsteadiness.

Involvement of the Vth and VIIth cranial nerves occurs late in the disease.

ACROMEGALY

- See: *Gigantism and acromegaly.*

ACROMIOCLAVICULAR SUBLUXATION

Usually caused by falling on the shoulder, elbow, or outstretched arm. Patients present, on the affected side, with:

- shoulder pain
- minimal arm elevation
- the hand of the unaffected side supporting the arm
- elevation of the distal end of the clavicle.

Analgesics and a St John arm sling with mobilization as soon as possible in cases of partial separation. Complete separation requires repositioning and bandaging.

ACUTE IRITIS (ANTERIOR UVEITIS)

Patients present with:

- a red painful eye
- photophobia
- decreased vision
- a constricted pupil
- a sluggish direct light reflex.

ADENOMYOSIS

Uterine endometriosis presents with:

- menorrhagia
- congestive dysmenorrhea:
  - pain starts about 7 days before the next menses
  - heavy, dull pain in the lower abdomen
  - pain progressively worsens until the onset of menses
  - pain is felt in the pelvis and lower back.
- anemia
- infertility.

ADHESIVE CAPSULITIS (FROZEN SHOULDER)

Subacute inflammation of the rotator cuff results in:

- pain which:
  - is constant, deep, and throbbing
  - is located around the shoulder and radiates to the outer arm
  - worsens so that the patient cannot sleep on the affected side
  - disappears with ankylosis of the shoulder joint
- progressive limitation of active and passive shoulder movement
- associated muscle atrophy.

ADRENOGENITAL SYNDROME

In addition to adrenal hyperplasia and/or tumors, syndromes of androgen excess may result from ovarian, placental, and hypothalamic–pituitary disorders. Clinical manifestations include:

- menstrual disorders
- hirsutism
- acne
- balding
- hoarse voice
- clitoral enlargement
- laboratory findings include elevated levels of 17-ketosteroids.

AGRANULOCYTOSIS

Leukopenia renders patients susceptible to infection. Agranulocytosis presents with:

- fever, chills, weakness
- painful oral lesions:
  - sore throat
  - oral ulcers

- skin lesions:
  - macules
  - papules
  - bullae
- a raised erythrocyte sedimentation rate (ESR)
- low white cell count.

Drugs, irradiation, hypersplenism, and bone marrow disorders are all possible causes of agranulocytosis and bone marrow suppression.

AIDS

- Human immunodeficiency virus (HIV) (a retrovirus) replicates in CD4 (T-helper (Th)) lymphocytes, macrophages in the brain, and dendritic cells of the skin. HIV alters the cytokine system, destroys CD4 cells and sets up autoimmune reactions. HIV infection is followed by:
- A cell-mediated reaction. The Th1 reaction involves γ-interferon, cytokines interleukin-2 and interleukin-12, and causes release of CD8 lymphocytes and cytotoxic killer cells. This response dominates during the phase that the patient is well.
- A humeral response. The Th2 reaction involves interleukins-4, -5, -6, and -10, and antibody production.

Primary infection presents clinically with:

- lymphadenopathy
- a trunkal maculopapular rash
- depression, irritability
- anorexia, weight loss
- retro-orbital pain
- headaches, photophobia
- fever and sweats
- lethargy, malaise
- arthralgia
- diarrhea
- a sore throat.

Onset is sudden and symptoms last 3–14 days. The sero-conversion illness is often mild, and patients seldom present for treatment. The presentation may be confused with glandular fever.

In those who progress to pre-AIDS, the presentation includes:

- persistent generalized lymphadenopathy
- localized fungal infection
- various cutaneous lesions (psoriasis, seborrheic dermatitis, molluscum contagiosum, herpes)
- night sweats
- weight loss and diarrhea.

Full-blown AIDS is characterized by:

- disseminated opportunistic infections
- unusual malignancies
- neurological disease, including dementia, myelopathy, and peripheral neuropathy.

AIDS cases are diagnosed on the following criteria:

- CD4+ T-lymphocyte count < 200 cells/mm^3 and HIV seropositive
  or
- the presence of an AIDS indicator disease
  or
- the presence of pulmonary tuberculosis, recurrent pneumonia, or invasive cervical cancer in a patient with laboratory evidence of HIV (seropositive) and the absence of another reason for immune system impairment.

If the polymerase chain reaction (PCR), which measures the amount of viral RNA in serum, becomes less expensive, this will become the preferred routine test for evaluating the progression of the disease. Tests currently used to assess the progression of the disease include:

- CD4/CD8 ratio
- p24 antigen (p24 like peptides used in immunization)
- p24 antibody
- neopterin (a protein secreted by HIV-infected macrophages)
- β_2 microglobulin (a protein secreted during lymphocyte activity).

ALCOHOLISM

The acute effect of alcohol is determined by the blood concentration:

- at a blood alcohol concentration of 0.05:
  - inhibitions are relaxed
  - judgement is impaired
  - mood is altered
- at a blood alcohol level of 0.1:
  - coordination is impaired
  - reaction time is delayed
  - peripheral vision is impaired
  - emotions are exaggerated.

Blood concentration of alcohol is determined by the amount consumed. However:

- Women reach a blood concentration of 0.05 after drinking less than men. Women absorb about one-third more alcohol from a similar size drink compared to males. The male stomach contains more alcohol dehydrogenase, which breaks down a percentage of the alcohol ingested. Once absorbed, alcohol is broken down by the liver.

- Carbonated alcohol passes more rapidly through the stomach. Drivers who drink champagne reach a blood concentration of 0.05 after drinking less ethanol than those drinking wine.

The liver can metabolize about 0.5 ounces of ethanol (one standard drink) per hour.

In general, regular consumption by men of less than 40 g/day is safe, 40–60 g/day is hazardous, and over 60 g/day is harmful. In women, regular consumption of less than 20 g/day is safe, 20–40 g/day is hazardous, and over 40 g/day is harmful. In pregnancy, 0–10 g/day is considered safe. Binge drinking may be just as damaging as a constant daily intake, although the clinical manifestations may differ.

At 10–20 g/day (1–2 standard drinks) alcohol improves the high density lipoprotein (HDL)/ total cholesterol ratio, but at 20 g/day men have an increased risk of pancreatic cancer. Habitual abuse of alcohol results in a clearly defined syndrome. Alcohol-related disorders include:

- Dietary deficiencies.
- Gastrointestinal complaints:
  - gastritis: persistent vomiting can cause esophageal tearing (Mallory–Weiss syndrome), with hematemesis
  - chronic diarrhea
  - hepatitis, cirrhosis, portal hypertension
  - pancreatitis with abdominal pain and malabsorption.
- Cardiovascular complaints:
  - hypertension
  - cardiomyopathy.
- Anemia due to:
  - bleeding attributable to liver disease
  - dietary deficiency of iron and vitamin B_{12} and folate
  - alcohol toxicity suppressing bone marrow.
- Central nervous system problems:
  - cognitive impairment
  - peripheral neuropathy
  - Wernicke–Korsakoff syndrome
  - epilepsy
  - cerebellar ataxia
  - coma in acute alcoholism, with slow stertorous respiration, a full pulse, and dilated pupils; the patient can usually be aroused.
- Proximal myopathy.
- Endocrine disorders, including:
  - hypoglycemia
  - pseudo-Cushing's disease
  - hypogonadism and feminization.

- Legal problems such as:
  - drink driving offences
  - motor vehicle accidents
  - assaults.
- Psychological problems such as:
  - anxiety
  - depression
  - suicide attempts.
- Family disruption.
- Declining work performance, including:
  - reduced productivity
  - frequent sick leave
  - lateness
  - ultimately, job loss.
- Economic difficulties due to:
  - gambling debts
  - outstanding personal loans
  - business failure.
- Changing habits and attitudes with increasing:
  - unreliability, procrastination
  - forgetfulness, excuses, and lies.

Alcohol withdrawal results in:

- tremors
- sweating
- nausea
- dry retching
- affective disturbances (fear, tension, anxiety, depression).

ALDOSTERONISM

See: *Hyperaldosteronism*.

ALOPECIA

Alopecia, or baldness, may be scarring or nonscarring.

Scarring alopecias are irreversible and permanent. They may result from trauma, severe infection, scleroderma, or chronic discoid lupus erythematosus.

Nonscarring alopecia may be attributable to diverse causes. It may be generalized (alopecia universalis), patchy (alopecia areata) or complete (alopecia totalis). Nonscarring alopecia may be drug induced or associated with various systemic diseases, such as lymphoma, endocrine disorders, or immunological diseases.

Alopecia areata presents with:

- patches of hair loss
- localized areas of complete hair loss anywhere on the body
- dystrophic nail changes, including:

- pitting
- opacification
- roughness (trachyonychia).

Male-pattern baldness is genetically determined.

ALVEOLAR CELL CANCER

See: *Lung cancer.*

AMEBIASIS

Entamoeba histolytica infection results in:

- abdominal pain and discomfort
- rectal pain and urgency
- dysentery (blood and mucus in the stool).

AMNESIA

Diffuse cerebral impairment or focal lesions can cause partial or total memory loss. Recent memory and the ability to form new memories can be markedly impaired when the limbic system is involved. Amnesia may be retrograde or post-traumatic.

AMPULLARY CANCER

Ampullary cancer presents with:

- intermittent jaundice due to sloughing of tumor
- intermittent occult blood or melena.

See: *Bile duct cancer.*

ANAL CANCER

Patients may present with:

- a hard persistent anal mass
- mucoid discharge and irritation.

Definitive diagnosis is made on biopsy.

ANAL FISSURE (fissure in ano)

Patients present with a history of constipation. The lesion starts with a transitory searing pain on defecation of a constipated stool, which becomes a throbbing/burning sensation and/or a dull ache. Pain lasts for minutes to hours and may interfere with normal activity and produce a fear of defecation. In addition to pain, patients describe:

- Bleeding on passing stool. A small quantity of red blood is passed and blood streaking on toilet paper is noted.
- Symptoms that may persist for weeks or months.

On examination:

- A midline anal fissure is noted on separation of the anal verge.
- A skin tag/sentinel pile may be noted at the lower end of the fissure.

The condition is characterized by spontaneous remissions and exacerbations.

ANALGESIC NEPHROPATHY

Patients have a prolonged history of analgesic ingestion of the order of three or more tablets each day over 5 years or more, or 1000 g of analgesics over 3 years. The presentation is one of:

- a history of chronic pain
- renal angle tenderness
- renal colic associated with the passage of sloughed papillae and clots
- nocturia, isosthenuria
- sterile pyuria (white cells with a negative urinary culture)
- hypertension.

ANEMIA

Depending on the severity of the anemia, patients present with:

- pallor
- tiredness
- dizziness
- dyspnea
- palpitations
- a low hemoglobin.

Megaloblastic anemia. Patients present with:

- pallor and the systemic effects of anemia
- a blood film with large red cells, hypersegmented polymorphs
- hypercellular megaloblastic bone marrow.

Two important, nutritionally correctable causes of megaloblastic anemia are: vitamin B_{12} deficiency anemia and folate-deficiency anemia.

Vitamin B_{12} deficiency anemia (pernicious anemia). Patients present with:

- tingling numbness in the extremities
- coldness in the extremities
- later stages, motor weakness and ataxia
- decreased serum vitamin B_{12}.

Vitamin B_{12} deficiency results in abnormalities in methyl or one carbon moiety metabolism. This may be responsible for a defect in myelin synthesis and the subsequent degeneration of the spinal cord.

Folate-deficiency anemia. Patients present with:

- glossitis
- insomnia, irritability
- skin and mucosal lesions
- a low serum folate level (this may be transitory)
- a low red cell folate level and a normal serum vitamin B_{12} level. The red cell folate level is reduced in both folate and vitamin B_{12} deficiency, as vitamin B_{12} is required for entry of folate into cells
- In diagnosing the cause of folate deficiency search for pregnancy, anticonvulsant therapy, poor diet in old age, alcoholism, and gastrointestinal disorders. Folate deficiency affects the intestinal epithelium, which in turn exacerbates the deficiency
- *Other causes of megaloblastic anemia.* Other causes are liver disease, alcoholism, and hypothyroidism. In these cases the bone marrow is not megaloblastic.

Iron-deficiency anemia. Clinical manifestations of severe iron deficiency include:

- pallor and the systemic effects of anemia
- a smooth tongue
- brittle nails
- cheilosis
- dysphagia (attributable to esophageal webs)
- impaired resistance to infection (depressed cell-mediated immunity)
- abnormalities in thermoregulation
- impaired cognitive and work performance (iron is an important mineral in enzymes)
- pica (food craving)
- pruritus.

Corroborating evidence to confirm the presence of an iron-deficiency anemia includes:

- Serum ferritin of less than 15 µg/l. Women with serum ferritin levels of 20 µg/l may have very low iron stores and, although not anemic, can be iron deficient.
- Increased total iron binding capacity. In iron deficiency there is reduced saturation of transferrin.

- Decreased serum iron levels.
- Increased free protoporphyrin in erythrocytes.

A confirmatory therapeutic test is based on the patient's response to iron therapy. In chronic iron-deficiency anemia hemoglobin releases oxygen more readily and tissue hypoxia may worsen in the initial phases of blood transfusion in chronic iron-deficiency states as the hemoglobin–oxygen affinity is restored more readily than the hemoglobin–tissue oxygenation balance. Oral replacement of iron is therefore preferred in chronic cases. The response to therapy may be monitored by weekly reticulocyte counts.

A therapeutic trial of oral iron supplements will confirm a diagnosis of anemia if reticulocytosis is detected within 7 days and the hemoglobin increases by 0.5–1.0 g/week. An early acceptable hemoglobin response is an increase of 2 g/dl over the first 3 weeks. A normal hemoglobin level should be achieved in 8 weeks. Iron stores may be corrected over 3–6 months. In premenopausal women, treatment to replenish iron stores may be continued for 2 years.

Pancytopenia (aplastic anemia). Anemia attributable to bone marrow failure presents with:

- red cell deficiency:
  - pallor
  - the systemic effects of anemia
- platelet deficiency:
  - ecchymoses and petechiae
  - hemorrhage, epistaxis, menorrhagia, melena, and occult blood in the stool may also be found
- white cell deficiency:
  - fever
  - reduced resistance to infection.

The definitive diagnosis of pancytopenia is made on bone marrow biopsy.

Hemolytic anemia. Hemolysis presents with:

- pallor and the systemic effects of anemia, as listed above
- mild jaundice (a pale yellow tinge)
- splenomegaly, hepatomegaly
- cholelithiasis in chronic cases.

Laboratory investigations reveal:

- a reticulocytosis
- a raised unconjugated bilirubin
- increased urinary urobilinogen
- methemoglobinemia and low haptoglobins in acute cases; in chronic cases, hemosiderinuria.

ANEURYSMS

Ballooning of the arterial wall may result from atherosclerosis or degeneration of the media. Structurally, aneurysms may be dissecting, fusiform, or saccular.

Dissecting aortic aneurysms present with:

- Excruciating midline pain which is sudden in onset and usually experienced in the retrosternal and midscapular area.
- Pain radiates to the abdomen, flank, and legs.
- Unequal pulses. This is diagnostic, and an absent femoral pulse should always be sought.
- A drop in blood pressure.

Complications include:

- shock (note a cold, clammy skin)
- hemiplegia
- aortic incompetence.

If the blood tracts out of the aorta, death results; if the blood re-enters the lumen the patient may reach emergency surgery.

Fusiform aortic aneurysms present with persistent pain which is:

- described as boring or penetrating
- relieved by leaning forward
- worst at night.

The clinical presentation of an aneurysm is influenced by its structure and its site. The clinical importance of an aneurysm is often related to its local pressure effects and its propensity to hemorrhage.

Femoral aneurysms may:

- be asymptomatic
- present as a pulsatile mass in the groin
- be associated with a bruit.

Abdominal aneurysms may present with:

- backache
- a pulsatile abdominal mass
- progressive back or abdominal pain (this is a serious prognostic symptom).

Thoracic aneurysms present with:

- an asymptomatic lesion seen on a radiograph
- substernal, back, or neck pain
- local pressure effects:
  - tracheal pressure presents with dyspnea and a brassy cough
  - esophageal pressure presents with dysphagia

- superior vena cava pressure is detected as distended neck veins and edema
- left recurrent laryngeal nerve pressure causes hoarseness.

Prior to rupture *intracranial aneurysms* are often asymptomatic, but may present with:

- headache on effort
- disorders of cranial nerves II, III, and V
- a cranial bruit.

After rupture intracranial aneurysms present as *subarachnoid hemorrhages* with:

- a severe headache of sudden onset
- nuchal rigidity
- blood in the cerebrospinal fluid.

Consciousness is often only briefly disturbed.

All patients with suspected aneurysms should be referred.

ANGINA PECTORIS

Angina pectoris, a condition of transient localized myocardial ischemia, presents clinically with:

- Chest pain which:
  - is experienced as a constricting substernal tightness
  - may radiate to the angle of the jaw, neck, back, left shoulder, or inner aspect of one or both arms
  - lasts less than 15 minutes, usually a few seconds to 2–10 minutes
  - is relieved by sublingual glyceryl trinitrate or rest
  - is precipitated by and clearly related to physical exertion (exercise, lifting weights), cold weather, and/or emotional stress.
- Dyspnea.
- No abnormalities on examination of the cardiovascular system.
- Unaltered cardiac enzymes.
- T-wave abnormality on the electrocardiogram (ECG).

If diagnosis is in doubt referral for an exercise stress test may be considered in patients who *do not* present with:

- unstable symptoms
- high blood pressure
- heart failure
- severe valve disease (e.g. severe aortic stenosis)
- an inability to walk briskly
- serious cardiac arrhythmia
- acute pericarditis, myocarditis, or endocarditis.

Very elderly patients are also excluded.

Variants of angina include:

- *Stable angina*:
  - pain occurs on exertion
  - pain is predictable
  - transient ST segment depression.
- *Nocturnal angina*:
  - pain occurs at night.
- *Decubitus angina*
  - pain occurs when lying flat and is relieved by sitting up.
- *Spasm angina*:
  - pain occurs at rest
  - transient ST segment elevation.

Coronary artery spasm may cause arrhythmias and lead to infarction.

- *Unstable angina*:
  - pain at rest
  - more frequent episodes of pain
  - painful episodes of longer duration.

The patient with unstable angina is at increased risk of infarction.

In *acute coronary insufficiency*:

- the constricting chest pain lasts for over 15 minutes
- pain is often precipitated by a cardiac arrhythmia
- the ECG and cardiac enzymes are normal.

Failure to respond to nitrite spray within 90 seconds indicates an incorrect diagnosis and flags the need for an intensive care ambulance.

ANKYLOSING SPONDYLITIS

Patients present with:

- Changes in the axial skeleton such as:
  - the insidious onset of back discomfort, which persists for more than 3 months
  - low back pain (the sacroiliac (tenderness) and vertebral joints are involved)
  - morning stiffness
  - decreased anterior flexion
  - thoracic spinal fusion (bamboo spine).
- Hip and shoulder, and knees and ankles may also become involved.
- Changes affecting the chest including:
  - irritation of the ribs at the vertebral insertion, with pain radiating to the anterior chest wall

  - swelling of manubriosternal joints
  - chest expansion, which is restricted to 3 cm or less.
- Pain exacerbated by coughing, sneezing, or changing position.
- Laboratory results that show a positive HLA-B27, negative rheumatoid factor, and often a raised erythrocyte sedimentation rate (ESR).
- Associated findings include:
  - fatigue, fever, weight loss
  - plantar fasciitis, Achilles tendonitis, iritis
  - chronic anemia.

ANORECTAL ABSCESS

A superficial or perianal abscess presents with:

- throbbing anal discomfort
- painful swelling
- local redness and tenderness.

Deeper abscesses present with:

- toxic symptoms
- less pain
- tender swelling on rectal examination.

ANTERIOR UVEITIS

See: *Acute iritis.*

ANTIBIOTIC DIARRHEA

Patients who have been on antibiotics, usually broad-spectrum antibiotics, may present with self-limiting diarrhea which develops within 21 or 28 days of antibiotic therapy. When on antibiotics, dietary supplementation with a yoghurt rich in bifidus and acidophilus is recommended.

ANXIETY DISORDER

- A number of disorders have been described that are characterized by anxiety. These include the following.

  Generalized anxiety. The individual experiences:

- A pervading persistent sense of anxiety.
- Excessive worry about trivial or unrealistic problems.
- Free-floating anxiety, which is unrelated to any specific event or situation.

- At least six of the following:
  - feelings of apprehension, an exaggerated startle response, hypervigilance
  - irritability, impatience, sensitivity to noise
  - difficulty concentrating, mental 'blanks'
  - sleep disturbance
  - autonomic dysfunction (palpitations, dizziness, dysphagia, diarrhea, hyperventilation, urinary frequency, clammy skin)
  - motor tension (restless, tremble, myalgia, headache, fatigue).

Phobic disorder. Fear is associated with particular situations or objects. The individual attempts to avoid the anxiety-provoking situation or object and becomes anxious when this is not possible. Simple phobias include fear of snakes, thunder, spiders, or cancer. Agoraphobia, defined as a fear of open spaces, may cause marked incapacity, with the individual confining themselves to their home and unable to use public transport, enter confined spaces, or enter crowded shops.

Panic attack. Panic attacks are experienced as recurrent, unexpected episodes of intense anxiety. *Panic disorder* is diagnosed when:

- No realistic anxiety trigger can be identified.
- A single attack is followed by 4 weeks during which fear of a second attack is experienced, or when four attacks occur in a 4-week period.
- Four of the following are present during an attack:
  - acute dyspnea
  - dizziness
  - palpitations
  - trembling
  - flushes, chills, or sweating
  - paresthesia
  - depersonalization.

Post-traumatic stress disorder. Persons who have experienced an intensely stressful event may revisit the event during sleep (dreams) and waking. Emotionally, they may feel as if the event is recurring, and strive to avoid triggers that remind them of the event. They are prone to the psychological symptoms of generalized anxiety.

Obsessive–compulsive neurosis. This disorder is associated with an inability to control or prevent recurrent intrusive thoughts. It is associated with ritual behavior.

See: Stress, *Hyperventilation syndrome*; Anxiety (Ch. 6).

AORTOILIAC ATHEROSCLEROSIS

See: *Arterial occlusion/insufficiency.*

APHTHOUS ULCERS

The progression of aphthous ulcers is from:

- a tingling hyperesthesia, which lasts for 1 day
  to
- moderately painful erythematous macules or papules with a red halo, which last up to 3 days
  to
- discrete painful oval ulcers, usually less than 10 mm in size
  to
- healing, which occurs within 10 days, without scarring.

In contrast to minor aphthae, major aphthae are larger than 10 mm, associated with submandibular lymphadenopathy and take longer to heal.

Aphthous ulcers are found on nonkeratinizing oral mucosa, and may follow minor trauma. Aphthous ulceration has been associated with: a deficiency of iron, folate, or vitamin B_{12}; dietary allergy; stress; and the luteal phase of menstrual cycle.

APPENDICITIS

Acute appendicitis presents with:

- Abdominal pain which:
  - presents as periumbilical colicky abdominal pain in the early stages
  - progresses to right iliac fossa tenderness
  - is continuous (if pain suddenly ceases, suspect perforation)
  - unrelated to the passage of unformed stool.
- Low-grade fever (98.6–100°F).
- Tachycardia (>100 beats/min) as the disease progresses.
- Vomiting (one or two episodes is more characteristic than continued vomiting).
- Depending on the position of the inflamed appendix:
  - frequency and dysuria due to bladder irritation
  - diarrhea due to large-bowel irritation
  - psoas spasm due to psoas muscle irritation
  - abdominal rigidity, guarding due to irritation of the anterior abdominal wall.

Patients may complain of 'flu-like' symptoms. Patients frequently have a history of previous attacks of abdominal pain.

ARRHYTHMIAS

See: *Palpitations* (Ch. 44).

ARTERIAL OCCLUSION/ INSUFFICIENCY

The clinical presentation of arterial occlusion depends on the artery involved. In cases of partial occlusion of the:

- Carotid bifurcation, the patient may present with:
  - transient weakness of an extremity
  - monocular blindness
  - mental confusion
  - occasionally, loss of consciousness.
- Vertebral artery, the patient may complain of:
  - dizziness
  - motor instability (basilar ischemia).
- Coronary artery, the patient complains of chest pain, which may radiate to the neck, jaw, and arm.
- Brachial artery, arm pain may be experienced.
- Intestinal circulation, abdominal pain is experienced.
- Renal artery, systemic hypertension may be precipitated.
- Aortoiliac artery, the patient may complain of:
  - pain in the buttock and hip
  - thigh pain precipitated by calf extension
  - pain that is aggravated by exercise and relieved by rest
  - impotence, in males.
- Femoropopliteal artery, patients experience intermittent claudication of the calf and foot.

Diseases attributable to atherosclerosis which are particularly prevalent are those affecting the coronary and lower limb vasculature. Occlusive peripheral vascular disease differs from functional arterial disorders in that, in the latter, the pulse is always present.

The clinical presentation of occlusive arterial disease is determined by:

- the extent of occlusion
- the collateral circulation
- the functional demands of the area.

Patients present with impaired limb perfusion and evidence of ischemia.

Impaired limb perfusion. Blood flow is determined by:

- Palpation of pulses (femoral, popliteal, dorsalis pedis, posterior tibial). Absent pulses are highly suggestive of atherosclerotic vascular disease.
- Testing pedal color change. Clinical findings suggesting impaired perfusion include:
  - pallor developing in a leg that is only slightly raised
  - pallor developing rapidly on high elevation of the leg or foot
  - dependency rubor (beefy redness) developing when the foot is returned to a dependent position

  - a flushing time that exceeds 20 seconds. (Elevate the lower limb for 2 minutes. Return the limb to the dependent position, and note the time taken for the leg to flush.)
- A venous filling time of 30 seconds. In patients with an intact saphenous system, the time taken for venous filling after elevating the leg for 2 minutes provides information about limb perfusion. A normal venous filling time is 7 seconds.

More accurate estimates of limb perfusion can be achieved using Doppler ultrasonography. The level of occlusion can also be determined by identifying:

- the pulse and pulseless zone
- a zone of temperature change
- spasm or tenderness overlying the occlusion.

Evidence of ischemia. Chronic hypoxia affects all limb tissues, resulting in:

- patchy cyanosis and pallor
- ischemic neuritis (shooting pains, paresthesia)
- muscle changes (cramps, weakness, atrophy)
- subcutaneous tissue changes (edema, atrophy, calcification)
- deformed, slow-growing nails
- shiny atrophic skin
- hair loss.

The condition is graded both with respect to muscular (intermittent claudication) and nutritional ischemia.

Nutritional ischemia is graded as follows:

- Grade I, a normal finding in the elderly, is associated with pedal changes that include:
  - minor color change
  - minor temperature changes
  - loss/absence of hair
  - atrophy of the pulps of the toes
  - toenails need to be cut less frequently.
- Grade II is characterized by:
  - definite temperature changes
  - moderate color changes
  - mild resting pain at night
  - mild erythralgia. (Erythralgia, or ischemic neuritis, which is most marked when the lower limbs are warm (in bed), is usually experienced as a burning discomfort of the feet.)
- Grade III (pregangrene) presents with:
  - severe temperature changes
  - marked color changes
  - marked skin atrophy
  - notable discomfort of the feet, pain in previously painless bunions and corns.

- Grade IV presents as:
  - gangrene with tissue necrosis
  - ulcers on the dorsum of the foot and/or anterior aspect of the leg which fail to heal.
- Muscle ischemia or intermittent claudication presents as pain in the calf, buttock, thigh, or feet. The pain is exaggerated by exercise and the distance a patient can walk without needing to stop and rest is used as an indication of the severity of the disease:
- Mild ischemia: pain after walking 500 m or more.
- Moderate ischemia: requiring a rest after 250 m.
- Severe ischemia: pain that stops the patient walking more than 125 m.
- Rest pain: a persistent gnawing ache, often aggravated at night when the cardiac output drops.

See: *Claudication.*

ARTERITIS

A condition of arterial inflammation and cellular infiltration, the clinical presentation of arteritis includes:

- pain over the involved area
- pulseless arteritis presenting as firm tender nodes
- arthralgia
- low-grade fever
- fatigue
- headaches
- organ involvement:
  - blindness
  - cerebral infarction
  - myocardial infarction.

ARTHRITIS

In the differentiation of joint pain consideration is given to discriminating between arthritis (joint inflammation) and arthralgia (painful joints).

Arthritis is an inflammatory process affecting the joints, and is characterized by:

- pain worst at rest (at night), improved by activity
- local pain with some spread
- localized joint swelling, effusion and warmth
- prolonged stiffness tending to ease with usage and responding to rest
- associated systemic illness.

See: *Gout; Osteoarthritis*; *Rheumatoid arthritis*; *Septic arthritis*; Table I.

Table 1
The clinical presentation of prevalent joint diseases

Variable	Rheumatoid arthritis	Gout	Osteoarthritis	Septic arthritis	Disc degeneration*
Prevalence	Female	Familial, male	> 50 years	Young males	Increases with age and occupation
Pain	+	+++	++	+++	+
Morning stiffness	++	–	–	–	–
Muscle weakness	+++	–	–	–	–
Swelling	Warm	Red, hot	–	Red, hot	–
Wasting	+++	–	+++	–	–*
Loss of movement	++	+++	+++	+++	+
Prevalent sites	Small joints, wrists, metacarpophalangeal, interphalangeal	Monoarticular metatarso-phalangeal joints (big toe)	Large joints, knee; interphalangeal, first carpal joint	Monoarticular joints	Spine
Etiology	? Immunological	Metabolic (purine metabolism)	Trauma, wear and tear	Infection (bacterial)	Trauma, wear and tear
Additional factors	Rheumatoid nodules	Acute, transient	Heberden's nodes†, bony spurs, lipping of spine	Organisms on culture	Wasting*
Laboratory investigations	Rheumatoid factor	Hyperuricemia	Often not applicable	Blood culture	Normal

*Disc prolapse.
†Spurs at the base of the terminal phalanx.

Acute viral arthritis. Acute polyarthritis is frequently of viral origin. It presents with:

- symmetrical inflammation, especially of the hands and feet
- joint pain
- fever
- skin rash.

The condition is of short duration and resolves spontaneously. Various viruses are involved, ranging from influenza, hepatitis A and B, and viruses responsible for the exanthemata of childhood, to epidemic Ross River fever in Australia.

Spondyloarthropathies. This group of disorders affects the whole spine. In general, the spondyloarthropathies present with:

- sacroiliitis, with or without spondylitis (vertebral joint inflammation)
- arthritis, especially of the larger joints
- tendonitis, fasciitis, chondritis
- systemic lesions (iritis, conjunctivitis, urethritis)
- serological picture of a negative rheumatoid factor and increased prevalent HLA-B_{27}
- a family predisposition.

Important conditions amongst this group are:

- *Ankylosing spondylitis.* This is characterized by an insidious onset, in which spinal stiffness dominates. Young males are particularly prone. Symptoms must have persisted for at least 3 months before a diagnosis is made.
- *Psoriatic arthritis.* In this condition, systemic polyarthritis is associated with recurrent scaly skin lesions and nail changes. See: *Psoriasis.*
- *Reiter's syndrome.* This is a form of reactive arthritis following specific venereal or intestinal infection. It presents with non-septic arthritis (often sacroiliitis), nonspecific urethritis, conjunctivitis and, possibly, iritis. Enteropathic arthritis with sacroiliitis and peripheral arthritis may develop in persons with inflammatory bowel disease (ulcerative colitis, Crohn's disease).

In contrast, rheumatoid arthritis affects the cervical spine and is seropositive.

Connective tissue disorders. In general, these conditions present with:

- Arthritis, particularly involving the small joints of the hand
- A raised erythrocyte sedimentation rate (ESR)
- Positive serology. One or more serological tests demonstrating circulating antibodies, such as rheumatoid factor, antinuclear antibodies, or other cellular components is frequently positive.

Conditions in this group seem to share an underlying inflammatory or immunological activity. Systemic lupus erythematosus and systemic sclerosis need to be differentiated from rheumatoid arthritis in the early stages. At a later stage skin rashes and Raynaud's phenomenon are helpful in diagnosis. Polymyositis and dermatomyositis present with muscle weakness and wasting of the proximal muscles of the shoulder and pelvis.

ASTHMA

In children, wheezing after exercise or at night is strongly suggestive of asthma. In simple allergic asthma a personal or family history of hay fever or eczema is common. Onset usually occurs in childhood or young adulthood. Asthma presents as episodes of acute respiratory distress manifest by:

- Recurrent episodes of:
  - wheezing
  - chest tightness
  - dyspnea (mainly expiratory)
  - coughing. This precedes dyspnea, is worst at night, and is thick and gelatinous if productive. Some relief is experienced by coughing up sputum.
- Attacks that last for hours or days.
- Reduced air entry on auscultation associated with prolonged expiration, scattered, or generalized wheezing.

Asthma is definitively diagnosed on lung-function tests (spirometry) when:

- bronchodilator treatment results in an increase in forced expiratory volume (FEV_1) of 15%, provided the baseline FEV_1 is more than 1.3 l
- bronchodilators cause an increase of 20% or more when the baseline peak flow is 300 l/min
- peak flow over 14 days varies by 20% or more in adults, or 30% or more in children.

Asthma may be categorized as mild, moderate, or severe according to the frequency of attacks.

Mild asthma:

- symptoms occur no more than once a week or on exercising.
- nocturnal asthma is absent.
- the FEV_1 is more than 75%.
- the mean peak flow rate does not vary by more than 20% over 14 days.
- bronchodilators are infrequently required.

Moderate asthma:

- mild attacks occur more than once a week.
- patients experience tightness and wheezing on most days.

- patients wake with asthma or have nocturnal asthma less than once a week.
- bronchodilators are needed on most days.
- the FEV_1 is 50–75%.
- the mean peak flow varies by 20–30% over a 14-day period.

Severe asthma:

- attacks occur daily, or regularly wake the patient at night.
- bronchodilator use is necessary more than 3 or 4 times a day.
- the FEV_1 is less than 50%.
- the mean peak flow variability exceeds 30% over 14 days.

The mean peak flow variability is calculated as:

$$\frac{(\text{Highest flow} - \text{Lowest flow}) \times 100}{\text{Highest flow}}$$

Chronic asthmatic bronchitis in persons over 35 years of age is a form of asthma with a more serious prognosis. Asthmatics may develop cor pulmonale and emphysema.

When monitoring an asthma patient it is important to keep a record of:

- Symptom frequency: both the number of attacks per month and the frequency of use of bronchodilator inhalation should be noted.
- Symptom severity: patients should be asked about symptoms that interfere with normal activities and/or disturb sleep.

Patient self-assessment can be refined through use of a peak flow meter. The patient records the best of three forced expiration readings and the peak flow following use of a bronchodilator. Peak flow meters are used to detect changes rather than make a diagnosis. In males the peak flow rate is 400–800 l/min; in females it is 200–600 l/min.

- Referral criteria for further medical assessment of asthmatics include:
- Athletes with exercise-induced asthma.
- Worsening symptoms such as:
  - waking twice or more with asthma
  - needing bronchodilator relief more than six times daily
  - attacks occurring every 4–6 weeks (episodic asthma)
  - a wheeze that is loud or becoming quiet
  - increasing frequency or severity of coughing, chest tightness, or dyspnea.
- Severe bronchial asthma presenting with:
  - medication being required more often than every 4 hours
  - dyspnea when sitting
  - speech limited to words (patients cannot manage phrases or sentences due to dyspnea; an inability to eat or talk during an attack is a very serious sign)

- sudden attacks
- attacks with notably reduced air entry (a silent chest)
- cyanosis
- use of accessory muscles of respiration
- sternal retraction in young children
- confusion or altered consciousness
- pulsus paradoxus
- peak flow meter reading of < 50 l/min in children or < 200 l/min in adults
- mean peak expiratory flow (PEF) variability > 30%

$$\frac{\text{Best PEF} - \text{Lowest PEF}}{\text{Best PEF} \times 100\%}$$

- exhaustion.

- Signs of hypoxia, such as:
  - restlessness
  - tachypnea
  - a pulse rate of > 140 beats/min in children or > 110 beats/min in adults.
- Evidence of complications, including:
  - cardiac asthma
  - failure of an intermittent therapy regimen.
- Continuous drug therapy is indicated in patients who:
  - have more than one attack per month
  - suffer severe attacks (require hospitalization)
  - use a β_2 stimulant inhaler more than once a week
  - wheeze continuously
  - have persistently low peak flow readings
  - have associated chronic obstructive airways disease (COAD)
  - have previously used steroids.

Bronchial asthma should not be confused with cardiac asthma. *Cardiac asthma* presents with:

- a heart problem
- attacks of dyspnea and wheezing, worst at night or on lying down
- pulmonary edema.

ATAXIA

- See: *Cerebellar dysfunction*; *Posterior column dysfunction*; *Vestibular dysfunction.*

ATELECTASIS

- See: *Pulmonary atelectasis.*

ATHEROSCLEROTIC HEART DISEASE

Atherosclerotic heart disease, the result of chronic focal ischemia scattered throughout both ventricles, presents with:

- a history of recurrent chest pain
- chronic cardiac failure
- acute and chronic arrhythmias, as fibrosis impairs the conduction system
- sudden death attributable to massive necrosis or a serious conduction defect.

ATRIAL FIBRILLATION

As ectopic impulses arise in the atria, the heart rate is determined by the state of polarization of the atrioventricular node. Atrial stimuli may reach 600 beats per minute.

Patients with atrial fibrillation present with:

- an irregular pulse rate (the irregularity is more pronounced on exercise)
- a variable pulse volume
- a rapid pulse (120–170 beats/min)
- a first heart sound of varying intensity
- a pulse deficit (a discrepancy between the pulse and heart rate is frequently found)
- no fourth heart sound.

Carotid sinus pressure slows the heart rate but does not effect the arrhythmia.

The patient tap test, in which the patient uses a finger to beat out their heart rhythm, is characterized by irregular tapping all over the place.

Variants of atrial fibrillation include:

- *paroxysmal/recurrent atrial fibrillation.* This variation is precipitated by alcohol and binge eating. The major complication is palpitations.
- *transient/acute atrial fibrillation.* Underlying pathology that needs to be explored in this form of atrial fibrillation includes: mitral stenosis, myocardial infarction, pericarditis, pulmonary embolus, and acute bacterial pneumonia.
- *sustained/chronic atrial fibrillation.* Sustained atrial fibrillation is usually attributable to cardiac failure, ischemic heart disease, hypertension, mitral valve disease, cardiomyopathy, or chronic obstructive airways disease (COAD). An important complication is emboli, which may cause a stroke.

Referral is indicated for:

- Echocardiography to investigate the cause.
- Possible cardioversion.
- Assessment of stroke risk and prophylaxis. The risk of stroke is 3–5 times higher in persons with atrial fibrillation. About 1 in 4 patients with ischemic stroke has atrial fibrillation.
- Re-evaluate current drug therapy. Digoxin, the drug most commonly used to control ventricular rate in patients with atrial fibrillation, may itself favor the onset of atrial fibrillation.

ATRIAL TACHYCARDIA (paroxysmal atrial (supraventricular) tachycardia)

A disorder of unknown etiology, atrial tachycardia is found in apparently healthy adults. The clinical presentation is:

- a regular pulse
- a rapid pulse (>120 beats/min)
- the sudden onset of palpitations
- dyspnea
- a history of previous attack
- predisposing factors in susceptible individuals:
  - anxiety
  - smoking
- attacks may be terminated by vagal stimulation.

Certain cases may be alleviated by normalizing spinal function. In the absence of organic heart disease, dysfunction of the upper thoracic spine (especially T4, T5) has been linked with paroxysmal supraventricular tachycardia.

ATROPIC VAGINITIS

See: *Menopause*.

ATYPICAL FACIAL PAIN

Patients present with pain that is:

- chronic and persists without interruption all day
- dull, boring, or pressing in character
- often vaguely localized over one cheek.

Family life is dominated by the patient's pain. A history of doctor shopping is common. The pain, which may have originated with a physical cause, becomes a psychological problem.

PART THREE

AUTONOMIC NEUROPATHY

Patients present with:

- postural dizziness, reduced heart rate variability, blackouts
- abdominal distension, borborygmus, persistent diarrhea, constipation
- impotence
- sweating abnormalities
- a sluggish pupillary reaction to light
- drying and cracking of skin.

BACTERIAL VAGINOSIS

Bacterial vaginosis attributable to anaerobic bacteria may be the precursor of pelvic inflammatory disease. Replacement of the normal vaginal lactobacilli with a mixed flora, usually including *Gardnerella vaginalis*, results in:

- vulval soreness
- burning
- a fine filmy white-gray discharge with a few bubbles
- a 'fishy' odor
- pH > 4.5.

Male partners are asymptomatic and should be treated.

BALANITIS

Males present 48–72 hours after intercourse with:

- soreness of the prepuce
- a subpreputial discharge
- phimosis (constriction of the foreskin) due to edema of the glans and prepuce
- tender inguinal lymphadenopathy.

BASAL CELL CARCINOMA

Basal cell carcinoma is the most common of the skin cancers. It is a slow-growing malignancy and may spread locally over many years. It is usually found in persons over the age of 35 years.

Findings suggesting basal cell carcinoma include:

- a slow-growing, small, smooth-surfaced, well-defined pink/red nodule
- the nodule has a pearly or translucent border (this is best seen by stretching the skin over the nodule)

- overlying telangiectatic vessels
- over time, central ulceration and crusting results in the typical 'rodent ulcer' with its rolled edge.

Lesions most commonly occur around the orbit or at the side of the nose.

BEHÇET'S SYNDROME

Postulated to result from an underlying autoimmune condition, Behçet's syndrome presents with:

- Shallow painful ulcers surrounded by a red areola. When ulcers are limited to the oral cavity they are termed aphthous ulcers. See: *Aphthous ulcers.*
- Genital ulcers on the scrotum or labia majora.
- Conjunctivitis or uveitis.
- Skin pustules or nodules.
- Thrombophlebitis.

Meningoencephalitis and brainstem syndromes may be found.

BELL'S PALSY

This is the sudden onset of unilateral facial paralysis. The cause is unknown. Patients present with unilateral:

- pain behind the ear
- facial weakness which develops over 12–48 hours
- flattening of facial grooves
- a lack of expression.

In severe cases, patients are unable to close their eye. Full recovery usually occurs within several weeks or months.

BENIGN PEPTIC STRICTURE

Benign peptic stricture is a complication of chronic severe reflux esophagitis. It presents with:

- Dysphagia when eating solid food.
- Dysphagia that slowly worsens over months.
- A history of reflux esophagitis:
  - burning substernal pain
  - pain may radiate to the neck, jaw, and arms
  - a pain–meal relationship
  - a long history of heartburn
  - pain relieved by assuming an upright position and taking alkali
  - waterbrash.

BICIPITAL TENDONITIS

Within 30 hours of excessive use, the biceps muscle may present with:

- pain which:
  - is dull in front of the shoulder
  - may radiate to just below the elbow
  - is sharp on resisted supination of the forearm with a flexed elbow
- tenderness along the bicipital groove with the arm externally rotated
- limited elevation of the arm with 90° abduction.

BILE DUCT CANCER

Cancer of the biliary tract is less common than pancreatic cancer and presents with:

- obstructive jaundice (jaundice may be intermittent due to sloughing of tumor when the cancer is periampullary)
- pruritus
- pain in the right upper quadrant
- nausea, anorexia, weight loss
- a palpable gallbladder (back-pressure may cause a healthy gallbladder to enlarge and a mass may be detected in the right upper quadrant).

Biliary tract cancer may involve:

- the bile duct epithelium (*cholangiocarcinoma*)
- the insertion of the bile duct into the duodenum at the ampulla or papilla of Vater. *Ampullary cancer* presents with intermittent jaundice and melena (bleeding) as the tumor necroses, and sloughs off into the intestine.

BILIARY COLIC

See: *Cholelithiasis.*

BLADDER CANCER

Vitamins A, B_6, C, and E reduce the recurrence of bladder cancer. The presentation includes:

- Terminal hematuria (bleeding at the end of micturition).
- Painless intermittent hematuria.
- Obstructive uropathy. As tumor grows:

- ureteric obstruction causes hydronephrosis
- bladder neck obstruction causes prostatism.

BLADDER PAPILLOMA

The clinical presentation is:

- terminal hematuria (bleeding at the end of micturition)
- painless recurrent hematuria.

BLADDER STONES

The clinical presentation is:

- Pain:
  - which is worst at the end of micturition
  - referred to the suprapubic and perineal area, or the tip of the penis in males.
- Terminal hematuria.
- Frequency.
- Obstructed bladder outflow. An impacted stone may have a ballvalve effect.

BLOOD DYSCRASIA

An abnormal and unhealthy blood picture.
See: *Agranulocytosis*; *Anemia* (Aplastic anemia); *Leukemia.*

BONE MARROW FAILURE

Bone marrow failure may result from:

- drug-induced bone marrow depression
- metastatic replacement of bone marrow
- fibrous replacement of bone marrow (myelofibrosis).

The underlying pathological process may affect any or all of these cellular elements. The homeostatic response determines the extent of involvement of cellular replenishment.

The clinical presentation includes:

- anemia, which presents as pallor
- neutropenia, which presents clinically as susceptibility to infections
- thrombocytopenia, which presents as easy bruising
- hepatosplenomegaly unassociated with lymphadenopathy (hepatosplenomegaly is due to extramedullary hemopoiesis).

The blood picture reflects the success of hemopoiesis in the liver and spleen. Diagnosis depends on marrow biopsy. In practice, these conditions are most likely to present as an anemia.

BOTULISM

Food poisoning caused by *Clostridium botulinum* presents 18–36 hours after ingestion of the toxin, with:

- nausea, vomiting, and abdominal cramps
- neurological symptoms, including:
  - dry mouth
  - diplopia
  - ptosis
  - loss of accommodation and pupillary reflexes
  - bulbar paralysis (detected as dysarthria, dysphagia, nasal regurgitation).

BRACHIAL NEURALGIA

Although self-limiting in most cases, the outcome depends on the cause. Brachial neuralgia may be experienced as a result of:

- Lesions of the lower cervical spine.
- Thoracic outlet syndrome. The brachial plexus may be under tension due to:
  - shoulder sagging (e.g. from carrying heavy bags)
  - a cervical rib.
- Pressure from a space-occupying lesion (e.g. Pancoast's tumor (cancer of the lung apex)).

Patients present with:

- repeated attacks of shoulder or neck pain
- episodes of shoulder or neck stiffness
- tingling numbness in the hand and fingers
- symptoms altered by postural changes
- weakness of hand grip
- muscle wasting.

BRAINSTEM LESION

The presentation of vascular lesions or tumors of the brainstem depends on the site of the lesion. Patients may experience an impaired respiratory drive.

Lesions affecting the top of the midbrain present with:

- paralysis of upward gaze
- convergence nystagmus

- miosis
- IIIrd nerve palsy.

Lesions of the pontomedullary junction present with:

- contralateral hemiplegia
- contralateral hemianesthesia of the body
- ipsilateral loss of pain sense on the face
- lesions of the VIth and VIIth cranial nerves.

Lateral medullary lesions present with:

- vertigo
- ipsilateral ataxia
- nystagmus
- miosis, ptosis, and anhydrosis
- contralateral hemianesthesia of the body
- loss of pain on the face
- hiccups, dysphagia.

BREAST ABSCESS

This is most likely to occur during or shortly after lactation. Patients present with:

- breast pain
- a tender mass.

BREAST CANCER

Breast cancer is the third major cause of death in adult women, after motor vehicle accidents and coronary artery disease. Its prevalence increases with age. Although the cause is unknown, the following links have been identified:

- *Inherited susceptibility.* About 1 in 20 breast cancers are inherited. Cardinal features of inherited breast cancer are:
  - early age of onset
  - bilateral disease
  - multiple primaries in the same individual
  - multiple affected relatives.

Women are at high risk of breast cancer if they have a family history of ovarian cancer, early onset of breast cancer (under 45 years) or at least three close relatives, all from the same side of the family, who have breast cancer.

- *Hormonal changes of menstruation.* Women who menstruate for more than 40 years run twice the risk of breast cancer compared with those who menstruate for less than 30 years. The number of ovulatory cycles before the first pregnancy determines the women's lifetime risk of developing breast cancer. It appears that the breast's susceptibility to carcinogens occurs during a relatively short period (probably in the teens).

- *Diet.* An increased risk of breast cancer appears to correlate with a diet rich in saturated fat, alcohol, and animal protein.
- *Smoking.* Smoking is possibly an initiator or early-stage promoter for breast cancer.

Breast cancer is diagnosed:

- By detecting abnormal mammography in women with no palpable mass in about 1 in 3 cases.
- Due to the presence of a palpable breast mass, which is located in the upper outer quadrant or axillary tail in up to 60% of cases. The patients present with:
  - a lump that is nontender, fixed, and hard
  - a deformity or alteration to the shape of the breast (nipple or breast elevation, nipple retraction, dimpling of skin (peau d'orange), localized skin rash).
- Axillary lymphadenopathy.
- Evidence of distal metastases (e.g. bone pain).
- Systemic symptoms (e.g. anorexia, weight loss).

Regularly performed breast self-examination can facilitate early diagnosis and significantly improve the 5-year survival rate. Women untrained in breast self-examination can detect lumps of approximately 1.5 in (3.8 cm) in size. Women who occasionally do breast self-examination are likely to detect a 1 in (2.5 cm) mass. Women who regularly do breast self-examination are expected to be capable of detecting lumps of 0.5 in (1.27 cm) in size. Mammography can detect lesions less than half this size.

BRONCHIECTASIS

Bronchiectasis is infection of localized dilated bronchi with underlying destruction of bronchial muscle and elastic tissue. Persons with localized bronchial obstruction (e.g. a foreign body), tenacious sputum (as in cystic fibrosis), chronic sinusitis, or pulmonary infection (e.g. pneumonia, whooping cough) are prone to develop bronchiectasis.

Bronchiectasis is most common in men and presents with:

- A chronic productive cough, worst on waking.
- Profuse production of purulent sputum, occasionally hemoptysis. Sputum production is related to changes in posture. Postural drainage by lying the head and thorax down off the side of the bed for 20 minutes three times a day may be helpful.
- Intermittent pyrexia.
- Persistent halitosis.
- Malaise, weight loss.
- Crackles, rhonchi.

Clubbing, dyspnea, and cyanosis are late signs. Identification of complications such as chronic suppuration, progressive pulmonary insufficiency with cor pulmonale, and hemoptysis indicate the need for medical attention.

BRONCHIOLITIS

Bronchiolitis is a lower respiratory disease affecting children between the ages of 3 months and 3 years. The child presents with:

- marked respiratory distress
- dyspnea with rapid shallow respiration
- inspiratory retraction of intercostal and suprasternal spaces
- prolonged expiration
- expiratory wheezing and rhonchi
- lung overinflation, detected as hyperresonance on chest percussion and diaphragm depression
- cyanosis.

Medical attention is required for children suspected of having bronchiolitis. (See Table II.)

Table II
Comparison between asthma and bronchiolitis

	Bronchiolitis	**Asthma**
Differences Age of onset	3 months to 3 years	Infancy to adulthood
Respiratory obstruction	Inspiratory and expiratory	Expiratory
Respiratory distress	Marked	Mild to marked
Auscultation	Wheezing and rhonchi	Wheezing
White cell count	Lymphocytosis	Eosinophilia
Similarities Expiration	Prolonged	Prolonged
Percussion	Hyperresonant	Hyperresonant
Radiograph	Hyperaeration	Hyperaeration

BRONCHITIS

Acute bronchitis presents with:

- a cough of short duration
- an irritating cough, which is initially dry but may later become productive and is occasionally an hemoptysis
- burning retrosternal discomfort
- dyspnea, often with wheeze

- fever
- scattered rhonchi
- episodic dyspnea, which may become progressive
- occasional crackles, altered by coughing.

Patients should be referred for medical attention if:

- they are very old or very young
- repeated attacks occur
- the condition worsens (it normally clears in 4–8 days)
- they develop:
  - dyspnea, wheezing, and chest pain
  - a purulent or bloodstained sputum
  - otitis media, sinusitis, rashes
  - a pyrexia which persists for longer than 36 hours
  - a temperature above 39°C
  - white spots appear on the throat
  - worsening pharyngitis.

Chronic bronchitis is defined as a cough productive of sputum, on all or most days for a continuous period of 3 months of the year, occurring for 2 years or more in succession, in the absence of a specific cause. Persistent irritation results in hypertrophy of bronchial mucosa. Irritated mucosa, due to its increased number of goblet cells and mucous glands, secretes excess mucus, resulting in mucous plugs, a productive cough, and a predisposition to infection. Predisposing factors are a history of smoking, viral and/or bacterial infection, air pollution, and food or pollen hypersensitivity.

Patients present with:

- episodic dyspnea or mild persistent dyspnea (both may be present)
- a productive cough (this is the dominant symptom)
- reduced exercise tolerance
- persistent rhonchi
- early onset of cor pulmonale.

Central cyanosis develops late.

Referral is indicated when complications are detected:

- superimposed infection (purulent sputum)
- cor pulmonale (right heart failure).

BRONCHOGENIC CARCINOMA

See: *Lung cancer.*

BRONCHOPNEUMONIA

See: *Pneumonia.*

BULBAR PALSY

See: *Motor neuron disease.*

BULIMIA

See: *Eating disorders.*

BURSITIS

Bursitis is inflammation of the thin-walled sac surrounding tendons and muscles where they pass over bony prominences. Acute bursitis presents with:

- Pain.
- Localized tenderness.
- Limitation of movement. The limitation depends on the bursa involved:
  - limitation of all shoulder movements, especially rotation in subacromial bursitis
  - a painful abduction arc at 40° in supraspinatus tendonitis
  - tenderness over the bicipital groove aggravated by resisted flexion of the elbow in bicipital tendonitis.
- Swelling and redness if the bursa is superficial:
  - swelling at the front of the knee in prepatellar bursitis
  - swelling at the back of the elbow in olecranon bursitis.

Chronic bursitis presents with:

- pain
- swelling
- tenderness
- muscle atrophy
- limited movement.

CAFFEINISM

Caffeine consumption levels are sufficient to cause pharmacological effects in most, and toxic effects in some, people. Approximate caffeine concentrations are:

- cola drinks contain about 50 mg in a 375-ml can
- a 150-ml cup of brewed coffee contains 88 mg
- a cup of instant coffee contains 70 mg
- brewed tea contains 40 mg
- a 150-ml cup or a 28-g chocolate bar contain 7.7 mg.

Chronic ingestion of caffeine is associated with tolerance, but no effect on blood pressure, blood glucose, or catecholamine levels is reported. The cardiovascular impact of coffee may, however, be related to its method of preparation. Boiled coffee raises blood cholesterol levels, but filtered and instant coffee have no effect on total or high density lipoprotein (HDL) cholesterol or blood pressure. Caffeine had no significant effect on bone loss in women who get the daily recommended calcium allowance of 800 mg/day. However, women with a low calcium intake and who drink two or three cups of coffee a day are at risk of increased bone loss.

Caffeinism, a toxic overdose of caffeine, occurs when over 7 mg/kg of caffeine is ingested per day. Symptoms include:

- anxiety and tension
- headaches
- insomnia
- irritability
- anorexia
- dizziness.

Flushing and arrhythmia as well as epigastric pain, diarrhea, and vomiting have been described.

Caffeine withdrawal is associated with side-effects such as:

- drowsiness
- headaches
- restlessness
- nervousness.

A double-blind placebo controlled trial using capsules containing 235 mg caffeine or placebo detected headache, fatigue, and mood disturbances in patients on placebo suffering caffeine withdrawal from their usual 2–3 cups of coffee per day (235 mg). Other studies have reported headache, lethargy, fatigue, muscle pain, or stiffness after withdrawal of 100 mg caffeine per day. This is the equivalent of one cup of coffee, two cups of tea, or three cans of caffeinated soft drink.

CALLUS

Clinical features are:

- a superficial circumscribed area of hard thickened skin (hyperkeratosis)
- lesions in sites of repeated trauma, especially on the hands and feet
- on paring:
  - heaped keratin
  - preservation of the skin markings.

CANDIDIASIS (moniliasis)

Candidiasis affects up to 75% of women. In 10% it is a recurrent problem. Candida can cause:

- Onychia: the nail is ridged and the lateral aspect is discolored.
- Paronychia: pustules develop at the nail fold.
- Intertrigo: well-defined, red, moist patches are detected in the submammary, groin, interglutate, and axillary folds.
- Perleche: fissuring, maceration, and crusting at the corners of the mouth.
- Thrush: whitish exudates form on the oral mucous membrane.
- Superficial glossitis, presenting as a beefy red tongue.
- Genital candida, presenting with:
  - Intense erythema: vulva, crural, perianal regions.
  - Pruritus: patients often complain of an intense itch.
  - Vaginal candidiasis: this is often associated with pregnancy and the use of oral contraceptives. Dyspareunia may occur. Patients have: a thick white 'cottage cheese' vaginal discharge and white patches appear attached to the vaginal mucosa.
  - Patches on the glans, penile shaft, labia, or vulva.
  - Predisposing factors include diabetes, oral contraceptives, systemic antibiotics, pregnancy, and immunosuppression.

Management of genital candida:

- Change the vaginal environment by:
  - vaginal douches with lactobacilli
  - changing the bowel environment to one less favorable to candida proliferation, through dietary change and normalizing the intestinal flora.
- Patients should avoid tight-fitting clothing and nylon underwear. Undergarments should be washed in fungicidal solutions, such as peroxides or bleaches.
- Avoid cosmetic preparations, which may cause allergies and promote growth of *Candida albicans*.
- Ensure good hygiene:
  - wash the genital area daily with lukewarm water and pat dry
  - after toileting, wipe the genital area from front to back
  - vaginal intercourse should not follow anal intercourse.

Asymptomatic partners need not be treated.

CARCINOID SYNDROME

Slow-growing tumors of argentaffin cells that secrete various vasoactive substances may be found in the ileum, stomach, or bronchus. Carcinoid syndrome should be investigated in patients presenting with:

- facial flushing
- abdominal cramps and diarrhea
- wheezing and dyspnea
- telangiectasis.

CARDIAC ASTHMA

Pulmonary edema is differentiated from bronchial asthma by:

- lung signs dominated by crackles
- dyspnea, which is mainly inspiratory
- pink frothy sputum
- cough follows dyspnea
- relief being obtained by standing by an open window.

Wheezing may be present.

CARDIAC FAILURE

See: *Heart failure.*

CARDIOMYOPATHY

Viral infections, alcoholism, thiamine deficiency, thyroid disease (thyrotoxicosis and myxedema), leukemia, and muscular dystrophy are all causes of cardiomyopathy.

Regardless of the cause, the clinical presentation includes:

- insidious left ventricular failure in a patient with an enlarged heart
- chest pain
- weakness
- dizziness
- dyspnea.

Management is influenced by the cause. Vitamin B_1 (100 mg/day) supplementation in appropriate cases can produce dramatic results. Daily coenzyme Q (100 mg) is also helpful, as is abstinence from alcohol.

CAROTINEMIA

This is a benign condition attributable to excess ingestion of carotene-rich foods, such as carrots, pumpkins, or pawpaw. The individual:

- feels well
- develops yellow discoloration of the skin

- the sclera remains white (this allows clinical differentiation from jaundice, in which the sclera is yellow)
- liver function tests are normal.

CARPAL TUNNEL SYNDROME

See: *Nerve entrapment.*

CATARACT

A cataract is an opacity of the lens. Cataracts are prevalent:

- in the elderly (very common in persons aged over 50 years)
- in persons with diabetes mellitus
- in persons on steroid therapy
- in children with the congenital rubella syndrome
- following eye trauma.

Clinical presentation:

- Visual impairment. Patients complain of gradually diminishing vision in one or both eyes.
- Eyesight deteriorates gradually and progressively, over months or years.
- Radial, hazy opacities are detected when light is focused on the lens. The ophthalmoscope aperture is usually set at +12 diopters for this procedure.
- An altered red reflex. Black shadows are detected against a red background in an immature cataract. The red reflex is lost in mature cataracts.
- In severe cases the pupil may appear white to the naked eye.

In persons with 6/18 vision or better, referral for surgery may be delayed until further visual deterioration has occurred. The major causes of blindness in developed countries are cataracts, glaucoma, diabetes mellitus, and age-related maculopathy.

CAUDA EQUINA SYNDROME

Cauda equina presents with:

- low back pain
- paresthesia or pain in the thighs and legs
- lower limb sensory changes, progressing to numbness of the:
  - buttocks (saddle anesthesia)
  - back of the legs
  - soles of feet
- a lower limb motor deficit, detected as paresis or paralysis of legs and feet

- calf atrophy
- bowel dysfunction
- bladder dysfunction.

CELIAC DISEASE

Patients with celiac disease are gluten sensitive. Patients with celiac disease who do not adhere to a gluten-free diet increase their lifetime risk of lymphoma. Patients should avoid gliadin-rich foods such as wheat, barley, and rye. They should also avoid oats and millet.

Celiac disease is characterized by:

- chronic mild diarrhea, steatorrhea
- bloating, flatulence, and a distended abdomen
- nausea
- chronic fatigue
- weight loss
- anemia attributable to folate, iron or, rarely, vitamin B_{12} deficiency
- severe recurrent aphthous ulceration of the oral mucosa
- mineral deficiency may cause paresthesia (calcium or magnesium deficiency), arrhythmias, muscle weakness, and low blood pressure (potassium deficiency). Tetany may result from hypocalcemia.
- biopsy demonstrates a 'flat' mucosa due to villous atrophy
- complications include osteomalacia, osteoporosis and, rarely, arthropathy.

CENTRAL RETINAL ARTERY OCCLUSION

Sudden blindness, particularly in elderly persons, may be the result of arterial occlusion due to spasm, degenerative changes or, more rarely, embolization to the central retinal artery. The clinical picture involves:

- sudden blindness
- on ophthalmology:
  - a milky white edematous retina
  - extremely narrow thread-like arteries
  - a 'cherry-red' spot (this is the rubor of the macula, which shines through the transparent retina).

CENTRAL RETINAL VEIN OCCLUSION

Occlusion of the central retinal vein is most prevalent in elderly persons. It may also be found in young females. The clinical presentation is:

- Sudden unilateral loss of vision.
- On ophthalmoscopy:
  - an engorged retina
  - tortuous vessels
  - hemorrhages.

CEREBELLAR DYSFUNCTION

The cerebellum integrates muscle contractions for the maintenance of posture. Cerebellar disorders result in:

- Dyssynergia. Muscle coordination is impaired and clumsiness results. Coordination is poor. Decomposition of movement results in normally smooth movements being performed in several parts.
- Intention tremor.
- Dysdiadochokinesia. The individual has difficulty in rapidly alternating supination and pronation of the hand.
- Dysmetria. Disturbance in the ability to stop movements results in past pointing when doing the finger–nose–finger test.
- Hypotonia.
- Nystagmus on lateral gaze.
- A broad-based gait. The trunk and head are rigid, the legs bent at the hips and the feet are widely spaced. Arms and stride are not coordinated. The individual lurches, and may fall.
- Ataxia. Unsteadiness is present when the eyes are open and is unchanged by closing the eyes.
- Dysarthria, manifest as slow, hesitant, scanning speech.

CEREBRAL TUMOR

Patients present with evidence of:

- raised intracranial pressure. See: *Intracranial pressure*
- seizures
- mental symptoms, including:
  - personality changes
  - drowsiness
  - impaired mental alertness/ability
  - depression
  - psychotic episodes.

Localizing signs on physical examination provide information on the site of the lesion:

- *Frontal lobe* involvement: personality changes, progressive hemiplegia, and speech defects are detected. Signs of an upper motor neuron lesion are present.
- *Parietal lobe* involvement: generalized or focal sensory seizures, contralateral impairment of position sense and two-point discrimination, speech disturbances, and denial of illness. Signs of an upper motor neuron lesion are detected.
- *Temporal lobe* involvement: quadratic hemianopia and peculiar behavior may result. The lesion may be silent if located in the nondominant hemisphere.
- *Occipital lobe* tumors: cause changes in the visual field.
- *Internal capsule* involvement: contralateral hemiplegia may result. Signs of an upper motor neuron lesion are present.
- *Thalamic lesions*: contralateral sensory impairment may result.
- *Basal ganglion* lesions: athetosis and dystonic postures.
- *Cerebellum* involvement: hypotonia, poor muscle coordination, nystagmus, and dysdiadochokinesia.
- *Cerebellopontine angle* tumor: unilateral deafness and tinnitus.
- *Pituitary fossa* involvement: hormonal changes and bitemporal hemianopia.
- *Brainstem* involvement: somnolence, vomiting, difficulty with swallowing and speech.

An upper motor neuron lesion presents with:

- muscle weakness, possible paralysis
- deep tendon hyperreflexia, possibly clonus
- increased muscle tone or spasticity (clasp-knife rigidity is noted)
- an extensor plantar reflex (Babinski sign).

CEREBROVASCULAR ACCIDENTS

See: *Stroke*.

CERVICAL CARCINOMA

Cervical cancer is most likely to arise at the squamocolumnar cell junction, the transformation zone of the cervix. Behaviors believed to be associated with an increased risk of cervical dysplasia and cervical cancer include:

- first intercourse at an early age
- multiple sexual partners
- herpes type 2 exposure
- human papilloma virus
- a high-fat diet
- smoking (doubles or triples the risk of cervical dysplasia).

Current thinking suggests that the disease progresses as follows:

- *Cervical intraepithelial neoplasia (CIN) stage 1.* Mild cervical dysplasia is detected in the outer third of the epithelium.
- *CIN stage 2.* Moderate dysplasia involves two-thirds of the epithelium.
- *CIN stage 3.* Severe dysplasia or carcinoma in situ is diagnosed. The patient is asymptomatic and diagnosis is made on a Pap smear.
- *Carcinoma of the cervix.* This presents with:
  - vaginal discharge (offensive, watery, brown or clear)
  - postcoital bleeding
  - dyspareunia
  - abnormal vaginal blood loss
  - a bulky uterus
  - on examination:

    Stage I: the cancer is confined to the cervix, which is freely mobile

    Stage II: the cervix is mobile, but the tumor has spread to involve a larger area of the cervix, parametrium, broad ligament, and/or the upper vagina

    Stage III: the cervix is fixed and the tumor involves the pelvic wall and/or lower vagina

    Stage IV: metastases involve the bladder, rectum, and/or pelvic structures.

CERVICAL DISC LESION

- See: *Spinal dysfunction.*

CERVICAL SPONDYLOSIS (osteoarthritis)

Cervical osteoarthritis presents with:

- neck stiffness, improved by exercise
- some restriction of neck movement
- secondary muscle contraction headaches:
  - a mild to moderate suboccipital ache
  - the pain is described as a nagging ache
  - pain occurs daily, being worst in the morning, but improves with gentle activity
  - pain that is aggravated by: initiating neck movement (pain does, however, improve with exercise); heavy activity
  - pain relieved by heat and muscle relaxation
- paresthesia (the patient may be woken at night with arm paresthesia)
- vertigo precipitated by a change in head movement

- tinnitus
- dysphagia
- earache.

Acute attacks may be superimposed upon the chronic underlying problem.

CERVICITIS

Cervical erosions may progress to chronic cervicitis, which presents with:

- a dull ache in the lumbosacral region
- low sacral backache, aggravated premenstrually
- lower abdominal or suprapubic pain
- a chronic profuse vaginal discharge (the mucoid discharge of cervical erosions may become mucopurulent in infected chronic cervicitis)
- urinary symptoms, particularly burning on micturition
- metrorrhagia.

Patients should have a Pap smear and be referred for electrocautery.

CHALAZION (external hordeolum)

Inflammation of the meibomian gland in the acute phase presents with a red painful swelling, which points to skin or bulbar conjunctiva. Chronic inflammation causes a painless swelling on the inner surface of the eyelid below the cartilage plate. Surgical drainage is required.

CHANCROID

Haemophilus ducreyi is the cause of a chancroid, or soft sore. After an incubation period of up to 14 days (usually 2–5 days), chancroid presents with:

- multiple tender ulcers
- ulcers that are ragged, with a necrotic base and an undermined edge
- moderate, matted tender lymphadenopathy.

Lesions are found on the penis, vulva, and thigh.

CHICKEN POX (varicella)

Chicken pox is a viral disease spread by droplets. The incubation period is 2–3 weeks and the virus is transmitted from 5 days before appearance of the rash to 6 days after eruption of the first crop of vesicles. Chicken pox presents clinically with:

- A mild 24–72 hour prodrome of slight malaise, fever, and myalgia. No prodrome occurs in children.
- A rash which develops on the trunk, face, scalp, and proximal aspects of the limbs.
- A rash which:
  - starts as tiny vesicles on an erythematous macular base and appears in crops over 2–5 days
  - may progress from macules through vesicles to pustules in a few hours
  - simultaneously has lesions in different stages of evolution (vesicles, pustules, and crusted erosions are present in the same patient)
  - scabs, which fall away between days 9 and 13 (a patient with scabs is not contagious)
  - heals over 7–21 days.
- Severe pruritus during the pustular phase.
- Complications:
  - Secondary infection of skin lesions, with scarring. Scarring occurs as punched-out pit-like depressions, often on the face, or firm whitish papules, found on the trunk. Trunkal scarring may only develop months after the acute exanthem.
  - Interstitial pneumonia.
  - Encephalitis.

The simultaneous presence of maculopapular lesions, vesicles, and scabs in a centripetal distribution clinically distinguishes this disease from smallpox.

CHILBLAINS (pernio)

Chilblains are precipitated by cold exposure. They present as:

- areas of blotchy red skin
- itchy, painful skin lesions
- lesions on the heels, toes, and fingers.

CHLAMYDIA

In women, chlamydia are involved in:

- over 20% of cases of cervicitis
- up to 50% of cases of pelvic inflammatory disease in those under 35 years of age.

Up to 50% of cases of females who have had contact with a male diagnosed as having nongonococcal urethritis acquire the organism.

In women, chlamydial infection:

- is usually asymptomatic
- may present with:
  - vulva irritation
  - a vaginal discharge (thick, yellow-white, and seen oozing from the cervical os)
- can also cause:
  - urethritis
  - mucopurulent cervicitis
  - endometritis
  - acute, subacute, or chronic salpingitis
  - perihepatitis
  - conjunctivitis
  - pharyngeal colonization
  - proctitis
  - seronegative arthritis.

In men, genital chlamydial infection presents with:

- urethritis (chlamydia is an important cause of nongonococcal urethritis in men)
- can also cause:
  - epididymitis
  - conjunctivitis
  - pharyngeal colonization
  - seronegative arthritis
  - proctitis.

Asymptomatic persons at risk of chlamydial infection are patients who:

- make inconsistent use of a barrier contraceptive (condom or diaphragm)
- have sexual contact with infected persons
- have another sexually transmitted disease
- have changed sexual partners in the last 6 months
- are female, are under 25 years old, and show
  - inflammatory cervical cytology
  - cervical ectopy.

Detection of the antigen using microimmunofluorescence confirms the diagnosis.

CHOLANGITIS

Ascending infection of the bile duct presents with:

- upper abdominal pain
- jaundice
- fever, often with rigors.

These patients usually have some underlying abnormality of the biliary system, such as stricture, neoplasia, or stones. Urgent referral is necessary, particularly in older patients, in view of the risk of Gram-negative septicemia and septic shock.

CHOLECYSTITIS

Patients with cholelithiasis may present with an attack of acute cholecystitis. The clinical picture of acute cholecystitis is determined by:

- Gallstone colic. (See: *Cholelithiasis.*)
- Chemical irritation of the gallbladder, which results in:
  - severe continuous pain, which may be largely localized to the right upper quadrant or radiate into the back
  - gallbladder tenderness and a positive Murphy's sign
  - a low-grade fever
  - a patient who resists any change in posture.

Women, especially obese women aged over 40 years, are at particular risk of *chronic cholecystitis.* Chronic cholecystitis is a syndrome characterized by:

- gallstone dyspepsia
- a tendency to gallstone formation
- a chronically inflamed gallbladder.

Patients with chronic cholecystitis may have attacks of acute cholecystitis.

Patients with chronic cholecystitis should be referred for medical evaluation and management, as obstruction of the cystic or common bile duct can have potentially serious repercussions.

CHOLELITHIASIS

Stones in the bile duct may be asymptomatic or present with:

- Pain, which:
  - is severe and lasts for hours
  - typically occurs postprandially or at night
  - may start in the back
  - radiates to the interscapular region
  - recurs as attacks of right hypochondrial pain
  - is associated with restlessness, nausea, and vomiting.
- A positive Murphy's sign. The patient is asked to inspire deeply, with the examiner's fingers under the right costal margin below the lower border of the liver. This sign is positive when inspiration is arrested due to tenderness caused by moving the inflamed gallbladder against the examiner's fingers.

- Jaundice.
- Chills, fever.

Biliary colic lacks the periodicity of renal or intestinal colic.

CHOLERA

Cholera is an infectious diarrhea caused by a Gram-negative organism, *Vibrio cholerae*. Patients may present with:

- Mild subclinical episodes of diarrhea. These patients act as carriers and spread the organism.
- Fulminant diarrhea, with:
  - rice-water stools
  - vomiting
  - muscle cramps and weakness
  - rapid dehydration, oliguria, and renal failure.

CHOLESTATIC JAUNDICE

Cholestatic jaundice results from impaired bile flow. It may result from obstruction to bile flow anywhere between the bile canaliculi and the entry of the bile duct into the duodenum at the ampulla of Vater. Intrahepatic causes are viral hepatitis, alcoholic cirrhosis, drugs (e.g. oral contraceptives), and primary biliary cirrhosis. Extrahepatic causes include pancreatic cancer, stones in the common bile duct, and ductal cancer. Patients present with:

- jaundice
- pruritus
- hypercholesterolemia and xanthomatosis
- impaired fat absorption, presenting as:
  - steatorrhea
  - prolonged prothrombin time
  - malabsorption of vitamins A, D, and K.

CHONDROMALACIA PATELLAE

See: *Patellofemoral pain syndrome.*

CHRONIC BRONCHITIS

See: *Bronchitis.*

CHRONIC FATIGUE SYNDROME

The etiology of chronic fatigue syndrome remains disputed, but immune dysfunction, either following viral infection, or food and/or chemical hypersensitivity, is postulated. Impaired blood flow to the central nervous system has also been demonstrated in patients with chronic fatigue syndrome. Impaired cell-mediated immunity is also often found in chronic fatigue syndrome patients. It has yet to be demonstrated whether this immune dysfunction is the result of a common organic cause or whether the immune dysfunction is a consequence of psychic stresses.

The three dominant criteria for categorization as chronic fatigue syndrome are:

- Unexplained persisting or relapsing fatigue which is:
  - generalized
  - new or of definite onset (not life-long)
  - present for more than 6 months
  - exacerbated by minor exercise and not the result of ongoing exertion
  - associated with significant disruption of usual daily activities. Fatigue results in a substantial reduction (> 50%), over at least 6 months, in previous levels of daily activity both occupational and social
  - not substantially relieved by rest.
- Neuropsychiatric dysfunction, including:
  - impairment of concentration (difficulty is experienced in completing mental tasks that were easily accomplished before the onset of the condition)
  - the recent onset of short-term memory impairment. (Impaired cognition is present in 90% of cases.)
- The absence of an alternative diagnosis, despite having been assessed over a 6-month period.

Attempts to define criteria for diagnosing chronic fatigue syndrome include requiring that two major and a number of minor criteria are present. The major criteria are:

- The new onset of persistent or relapsing, debilitating fatigue in a person:
  - with no previous history of similar symptoms that does not resolve with bed rest
  - that decreases daily activity by more than 50% for 6 months or longer.
- The absence of other clinical conditions that may produce chronic fatigue, as ruled out by history, physical examination, and selected laboratory tests.

Minor criteria, 4–8 of which need to be met depending on the classification, are:

- mild fever (< 38.6°C orally or 38.8°C rectally) or chills
- a sore throat (nonexudative pharyngitis is found in 75% of cases)
- palpable (< 2 cm) or tender cervical or axillary lymphadenopathy (lymphadenopathy is found in 50% of cases)

- unexplained generalized muscle weakness
- myalgia (present in 80% of patients)
- postexertional malaise lasting more than 24 hours after levels of exercise that were easily tolerated previously (this is found in 85% of patients)
- generalized headaches (3 out of 4 patients complain of a new pattern of headache or increased severity)
- migratory arthralgia without arthritis (found in 85% of patients)
- neuropsychologic complaints, such as photophobia, transient visual scotomata, forgetfulness, irritability, confusion, difficulty in thinking, inability to concentrate, and depression
- unrefreshing sleep (75% of patients experience hypersomnia or insomnia)
- an onset of the symptom complex over a few hours to days.

Cases that fail to meet the criteria of unexplained chronic fatigue are categorized as idiopathic chronic fatigue rather than chronic fatigue syndrome. Depression and fever are encountered in 85% and muscle weakness in 75% of cases.

Laboratory tests are largely unhelpful in diagnosing chronic fatigue syndrome. Baseline data, all of which should be normal, include urinalysis, complete and differential blood count, blood chemistry (glucose, calcium), erythrocyte sedimentation rate (ESR), and renal (creatine), liver (enzymes), and thyroid tests. A metabolite CFSUM1 (CFSomeone) has recently been identified in the urine of chronic fatigue sufferers. It may become a diagnostic marker.

As chronic fatigue syndrome lacks a definitive diagnostic marker, diagnosis of this syndrome requires that a number of conditions be specifically excluded. It is therefore prudent to refer patients with limited psychosocial functioning who have an illness of insidious onset and to exclude physical conditions such as:

- hypothyroidism
- chronic hepatitis
- chronic anemia
- neuromuscular disease
- occult malignancy.

These findings suggest a chronic physical or psychiatric disorder. In addition, patients should be referred for investigations in order to adequately explain:

- weight loss in excess of 10% of body weight
- significant pyrexia
- snoring and daytime somnolence (check for sleep apnea)
- specific symptoms (e.g. tarry stool, dyspepsia).

A current or previous history of the following excludes a diagnosis of chronic fatigue syndrome:

- drug or alcohol dependence
- psychotic disorders
- manic–depressive disorder.

Chronic fatigue syndrome has been variously termed: myalgic encephalomyelitis; chronic neuromuscular viral syndrome; postviral syndrome; chronic Epstein–Barr viral syndrome; viral fatigue state; epidemic neuromyasthenia; neurasthenia; Icelandic disease; Royal Free disease; Tapanic disease; chemical AIDS; and APICH syndrome (autoimmune polyendocrinopathy, immune dysregulation, candida hypersensitivity).

CHRONIC OBSTRUCTIVE AIRWAYS DISEASE (COAD)

See: *Obstructive airways disease.*

In COAD the dominant picture is one of expiratory airflow obstruction. Irritation and inflammation result in mucous plugs and fibrosis at the level of the bronchioles. In some patients bronchial involvement is marked and the clinical picture favors chronic bronchitis. In other patients alveolar involvement is marked and the clinical picture favors emphysema.

CHRONIC VENOUS INSUFFICIENCY

See: *Vascular insufficiency.*

CIGUATERA

Fish ingestion of dinoflagellates, notable after disturbance of coral reef, may result in fish poisoning. Persons eating tropical water fish such as Spanish mackerel, spotted mackerel, red and sweetlip emperor, red bass and coral trout may present within 5–6 hours of eating with:

- abdominal pain
- nausea
- diarrhea
- reversed temperature sensation
- pruritus
- paresthesia
- arthralgia.

CIRRHOSIS

Liver cirrhosis is a chronic destructive process in which fibrous replacement of parenchymal cells progressively impairs liver function. The most common causes of cirrhosis are alcohol abuse and as a complication of hepatitis B infection.

The clinical presentation includes:

- Evidence of the underlying cause:
  - a history of alcohol abuse, confirmed by current peripheral neuropathy
  - a history of acute hepatitis B infection.
- Evidence of impaired liver function:
  - weakness, fatigue, weight loss
  - pain in the right hypochondrium
  - a firm to hard hepatomegaly with a blunt or nodular edge
  - impotence, testicular atrophy, gynecomastia
  - clubbing
  - late onset of jaundice
  - liver failure, detected as a flapping tremor, confusion, encephalopathy.
- Evidence of portal hypertension. Hepatic fibrosis impairs portal blood flow, resulting in:
  - congestion of the gastrointestinal tract with:
    nausea
    anorexia
    flatulence
    vomiting
  - back-pressure on the portal system with:
    splenomegaly
    ascites
  - the development of a collateral circulation presenting as:
    esophageal varices (rupture leads to hematemesis and melena)
    caput medusa (periumbilical varices)
    hemorrhoids.

Persistent alcohol ingestion is an indication for referral.

CLAUDICATION

Pain in the lower limb may be attributed to arterial, neurological, venous, or rheological factors.

Arterial claudication presents with:

- intermittent claudication, in which pain relief is achieved by standing still
- pain in the calf
- absent distal pulses
- an ankle/arm systolic ratio of less than 0.8.

Neurological claudication presents with:

- pain along the distribution of a dermatome
- pain relieved after lying down for at least 30 minutes

- abnormal neurological signs following exercise
- a working diagnosis confirmed by myelography.

Venous claudication presents with:

- calf pain
- pain relieved by elevating the edematous leg
- a diagnosis, which may be confirmed by venography.

Rheological claudication occurs in patients with gross hyperviscosity, as in polycythemia. Patients present with:

- pain:
  - usually involving the whole leg
  - relieved by standing still
  - associated with bounding pulses
- confirmatory tests are a full blood count and erythrocyte sedimentation rate (ESR).

CLUSTER HEADACHE

Males aged 20–40 years are at particular risk. Patients present with:

- head pain, which is:
  - unilateral, starting around the eye (may involve the whole hemicranium)
  - sudden in onset
  - constant and severe.
- attacks of headache:
  - which occur in bouts lasting for up to 24 weeks
  - with up to three attacks in a 24-hour period
  - with each attack lasting 30–120 minutes.
- associated findings include:
  - a red, lacrimating eye
  - a blocked nostril on the same side as the headache
  - nausea
  - myosis, ptosis.
- glyceryl trinitrate will precipitate an attack within 30–90 minutes.
- smoking and alcohol may trigger an attack.

COAGULATION DEFECTS

Patients on anticoagulants and those with coagulation defect present with:

- hemarthoses
- hematomas
- purpura

- delayed but profuse postoperative bleeding
- a prolonged prothrombin time.

COLORECTAL CANCER

The incidence of colorectal cancer is very low before the age of 50 years. All persons over the age of 40 years with colonic symptoms should have cancer actively excluded. The clinical presentation of colorectal cancer includes:

- A persistent change in bowel habit. In colon cancer, constipation predominates; in rectal cancer, diarrhea is more common.
- Pain which is:
  - a vague abdominal discomfort (in colon cancer, colicky pain is common; in rectal cancer, tenesmus is prevalent)
  - precipitated by eating, due to the gastrocolic reflex stimulating peristalsis
  - may be relieved by defecation.
- A nontender palpable mass. At best a mass is detectable in 34% of colon cancers and in 75% of rectal cancers. Digital rectal examination detects only 50% of rectal and 10% of colon cancers. Abdominal examination for a palpable mass is usually negative.
- Rectal passage of blood and mucus.
- Anemia.
- Anorexia.
- Weight loss.
- A clinical course which is progressive and unremitting.

The site of the lesion influences the presentation:

- Lesions of the ascending and transverse colon present predominantly with:
  - abdominal colic
  - anemia due to occult blood loss.
- Lesions of the descending colon present predominantly with abdominal colic.
- Lesions of the sigmoid colon and rectum present predominantly with:
  - abdominal pain
  - diarrhea
  - rectal bleeding.

Factors predisposing to colorectal cancer include:

- The presence of pre-existing polyps. The majority of large-bowel cancers arise from benign polyps. Villous adenomas have the highest risk of neoplastic change, followed by tubular adenomas. Metaplastic polyps are not considered a cancer risk.

- Dietary choices. High alcohol, particularly beer, intake has been linked to rectal cancer, while a high-fat, high-energy, low-fiber diet has been linked to an increased risk of colon cancer. Diets rich in insoluble fiber and indigestible starch are protective. Green bananas and cold boiled potatoes are good sources of indigestible starch.
- Chronic inflammatory bowel conditions.
- A sedentary lifestyle and high body mass index (increased waist/hip ratio) have recently emerged as independent risk factors for colon cancer.

Regular aspirin ingestion of 4–6 tablets per week over 20 years has been shown to reduce the risk of colorectal cancer by 50% in women. Persons with multiple risk factors for colorectal cancer should take aspirin (300 mg; one tablet) daily. This is higher than the dose (80 mg/day) required for cardiovascular protection.

COMMUNICATING HYDROCEPHALUS (normal pressure hydrocephalus)

Cortical atrophy in elderly patients may result in:

- dementia
- gait disorders
- urinary incontinence.

CONDYLOMA ACUMINATA

Venereal warts result from benign infection with the papilloma virus. The warts:

- are painless
- present as thin flexible papules
- may become confluent and form a cauliflower lesion.

Condylomata acuminata must be differentiated from condylomata lata, the flat coppery wart of secondary syphilis.

CONGENITAL HEARING LOSS

Rubella, anoxia during delivery, and ototoxic drugs may cause congenital deafness. Babies present with:

- failure to show a startle response when exposed to a loud noise
- failure to develop normal speech.

CONGENITAL HEART DISEASE

Central cyanosis in a neonate may be due to cerebral, respiratory, or cardiac disorders. Depending on the lesion, patients with congenital heart disease may present with:

- a cardiac murmur
- cyanotic spells without respiratory distress
- tachycardia
- congestive heart failure
- hypoxic episodes characterized by irritability, dyspnea, and marked cyanosis.

CONGENITAL HIP DISLOCATION

The baby or young child presents with:

- asymmetrical skin creases in the thigh
- a thigh which cannot be completely abducted to meet the examination table when the hip and knee are flexed
- adductor spasm
- a painless limp on walking.

CONJUNCTIVITIS

Conjunctivitis may be due to an allergy or infection.

Spring catarrh (hay fever). This is believed to be associated with the rise in temperature accompanying spring and summer. Preliminary management includes reassurance and wearing dark glasses when outside. Spring catarrh presents with:

- severe itching
- a thick white discharge
- brownish or milky discoloration of exposed conjunctiva
- cobblestone appearance (rough papillae) to the conjunctiva lining the upper eyelid
- exposed conjunctiva thickened with silvery scales in severe cases.

Allergic conjunctivitis. The patient may be allergic to eye make-up, eye medication, pollens, grasses, and animal dander. In these cases blepharitis is often noted. Normal saline eyedrops may provide some relief. The action of eyedrops may be prolonged by closing the eyes and occluding the opening of the lachrymal ducts by pinching on either side of the nose with the thumb and forefinger for 30–60 seconds. Allergic conjunctivitis presents with:

- itching
- lacrimation

- photophobia
- normal or slightly reddened conjunctiva
- chemosis (conjunctival edema) in severe cases.

Infection. All persons with bilateral red eyes should be referred unless diagnosed as having either spring catarrh or allergic conjunctivitis. When the red eyes are due to infective conjunctivitis, ocular crusts and any discharge should be removed with saline drops and warm water. Patients should not share towels, face cloths, or pillows. They should also be advised to wash their hands before and after touching their eyes. Infective conjunctivitis may be:

- *Viral conjunctivitis.* Adenovirus or pink eye presents with:
  - bilateral diffuse conjunctival injection
  - gritty irritation
  - watery discharge
  - preauricular lymphadenopathy (finding a small, tender node just below the zygomatic arch in front of the ear is highly suggestive of a viral cause).

(See: *Herpes* (*Herpes keratoconjunctivitis*).)

- *Bacterial conjunctivitis.* This presents as:
  - a gritty irritation
  - a purulent exudate (eyelids are stuck together in the mornings)
  - diffuse injection of the conjunctiva.

Infection usually starts in one eye and spreads to the other.

CONNECTIVE TISSUE/ COLLAGEN DISORDERS

This is a heterogeneous group of multisystem disorders that have in common:

- inflammation, often involving skin, joints, and other tissues rich in connective tissue
- an altered pattern of immune regulation.

Diseases included in this group are:

- systemic lupus erythematosus
- rheumatoid arthritis
- scleroderma (the focus is on the skin and viscera)
- mixed connective tissue disease
- Sjögren's syndrome (the focus is on exocrine glands, leading to ocular and mucosal dryness).

Patients with connective tissue disorders often have:

- serological changes (e.g. antinuclear antibody, rheumatoid factor)
- Raynaud's phenomenon
- exacerbations and remissions.

CONSTIPATION

Constipation is considered to encompass:

- infrequent stools
- excessively hard stool
- tenesmus.

Functional constipation. See dyschezia.

Iatrogenic constipation may result from drug ingestion. Drugs causing constipation include:

- calcium supplements
- iron supplements
- opioid analgesics (codeine)
- antacids (aluminum hydroxide)
- laxative abuse
- muscle relaxants
- ganglion blocking agents
- antidepressants (monoamine oxidase inhibitors, tricyclic anti-depressants)
- barbiturates
- phenothiazines
- diuretics
- cytotoxic drugs
- vasodilators.

CONSTRICTIVE PERICARDITIS

See: *Pericarditis.*

CONVULSION

See: *Epilepsy.*

Febrile convulsion. Certain children are prone to convulsions when they have a high temperature. The commonest cause is an upper respiratory tract infection. Immediate intervention involves maintaining an airway and preventing self-injury. It is helpful to lie the child on their side with their head down, to prevent aspiration. Lowering the child's temperature is a priority. Prevention of future occurrences may be achieved by tepid sponging, a cool fan, and stripping the child to their underwear. Paracetamol may be necessary to adequately control the temperature.

CORN

Patients present with:

- a hyperkeratotic area resulting from pressure and friction
- conical masses of keratin which may be flattened due to pressure (e.g. on the sole)

- lesions are found in areas of thin skin:
  - over toe joints (hard corns)
  - between the toes (soft corns)
- tenderness on pressure
- on paring, a sharply outlined translucent core is seen to interrupt the normal skin markings.

CORYZA (common cold)

The common cold presents predominantly with nasal symptoms and signs. The incidence in children is 4–8 per year, and in adults 2–6 per year.

Ranked in order of frequency, the clinical presentation includes:

- nasal catarrh, presenting as a clear watery discharge which becomes mucopurulent in 24–48 hours
- sneezing
- mild diffuse erythema of the pharynx, which lasts 3–5 days and is associated with nasal obstruction and a mildly sore throat
- hoarseness (see: *Laryngitis*)
- cough (present in less than half of patients)
- lethargy, malaise
- headache, myalgia
- mild fever and chills
- tearing (epiphora).

Coryza differs from influenza in that in the common cold:

- myalgia is rare
- fever is mild
- nasal and throat symptoms dominate.

COSTOSTERNAL AND COSTOCHONDRAL SYNDROME

Patients present with:

- diffuse pain in the anterior part of the chest wall
- pain radiation to the whole chest that may extend into the arm
- tenderness on palpation of the costosternal junction
- tenderness along contiguous intercostal muscles
- pain is reproduced by palpation of affected costochondral joints (Tietze syndrome involves second or third costochondral joints on the left)
- severity which varies from dull ache to throbbing

- pain which is worsened by movement, especially deep inspiration
- the condition may be associated with anxiety and hyperventilation and a history of overuse, trauma, or upper respiratory infection. The disorder may disappear spontaneously in a few days and may recur intermittently for months or years.

CRACKED SKIN

Patients with very dry skin may present with:

- fissures on the fingertips next to the nail fold, the heels, or lips
- local pain.

Protection against irritants, detergents, and drying soaps with gloves and socks plus emollient creams may relieve the problem.

CRAMPS

Muscle cramps may result from inadequate perfusion, electrolyte imbalance, or may be of undetermined cause. The patient presents with:

- severe limb pain associated with strong muscle contraction
- abrupt onset
- episodic muscle spasms.

CROHN'S DISEASE

See: *Inflammatory bowel disease.*

CROUP (laryngotracheobronchitis)

- Croup is a condition encountered in young children and is characterized by inspiratory stridor. Viral croup is usually caused by parainfluenza viruses, but may also be caused by respiratory syncytial and influenza type A viruses. It is a self-limiting condition which develops gradually over 48–72 hours. Children between the ages of 3 and 36 months are most at risk. Viral croup presents with:
  - inspiratory stridor
  - a barking cough
  - low-grade fever
  - moderate hoarseness
  - minimal cyanosis, if present
  - a normal white cell count
  - subglottic narrowing on an anteroposterior radiograph.

(See: *Laryngotracheobronchitis.*)

Bacterial croup (epiglottitis) is caused by *Haemophilus influenzae* and is more common in children aged 2–5 years. It is a more serious condition than viral croup and can rapidly progress, within 4–12 hours, to respiratory arrest if left untreated. Bacterial croup presents with:

- inspiratory stridor
- cyanosis
- marked dysphagia
- fever (38.5°C)
- marked hoarseness
- a markedly raised white cell count
- a swollen epiglottis on a lateral film.

Spasmodic croup is of idiopathic etiology and is a recurrent disease of short duration. Children aged 1–4 years are prone to sudden attacks of spasmodic croup, usually at night. The presentation includes:

- inspiratory stridor
- a barking cough
- no fever
- mild or no hoarseness
- no dysphagia
- no cyanosis
- normal radiographic findings
- normal white cell count.

Other conditions that may cause inspiratory stridor are tracheitis and inhalation of a foreign body.

CUSHING'S SYNDROME

A condition of excess glucocorticoids, Cushing's syndrome presents with:

- sudden onset of centripetal obesity characterized by:
  - a 'moon' face (increased facial fat)
  - a 'buffalo' hump (a dorsocervical fat pad)
- hirsutism
- acne
- a thin atrophic skin (other skin changes include spontaneous ecchymoses, purple striae, and delayed wound healing)
- osteoporosis, often with low-back pain
- hypertension, fluid retention
- weakness, muscle wasting
- mood lability varying to psychosis (depression, euphoria, irritability, insomnia)
- decreased libido

- oligomenorrhea or amenorrhea
- laboratory findings include:
  - raised serum cortisol and urinary 17-hydroxysteroids
  - glycosuria
  - low serum potassium and chloride
  - hyperglycemia.

Recent studies have shown that steroid-induced spinal, but not radial and femoral, osteoporotic fractures may be reduced by calcium (1000 mg/day) plus calcitriol (0.5–1 mg/day).

CYSTIC FIBROSIS

Cystic fibrosis is an autosomal recessively inherited condition which results in the production of abnormally viscid glandular secretion. The condition usually begins in infancy. Patients are troubled by:

- Chronic respiratory problems:
  - persistent cough (coughing is related to posture)
  - recurrent infection
  - bronchitis
  - bronchiectasis.
- Pancreatic insufficiency:
  - malabsorption
  - steatorrhea
  - weight loss, failure to thrive.
- infertility.

CYSTITIS

The clinical presentation of bladder irritation (cystitis) is:

- frequency
- urgency
- dysuria or burning on micturition.

Hemorrhagic cystitis also presents with:

- terminal hematuria (bleeding at the end of micturition)
- suprapubic tenderness
- a positive urine culture.

Honeymoon cystitis presents with:

- dysuria
- a high level of sexual activity
- sterile urine.

CYTOLYTIC VAGINOSIS

This condition is believed to be the result of overgrowth by lactobacilli. Cytolysis of the vaginal epithelium is associated with:

- A frothy white discharge.
- Symptoms that increase during the second half of the menstrual cycle include:
  - dyspareunia
  - vulval pruritus
  - dysuria.

These patients are often misdiagnosed as having a yeast infection. A wet mount is required to exclude *Candida.*

DACRYOCYSTITIS

Infection of the lacrimal sac secondary to obstruction of the nasolacrimal duct presents with:

- localized tender swelling of the lower lid over the medial canthus
- a history of a watery eye
- palpebral injection
- a mucopurulent discharge.

DANDRUFF

This presents as dry flaky skin. (See: *Seborrheic dermatitis.*)

DEEP VEIN THROMBOSIS

Obstruction of the deep venous system of the lower limb by thrombosis may result in venous insufficiency. The clinical presentation of deep vein thrombosis (DVT) varies. It may be asymptomatic or present with:

- an aching tight calf
- calf tenderness and muscle spasm
- pitting ankle edema
- tender limb induration distal to the occlusion
- failure of venous drainage on limb elevation
- pain induced in the calf on dorsiflexion of the foot (Homan's sign). (*Note*: The risk of dislodging thrombus and precipitating pulmonary embolization makes this procedure dangerous and it should not be used, particularly as it is an unreliable diagnostic test.)

The complications of DVT include:

- varicose veins following valve destruction (see: *Varicose veins*)
- pulmonary embolism (see: *Pulmonary embolism*), which may be the first clinical evidence of DVT in asymptomatic disease
- ankle blow-out syndrome due to damage to ankle perforators
- a postphlebitic leg, in which thrombosis involves major deep veins
- venous gangrene following extensive thrombosis
- chronic venous insufficiency.

Ankle blow-out syndrome. When the high pressure within the deep venous system is transmitted through incompetent perforators into the superficial veins around the ankle, venous congestion around the medial malleolus occurs. Patients with ankle blow-out syndrome present with pedal:

- edema
- cyanosis
- fat necrosis
- fibrosis, causing a bottle-shaped leg
- persistent deep ulceration.

Chronic venous leg ulcers improve when use of standard compression bandages is combined with 300 mg/day enteric-coated aspirin orally.

Postphlebitic leg. Proximal extension of the ankle blow-out syndrome presents with:

- a bursting pain aggravated by standing
- edema extending proximally up the leg
- cyanosis extending proximally up the leg
- the features of the ankle blow-out syndrome.

Venous gangrene. Extensive venous thrombosis resulting in inadequate limb perfusion with tissue anoxia and necrosis. Venous gangrene presents with:

- swelling
- fibrosis
- deep necrotic ulcers
- superimposed infections.

Chronic venous insufficiency. (See: *Vascular insufficiency*.) In addition to the more specific syndromes, any obstruction to venous draining is accompanied by varying degrees of chronic venous insufficiency. The mildest form is minimal edema upon prolonged standing. More clinically relevant is chronic venous insufficiency, which presents with:

- progressive leg edema
- atrophic skin (skin is thin and shiny)
- a cyanotic limb (brown ankle or leg pigmentation is due to red cell extravasation and hematin denaturation)
- fibrotic subcutaneous tissue
- pruritic lesions
- chronic recurrent ulceration.

DELIRIUM (acute organic brain syndrome; acute confusional state)

Patients with infections, particularly those with high fevers, or drug toxicity may present with delirium. Patients with dementia are at particular risk of delirium in such circumstances. Delirium is characterized by:

- a rapid onset
- reduced or clouded consciousness
- disorientation and impaired attention or memory impairment
- two or more of:
  - misperceptions, which may lead to visual and/or auditory hallucinations
  - incoherent speech
  - a sleep disturbance (symptoms worst at night)
  - altered psychomotor activity
- a fluctuating course over hours or weeks.

DEMENTIA

Dementia affects 5% of the population over 65 and 20% over 80 years of age. It is characterized by progressive deterioration in mental, particularly cognitive, functioning. Senile and presenile (Alzheimer-type) dementia may be due to a degenerative process. Atherosclerotic dementia may be due to multiple cerebral infarcts. Infections can cause an acute-onset dementia. Various systemic disorders (e.g. myxedema), local brain tumors, nutritional deficiencies (e.g. vitamins B_{12} or B_3), alcoholism, and collagen diseases may also be causes of dementia.

Patients present with:

- Gradually progressive deterioration over months and years.
- Memory impairment characterized by:
  - Poor short-term memory: recent events, occurring hours or moments before, are forgotten.
  - Better retention of long-term memory: familiar tasks are well performed, but learning new tasks is very difficult.
  - Poor concentration.
- Gradual personality disintegration with:
  - blunting of affect
  - tactlessness and increasing coarseness
  - social withdrawal
  - apathy and loss of initiative.
- Progressive intellectual impairment with:
  - diminished problem-solving skills
  - poor judgement and insight
  - a rigid outlook
  - poverty of thought.

- Language deterioration with:
  - difficulty in reading and writing
  - disordered speech.
- Mood changes, including depression, anxiety and, in some cases, elation.
- A normal level of consciousness, although patients are inattentive.
- Normal blood count, biochemistry, cerebrospinal fluid, and brain scans (early).

DENGUE

Dengue is a mosquito-borne viral disease. It presents with a prodrome of:

- high fever
- severe headache and ocular pain
- vomiting and abdominal pain
- myalgia and bone pain
- a maculopapular rash

This may be followed by dengue hemorrhagic fever in which:

- a continuous fever persists for 2–7 days
- hemorrhagic manifestations include petechiae, purpura, and epistaxis.

Dengue shock syndrome, which is characterized by marked hypotension, may develop.

DENTAL CARIES

Dental caries present with pain which:

- is often localized to the affected tooth
- may be diffuse over the maxilla or mandible
- may be referred over the superior and anteromedial surface of the pinna and anterior surface of the eardrum
- is aggravated by:
  - cold, if dental pulp is vital
  - heat, if dental pulp is necrotic
- does not cross the midline.

A periapical abscess has a similar presentation. Gum redness and swelling may be detectable.

DEPRESSION

Depressed persons experience lack of motivation and mood changes, with emotional, physical, and social repercussions.

Laboratory tests are normal. Depression may be overt or masked.

Major depression is diagnosed when for a period in excess of 14 days patients complain of:

- A pervasive depressed mood.
- Loss of interest or pleasure.
- Three or more of the following are present:
  - significant loss or gain of appetite or weight
  - sleep disturbance (early morning waking, difficulty falling asleep, hypersomnia)
  - psychomotor retardation or agitation
  - feelings of worthlessness or guilt
  - impaired thinking or concentration, indecisiveness, pseudo-dementia.
- Autonomic nervous system problems:
  - change in bowel habit (constipation)
  - palpitations
  - dry mouth
  - menstrual disorders.
- Psychosomatic problems:
  - arthralgia
  - chest pain
  - weakness
  - nausea
  - psychogenic vomiting.

Masked depression may be present when the patient displays:

- flatness of mood
- lack of interest in work and hobbies
- loss of self-worth
- avoidance of people
- loss of physical energy, lethargy
- an inability to cope with stress
- a disturbed sleep pattern
- an all-pervading anxiety
- suicidal thoughts.

Medical depression may result from or be associated with:

- viral disease:
  - influenza
  - viral hepatitis
  - infectious mononucleosis.
- Connective tissue disorder:
  - rheumatoid arthritis
  - systemic lupus erythematosus.
- Endocrine disorder:
  - myxedema
  - Cushing's disease
  - Addison's disease.

- Nutritional deficiency:
  - vitamin B_{12} deficiency
  - vitamin B_3 deficiency.
- Drugs:
  - alcohol
  - sedative hypnotics
  - certain antihypertensive agents
  - oral contraceptives.
- Cancer of the pancreas.

DERMATITIS (eczema)

More than half of all skin diseases can be classified as dermatitis or eczema. The terms are interchangeable. Dermatitis is widespread and present in various forms, including:

- erythema and edema
- vesicles which change to red weeping crusted lesions or scaling papules
- itching or burning areas which thicken with persistent scratching.

Dermatitis may be acute, subacute, or chronic. Two elements are important in dermatitis: a genetic predisposition, which dominates in persons with atopic eczema; and a trigger factor, such as an emotional upset, trauma, or an irritant.

In *contact dermatitis (exogenous eczema)* the external trigger is all important. Contact dermatitis is triggered by direct skin contact with an irritant. It presents with:

- red scaly or weeping patches (at the site of contact with irritant)
- mild to moderate pruritus.

When internal causes dominate, dermatitis may take one of the following forms:

Atopic dermatitis/eczema. This has been described as an 'itch that rashes'. The presentation includes:

- A history of atopy. Patients often also have other evidence of a tendency to allergy (e.g. hay fever, asthma, urticaria (pruritic wheals)).
- Pruritus.
- A variation with age.
  - In infantile eczema, a red skin with small vesicles and small oozing cracks are noted. Lesions are frequently found on the face, wrists, flexures, and in a nappy distribution around the buttock.
  - In childhood eczema, papules and skin thickening is found in the flexures.

- In adults, papules, and crusted thickened lesions may weep as a result of scratching. Lesions are found in flexures, on the neck, face, and legs and feet, back of the hands, and anogenital region.

Discoid eczema. Anxious middle-aged individuals are prone to this form of eczema, which presents with:

- pruritus
- small vesicles that burst leaving crusts
- lesions that coalesce to form plaques
- coin-shaped lesions
- lesions commonly found on the back of the hands and forearms, and the legs and thighs.

Pompholyx. This presents with:

- excessive sweating in affected areas
- an itchy burn
- vesicles resemble sago grains
- brownish scales develop after the vesicles rupture
- lesions are found on the palm, soles, and fingers.

Seborrheic dermatitis. This presents as:

- macular lesions or pinhead papules
- yellow scales
- itchy in adults, less so in children
- scaly disease of hairy areas, causing dandruff when affecting the scalp, and blepharitis when involving eyelashes.

Dermatitis herpetiformis. This presents with:

- the gradual onset of clusters of tiny vesicles, papules, and macules
- intensely pruritic lesions (scratching may obscure the lesions)
- lesions are often symmetrically distributed on extensor surfaces.

Immunological abnormalities are common in these patients.

DIABETES INSIPIDUS

Deficiency of antidiuretic hormone (ADH) produced or released from the posterior pituitary or failure of the kidney tubules to respond to ADH leads to an ability to concentrate urine and conserve water. Patients with diabetes insipidus present with:

- polydipsia
- polyuria (more than 6 liters of urine may be passed each day)
- an inability to concentrate urine on fluid restriction (even when dehydrated the urinary specific gravity is persistently less than 1.006).

DIABETES MELLITUS

Diabetics are categorized as insulin or non-insulin dependent. The typical clinical picture of the *insulin-dependent diabetes mellitus* (IDDM) is that of a lean individual, under 30 years of age, who over recent days or weeks has experienced thirst, polyuria, and weight loss. The patient with *noninsulin-dependent diabetes mellitus* (NIDDM) is likely to be over 40 years of age with a family history of diabetes. They are often overweight and complain of having gradually experienced increasing fatigue, susceptibility to infections, and vascular disease. Pacific islanders, Australian Aboriginals, Mauritians, southern Europeans, Asian Indians, and Chinese show a particularly high prevalence of NIDDM.

A definitive diagnosis of diabetes mellitus is made on finding:

- Raised blood glucose on two separate occasions in an asymptomatic individual. Raised blood glucose may be detected as a:
  - Random blood glucose in excess of 11 mmol/l.
  - Fasting venous plasma glucose equal to or exceeding 7.8 mmol/l.
  - Venous plasma glucose in excess of 11.0 mmol/l at 2 hours during a standard oral glucose tolerance test. Impaired glucose tolerance, rather than diabetes, is diagnosed when fasting venous plasma glucose is less than 7.8 mmol/l and venous plasma glucose is in the range 7.8–11.0 mmol/l at 2 hours in the standard oral glucose tolerance test.
- Raised blood sugar on one occasion in a symptomatic individual. Symptoms suggestive of diabetes mellitus include:
  - Thirst and polyuria. Nocturnal polyuria is an important indication of faltering glycemic control.
  - Polyphagia and weight loss.
  - Unexplained fatigue or weakness.
  - Vulvovaginitis or pruritus.
  - Recurrent blurred vision.
  - Muscle weakness, often involving clawing of the toes.
  - Peripheral neuropathy in the form of glove and stocking paresthesia.
  - Recurrent infections.

Complications in diabetes increase with age. Tight blood sugar control delays the onset and progression of complications.

Acute complications include:

- Ketoacidemic or hyperglycemic coma. This is associated with insulin underdose or a preceding infection. The patient with diabetic acidosis presents with:
  - slow deep or rapid breathing
  - thirst and dehydration

- nausea and vomiting
- the absence of sweating
- fruity breath
- a weak pulse, which may be irregular
- polyuria, glycosuria, and ketonuria.

- These findings develop over hours or days.
- Hypoglycemic coma. This results from a skipped meal, insulin overdose, or exercise. Within minutes the patient demonstrates:
  - stertorous breathing
  - marked sweating
  - palpitations, tachycardia
  - slurred speech
  - normal hydration
  - central nervous system changes (e.g. a Babinski response, dilated pupils).

Chronic complications. These range from macrovascular disease to microvascular disease. Aberrant lipid metabolism is more closely linked to macrovascular disease, and impaired glycemic control predisposes to microvascular disease. Chronic complications include:

Eye problems. Ocular manifestations of diabetes include:

- Blurred vision:
  - Transient myopia may occur during periods of poor control. Visual change is due to the osmotic effect of glucose on the crystalline lens.
  - Unclear vision. Blurred vision may result from closure of capillaries with focal axon swelling and macular edema. Along with microaneurysms, cottonwool exudates, and hemorrhages, these changes are encountered in nonproliferative diabetic retinopathy.
- Blindness. Each year in the USA almost 6000 new cases of blindness are attributable to diabetes. Four out of five cases of blindness due to diabetes are attributable to diabetic retinopathy. With laser therapy diabetic retinopathy is a treatable condition. Significant risk factors for diabetic retinopathy include: treatment with insulin or oral hypoglycemic drugs, diabetes of 7 years or more duration, an albumin excretion rate of 21 μg/min or more and age of 50–66 years. Blindness is attributable to:
  - Cataracts.
  - The complications of neovascularization in patients with proliferative retinopathy. Neovascularization increases the tendency to bleeding and fibrosis resulting in vitreous hemorrhage and retinal detachment.

Renal disease. Retinopathy is likely to precede nephropathy in diabetics. One in 10 adult-onset diabetics has evidence of renal disease within 20 years of the initial diagnosis. Renal complications of diabetes include:

- Diabetic nephropathy. Predictors of diabetic nephropathy are:
  - Microalbuminuria. Microalbuminuria, the passage of 30–300 mg/day, is an early sign of nephropathy. In insulin-dependent diabetics, microalbuminuria of more than 50 mg/24 hours on more than one occasion is predictive of clinical diabetic nephropathy within 10 years. In noninsulin-dependent diabetics, it is strongly linked with cardiovascular risk. Albuminuria detected on dipstick testing (> 550 mg/24 hours) is predictive of future renal failure.
  - Hypertension.
  - Hyperfiltration (glycosuria).
  - Poor glycemic control. Intensive control of blood glucose reduces albuminuria by 60%.
- Urinary tract infection. Vigorous treatment of any urinary tract infections is necessary.
- Papillary necrosis.
- Bladder dysfunction. Associated with diabetic neuropathy, diabetics may experience a reduced sensation of bladder fullness, a poor stream, hesitancy, and straining.

Neuropathy. Tall individuals with poor glycemic control and a long history of diabetes are most at risk. After 25 years of diabetes, 50% have evidence of neuropathy. Patients with neuropathy present with:

- Sensory neuropathy. Patients may have:
  - An asymptomatic sensory neuropathy.
  - Chronic progressive sensory neuropathy. This is irreversible and may result in: painful paresthesia, foot ulcers, or neuropathic joints.
  - Acute reversible neuropathy. Acute burning pain is self-limiting and may coincide with poor metabolic control.
- The peripheral sensory neuropathy of diabetes is described as having a glove and stocking distribution of:
  - numbness
  - pain which is worst at night
  - dysesthesiae, which is often burning in nature and worst at night
  - reduced touch and vibration sense, indicating involvement of the large fibers
  - reduced pin prick sensation, indicating involvement of the small fibers.
- Motor neuropathy. Small nerve fibers are affected, and patients present with:
  - muscle cramps
  - weakness
  - atrophy of small muscles of the foot
  - imbalance between pedal flexors and extensors
  - clawing of the toes, forward migration of the fibrofatty foot pads

- abnormal bony prominences and prolapsed metatarsal heads
- callus formation
- ulceration.

- Focal neuropathy:
  - Foot drop due to a common peroneal nerve palsy.
  - Cranial nerve palsies. These mononeuropathies usually resolve spontaneously within 3 months. The third, sixth, and seventh cranial nerves are most commonly involved. Diabetic neuropathy of the third cranial nerve spares the parasympathetic innervation of the pupil, so pupillary constriction to light is retained. This differs from an oculomotor lesion attributable to an aneurysm of the posterior communicating artery.
  - Diabetic amyotrophy due to infarction of the femoral nerve, with pain and weakness in the quadriceps.
  - Carpal tunnel syndrome.
- Autonomic neuropathy presents with:
  - postural dizziness, blackouts
  - persistent diarrhea, constipation
  - impotence
  - sweating abnormalities
  - sluggish pupillary reaction to light
  - dry cracking skin.
- Diabetics with neuropathy are at risk of:
  - Failing to recognize and/or experience the early signs of hypoglycemia normally mediated through the autonomic nervous system.
  - Foot problems. Macrovascular peripheral vascular disease (the risk of atherosclerosis is more than doubled in diabetics) coupled with sensory and motor changes predisposes diabetics to major foot problems. Referral to a podiatrist for pedal hygiene is recommended.

DIETARY INTOLERANCE

Dietary intolerance or malabsorption of lactose, sucrose, or sorbitol may result in:

- bloating
- flatulence
- diarrhea.

Disaccharide intolerance presents with various combinations of:

- frothy stools
- abdominal pain
- abdominal distension
- recurrent abdominal pain in older children.

Symptoms usually occur 30 minutes after a milk feed. Lactose intolerance should be differentiated from cow's milk protein allergy, which presents with:

- esophageal reflux
- vomiting
- colic
- irritability
- loose stools.

(See: *Lactase deficiency*; *Celiac disease*, for information about gluten intolerance.)

DIPHTHERIA

Corynebacterium diphtheriae is spread by droplets. After an incubation period of 7 days, diphtheria presents with:

- pain on swallowing
- a thick gray membrane over the tonsils, pharynx, or larynx
- a mild temperature (<38°C).

The disease can be prevented by immunization.

DISCOID LUPUS ERYTHEMATOSUS

Discoid lupus erythematosus is a chronic recurrent disorder which primarily affects the skin. Patients present with:

- sharply circumscribed erythematous macules and plaques
- follicular plugging
- scales
- telangiectasia.

Lesions may be limited to above the chin or may be widespread.
Systemic lupus erythematosus must be excluded.

DISC PROTRUSION OR PROLAPSE

See: *Spinal dysfunction*.

DISLOCATION

Posterior elbow dislocation presents with:

- a history of falling on an outstretched arm
- an unusually prominent olecranon process
- an immovable joint
- the arm flexed at 40°.

In contrast to a supracondylar fracture, in elbow dislocation the:

- forearm is not supported by the opposite hand
- the altitude of the bony triangle is shortened.

Shoulder dislocation presents with:

- anteromedial displacement of the humerus
- disruption of the bony shoulder triangle, with flattening of the shoulder profile
- the arm is minimally elevated with and supported by the opposite hand.

Rarely, posterior dislocation occurs and presents with painful restriction of external rotation.

DIVERTICULITIS

Colonic diverticulae are mucosal outpouchings at sites where the bowel wall is weakened by entry of the neurovascular bundle through the muscle layer. Inflammation of these outpouchings results in diverticulitis, which presents clinically with:

- colicky abdominal pain (diverticulitis is sometimes referred to 'left-sided appendicitis', as the sigmoid colon is most frequently involved)
- alterations in bowel habit
- tenesmus (straining at stool)
- mucus in the stool
- anorexia, nausea, vomiting
- a tender abdominal mass
- occasionally massive hemorrhage.

The clinical course is one of attacks and remissions.

A low-fiber diet is advocated during acute attacks, while a high-fiber maintenance diet is thought to reduce intraluminal pressure and the risk of diverticulum formation. Attacks can be minimized by avoiding foods such as nuts, seeds, hulls, or berries, which could be trapped in a diverticulum.

DONOVANOSIS

Donovania granulomatis, after an incubation period of 7–28 days, presents with:

- elevated, beefy, red, well-demarcated granuloma
- single or multiple lesions
- lesions with a friable base and a ragged, serpiginous edge
- mild to severe pain
- inguinal granulomas.

Lesions are usually found on the penis and labia.

DROP ATTACK

Patients fall without loss of consciousness. Drop attacks may result from bilateral leg weakness. (See: *Transient ischemic attack.*)

DRUG ERUPTION

A variety of drugs may give rise to skin lesions. Most drug reactions resolve when the drug is removed. Examples of drug eruptions include:

- Urticaria due to penicillin.
- Maculopapular rashes due to barbiturates.
- Mucocutaneous eruptions due to sulfonamides.
- Aciniform lesions due to corticosteroids.
- Photosensitivity due to phenothiazides.
- Purpuric eruptions due to anticoagulants.
- Exfoliation due to penicillin or sulfonamides.
- Fixed drug eruptions due to tetracyclines or phenolphthalein. Patients present with well-circumscribed purplish lesions that reappear each time the drug is taken. Lesions may be isolated.

DRUG REBOUND HEADACHE

Headaches may result from withdrawal of corticosteroids, caffeine, alcohol, analgesics, and amfetamines. Patients present with a dull headache following withdrawal of the drug. The headache persists for 5–7 days.

DRUG WITHDRAWAL

Drugs that produce dependence:

- Have a psychological effect: they reduce discomfort or increase pleasure.
- May induce physical tolerance: larger doses are required to achieve similar effects.
- Produce a withdrawal syndrome characterized by:
  - unpleasant physiological effects when the drug is discontinued abruptly
  - psychological craving
  - a clinical picture characteristic of the drug involved.

DRY EYES

Dry eyes may be attributable to local or systemic causes. They may be due to:

- lacrimal gland dysfunction attributable to age, drugs, lymphoma, or systemic connective tissue disorders
- impaired eyelid function due to trachoma scarring, exophthalmos, a nerve palsy (V or VII)
- mucin deficiency in hypovitaminosis A or trachoma
- excessive environment exposure, due to either dry conditions or exophthalmos.

Dry eyes present with:

- Ocular grittiness.
- A burning itching sensation.
- Difficulty in moving the eyelids.
- The sensation of a foreign body.
- Irritation, which worsens as the day progresses.
- A positive Schirmer test. Whatman No. 41 filter paper is used to test for aqueous deficiency. A 5 mm × 35 mm strip of filter paper is folded and hooked over the nasal end of the lower eyelid. The patient is instructed to look down and keep the eyes firmly closed. After 5 minutes, if less than 5 mm of the filter paper is wet, a dry eye is diagnosed.

In the absence of ocular disease, and with adequate therapy for the primary condition, ocular dryness may be reduced using a room humidifier to reduce environmental dryness and a trial of 'artificial tear substitutes'. Visulose (methylcellulose), Liquifilm (polyvinyl alcohol), or Ultra Tears (hydroxypropylmethylcellulose) may be instilled as often as necessary. A starting regimen is often two drops four times a day.

DUODENAL ULCER

See: *Peptic ulcer disease.*

DYSCHEZIA

Functional constipation (dyschezia) is attributable to poor dietary and bowel habits. Simple constipation presents with:

- straining at stool
- infrequent defecation (less than once per day)
- a full rectum on examination (fecal impaction)
- hard fecal masses
- staining due to inadvertent passage of feculent mucus

- predisposing factors:
  - persistent suppression of the call to stool
  - low-fiber diet
  - fear of painful defecation (anal fissure, thrombosed pile).

DYSENTERY

Blood and mucus in the stool may result from:

- infection (e.g. shigellosis (bacillary dysentery), amebiasis)
- inflammatory bowel disease (e.g. ulcerative colitis, Crohn's disease)
- malignancy (e.g. rectal cancer).

EATING DISORDERS

Eating disorders are most commonly encountered in young women who have a morbid fear of becoming fat.

Anorexia nervosa is characterized by radical restriction of energy intake and emaciation. Features of the condition include:

- Onset around puberty or before the age of 25 years.
- Anorexia with loss of 25% or more of original body weight. Emaciation is profound in the advanced cases.
- A distorted self-image. Sufferers fail to recognize they are extremely thin.
- A psychological abhorrence of food that overrides hunger.
- No known psychiatric or medical illness that provides an alternate explanation.
- At least two of the following:
  - amenorrhea
  - bradycardia
  - periods of overactivity, ritual exercising
  - episodes of bulimia
  - vomiting, which may be self-induced
  - lanugo hair.

Complications include hypokalemia, cardiac arrhythmias, and death.

Bulimia is characterized by massive binge eating followed by self-induced vomiting as a weight-control measure. Weight is usually relatively normal at the time of diagnosis. Features of the condition include:

- secretive eating habits
- mood swings
- preoccupation with weight control
- effortless vomiting
- laxative abuse

- binge eating
- food collection and hoarding rituals.

Complications include hypokalemia, cardiac arrhythmias, esophageal rupture, and aspiration.

ECTOPIC PREGNANCY

Patients who have a history of pelvic surgery, pelvic inflammatory disease, or a previous ectopic pregnancy are at risk of ectopic pregnancy. Ectopic pregnancy should be suspected in women who present with:

- Pregnancy:
  - a history of one or more missed period
  - a uterine size that is not consistent with the stage of pregnancy.
- A brownish vaginal discharge or vaginal bleeding.
- Pain:
  - unilateral cramping in an iliac fossa is followed by severe constant lower abdominal pain
  - may radiate to the rectum, vagina, or leg
  - is aggravated by movement.
- Exquisite tenderness is detected on cervical palpation.
- Shock.

ECZEMA

See: *Dermatitis*.

EMPHYSEMA

The major features of emphysema are breathlessness, lung hyperinflation, and airflow obstruction on pulmonary function tests. Emphysema may be due to:

- An α_1-antitrypsin deficiency. In this inherited condition the liver fails to produce α_1-antitrypsin, an enzyme normally produced in amounts just sufficient to neutralize the trypsin released during cleansing by inflammatory cells.
- Alveolar macrophages and other inflammatory cell products. Dying phagocytes release digestive enzymes (including trypsin) which damage the surrounding tissue. Macrophages may be destroyed attempting to engulf smoke particles and other air pollutants.

Enzymatic destruction of lung tissue results in loss of elastic recoil and alteration to the alveolar surface tension. Progressive thinning of alveolar walls leads to air trapping due to reduced elastic recoil and collapse of small intrapulmonary airways during expiration. The severe small airways obstruction in emphysema is attributable to this lesion. Breakdown of thinned alveolar walls results in bullae formation and diminishes the surface area for gaseous exchange. Hypoxemia results.

The patient presents clinically with:

- gradually progressive dyspnea (the dominant symptom)
- poor exercise tolerance
- a barrel chest
- use of accessory muscles of respiration
- pursed lip breathing
- increased resonance on percussion
- diminished breath sounds on auscultation
- vesicular breath sounds with prolonged expiration
- occasional wheezes
- minimal cough with scanty sputum
- polycythemia (pink puffers have a stronger ventilatory drive than those emphysematous patients who are cyanosed).

EMPYEMA

Empyema is infection within the pleural cavity. Infection of a pleural effusion may result from underlying lung pathology, traumatic penetration of the pleural cavity, or transdiaphragmatic spread of a subphrenic abscess. The patient presents with:

- fever and leukocytosis
- impaired local chest movement
- possible mediastinal shift (the trachea is displaced to the side away from the empyema)
- stony dullness on percussion
- reduced or absent breath sounds.

Pleural aspiration is diagnostic. Patients suspected of empyema should be referred for drainage and antibiotics.

ENCEPHALITIS

Inflammation of the brain presents with:

- Fever.
- Acute onset of headache.
- An altered level of consciousness:
  - drowsiness (this carries a good prognosis)
  - confusion
  - coma (the prognosis is bad)
  - fits (the prognosis is poor).

- Behavioral changes.
- Focal central nervous system lesions.
- Skin lesions may be present, depending on the cause.

ENDOCARDITIS

Inflammation of the inner lining of the heart can distort valves and act as a site for vegetation (clot) formation. Patients present with:

- Heart murmurs.
- Embolic phenomena. Infarction may follow peripheral lodging of bland emboli:
  - microscopic hematuria (renal failure may develop)
  - splinter hemorrhages in the nail bed
  - petechial hemorrhages in skin and mucous membranes
  - raised painful nodules (Osler's nodes) as a result of emboli to subcutaneous tissues of the fingers, toes, palms, soles.

In patients with septic emboli, additional findings include:

- fever
- clubbing
- anemia
- splenomegaly
- a positive blood culture.

Subacute bacterial endocarditis is a particular problem in patients with valvular disease. Evidence of embolic phenomena and changing heart murmurs are indications for medical management.

ENDOMETRIAL CANCER

Endometrial cancer is usually diagnosed in postmenopausal women. Women with diabetes are at increased risk. Risk factors associated with the development of endometrial carcinoma include prolonged estrogen exposure, endometrial polyps, menorrhagia, obesity, and hypertension. The clinical presentation includes:

- abnormal uterine bleeding
- a brown offensive vaginal discharge
- a bulky uterus.

Occlusion of the cervix by tumor may result in a uterine cavity distended by pus (pyometra) or blood (hematometra).

ENDOMETRIOSIS

Endometriosis is a disorder of uncertain etiology which occurs in at least 8% of women. It is the most common cause of chronic pain in women in the reproductive age group and is found in 20% of infertile women. Regular aerobic exercise of 5 hours per week, smoking, and childbearing appear to reduce the risk of endometriosis. A diagnosis of endometriosis is often delayed. The average delay in women developing the disease as a teenager is 8 years. Endometriosis is clinically characterized by:

- The cyclical occurrence of pain:
  - ovulation pain
  - premenstrual pain
  - premenstrual tension
  - deep dyspareunia
  - dysuria
  - bowel pain.
- Congestive dysmenorrhea:
  - pain starts several days, often 7 days, before the next menses
  - a heavy, dull pain is felt in the lower abdomen
  - pain progressively worsens until the onset of menses
  - pain may also be felt in the pelvis and lower back.
- Menorrhagia.
- The cyclical occurrence of diverse symptoms:
  - change in bowel habits with menstruation
  - spotting between periods
  - bloating
  - tiredness.
- Infertility.
- Bulky uterus.

(See: *Adenomyosis*.)

Laparoscopy is useful in diagnosis, and a vaginal ultrasound scan may assist in assessing the severity of the disease by demonstrating a fixed ovary or endometriosis in the ovary.

ENURESIS

Enuresis is the involuntary discharge of urine in an individual over 5 years of age. Enuresis may be:

- *Primary.* Primary enuresis occurs when there has never been any significant evidence of bladder control.
- *Secondary.* Secondary enuresis follows one or more periods of full bladder control. There should have been at least one period of 12 months' duration of full bladder control before secondary enuresis is diagnosed.
- *Nocturnal.* Nocturnal enuresis, bed-wetting at night, has a prevalence of 10% at 5 years of age, when the stages of bladder development are usually complete. It declines as the child gets older, with 1–2% of adults having this problem. It is twice as common in males.

The stages of bladder development are:

- Reflex micturition in infancy.
- Awareness of a full bladder develops at 1–2 years of age.
- The ability to tense muscles of the pelvic floor and hold urine develops at around 3 years of age and results in increased bladder capacity.
- The ability to stop the urinary stream at will occurs at around 4 years.
- The ability to start and stop the urine stream at any stage of bladder filling develops by 6 years.

In patients with nocturnal enuresis it is necessary to exclude physical causes such as:

- Congenital malformation. Urethral stricture leads to urinary leaks by day and night. Spinal cord defects are associated with other neurological signs.
- Urinary tract infection, which presents as:
  - failure to thrive, anorexia, and vomiting in infancy
  - burning on micturition and 'hot' urine in children.
- Convulsions. Children who wake with a bitten tongue or lip and have disturbed bed clothes may be epileptic.
- Sexual abuse. This may be suspected in the presence of:
  - vaginal soreness, with or without bleeding, in young girls
  - onset of enuresis and/or encoporesis
  - behavior change
  - urinary signs (hematuria, pyuria).
- A stage 4 sleep disorder. Incontinence is a variable nightly occurrence and usually occurs in the first third of the night.

EPIDIDYMO-ORCHITIS

Acute epididymo-orchitis results from sexually transmitted pathogens in younger patients and urinary tract infections following obstructive uropathy or instrumentation in older patients. Acute epididymo-orchitis presents with:

- scrotal pain, which develops over several hours
- tender induration of testis and epididymis
- scrotal swelling
- a urethral discharge
- dysuria, frequency
- pyuria, bacteriuria.

An important finding that differentiates epididymo-orchitis from torsion is that in this condition elevation of the testis and epididymis decreases discomfort.

EPIGLOTTITIS

Haemophilus influenzae primarily affects children under the age of 2 years. Patients present with:

- an acute onset
- a sore throat
- hoarseness
- abrupt onset of acute fever
- dysphagia and drooling
- rapidly developing inspiratory stridor
- dyspnea and chest retraction
- a cherry-red, swollen epiglottis.

At the last stage, intubation is usually necessary to maintain an airway. Examination of the epiglottis may precipitate spasm, and emergency intubation may be necessary.

EPILEPSY

Epilepsy is characterized by a recurrent seizure pattern during which paroxysms of cerebral dysfunction present with brief attacks of altered consciousness, motor activity, sensory experience, or behavior. Seizures may be idiopathic or attributable to systemic disorders or local brain lesions. Patients may present with generalized seizures or partial or focal seizures.

Generalized seizures.

- Petit mal seizures:
  - loss of consciousness for 10–30 seconds
  - the patient stops any activity for the duration of the attack and then continues after the attack
  - attacks may occur several times a day
  - do not start after the age of 20 years
  - variations of petit mal may present as myoclonic jerks or a drop attack.
- Grand mal seizures:
  - a prodrome of mood change may be present
  - an aura of an epigastric sensation accompanied by a cry may immediately precede an attack
  - the attack lasts 2–5 minutes and presents with:
    falling, accompanied by a loss of consciousness
    tonic and clonic contractions affect the total body
    possible tongue biting and incontinence of urine and feces
    the postictal state is characterized by:
    headache
    a deep sleep
    muscle soreness.

Status epilepticus occurs when grand mal seizures recur without any intervening periods of consciousness.

Partial or focal seizures. The presentation is characterized by the region of the brain involved. Patients may present with:

- Alterations in consciousness, which vary from total loss of consciousness to confusion, during which the patient loses contact with the surroundings for up to 2 minutes.
- Focal manifestations.

Focal manifestations vary according to the site of the lesion:

- Frontal lobe (Jacksonian) epilepsy presents with localized muscle twitching, usually starting in the hand or foot and then involving the whole extremity.
- Parietal lobe epilepsy presents with numbness or tingling.
- Temporal lobe epilepsy (complex partial seizure) presents with:
  - Perceptual disturbance: hallucinations, especially for taste and smell (the patient may be observed smacking their lips and chewing); illusions (people and objects change size).
  - Disturbed consciousness: absent attacks (the patient may appear to be in a trance for 2–3 minutes); permanent short-term memory loss; patients may be unresponsive to commands.
  - Feelings of unreality, déjà vu (familiarity).
  - Unprovoked aggression, fear, or anxiety.

EPISTAXIS

Nosebleeds may be unilateral or bilateral. Causes range from local trauma to systemic disease such as hypertension, a blood dyscrasia, or chronic renal disease. Bleeding can often be controlled by pinching the nasal alae for 10 minutes.

EROSIVE ESOPHAGITIS

See: *Esophageal reflux.*

ERYSIPELAS

This is an acute inflammation of skin and subcutaneous tissue caused by streptococci. Erysipelas presents with patches:

- Which are circumscribed hot and erythematous. Vesicles or bullae may develop on the surface of the patch.
- With an advancing margin.
- Associated findings include malaise, fever, and pain.

ERYTHRASMA

A common chronic superficial skin infection caused by *Corynebacterium minutissimum*, erythrasma presents with:

- superficial red-brown scaly patches
- coral pink fluorescence with Wood's light.

ERYTHROMELALGIA

Vasodilatation of the extremities results in:

- Burning pain which:
  - starts in the palms or soles
  - may spread to involve the whole extremity
  - is precipitated by heat
  - is relieved by cooling the affected part.
- Swelling of the hands or feet after exposure to heat or exercise.

ESOPHAGEAL CANCER

Patients present with:

- Dysphagia which is:
  - steadily progressive
  - precipitated by swallowing
  - worsens over weeks
  - worst with solids.
- Substernal pain.
- Weight loss.
- Anemia (this occurs late).

A history of smoking and alcohol abuse is common.

ESOPHAGEAL DIVERTICULUM

Patients present with:

- Dysphagia precipitated by eating.
- Halitosis.
- Regurgitation.
- Substernal pain.
- A palpable neck swelling which gurgles.
- Nocturnal aspiration, characterized by:
  - coughing
  - wheezing
  - dyspnea.

ESOPHAGEAL REFLUX

Reflux dyspepsia is the most common cause of dyspepsia in western societies. Persons with gastroesophageal reflux have symptoms that persist for weeks and years. Constitutional symptoms, such as fever or malaise, are absent. Reflux esophagitis causes dyspepsia, characterized by pain that is:

- Retrosternal.
- Usually burning in nature (pyrosis), but may rarely be cramping.
- Occasionally radiates to the neck or arms.
- Demonstrates periodicity both within a 24-hour period and over weeks and months. Nocturnal pain is common.
- Aggravated in circumstances that challenge the tone of the gastroesophageal sphincter, including:
  - bending and lying down, especially after a large meal
  - increasing intra-abdominal pressure (tight garments, corsets, or pregnancy all increase reflux)
  - dietary indiscretions that decrease the tone of the gastroesophageal sphincter (chocolate, coffee, alcohol, fatty meals, and smoking all enhance reflux); gastroesophageal sphincter tone seems to be augmented by high protein meals and gastric alkalinization.

Other characteristics of reflux esophagitis are:

- Regurgitation. Reflux of fluid into the pharynx creates the sensation of a salty or metallic liquid in the back of the throat, called waterbrash. Waterbrash has also been described as brisk salivation in response to acidification of the esophagus.
- Excessive belching.
- Rarely, by an angina-like chest pain, queasiness, and nausea.
- Chronic reflux esophagitis can lead to esophageal erosion, ulceration with hematemesis and, ultimately, fibrosis and stricture formation. Esophageal stricture is not uncommon in the elderly. Patients with gastroesophageal reflux should be referred for investigation and treatment when complications are suspected. Symptoms suggesting complications include:
- Odynophagia (pain on swallowing).
- Dysphagia. About one in three persons with reflux experience dysphagia. Difficulty with swallowing is intermittent and can occasionally be painful. It may result from: esophageal peristalsis, esophageal hypersensitivity or, more rarely, stricture formation. There is also a risk of carcinomatous change.
- Nocturnal coughing or choking. The cough is sudden in onset and may be precipitated by a change in posture.
- Hematemesis and/or anemia.
- A wheeze. Aspiration of refluxed gastric contents causes bronchial irritation.
- Angina-like chest pain.
- Weight loss.
- Onset after the age of 45 years.
- Throat symptoms. Symptoms are located behind the larynx or lower neck rather than the back of the throat. Symptoms may persist for weeks or years and present as:
  - a chronic sore throat
  - globus pharyngeus/hystericus
  - a chronic cough

  - hoarseness
  - chronic throat-clearing
  - halitosis.

The mechanisms postulated to explain throat symptoms in reflux esophagitis include:

- referred irritation from the distal esophagus
- inflammation of the laryngopharynx due to direct exposure to acid
- reflex contraction of the cricopharyngeus muscle secondary to distal esophageal acid exposure.

ESOPHAGEAL SPASM

Esophageal spasm presents with:

- Intermittent dysphagia.
- Substernal pain, which may be:
  - a constricting deep pain that radiates to the back
  - a colicky pain.
- Pain which:
  - lasts up to 6 hours
  - is unrelated to exercise
  - is precipitated when stimulating esophageal peristalsis by swallowing food or drinking.

ESOPHAGEAL TEAR

This may occur as a result of repeated vomiting. Patients often have a history of alcoholism and present with:

- hematemesis
- melena.

ESSENTIAL TREMOR

Benign essential or familial tremor is inherited as an autosomal dominant disorder with variable penetrance. There is usually little disability. Gait is normal. The tremor may start in adolescence or early adulthood. Patients present with an action tremor of around 8 cycles/s which:

- Starts in the hand.
- May spread to involve:
  - the head (titubation)
  - chin
  - trunk.

- Impairs writing.
- May affect speech.
- Interferes with the handling of full glasses, cups, or spoons.
- Is worsened by:
  - anxiety
  - alcohol.

EXERTIONAL HEADACHE

Headaches may be precipitated by exertion, including sexual intercourse. These headaches are benign, but serious causes of headaches associated with raised intracranial pressure must be excluded.

EXTRADURAL HEMATOMA

Fracture of the temporal bone may result in an extradural hematoma which presents with:

- Scalp edema above the ear.
- Concussion followed by recovery then drowsiness and deepening coma.
- Signs of intracranial temporal compression including:
  - motor or auditory aphasia
  - homonymous hemianopia
  - psychomotor epilepsy.
- Ipsilateral third nerve palsy due to herniation.
- Progressive contralateral hemiplegia.

EXUDATIVE TONSILLITIS

See: *Tonsillitis syndrome.*

FACET LESION

See: *Spinal dysfunction.*

FACET JOINT DYSFUNCTION

See: *Spinal dysfunction.*

FECAL IMPACTION

Patients with a history of constipation present complaining of:

- spurious diarrhea
- feces on rectal examination
- fecal incontinence or soiling.

FELON

A felon is an abscess of the terminal pulp space of a digit. It is characterized by:

- Swelling of the fingertip.
- Pain which:
  - is initially dull
  - becomes throbbing.
- The development of exquisite tenderness.
- Pus formation detected by:
  - induration of the pulp
  - loss of resilience.

The abscess may discharge, or osteomyelitis may develop.

FIBROADENOMA

See: *Fibrocystic breast disease.*

FIBROCYSTIC BREAST DISEASE

Fibrocystic breast disease is reported by one in five menstruating women. It has been suggested that this condition is an exaggeration of the normal breast tissue response to hormonal changes associated with the menstrual cycle.

Fibrocystic breast disease presents clinically with:

- Cyclical signs and symptoms. Signs and symptoms are:
  - most marked just before and during the early stages of menses
  - least marked some 5–7 days after the onset of menstruation
  - believed to be aggravated by methyxanthines (found in chocolate, cola, tea, and coffee).
- Breast tenderness.
- Lumpy breasts. Breast nodularity varies with the phase of the menstrual cycle. The lumpiness may present as:
  - Ropey thickening of breast tissue. This is most pronounced in the upper outer quadrant.
  - Cysts. Solitary or multiple cysts become more common as menopause is approached. Aspiration and cytology of the fluid is the treatment of choice.

  - Fibroadenomas. The most common breast masses in women under 25 years of age, fibroadenomas are rubbery, smooth, mobile, painless masses. For those other than the very small ones, which can be safely watched, excision is the treatment of choice. Fibroadenomas will not regress and often slowly enlarge, sometimes causing significant anxiety.
- Nipple discharge. This may be unilateral or bilateral. Cancer must be excluded.

Patients with lumpy breasts should be referred if:

- an uninvestigated lump persists 1 week after the onset of menstruation
- an undiagnosed nipple discharge is detected in a nonpregnant or nonlactating woman.

FIBROEPITHELIAL POLYP

Fibroepithelial polyps (skin tags) are usually asymptomatic. They are usually multiple and are most commonly found on the neck, axilla, and groin. These benign lesions are:

- small, soft, and pedunculated
- either flesh-colored or pigmented.

FIBROIDS

Back pain often results from cervical or intraligamentous fibroids. Pain may result from:

- red degeneration, torsion, hemorrhage, or infection of the fibroid
- attempted extrusion of a fibroid polyp from the uterine cavity.

Fibroids present with:

- Menorrhagia.
- Anemia.
- Dysmenorrhea:
  - cramping pain with the onset of menstruation
  - pain improves 48 hours after the onset of menstrual bleeding.
- Pressure symptoms. This varies depending on the position of the fibroid in relation to other structures. Variations include:
  - anterior fibroids causing bladder symptoms
  - posterior fibroids, causing dyspareunia and a change in bowel habit
  - pressure on nerves, causing neuralgia, backache, and vague abdominal pain
  - pressure on veins, obstructing venous return and resulting in pedal edema, varicose veins, and/or hemorrhoids
  - a vaginal discharge.

FIBROMYALGIA

Fibromyalgia, a condition associated with widespread chronic musculoskeletal pain and tenderness is characterized by a profound but reversible change in the pain modulating system. Fibromyalgia is a condition in which the pain threshold has been lowered. Two central features are enhanced perception of a distressing body sensation apparently unrelated to a diseased organ, and the presence of tender points. While regular aerobic exercise raises the pain threshold, increased psychological stress, insomnia, and anxiety reduce the pain threshold. Fibromyalgia has been defined as stress-associated muscle pain, which presents as a chronic pain syndrome of over 3 months' duration.

Fibromyalgia is clinically diagnosed on finding the core characteristics of:

- Diffuse generalized or localized pain, in the absence of local causes, which has persisted for 3 months or more. Pain is widespread, involving both sides of the body, above and below the waist, and includes the axial skeleton.
- More than five tender points. Some authors require pain in 11 of 18 defined tender-point sites. Tender-point sites include the:
  - occiput at the insertion of suboccipital muscles
  - low cervical region on the anterior aspect of intertransverse spaces C5–C7
  - midpoint trapezius along the upper border
  - the lateral epicondyle 2 cm distal to the epicondyles
  - supraspinatus above the scapular spine and close to the medial border
  - second rib along the upper lateral aspect of the second costochondral junction
  - gluteal region in the upper outer quadrant of the buttocks
  - greater trochanter, posterior to the trochanteric prominence
  - knee over the medial fat pad proximal to the joint line.

A tender point is painful, not just tender, to palpation using digital pressure of 4 kg or less. Tender points differ from trigger points in that pain is not referred on palpation.

- Normal laboratory tests and the absence of underlying disease.

In addition to the core characteristics, which are found in all cases, more than 75% of patients complain of:

- fatigue
- a sleep disturbance
- morning stiffness, which lasts for less than 30 minutes.

A number of patients also complain of:

- subjective swelling of the hands and/or elbows
- headaches
- dysesthesias.

FIBROSING (ALLERGIC) ALVEOLITIS

Moldy products contain antigens that may initiate allergic or fibrosing alveolitis. For example, an antigen in moldy hay causes 'Farmer's lung' and an antigen in pigeon droppings causes 'Pigeon fancier's disease'. Patients present with:

- progressive dyspnea
- cyanosis
- cough
- on lung auscultation, persistent generalized crackles unchanged by coughing
- fever
- weight loss
- clubbing.

FISH POISONING

Fish poisoning may result from natural toxins. In ichthyosarcotoxism the toxin is found in the flesh of fish, usually located in tropical waters. Four important examples of ichthyosarcotoxism are ciguatera, tetrodotoxism, clupeotoxism, and scombroid poisoning. These fish toxins are resistant to cooking, freezing, drying, and smoking. Ichthyosarcotoxic fish are not distinguishable by appearance or smell. No field test is available for recognition of these fish; neither is there an antidote to neutralize toxin. (See: *Ciguatera; Scombroid.*)

Tetrodotoxism presents 10–15 minutes after exposure to puffer, toad, or blow fish. Patients may present with:

- abdominal pain
- nausea and vomiting
- tingling of parts of the body which have been in contact with the poisonous fish
- generalized paralysis.

Clupeoid presents shortly after eating sardines, herring, or anchovies. Patients present with:

- a metallic taste
- a dry mouth
- gastrointestinal upsets
- cardiovascular collapse.

Outbreaks are sporadic, and the cause is unknown.

FOLLICULITIS

See: *Staphylococcal diseases.*

FOOD POISONING

Food poisoning results from ingestion of a preformed toxin. The clinical picture depends on the nature of the toxin.

Staphylococcal food poisoning presents with:

- an incubation period of 1–8 hours following ingestion of the suspect food
- abrupt onset of nausea and vomiting
- abdominal cramps
- slight diarrhea
- recovery within 1–2 days.

One to four days after eating suspect food, patients with *botulism* develop paralysis resulting in:

- diplopia
- dysphagia
- respiratory distress and ventilation failure.

Within 8–16 hours of ingesting food with *Clostridium perfringens* toxin, patients present with:

- diarrhea
- vomiting may be present
- recovery occurs in 1–4 days.

FOOT STRAIN

A common cause of podalgia (foot pain), foot strain may result from abnormal stress (e.g. an unfit athlete) or from normal stress on an abnormal foot (e.g. flat feet). Prolonged walking or standing causes:

- aching feet, with or without calf pain
- initially, tenderness along the medial border of the plantar fascia.

Acute foot strain is self-limiting, recovering rapidly with rest. Chronic foot strain requires correction of the underlying problem.

FOREIGN BODIES

The presentation of an *inhaled foreign body* depends on the size of the object and the site of obstruction. In general, foreign-body inhalation presents with:

- An explosive onset. Clinical findings occur within minutes of inhaling the foreign body.
- Evidence of obstruction:
  - a wheeze in cases of bronchial obstruction

- inspiratory stridor in cases of upper airway obstruction
- decreased air entry.
- Cyanosis, depending on the size of the inhaled object.

In chronic obstruction, recurrent chest infections are encountered.

Foreign bodies lodged in the nose may cause unilateral:

- epistasis
- nasal obstruction.

Foreign bodies in the ear may present with:

- Some conduction hearing loss.
- Discomfort. This depends on the foreign body (e.g. buzzing, in the case of a live insect, causes extreme discomfort).
  Removal of a live insect includes trying to:
  - lure the insect out with a bright light in a dark room
  - kill the insect by inserting alcohol ear drops or olive oil into the ear canal
  - dislodge the killed insect by pulling the pinna posteriorly and shaking the head with the affected ear facing downward
  - syringing, provided the drum is intact (a skilled operator is required).

Foreign bodies in the eye present with:

- A unilateral red eye.
- Pain:
  - a gritty irritation
  - aggravated by blinking.

Visualization of a foreign object is done as follows:

- *Under the eyelid.* If the foreign body is on the sclera or conjunctiva it may be removed with the corner of a piece of gauze or a cottonwool bud. Examination of the upper conjunctiva requires that the patient look down at all times while the practitioner everts the eyelid and examines the superior fornix by:
  - grasping the eyelashes of the upper lid between finger and thumb and pulling down.
  - simultaneously pressing down on the skin of the upper eyelid with a match held horizontally across the eyelid. The aim is to get above the cartilage in the upper eyelid.
  - flipping the eyelid upwards.
- *On the cornea.* By shining the light from the side. Fluorescein may be necessary. Foreign bodies which are detected on the cornea should be referred.

Indications for referral are:

- a clear history of injury, even in the absence of a visualized foreign body
- an eccentric pupil or shallow anterior chamber

- a foreign body which has lodged in the eye for more than 36 hours.

FRACTURED METACARPAL

Patients present with:

- A painful palm.
- A swollen palm.
- Depending on the fracture:
  - a painful palmar prominence in complete fracture
  - loss of knuckle prominence on clenching of the fist in spiral fracture of the metacarpal.
- A fist which cannot be clenched and a thumb which cannot be opposed to the little finger in oblique fracture through the base of the first metacarpal (Bennett fracture).

FRACTURED RIB

Patients present with:

- local tenderness
- pain on movement.

FRECKLES

Freckles are benign areas of hyperpigmentation. *Ephelides* are juvenile freckles, *lentigines* are senile freckles. Functioning melanocytes decrease with age. The loss is blotchy rather than uniform. Solar exposure may result in compensatory hypertrophy of some melanocytes, with senile freckle formation.

FUNCTIONAL ARTERIAL DISORDERS

Patients with digital ischemia attributable to functional arterial disorders have normal pulses. A palpable pulse helps to differentiate between functional and organic arterial disorders. Persons with functional arterial disorders or ulceration of the digits should be referred for investigation of a newly diagnosed Raynaud's phenomenon.

Functional arterial disorders. These may present as:

- *Raynaud's disease or phenomenon.* (See: *Raynaud's disease and phenomenon.*)
- *Livido reticularis.* This idiopathic vasospastic disorder causes:
  - skin mottling of the extremities (reticulated cyanotic areas surround pale areas)

- may be associated with occult malignancy
- is found particularly in young women.

- *Acrocyanosis.* Arteriolar vasoconstriction associated with dilatation of the venous plexus results in hands and feet that are:
  - cyanotic
  - damp
  - cold
  - symmetrically involved.
- *Erythromelalgia.* Vasodilatation of the extremities results in pain which:
  - is burning in nature
  - starts in the palms or soles
  - may spread to involve the whole extremity
  - is precipitated by heat
  - is relieved by cooling the affected part.
- *Causalgia.* This condition is characterized by:
  - vasomotor instability, resulting in changes of color, temperature, and skin texture
  - a burning aching pain which is more severe than warranted by the extent of trauma.
- *Sudek's atrophy.* (See: *Reflex sympathetic dystrophy.*)
- *Pernio.* Chilblains present with areas of:
  - blotchy red skin
  - itchy, painful skin areas on the heel, toes, fingers.

They are precipitated by cold exposure.

Frostbite. Tissue freezing follows cold exposure and results in:

- blistering
- deep ulceration.

GALLSTONE COLIC

Depending on the site of the stone the patient may present with gallstone colic or biliary obstruction. (See: *Cholecystitis.*)

Gallstone colic. Pain is severe and intermittent and lasts several hours following stone impaction. The stone may have impacted in the cystic or common bile duct. In either case, the smooth muscle of the gallbladder wall contracts against the obstruction, resulting in pain which:

- Is episodic. Episodes of pain:
  - are rapid in onset
  - are perceived as a fluctuating pain superimposed on a constant severe ache
  - gradually abate (there are no pain-free periods for 30- to 120-minute intervals).
- Is localized to the epigastrium and right upper quadrant.

- Radiates to the tip of the right scapula or, in instances when the stone is in the common bile duct, to the interscapular area. Pain may also radiate into the back.
- Sufficiently severe to:
  - cause restlessness
  - induce autonomic symptoms such as sweating and vomiting.

Gallstone colic is an indication for surgical referral.

Biliary obstruction. Varying degrees of biliary obstruction may occur, as evidenced by:

- transient jaundice
- dark urine with bilirubin and urobilinogen detected on dipstick testing
- pale stools.

GALLSTONE DYSPEPSIA

Patients with gallbladder dyspepsia should be investigated for the presence of gallstones. A glass or two of alcohol each day appears to reduce the risk of gallstones. Patients present with:

- Flatulence. Gallstone dyspepsia is characterized by flatulence. Unlike acid dyspepsia, alkalis do not provide relief, and the periodicity associated with ulcers is absent. Patients with flatulent dyspepsia are prone to:
  - postprandial fullness
  - belching and flatus
  - abdominal distension
  - increased borborygmi
  - aggravation of symptoms by fried or fatty foods.
- Pain:
  - is experienced as a deep ache in the right hypochondrium
  - radiates to the back, below the right scapula and the tip of the right shoulder
  - is precipitated when stimulating gallbladder contraction by eating fatty food.
- Indigestion.

Patients should be referred when symptomatic gallstones are suspected.

GALLSTONES

One in ten people over the age of 40 has gallstones. Half of the population with radiologically detectable gallstones never present with symptoms. Furthermore, a proportion of persons with dyspepsia and gallstones experience no relief of their dyspepsia after having their gallstones removed.

Bile is continuously produced by the hepatocytes and biliary ductules, at a rate of 500–1500 ml/day. Bile is composed of water, bile acids, cholesterol, phospholipid, and bile pigments such as bilirubin.

Gallstones may be:

- *Cholesterol.* Cholesterol stones are formed when the ratio of cholesterol to bile acid and phospholipid in the gallbladder exceeds 1.5. Cholesterol gallstones are associated with:
  - Obesity.
  - Fasting. This increases the bile saturation with cholesterol as the bile acid pool decreases.
  - Estrogens. The male/female ratio of gallstones is 1 : 4. Estrogen decreases chenodeoxycholic acid, a bile acid which enhances the solubility and excretion of cholesterol. Taurine in doses of 3–6 g/day is believed to increase the size of the bile acid pool and prevent gallstones.
- Bile pigment. Bile-pigment stones are prevalent in persons with disorders of hemolysis. Bile-pigment stones are predominantly composed of calcium bilirubinate.
- Mixed. Mixed stones, containing both cholesterol and bile pigments, are found in three out of four cases of gallstones.

GANGLION

Ganglia are deep subcutaneous cysts associated with joints or tendon sheaths. Cysts are located near any joint or tendon, particularly around the wrist, fingers, and dorsum of the foot. Clinical features are:

- an immobile translucent cyst
- associated arthritis and synovitis.

Recurrences are common.

GASTRIC CANCER

See: *Stomach cancer.*

GASTRITIS

Inflammation of the gastric mucosa may result in erosive or nonerosive gastritis. Gastritis is frequently asymptomatic.

Erosive gastritis is associated with aspirin, nonsteroidal anti-inflammatory drugs, alcohol, and severe stress. Patients may be asymptomatic or present with:

- epigastric discomfort
- nausea

- hematemesis
- melena.

Nonerosive gastritis may involve the:

- Fundus. Fundal gastritis is usually asymptomatic and is common in the elderly. Achlorhydria may be present in cases of atrophy.
- Antrum. Gastritis involving the antrum is superficial and caused by *Helicobacter pylori*. It may be asymptomatic or associated with dyspepsia.
- Pylorus. Pyloric gland gastritis results for duodenal regurgitation. It is generally asymptomatic, but may be associated with peptic ulcers.

GASTROENTERITIS

- Food poisoning and viral and bacterial infections can all cause gastroenteritis. Acute gastroenteritis presents with:
  - diarrhea, which lasts for 2–10 days (usually 3 days)
  - nausea and vomiting, which lasts for under 48 hours
  - colicky or cramping abdominal pain
  - anal soreness
  - fever
  - headache, myalgia
  - tiredness.

GASTROESOPHAGEAL REFLUX

See: *Esophageal reflux*.

GASTROPARESIS

Gastroparesis is found in one-third of cases with functional dyspepsia. Although usually idiopathic, gastroparesis may result from:

- neurological involvement of the gut in diabetes
- a connective tissue disorder
- medication (e.g. tricyclic antidepressants, opiates).

Gastroparesis presents with:

- epigastric discomfort
- nausea
- fullness
- early satiety.

Findings that suggest the need for referral for further investigation are:

- Weight loss. Endoscopic investigation is indicated when weight loss occurs and/or the first onset of dyspepsia is in late middle or old age.
- Nutritional impairment.

GIARDIASIS

This protozoan alternates between trophozoite and cyst forms in its lifecycle. It infects the new host in a cyst form. Spread is fecal–oral or via contaminated water. *Giardia lamblia* infection has both acute and chronic phases. The acute phase, which starts 9–15 days after exposure, lasts for 3–4 days and presents with:

- watery offensive explosive stools
- anorexia and nausea
- abdominal cramps, distension, and flatulence (this is most marked early in the day)
- fatigue.

The chronic phase, which smolders for months, is characterized by:

- intermittent diarrhea (this alternates with constipation)
- offensive steatorrhea
- flatulence and abdominal distension
- weight loss
- lassitude, fatigue
- myalgia
- headaches.

GIGANTISM AND ACROMEGALY

Excess production of growth hormone results in gigantism or acromegaly depending on the stage of epiphysial closure. The clinical manifestations are:

- excessive skeletal growth (gigantism) prior to epiphysial closure
- large hands and feet
- lower jaw protrusion
- headaches
- visual field loss
- amenorrhea
- weakness and sweating.

Confirmatory special investigations include:

- an enlarged sella turcica
- tufting of the terminal phalanx seen on the radiograph
- elevated serum growth hormone
- glucosuria
- normal thyroxine (T_4).

GINGIVOSTOMATITIS

Inflammation of the oral mucosa and gums may result from trauma, infection, malnutrition, or neoplasia. The presentation varies, depending on the underlying cause. In general, patients present with:

- Oral pain or discomfort.
- A mucosal lesion:
  - a white patch on a red background in candida
  - a painful ulcer in herpes
  - a raised fungating mass in malignancy.
- Halitosis. This may be present, depending on the cause.

GLAUCOMA

Acute angle closure glaucoma presents with raised intraocular pressure resulting from interference with the flow of aqueous fluid through the anterior chamber. The clinical presentation involves:

- a fairly sudden onset of severe ocular pain
- frontal headache
- blurred vision
- halos around light
- circumcorneal redness
- a dilated pupil (the pupil may be irregular)
- a serous discharge
- haziness of the cornea on ophthalmoscopy
- increased intraocular tension.

A definitive diagnosis is made on detecting raised intraocular pressure. Tonometry is a relatively simple technique and provides a reasonably accurate indication of raised intraocular pressure.

The features of *chronic glaucoma* are:

- Gradually failing vision. Peripheral vision is predominantly impaired, resulting in tunnel vision.
- A white, painless eye.
- Cupping of the optic disc on ophthalmoscopy. The cup/disc ratio is normally less than 1:2. Glaucoma should be suspected in patients with a large optic cup and in individuals in whom the optic-cup diameter differs between the two eyes.
- Raised intraocular pressure. This is initially detected on palpation of the eyeball and is confirmed on tonometry.

Unless treated, this disease will progress to blindness. Adults, particularly the elderly, are at risk of chronic glaucoma.

GLOBUS HYSTERICUS/ PHARYNGEUS

Globus hystericus is a term used to label patients presenting with functional dysphagia. The clinical presentation includes:

- A subjective sensation of a lump in the throat:
  - no cause–effect relationship to eating and drinking can be demonstrated
  - a sensation of difficulty in swallowing saliva is experienced.
- Dysphagia that is:
  - unrelated to any objective obstruction to solids or liquids
  - associated with the normal passage of liquids and solids (patients have no difficulty in swallowing food or drinks at mealtimes)
  - precipitated by anxiety.
- Evidence of psychosocial tension or anxiety (e.g. alert posture, muscle tension).

GLOMERULONEPHRITIS

Glomerulonephritis is the glomerular response to tissue injury. The mechanisms underlying glomerular injury include:

- Immunocomplex disease (see acute glomerulonephritis, below).
- The development of antibodies to glomerular basement membrane (autoimmunity).
- Complement activation via the alternate (properdin) pathway by triggers such as bacterial polysaccharides or aggregated immunoglobulin A (IgA).
- Other poorly described nonimmune mechanisms.

The histological responses associated with glomerulonephritis include: glomerular basement membrane thickening; glomerular hypercellularity due to proliferation of endothelial, epithelial, and mesangial cells; and hyalinization of glomeruli in cases of chronic injury. The six most prevalent histologically based diagnoses are:

- acute proliferative glomerulonephritis
- rapidly progressive glomerulonephritis
- membranous glomerulonephritis
- lipoid glomerulonephritis/minimal light-chain glomerulonephritis
- membranoproliferative glomerulonephritis
- chronic glomerulonephritis.

The value of the histological diagnosis lies in its usefulness as a prognostic tool both for progression of the disease and potential response to therapy, usually steroids. In many cases the condition develops insidiously, and the diagnosis is often first suspected following screening urinalysis.

Within the context of these major histological diagnoses are a number of clinical presentations. Glomerular damage may present clinically with any combination of:

- hematuria
- oliguria
- proteinuria
- azotemia (the retention of nitrogenous products is an integral aspect of uremia)
- edema
- hypertension.

Three important conditions are acute glomerulonephritis, the nephrotic syndrome, and chronic glomerulonephritis.

Acute glomerulonephritis presents with:

- Smoky urine.
- Oliguria.
- Malaise.
- Anorexia.
- Low-grade fever.
- Headache.
- Moderate hypertension.
- Periorbital edema.
- Proteinuria.
- A history of:
  - Infection in the previous 2 days. This suggests mesangial IgA nephropathy.
  - Impetigo or streptococcal throat in the previous 10–21 days. This is characteristic of acute poststreptococcal glomerulonephritis.

Over 90% of patients with acute streptococcal glomerulonephritis recover completely.

The *nephrotic syndrome* is characterized by:

- severe generalized edema
- marked proteinuria
- hypoalbuminemia
- lipiduria.

Chronic glomerulonephritis is diagnosed in the presence of:

- azotemia
- edema
- hypertension.

Persons in whom glomerular damage progresses present with renal failure. (See: *Renal failure*.)

PART THREE

GLUTEUS MUSCLE SYNDROMES

- **Gluteus maximus syndrome.** Trigger points in the gluteus maximus can cause buttock, posterior thigh, and coccyx pain.
- **Gluteus medius syndrome.** Gluteus medius trigger points refer pain over the sacrum, iliac crest, midbuttock, and upper thigh posteriorly.
- **Gluteus minimus syndrome.** Trigger points in the:
  - Posterior area of gluteus minimus refer pain over the lower buttock, posterior thigh and calf, iliac crest, midbuttock, and upper thigh posteriorly.
  - The anterior area of gluteus minimus refer pain over the lower buttock, the lateral thigh, and leg. The knee is spared.

GONORRHEA

Primary infection with *Neisseria gonorrhoeae*, a Gram-negative diplococcus, is asymptomatic in more than 25% of females but less than 10% of males.

As females form an asymptomatic reservoir of infection, it is important to treat both partners once the disease has been diagnosed. When symptomatic, females complain of:

- a discharge
- dysuria.

Some 2–10 days after sexual exposure, males present with:

- dysuria
- a purulent urethral discharge.

In both sexes:

- Local spread may cause abdominal and pelvic or scrotal pain.
- Systemic spread is associated with:
  - fever and chills
  - pustular or hemorrhagic skin lesion
  - tenosynovitis
  - migratory polyarthritis
  - septic arthritis.

GOUT

The natural history of gout includes stages of:

- asymptomatic hyperuricemia
- acute gouty arthritis (symptom-free periods occur between attacks)
- chronic gouty arthritis.

In acute gout the typical presentation is:

- A hyperacute onset. Within 24 hours patients develop intense pain, usually in the early hours of the morning, affecting one or two joints. The big toe is frequently involved.
- Affected joints, which are swollen, red, warm, and exquisitely tender.
- Warm, swollen, and erythematous soft tissue around affected joints.
- A history of acute attacks which last 2–21 days.
- Recurrent attacks which last longer than the initial attack.

Tophi are common in patients with chronic gout. Uric acid stones are also a particular problem in persons with an acid urine and low fluid intake. In addition to a high purine load due to endogenous purine production in gout patients, persons with high levels of nucleic acid breakdown are also at risk of uric acid stones. Purine breakdown is high in leukemia and multiple myeloma.

GUILLAIN–BARRE SYNDROME

Also termed postinfectious polyneuropathy. (See: *Neuropathy.*)

GYNECOMASTIA

Gynecomastia is a benign enlargement of tissue in the male breast. It develops in males due to an imbalance in the ratio of free estradiol to free testosterone. Up to 90% of newborn babies have gynecomastia due to the transplacental passage of estrogen. Gynecomastia is also common in pubertal boys, but the prevalence drops in adulthood.

Gynecomastia requires referral for causal diagnosis when:

- No cause is apparent. Although one-quarter of cases are idiopathic and another quarter attributable to puberty, causes that must be excluded are endocrine disorders, liver disease, and testicular tumors.
- It is unilateral.
- There are signs of malignancy (e.g. fixation to skin or chest wall, drainage lymphadenopathy).
- Symptoms persist.
- Psychological suffering is detected.

HABIT COUGH

This should be suspected when a well-looking patient has a cough which:

- is explosive, barking, or honking
- is dry
- is readily produced on request
- does not interfere with sleep
- often occurs in spasms.

HAY FEVER

Patients with seasonal allergies may present with hay fever. Clinical findings include:

- Allergic conjunctivitis:
  - itchy eyes
  - lacrimation
  - photophobia
  - normal or slightly reddened conjunctiva.
- Allergic rhinitis:
  - the allergic salute (rubbing the end of the nose)
  - sneezing
  - nasal stuffiness
  - a watery nasal discharge.
- Blue rings under the eyes ('shiners').
- Fatigue.

HEART BLOCK

Predisposing factors include: ischemic heart disease, myocarditis, cardiomyopathy, aortic stenosis, and digitalis. There are various levels of heart block.

First-degree heart block presents with:

- a slow pulse
- a first heart sound of varying intensity.

Second-degree heart block presents with:

- a slow pulse.

Only half or 1 in 3 sinoatrial impulses are transmitted to ventricles.

Complete heart block is characterized by:

- no increase in heart rate with exercise (impulses arising from the sinoatrial node do not reach the ventricle)
- syncope associated with ventricular asystole
- asystole (this is usually fatal if it lasts longer than 3 minutes).

If persons with heart block are not under medical management, refer them for assessment and intervention.

HEART FAILURE (cardiac failure)

The clinical presentation of cardiac failure is influenced by:

- the signs and symptoms attributable to the cause of the condition
- the results of an impaired cardiac output
- venous congestion due to the back-pressure of a failing ventricle.

The most helpful diagnostic signs of cardiac failure are frequently attributable to back-pressure resulting from a failing heart. In the case of left ventricular failure (LVF) the lungs, and in the case of right ventricular failure (RVF), the systemic venous system, provide important clues in diagnosis. Although both ventricles may be in failure, it is convenient to assess the patient for LVF and RVF separately.

Left ventricular failure. LVF can result from: myocardial infarction; increased resistance to outflow as in hypertension, aortic stenosis, or coarctation of the aorta; or volume overload, as found in valvular (aortic or mitral) incompetence.

The clinical presentation of LVF includes:

- Dyspnea. This is:
  - mild, when shortness of breath is experienced climbing stairs or walking uphill
  - moderate, when breathless on walking a moderate distance on the flat or doing routine housework
  - severe, when breathless at rest or on slow level walking.
- Orthopnea. This is defined as breathlessness which occurs when the patient lies flat. Patients may wake at night and feel the need to get up and go to a window. The pathogenesis of paroxysmal nocturnal dyspnea is similar to that of orthopnea, and reflects fluid redistribution in the lungs on assuming a recumbent position.
- In the absence of another explanation, LVF should be assumed in patients with orthopnea and exertional dyspnea.
- Cough. The cough is worst at night and, although initially dry, later becomes watery, frothy, and may become pink stained.
- Wheezing (cardiac asthma) is attributable to pulmonary edema of the respiratory tree.
- Basal crepitations attributable to edema of the alveoli. Initially confined to the bases, crackles later extend laterally and up the back.
- Palpitations following exercise or anxiety.
- Fainting and dizziness on exertion.
- Tachycardia, tachypnea.
- Gallop rhythm. S4 appears early, S3 is detectable later in the course of the illness.
- Inferolateral displacement of a forceful apex beat.
- Pansystolic murmur of mitral incompetence reflects ventricular dilatation.

- Cold extremities, such as the hands and nose, reflect poor vascular perfusion.
- Cyanosis, in severe cases.
- Pulsus alternans. The changing stroke volume in LVF results in an arterial pulse of varying amplitude.

Persons with systemic hypertension are at particular risk of left heart failure.

Right ventricular failure (RVF). RVF can result from: myocardial infarction; increased resistance to outflow, as in pulmonary hypertension, pulmonary stenosis, or chronic respiratory disease (cor pulmonale); or volume overload, as found in valvular (pulmonary or tricuspid) incompetence.

RVF presents with:

- Dependency edema.
  - in the early stages this is detected in the ankle in ambulatory patients or in the sacrum of bedrest patients
  - late in the disease edema may involve the thighs, scrotum, and abdomen
  - in severe cases, pleural effusion and ascites may be present.
- Anorexia and a sensation of epigastric or abdominal fullness.
- Tender hepatomegaly. Pain over the right hypochondrium is due to liver edema stretching the liver capsule.
- Oliguria by day and nocturia. Improved venous return on lying down enhances urinary excretion.
- Raised jugular venous pressure. With the patient at 30° to the horizontal, the vertical height of the jugular venous pressure is normally no more than 4 cm above the sternal angle.
- A parasternal heave.
- Pansystolic murmur of tricuspid incompetence.
- Proteinuria.
- Menorrhagia.

Patients with RVF attributable to lung disease are diagnosed as having cor pulmonale. In addition to the findings characteristic of right heart failure, these patients may also have warm cyanosed extremities and a bounding pulse due to poor oxygenation. Persons with chronic lung disease are at particular risk of right heart failure.

Bilateral ventricular failure. Conditions in which bilateral ventricular failure may be found include: myocardial infarction, myocarditis, cardiomyopathy, and conditions of high output failure, such as thyrotoxicosis and severe anemia.

Management review. Clinical findings suggesting the need to review management, including drug therapy, include:

- Worsening dyspnea especially in patients who are dyspneic at rest or following mild exertion.
- Intercostal recession.
- Central cyanosis.
- A diastolic blood pressure of 130 mmHg or higher.

- An elevated jugular venous pressure. As this sign is often difficult to detect refer on suspicion.
- Tachypnea of 30 beats/min.
- Tachycardia of 120 beats/min or bradycardia of 50/min. Refer at 60/min in patients on digoxin.
- Hemoptysis.
- Constricting chest pain.
- Albuminuria or hematuria which is unrelated to a urinary tract infection.
- Significant side-effects attributable to drug therapy (e.g. weakness, calf muscle cramps, nausea, and vomiting).
- The development of a pulse deficit. A discrepancy between the heart and pulse rate is termed a pulse deficit. Cardiac irregularity may result in a variable stroke volume. When the stroke volume decreases to a level insufficient to elicit a palpable arterial pulse, a pulse deficit is diagnosed.
- Pulsus paradoxus (i.e. a blood pressure fluctuation between inspiration and expiration which exceeds 15 mmHg). The development of pulsus paradoxus suggests that cardiac flow into the left side of the heart is impeded (e.g. chronic obstructive airways disease, constrictive pericarditis, pericardial effusion). The difference between the arterial pressure during systole and diastole is usually 30–40 mmHg. A physiological arterial pressure fluctuation is associated with respiration. The pulse pressure is higher during expiration and lower during inspiration. This difference is some 5–15 mmHg.

HEAT STROKE

Sunstroke or hyperpyrexia may be preceded by a prodrome of headache, vertigo, and fatigue. Patients present with:

- a hot, dry, flushed skin
- tachycardia, with a pulse rate reaching 160 or 180 beats/min
- a normal blood pressure
- disorientation which may precede loss of consciousness.

A core temperature of 41°C is a grave prognostic sign. Heat stroke is a medical emergency.

HEMANGIOMA

Hemangiomas are localized skin or subcutaneous lesions resulting from hyperplasia of blood vessels. Congenital hemangiomas include:

- A port-wine stain (nevus flammeus) which:
  - presents as a flat pink/purplish lesion
  - is present at birth

- commonly involves the neck
- does not usually fade, but may be obscured with cosmetics.

- A strawberry mark or capillary hemangioma which:
  - presents as a raised, bright red lesion
  - develops shortly after birth and enlarges slowly for several months
  - usually regresses and disappears within 48–60 months.
- A cavernous hemangioma which:
  - presents as a raised, red lesion composed of large vascular spaces
  - rarely regresses, and surgical excision may be warranted.

Spider nevi, the small bright red faintly pulsatile lesions with a central arteriole, are not congenital but acquired. Spider nevi are encountered during pregnancy and are common in patients with liver cirrhosis.

HEMATOCOLPOS

A virgin with an imperforate hymen may present with cyclic aggravation of backache. Menstrual blood accumulates proximal to the hymen, causing backache with each 'occult' period.

HEMOPHILIA

Hemophilia is a bleeding disorder inherited as a sex-linked recessive gene. The clinical presentation reflects defective production of clotting factors. Patients with this coagulation defect present with:

- bleeding after trivial injuries
- prolonged bleeding
- hemarthroses
- hematomas
- purpura
- postoperative bleeding is delayed in onset but profuse.

HEMORRHOIDS (internal hemorrhoids)

Patients often have a history of poor bowel habits. They present with:

- Bleeding on defecation. Blood may:
  - splatter the pan
  - be streaked on the toilet paper or the stool's surface.

- Varying degrees of protrusion of the anal mucosa. This is used as a basis for classification of hemorrhoids:
  - First-degree hemorrhoids do not prolapse. A bulge may be noted above the dentate line on anal examination.
  - Second-degree hemorrhoids do prolapse on defecation but reduce spontaneously.
  - Third-degree hemorrhoids prolapse on defecation and require digital replacement.
  - Fourth-degree hemorrhoids are associated with:
    persistent prolapse
    mucoid discharge
    pruritus
    medial lines on the protruding lesion (this differentiates the hemorrhoid from rectal prolapse, which has concentric lines on the protruding mucosa).
- Thrombosis. A complication is the development of a thrombosed internal pile. This presents with:
  - a swollen prolapsed hemorrhoid
  - severe, acute throbbing anal pain
  - an anal mass that has a velvety mucosal-lined internal surface and a shiny skin-covered external component
  - occluded venous return
  - painful defecation
  - fibrosis and spontaneous cure
  - suppuration and ulceration.

HEMOTHORAX

Blood in the pleural cavity presents clinically with:

- dyspnea
- dullness to percussion over the involved area
- decreased breath sounds
- shock (this depends on the volume of blood lost and the extent of cardiopulmonary embarrassment due to mediastinal shift).

HENOCH–SCHONLEIN PURPURA

Also known as allergic or anaphylactoid purpura, this condition involves vasculitis of skin, joint, intestinal, and renal vessels. Patients present with:

- purpura, which may be itchy
- joint pain
- abdominal pain
- fever and malaise
- hematuria and proteinuria.

HEPATIC FAILURE

When liver destruction reaches a stage at which the number of functional hepatocytes are unable to cope, liver failure results. Liver failure is recognized clinically by the impairment of normal liver functions. Manifestations of impaired liver function include the following.

Jaundice. This is evidence of bilirubin retention. Hepatocytes conjugate bilirubin (derived from the breakdown of red cell heme) with glucuronic acid, and excrete conjugated bilirubin in the bile. Unconjugated bilirubin is bound to albumin and transported to the liver. Jaundice may be:

- Prehepatic. This jaundice has a marked increase in unconjugated bilirubin.
- Posthepatic. In this form of jaundice a marked increase in conjugated bilirubin is present.
- Cholestatic. Conjugated bilirubin regurgitates into the serum and forms a complex with albumin. Once the biliary obstruction has been relieved, the patient's recovery from jaundice is slow, owing to the long half-life of this conjugated bilirubin–albumin complex.

Edema. Generalized edema results from both:

- Hypoalbuminemia. The damaged liver is unable to synthesize albumin adequately. Reduced serum albumin levels decrease oncotic pressure and reduce interstitial fluid resorption.
- Hyperaldosteronism. The damaged liver is unable adequately to catabolize and excrete aldosterone. Raised aldosterone levels enhance sodium retention.

Hypoalbuminemia. Plasma albumin levels are considered an index of the functional hepatic mass. Albumin is useful in assessing chronic liver disease, as its plasma concentration falls as the disease progresses. Once ascites develops the usefulness of this test is diminished. Serum albumin is a good guide to prognosis in liver disease.

Hemorrhage. Impaired production of clotting factors results in a prolonged prothrombin time when hepatic synthesis of vitamin K-dependent coagulation factors (II, VII, IX, X) is impaired. As an abnormal prothrombin time may result from vitamin K malabsorption, it is important to distinguish between hepatic dysfunction and malabsorption. Patients present with:

- purpura
- epistaxis
- melena
- menorrhagia.

Skin changes. These include:

- Pruritus. This is found in cholestatic jaundice due to obstruction to the excretion of bile salts.
- Changes due to impaired estrogen catabolism and excretion may result in:
  - spider nevi
  - telangiectasis
  - palmar erythema
  - pigmentation
  - clubbing.

Feminization. Due to impaired metabolism of sex hormones, males develop:

- gynecomastia
- testicular atrophy.

Halitosis. Fetor hepaticus is attributable to impaired metabolism of ammonia and other mercaptones.

Encephalopathy. Impaired detoxification of metabolites may cause:

- a flapping tremor
- confusion
- later, coma.

Development of collateral circulation. In cirrhosis with associated portal hypertension, varices develop due to altered hepatic vasodynamics. These include:

- hemorrhoids
- esophageal varices
- caput medusa (periumbilical varices).

Metabolic/hematological changes. Laboratory investigations may be conveniently considered as:

- Those which assess the functional capacity of the liver. Tests that assess hepatocyte function include:
  - serum bilirubin
  - serum albumin
  - prothrombin time.
- Those which serve as markers of hepatobiliary disease. The presence in the serum of intracellular liver enzymes provides a basis for ascertaining hepatobiliary disease. The enzymes used in liver function tests are, however, found in a number of tissues, and therefore are not specific indicators of hepatic disease.
  - Gammaglutamyl transferase/transpeptidase (GTT) is a very sensitive but nonspecific indicator of hepatobiliary disease. It is markedly raised in alcoholic cirrhosis and moderately raised in biliary obstruction, and also in hepatocellular hepatitis.
  - Alkaline phosphatase is markedly raised in biliary obstruction and moderately raised in liver infiltration.

- Transaminases reflect hepatocyte damage or necrosis. The serum level of these transaminases reflects the extent of hepatocellular necrosis, but does not correlate with the clinical outcome of liver disease. Both are markedly raised in hepatocellular hepatitis:

Alanine amino transferase is most sensitive for viral hepatitis (especially chronic hepatitis B or C), excess alcohol ingestion, and drug reactions
Aspartate amino transferase may be unusually low in uremia.

HEPATITIS

(See: *Viral hepatitis.*)

Various drugs may be toxic to the liver. In certain cases toxicity is the result of high doses (e.g. paracetamol causes liver disease when the dose exceeds 10 g, and mortality rises steeply when the dose reaches 25 g). Alcohol, niacin, and vitamin A are also hepatotoxic in high doses. In other cases, liver sensitivity to certain drugs is idiosyncratic. Drugs included in this category are phenothiazines, monoamine oxidase inhibitors, indometacin, oral contraceptives, and isoniazid.

Patients present with:

- Acute hepatitis:
  - anorexia, nausea
  - tenderness in the right upper quadrant
  - jaundice
  - abnormal liver function tests.
- Chronic hepatitis:
  - malaise, fatigue
  - abnormal liver function tests.

HEPATOMA

Primary liver or hepatocellular cancer is a common cancer and is a complication of chronic active hepatitis following hepatitis B infection. Patients present with:

- weight loss
- a dull abdominal pain in the right upper quadrant
- a palpable liver mass or a nodular liver
- occasionally, ascites, a liver bruit, or hepatic friction rub
- laboratory investigations showing:
  - a markedly raised alkaline phosphatase
  - raised 5-nucleotidase
  - a positive α-fetoprotein.

HERNIA

A hernia is a protrusion of abdominal contents through a weakness in the muscle or supporting tissue.

Inguinal hernia. These arise at the point where the spermatic cord leaves the abdomen. They may be direct or indirect.

Direct inguinal hernia. Abdominal contents protrude through the posterior wall of the inguinal canal. Patients present with:

- A mass in the groin medial to the epigastric vessels.
- A mass that appears and disappears rapidly with a change in position. The wide neck and direct route of protrusion facilitates rapid spontaneous reduction of the hernia. Strangulation is uncommon.
- A palpable cough impulse.

Indirect inguinal hernia. Abdominal contents herniate through the deep inguinal ring and follow the route of the tunica vaginalis along the inguinal canal into the scrotum. Patients present with:

- A mass in the groin and scrotum which:
  - disappears or decreases in size on lying down or with direct pressure
  - appears or the size increases on straining or when the patient stands
  - is resonant to percussion
  - cannot be 'got above' when examining the scrotum.
- Variable pain depending on the size of the aperture and the contents of the sac:
  - somatic pain is worst early but eases as the size of the aperture increases
  - visceral pain, attributable to the contents of the sac, disappears when the hernia is reduced.
- A cough impulse. The mass expands on coughing in uncomplicated cases. This characteristic is lost if the hernia becomes strangulated.
- Complications include:
  - Irreducibility. Adhesions or expansion of the sac's contents may prevent the hernia from reducing. Leisurely referral is indicated.
  - Strangulation. Obstruction to the blood supply requires emergency referral for surgery in order to prevent bowel necrosis. The patient presents with:

    acute local tenderness
    abdominal distension
    intestinal obstruction, with: colicky abdominal pain; constipation and failure to pass flatus.

Femoral hernia. These arise at the point where the femoral vessels leave the abdomen and push under the inguinal ligament. Femoral hernias are more common in females and:

- Bulge forward and then upwards.
- Emerge lateral to the pubic tubercle.
- Are usually small.
- Are liable to complications such as:
  - bowel obstruction
  - strangulation.

Hiatus hernia. These involve a portion of the stomach entering the thorax. Two variations of hiatus hernia are encountered:

1. *Rolling hiatus hernia.* A portion of the stomach rolls up into the thorax to produce a paraesophageal hernia. The gastro-esophageal junction remains in the abdomen. In rolling hiatus hernia, due to displacement of an abdominal viscus, patients present with symptoms of mechanical obstruction in the thorax:
   - cough
   - dyspnea
   - hiccups
   - palpitations
   - chest pain/pressure.
2. *Sliding hiatus hernia.* The gastroesophageal sphincter rides up into the thorax, with resultant impairment of sphincter tone. In sliding hiatus hernia, patients present with:
   - Symptoms of mechanical obstruction in the thorax.
   - Symptoms of esophageal reflux:
     - heartburn
     - regurgitation
     - dysphagia.
   - Complications attributable to chronic reflux esophagitis include:
     - esophageal erosion
     - esophageal ulceration with hematemesis
     - fibrosis and stricture formation (this is not uncommon in the elderly).

HERPES

Herpes may be encountered in various anatomical areas. The basic clinical presentation includes:

- An incubation period of 2–7 days.
- Crops of lesions which pass through the phases of:
  - localized paresthesia, 1–3 days
  - a red macule
  - vesicles that appear on day 3 or 4
  - pustule formation
  - ulceration with painful superficial ulcers with sharp edges
  - dry crusting.
- Painful multiple lesions.
- Tender bilateral inguinal lymphadenopathy.

Herpes genitalis. Genital herpes is very common. Only one-quarter of the infected population have a clinical history, and viral shedding and transmission occur in the absence of genital lesions. The annual risk of transmission of genital herpes from an infected partner in a heterosexual couple is 10%.

Primary genital herpes presents with:

- Extensive skin lesions on the penis, cervix, vulva, and/or thigh.
- Early herpes genitalis presents with:
  - umbilicated vesicles on an erythematous base
  - mild pain
  - moderate lymphadenopathy.
- Lesions progress to:
  - multiple painful ulcers of similar size
  - ulcers with a clean base and erythematous margin.
- Healing herpes genitalis presents with:
  - crusts on an erythematous base
  - mild pain
  - mild lymphadenopathy.
- Dysuria. This is found in 83% of infected females.
- Profuse watery vaginal discharge, found in 85% of infected women.
- Autonomic dysfunction:
  - paresthesia in the sacral area and thighs
  - urinary retention
  - constipation
  - impotence.
- Headache.
- Myalgia.
- Lethargy.
- A positive culture for herpes simplex virus 1 and/or 2.
- Serology is antibody positive.

Recurrent genital herpes:

- is less painful
- has a shorter duration than the primary lesion
- is associated with prodromal paresthesia (patients may experience sharp pain in the legs, hip, and perineum for 7 days or more).

Herpes keratoconjunctivitis. This is associated with:

- a corneal ulcer
- gritty irritation
- photophobia
- reflex lacrimation
- blurred vision, depending on the site of the lesion.

Herpes pharyngitis. This presents with:

- a diffusely red pharynx
- areas of focal ulceration.

Herpes proctitis. This presents with:

- severe rectal pain
- tenesmus (straining at stool may be present)
- myalgia
- fever
- headache
- constipation.

Herpes zoster. This presents with:

- burning pain in the distribution of intercostal nerves
- vesicle formation which usually, but not always, follows the initial pain.

HYDROCELE

A hydrocele is a collection of clear fluid in the tunica vaginalis surrounding the testis. Hydroceles may be primary or secondary to testicular infection, torsion, or tumor. Hydroceles present with:

- a sensation of scrotal heaviness
- a tense or fluctuant scrotal swelling (this can be transilluminated).

The testis may not be palpable, depending on the size of the hydrocele. Hydroceles are usually painless, but occasionally pain radiating to the back may be experienced. An unexplained acute hydrocele needs to be investigated and definitively diagnosed.

HYPERALDOSTERONISM

Conn's disease is due to excess production of aldosterone, an adrenocortical hormone. Clinical manifestations are:

- Polyuria and polydipsia.
- Muscular weakness.
- Hypertension.
- Laboratory findings include:
  - raised urinary aldosterone levels
  - reduced plasma renin levels
  - hypokalemia
  - hypernatremia
  - alkalosis.

HYPERCALCEMIA

Persistent hypercalcemia is commonly caused by primary hyperparathyroidism or malignancy, with or without bony metastases. It is particularly associated with solid tumors of the lung and kidney and hematological malignancies such as multiple myeloma, lymphoma, and leukemia. Drugs (calcitriol, vitamin A, calcium supplements with vitamin D, thiazides, and aluminum), immobilization, and hyperthyroidism are rare causes.

Clinical manifestations of hypercalcemia include:

- polyuria and polydipsia
- thirst, anorexia, nausea, and vomiting
- constipation
- corneal 'band keratopathy,' subcutaneous calcification
- pruritus
- occasionally, muscle fatigue, weakness
- occasionally, paresthesia.

Serum calcium is raised. Parathyroid hormone is usually raised in hyperparathyroidism and reduced in hypercalcemia due to malignancy.

HYPERPARATHYROIDISM

Primary hyperparathyroidism, which is characterized by hypersecretion of parathyroid hormone (PTH), is quite common in the elderly. It is four times more common in women than men, and occurs most frequently in postmenopausal females. Most patients have mild hypercalcemia and are asymptomatic. Reduced cortical bone density is a frequent result. Excessive hyperparathyroid hormone levels due to tumor or hyperplasia of the parathyroid glands results in hypercalcemia, calciuria and, in the absence of adequate calcium supplementation, bone disease.

Clinical manifestations include:

- Hypercalcemia.
- Anemia.
- Memory impairment.
- Renal findings:
  - polyuria, polydipsia
  - renal stones, nephrocalcinosis
  - uremia.
- Bone lesions:
  - bone pain
  - cortical osteopenia
  - cystic bone lesions
  - occasionally pathological fractures.
- Proximal myopathy, weakness.
- Drowsiness, depression, delirium.
- Possible associations:
  - hypertension
  - intractable peptic ulceration
  - chondrocalcinosis
  - gout

  - glucose intolerance
  - pancreatitis.

Confirmatory laboratory findings include:

- raised serum and urinary calcium levels
- low or normal serum phosphate, high urinary phosphate
- alkaline phosphatase normal or raised.

Ionized serum calcium must be specifically requested (total calcium is routinely reported) and ionized calcium must be adjusted for albumin. Serum calcium and creatinine should also be screened at 6-monthly intervals.

Referral should be considered in primary hyperparathyroidism when:

- Serum calcium exceeds 2.75 mmol/l
- The patient is over the age of 50 years
- Skeletal problems are present, when:
  - bone density exceeds two standard deviations below the normal mean
  - rapid bone loss is detected on obligatory 6-monthly screening
  - osteitis fibrosa is detected.
- Renal risk is increased. Problems are imminent:
  - when the glomerular filtration rate is low for the patient's age
  - when nephrolithiasis or nephrocalcinosis is detected.
- There is evidence of pancreatitis.

HYPERTENSION

See Chapter 1, pp. 13–18.

HYPERTENSIVE ENCEPHALOPATHY

In mild hypertension, headaches may be present. In malignant hypertension, hypertensive encephalopathy presents with:

- nausea
- severe headache
- transient disturbances of speech, vision, sensation, and/or paresis
- disorientation and convulsions may occur.

HYPERVENTILATION SYNDROME

Hyperventilation is a feature of anxiety. Immediate intervention involves attempting to:

- control the rate and depth of respiration
- raising the blood carbon dioxide level (rebreathing from a paper bag is often effective).

The patient should be reassured and the cause identified. Patients present with:

- Dizziness or light-headedness.
- Air hunger and dyspnea.
- Dry mouth and sweating.
- Palpitations.
- Agitation.
- Fatigue.
- Peripheral and perioral paresthesia.
- In extreme cases:
  - Carpopedal spasm. Loss of carbon dioxide due to over-breathing tends to distort the acid–base balance towards alkalemia, which in turn causes neuromuscular irritability.
  - Syncope. Loss of consciousness may be partial and relatively prolonged compared with the rapid recovery of vasovagal attacks.

HYPOCHONDRIASIS

Hypochondriasis is defined as an abnormal form of illness behavior in which the individual experiences and manifests a degree of concern over their state of health which is out of proportion to the degree of objective evidence of disease. An alternate definition suggests a transient or persistent tendency to experience and communicate psychological distress in the form of somatic symptoms (somatization).

Hypochondriacs demonstrate:

- disease fear
- disease conviction
- bodily preoccupation
- somatic symptoms.

Patients may be categorized as having:

- *Somatization disorders*, which may present as:
  - Augmentation and amplification of normal body sensations.
  - Misinterpretation of body sensations as serious disease.
  - Illness behavior in order to elicit care. Patients may have difficulty in verbalizing emotions and resort to physical expressions of disease.
  - Anxiety and/or depression.
  - Two or more of the following:

  pain in the extremities
  dysmenorrhea

dyspnea at rest
dysphagia
amnesia
vomiting (in nonpregnant patients)
burning sensation in sexual organs or rectum (other than during intercourse).

- *Psychopathological hypochondriacal ideas*, including:
  - phobias (irrational/exaggerated fears)
  - obsessions (repetitive and intrusive thoughts)
  - delusions (false unshakeable beliefs).

It is important to exclude organic disease and depression in hypochondriac patients. Management requires a detailed psychosocial history and involvement of the patient's significant other. Recognition of the patient's distress is fundamental, as bland reassurance is seldom, if ever, effective. Regular appointments and avoidance of medication are important aspects of patient care.

HYPOGLYCEMIA

Hypoglycemia may occur in persons with diabetes mellitus or it may be functional. There is no single threshold blood glucose level that triggers hypoglycemia. Symptomatic hypoglycemia appears to be related to:

- the rate of fall of blood glucose
- the actual blood glucose level
- the intensity of the homeostatic responses attempting to normalize blood glucose levels.

When the blood glucose level reaches:

- 4–5 mmol/l, epinephrine and glucagon are secreted to increase blood glucose levels.
- 4 mmol/l, sophisticated tests can detect early cognitive changes.
- 3–4 mmol/l, more cognitive changes occur and neurogenic features appear. These symptoms should alert the diabetic to immediately increase their sugar intake.
- Below 3 mmol/l neuroglycopenic symptoms predominate and drowsiness is noted.
- Below 2.5 mmol/l there is a substantial risk of coma and seizures.

Persons suspected of hypoglycemia may require referral if:

- Adult-onset diabetes is suspected (postprandial hypoglycemia 3–5 hours after eating is suggestive).
- Spontaneous or fasting hypoglycemia occurs.
- Alcohol abuse appears to be a factor. Persons who become hypoglycemic within 24 hours of a binge unaccompanied by food require specialized assistance.

Diabetic hypoglycemia. This is diagnosed at blood glucose levels of less than 3.5 mmol/l. Diabetic hypoglycemia presents with:

- Neuroglycopenic symptoms including:
  - confusion (hypoglycemic syncope is characterized by muscle weakness and mental confusion rather than loss of consciousness)
  - lethargy
  - impaired performance
  - visual disturbances, diplopia
  - behavioral changes (irrational behavior, anger, aggression).
- Catecholamine-mediated symptoms, such as:
  - anxiety
  - headaches
  - palpitations, tachycardia
  - sweating
  - tremors and restlessness
  - transient episodes of dizziness
  - poor concentration.

Functional hypoglycemia. The underlying mechanism of functional hypoglycemia remains disputed. Enhanced insulin sensitivity, impaired glucose homeostatic mechanisms, and food and chemical sensitivity have all been postulated. In functional, or reactive, hypoglycemia the presentation includes:

- Catecholamine-mediated symptoms.
- Neuroglycopenic symptoms, especially:
  - chronic or intermittent fatigue
  - episodic tiredness, often within 1 hour of eating
  - a sleep disturbance.
- Symptoms which usually occur 2–4 hours after a meal.

Patients often consume large quantities of coffee, tea, alcohol, or tobacco and have a sweet tooth.

HYPOPARATHYROIDISM

Transient hypoparathyroidism may be encountered in infancy due to magnesium deficiency or as a result of excessive phosphate ingestion (cow's milk tetany). In adults, hypoparathyroidism may follow thyroidectomy and has been diagnosed in a number of autoimmune disorders.

Clinical manifestations of hypoparathyroidism are:

- Tetany, carpopedal spasm.
- Stridor, wheezing, dyspnea.
- Cramps, of both the skeletal musculature and abdomen.
- Urinary frequency.
- Brittle, thin nails.

- Cataracts.
- Photophobia, diplopia.
- Mental sluggishness, personality change.
- Chvostek's sign: tapping of the facial nerve near the angle of the jaw causes contraction of the facial muscle.
- Trousseau's phenomenon: application of the baumanometer cuff precipitates carpal spasm.
- Confirmatory laboratory findings include:
  - low serum calcium
  - high serum phosphate, with a normal alkaline phosphatase
  - reduced urinary calcium excretion.

HYPOTENSION

Postural or orthostatic hypotension is an excessive drop in blood pressure on standing. Postural hypotension is usually a complication of drug therapy for hypertension or excessive diuretic use. Hypotension may result from:

- An inability to maintain an adequate circulating volume (e.g. adrenal disease, dehydration).
- Impairment of the normal sympathetic tone of the vasculature (e.g. alpha blockers).
- Peripheral vasodilatation (e.g. exercise causing metabolite-induced hypotension; or drug-related vasodilatation, as with hydralazine therapy).

Low blood pressure is not considered a problem, unless it is symptomatic. Persons with hypotension (diastolic < 60 mmHg, systolic <100 mmHg) may be troubled by:

- light-headedness, faintness
- visual blurring
- mental confusion
- syncope.

Impaired cerebral perfusion and autonomic homeostatic adjustments to restore cardiovascular competence are responsible for the early clinical presentation of symptomatic low blood pressure. If hypotension persists, shock supervenes.

HYPOTHYROIDISM

See: *Thyroid disease.*

HYSTERIA

Patients are often young and female. They present with:

- An hysterical personality. These persons are:
  - self-centered
  - have shallow dialogue
  - demonstrate exaggerated emotional responses
  - demand attention.
- Hysterical syncope. Fainting:
  - occurs in the presence of others
  - is accompanied by a graceful fall which does not cause injury
  - is associated with a normal blood pressure, pulse, and color.
- Bizarre gait.

IATROGENIC DEAFNESS

Drug-induced deafness may result from ingestion of:

- aminoglycoside antibiotics
- salicylates
- certain diuretics (e.g. frusemide).

Depending on the drug involved, deafness may be temporary or permanent, and associated with tinnitus and vertigo.

ICE-PICK HEADACHE

Contact between cold foods or drinks and the oropharyngeal mucosa may, in susceptible individuals, precipitate a headache. The 'ice-pick' or 'ice-cream' headache:

- Presents as a sharp pain in the region of the forehead, temple or ear. The pain is often described as a deep headache.
- Is a transient pain which lasts for up to 2 minutes.
- Occurs within 25–60 seconds of cold food contacting the oral mucosa or roof of the mouth.

IDIOPATHIC EDEMA

In health, upright posture causes venous pooling in the legs and a reduced circulating volume. Compensatory sodium retention of water resorption can result in weight gains of up to 1.5 kg. In idiopathic edema this process is exaggerated in otherwise fit menstruating women who present with:

- marked peripheral edema of the hands, ankles, and abdomen
- substantial premenstrual weight gain.

IMPACTED MOLAR

Pain may be:

- Localized to the mandible or maxilla.
- Radiate to the:
  - superior and anteromedial surface of the pinna
  - anterior surface of the eardrum.

IMPACTED WAX

Cerumen forms a protective layer on the skin of the external canal. Excess wax may cause:

- a conduction hearing loss
- a feeling of aural fullness or earache
- tinnitus (wax impacted on the eardrum may cause tinnitus). If an attempt is to be made to remove the wax:
- Soften the wax using sodium bicarbonate drops. Visualize the eardrum to ensure that it is intact before putting drops in the ear.
- Soothe dryness and itching with drops of olive oil.
- Insert ear drops. This is preferably not attempted by the patient. Proceed by:
  - flexing the patient's head to one side so that the ear to receive the drops is facing upwards
  - insert the drops
  - compress the tragus for a few seconds to encourage drainage of drops into the ear canal.
- Syringe the ear. Soften the wax using sodium bicarbonate, glycerine, or mineral oil drops for several days prior to syringing. Syringing is contraindicated in ears with perforated drums. In patients with an intact eardrum:
  - cover the patient with a plastic sheet and have a container available to catch the water
  - use tepid water (water should be close to body temperature)
  - do not insert the nozzle too far into the external meatus
  - pull the auricle upward, back and slightly outward
  - direct the stream superoposteriorly along the auditory canal
  - dry the ear afterwards to ensure no residual water remains.

Damage to the eardrum during syringing presents with:

- Acute transient pain at the moment of rupture. Patients should be referred. A healthy eardrum does not rupture.
- Deafness.
- Tinnitus.
- Rarely, vertigo.

Blood in the ear canal and a tear in the eardrum may be noted.

IMPETIGO

Two organisms, *Staphylococcus pyogenes* and *Streptococcus pyogenes*, give rise to:

- superficial vesicles
- golden crusts.

See: *Glomerulonephritis*; *Rheumatic fever*; *Tonsillitis syndrome*.

INCONTINENCE

Urinary incontinence is attributed to factors that raise intra-vesical pressure and/or lower urethral resistance. Incontinence is a problem to 1 in 10 people over 65 years of age living in the community. In the nursing home population the prevalence rises to 60%. One in three women have occasional small leakage. Until the age of 60 years the incidence in women outnumbers men by 7:1. Aging tends to be associated with an increase in unstable contractions, smaller bladder capacity, lower flow rates, and increased residual volume.

The character of urinary leakage may be broadly described as:

- Urge incontinence: the involuntary loss of urine associated with a strong desire to void.
- Stress incontinence: involuntary loss of urine is associated with a rise in intra-abdominal pressure in the absence of detrusor activity.

In *urge incontinence* the bladder is unstable. Urge incontinence is characterized by:

- Precipitancy. This results from a combination of:
  - motor urgency, where the urgency is attributable to a fear of leakage
  - sensory urgency, where the urgency is due to discomfort.
- Evidence of the underlying problem. The presentation varies depending on the nature of the problem. In:
  - Acute urinary cystitis with its intense irritation, the patient experiences: frequency; dysuria; sensory urgency (due to discomfort).
  - Detrusor instability, the presentation is: frequency; nocturia; motor urgency due to fear of leakage.
  - Uterovaginal prolapse, the woman complains of: sacral or low back pain; symptoms that worsen as the day progresses; a sensation of 'something coming down'; a vaginal discharge.
- Drug aggravation of the problem. This may be attributable to:
  - Increased bladder excitability in the case of caffeine or cholenergic drugs.
  - Decreased bladder awareness as a result of alcohol or sedatives, including hypnotics, antihistaminics, antidepressants, and tranquilizers.

– An increased bladder-filling rate due to increased filtration in persons on loop diuretics, or polydipsia in persons on lithium.

Stress incontinence is associated with sphincter weakness. Stress incontinence presents with:

- Uncontrolled leakage of small volumes of urine from a full bladder due to urethral sphincter incompetence.
- Incontinence precipitated by an increase in intra-abdominal pressure, as in coughing, sneezing, or straining.
- One or more predisposing factors:
  - factors predisposing to raised intra-abdominal pressure include: obesity; abdominal tumors; urinary tract infections; a chronic cough, as in smokers.
  - Conditions predisposing to weakened bladder neck support include: menopause; parturition; hysterectomy.
  - Iatrogenic precipitating factors include drugs which relax the sphincter (e.g. α-adrenergic blockers used in the treatment of hypertension).

Patients with stress incontinence may be helped by simple measures such as pelvic floor exercises (Box I) and postural changes such as crossing the legs and bending forward prior to

Box I
*Pelvic muscle exercises**

Stage 1: Identify the correct muscle to exercise

1. Identify the muscles around your back passage or rectum:
   - sit or stand comfortably
   - imagine that you are trying to control diarrhea by consciously tightening the ring of muscles around the back passage
   - hold this squeeze for four seconds each time
2. Strengthen bladder support:
   - go to the toilet and commence passing urine
   - try to stop the flow of urine in midstream
   - recommence voiding until the bladder has emptied

The muscles used to slow or stop the flow of urine are the front pelvic muscles, which help support the bladder

3. Check you are strengthening the correct muscles by inserting a finger into the vagina
   Squeeze the finger by contracting the pelvic muscles

If the finger cannot be felt to be squeezed then either the wrong muscles are being exercised or the muscles are still very weak

Don't

- Bear down as if trying to pass a bowel motion
- Bear down as during childbirth

Box continues

*Pelvic muscle exercises**

This strengthens the wrong muscles and may make the incontinence worse

Do

- Exercises to identify the correct pelvic muscles for at least one week

Stage 2: Exercises to strengthen pelvic muscles

Slow and quick exercises are important to strengthen the pelvic muscles properly

Slow exercises

While sitting or standing with thighs slightly apart:

- contract the muscles around the back passage (rectum)
- contract the front muscles around the vagina
- hold this contraction while counting to five slowly
- relax these muscles
- repeat this four times

Try to be aware of the squeezing and lifting sensation on the pelvis that frequently occurs when these exercises are done correctly

Quick exercises

While sitting or standing:

- tighten the muscles around the front and back passage, together
- hold this contraction for 1 second and relax
- repeat this exercise five times in quick succession

With practice the exercises should be quite easy to master. They can be carried out at any time

Do

- Pelvic exercises every day while going about your daily chores
- Ideally, do the exercises every hour, but certainly no less than four times every day
- Each 7–14 days, return to Stage 1 to check that the correct muscles are being used

Don't

- Do these exercises while passing urine

*Reprinted with permission from Fonda D, Wellings C 1988 Incontinence of urine. Australian Family Physician 17(8): 657

coughing or sneezing. While these exercises are particularly useful for women, they may also be helpful for men, particularly those suffering from dribbling or urgency.

In addition to characterizing the nature of the urinary leakage, incontinence has also been classified as:

- *Overflow incontinence.* This refers to the involuntary loss of urine associated with excess bladder distension. Overflow incontinence is associated with:
  - Uncontrolled leakage of small amounts of urine.
  - Mixed urge and stress incontinence.
  - An enlarged bladder (the percussion note over the symphysis pubis is dull).
  - Bladder outflow obstruction as encountered in those with: a long history of prostatism; a history of urolithiasis or bladder cancer.
  - Atonic bladder, as in: chronic urinary retention; anti-cholinergic therapy, which relaxes the bladder, thus precipitating overflow incontinence.
- *Senile incontinence.* This is diagnosed in elderly patients who present with:
  - incontinence
  - confusion and/or dementia
  - a normal genitourinary system.
- *Neurogenic bladder.* A neurogenic bladder is diagnosed in the presence of:
  - an overdistended flaccid bladder
  - incomplete bladder emptying
  - a urinary dribble
  - a history of diabetes, spinal cord injury, multiple sclerosis, or a disc lesion.
- *Bladder instability.* This is strongly associated with urge incontinence, and presents with:
  - urinary frequency
  - urgency due to motor instability (the patient's urgency is due to their fear of leakage)
  - nocturia
  - nocturnal enuresis.
- *Enuresis.* This is the involuntary discharge of urine in persons over 5 years old. (See: *Enuresis.*)

Referred or specific therapy is indicated in patients with incontinence associated with:

- Obstructive symptomatology. This should be suspected in patients with:
  - hesitancy
  - a poor stream
  - a terminal dribble
  - incomplete emptying.
- Inflammation or infection. This is suggested by:
  - dysuria
  - frequency
  - sensory urgency.
- Abdominal masses. Suspect masses in cases of:
  - female genital, particularly uterine or ovarian, pathology

- chronic urinary retention with overflow
- fecal impaction.

INFANTILE COLIC

During early infancy, colic presents with:

- paroxysms of crying
- aerophagia, flatulence, and abdominal distension
- adequate weight gain.

INFECTIOUS MONONUCLEOSIS

Usually found in older children and teenagers, Epstein–Barr virus infection, or glandular fever, presents with:

- High fever.
- Tonsillitis.
- Exudative pharyngitis in which the tonsillar exudate fails to resolve within 7 days.
- Malaise.
- Generalized lymphadenopathy.
- Splenomegaly.
- Skin rash. A maculopapular rash may develop between days 4 and 7 of the illness and last up to 10 days. The rash may be urticarial or purpuric.

The diagnosis is confirmed on finding an atypical lymphocytosis on laboratory investigation.

INFLAMMATORY BOWEL DISEASE

See: *Arthritis*, under which spondyloarthropathies are considered.

The etiology of ulcerative colitis and Crohn's disease remains uncertain, and postulates range from an autoimmune disorder to psychosomatic dysfunction. Developments in the field of psychoneuroimmunology have linked emotion with immune status, and a biochemical explanation involving immune-based inflammatory responses of the gut mucosa to neurotransmitters and neurohumoral peptides has been postulated.

The clinical picture of *inflammatory bowel disease* is that of:

- Bloody diarrhea.
- Mucopus in the stool.
- Nocturnal diarrhea.
- Diarrhea with urgency, accidents.
- Cramping, lower abdominal pain associated with diarrhea.

- Constitutional findings:
  - fever
  - malaise
  - weight loss.
- Extraintestinal manifestations:
  - migratory, large joint arthropathy, sacroiliitis, spondylitis
  - iritis and/or episcleritis
  - skin lesions (erythema nodosum, aphthous stomatitis)
  - sclerosing cholangitis
  - anemia.
- Relapses and remissions. The severity of relapses is ascertained by the:
  - frequency of loose stools
  - presence of abdominal pain
  - bleeding
  - pulse and temperature.

Crohn's disease invariably involves the ileum, but any part of the bowel can be affected. In Crohn's disease (regional enteritis, granulomatous colitis) patients present with:

- Colicky abdominal pain.
- Recurrent dysentery (blood and mucus is found in the stool).
- Complications such as:
  - partial bowel obstruction (transmural inflammation results in marked fibrosis with stricture formation)
  - a lower abdominal mass.

Histology shows marked macrophage infiltration, suggesting an underlying cell-mediated immune process.

Definitive diagnosis of both Crohn's disease and ulcerative colitis depends on finding characteristic changes on procto-sigmoidoscopy and colonoscopy. Barium enema is also useful in ulcerative colitis.

In *ulcerative colitis* plasma cell infiltration is marked, suggesting an underlying humeral immunity process. The lesions in ulcerative colitis are limited to the colon and involve the superficial layers of the epithelium. The rectum is invariably involved, with superficial inflammation of the bowel mucosa spreading proximally.

In mild ulcerative colitis patients present with:

- slight left-sided abdominal colic
- two or three bowel evacuations in the morning
- no rectal bleeding.

In severe ulcerative colitis the presentation is one of:

- frequent bloody motions
- moderate or severe abdominal cramps
- pain relieved by defecation

- nocturnal diarrhea
- tenesmus.

Ulcerative colitis restricted to the rectum or sigmoid colon has a more favorable prognosis. The 10-year survival rate is 75%, and there is an increased risk of colon cancer after 10 years. The prognosis of ulcerative colitis is better than Crohn's disease.

Management of active inflammatory bowel disease includes:

- Dietary intervention that:
  - favors high-protein, high-energy foods (egg flips, fortified milk, sustagen)
  - avoids high-fiber, poorly digested foods (nuts, grapes, multigrain bread)
  - uses medium-chain triglyceride oils in patients with fat malabsorption.
- Drug therapy. Corticosteroids are used during acute exacerbations. Aminosalicylates (sulfasalazine) are used indefinitely to reduce the likelihood of recurrence.
- Psychotherapy. The psychosomatic nature of this disorder requires that the patient's needs are identified and that any distorted beliefs about their illness are addressed. Criteria indicating the desirability for psychiatric referral include:
  - the presence of an obvious psychological precipitating event
  - sustained depression, anxiety, or undue dependency on carers
  - evidence of anger or the use of rage to manipulate others
  - an expressed wish to become more independent of family.

INFLUENZA

After an incubation period of 1–3 days, both influenza A and influenza B present as a mildly debilitating illness. Before a diagnosis of influenza is made, six of the following must be present:

- Sudden onset (less than 12 hours).
- High fever.
- Chills or rigors.
- Close contact with cases.
- Constitutional symptoms, which occur within 48 hours of onset of illness and overshadow respiratory symptoms, include:
  - malaise, prostration or weakness
  - myalgia (generalized muscle aching is characteristic)
  - headache.
- Absence of respiratory signs, except for:
  - redness of nasal mucous membranes
  - a red throat
  - a cough, which may be painful.

As influenza is a viral disease, management is largely limited to bedrest, lots of fluids, and 4-hourly aspirin or paracetamol. Antibiotics may be indicated to reduce the risk of superinfection in those at particular risk.

Annual immunization against influenza is indicated in high-risk groups such as:

- adults or children with chronic debilitating cardiac, pulmonary, renal, or metabolic disease such as diabetes mellitus
- children with immunosuppressive disorders or asthma
- recipients of immunosuppressive therapy
- persons over 65 years of age
- residents of nursing homes.

INGROWING TOENAIL

Onychocryptosis, or an ingrowing toenail, is:

- Usually located along the lateral edges of the great toe.
- Exacerbated by:
  - tight shoes
  - poor hygiene
  - faulty nail clipping.
- Associated with penetration of the edge of the nail plate into the tissue of the lateral nail fold, causing breaching of the skin and resulting in pain, inflammation, and swelling.

INSOMNIA

See: *Sleep disorders.*

INTERSTITIAL FIBROSIS

See: *Restrictive lung disease.*

INTESTINAL OBSTRUCTION

Intestinal obstruction may be mechanical or functional (paralytic ileus).

Paralytic ileus presents with:

- widespread tenderness
- marked generalized distension
- a silent abdomen.

Functional intestinal obstruction may occur as a result of irritation of the peritoneal cavity or be attributed to ischemia due to impaired perfusion of the bowel by the mesenteric artery.

PART THREE

The clinical presentation of *mechanical intestinal obstruction* is largely determined by the level and cause of the obstruction. Small bowel obstruction presents with:

- colicky epigastric or central abdominal pain
- mild to moderate central abdominal distension
- loud bowel sounds
- vomiting (this is an early sign)
- marked dehydration.

Small bowel obstruction may occur as a result of adhesions following surgery, in an irreducible hernia, or the bowel may telescope in children, causing intussusception.

Large intestinal obstruction, which is frequently attributable to neoplastic or diverticular disease, presents with:

- the gradual onset of central or lower abdominal pain
- colicky abdominal pain (pain increases in intensity for 5–10 minutes then decreases till pain is minimal or absent)
- loud bowel sounds as peristalsis attempts to overcome the obstruction
- diarrhea, later followed by absolute constipation
- mild to moderate distension most marked in the periphery of the abdomen
- vomiting is moderate and occurs late.

Sigmoid volvulus, in which the mesentery of the sigmoid colon is twisted, presents with evidence of bowel obstruction and pain in the left iliac fossa.

INTRACRANIAL PRESSURE

Increased intracranial pressure presents with:

- Headaches which:
  - occur daily
  - get progressively worse over days, weeks, and months
  - are worst on waking
  - ease as the day progresses
  - are initially localized, later become diffuse
  - are exacerbated by head-low position and/or exertion.
- Vomiting without associated nausea.
- Nausea.
- Papilledema.

INTUSSUSCEPTION

See: *Intestinal obstruction.*

This condition is a prevalent cause of intestinal obstruction in preschool children especially those between 5 and 48 months.

One portion of the bowel telescopes into a second portion of bowel causing:

- severe intestinal colic (babies give a shrill cry)
- vomiting
- redcurrant jelly in the stool
- a sausage-shaped mass in the right upper quadrant
- alternating high-pitched and absent bowel sounds.

The child is pale, anxious, and clearly ill.

IRITIS

See: *Acute iritis.*

IRRITABLE BOWEL SYNDROME (spastic or mucous colitis)

Although more prevalent in females, about one in every five apparently healthy people suffer from this condition. Although irritable bowel syndrome is a chronic disorder found in over 15% of the population, only one in five sufferers seeks professional advice. Persons with this condition who do seek professional assistance usually do so because of the severity of the abdominal pain or the coexistence of anxiety and depression. Irritable bowel syndrome is a disorder of bowel motility, and patients are in excellent general health. Motility studies have found:

- an exaggerated colonic motor response to a variety of stimuli
- abnormal esophageal motility and low esophageal sphincter pressure.

Irritable bowel syndrome is defined as at least 3 months of continuous or recurrent symptoms such as:

- Abdominal pain. The abdominal pain is recurrent and varies in nature, duration, and location. It has been described as:
  - A tender gut, colicky or aching in nature.
  - Occurring in various locations and may shift in the same patient. Recurrent pain in the right iliac fossa or right hypochondrium is more likely to be irritable bowel than appendicitis or gallbladder disease.
  - Having a varying duration, with painful episodes lasting minutes, hours, or days.
  - Being relieved by defecation.
  - Being associated with a change in bowel frequency and/or stool consistency.
- Abdominal distension. The sensation of abdominal distension, which occurs in 90% of patients, is often described as

involving the lower abdomen and worsening during the day. It is probably due to involuntary lowering of the diaphragm and an exaggerated lumbar lordosis. Patients experience:
  - A sensation of being unable to bear pressure on the abdomen, including tight clothing.
  - Flatulence, which is aggravated by baked beans, cabbage, or Brussels sprouts.
  - Bloating, which may be aggravated by fatty meals.
  - Belching and/or heartburn.
- Altered bowel function with respect to stool:
  - Frequency (patients experience an increased desire to defecate).
  - Formation (stools may be soft or hard pellets, or flattened ribbons).
  - Passage. Passing a stool may be associated with: tenesmus (one in five patients strains at stool); a sensation of incomplete evacuation; urgency.
  - Mucus. One in five patients passes rectal mucus. The presence of blood excludes a sole diagnosis of irritable bowel syndrome.

The disordered bowel habit often tends to divide patients into subgroups, described as:

- Pain with alternating diarrhea and constipation.
- Painless diarrhea. In these patients a 'morning rush syndrome' is common, with the patient needing to defecate several times in the morning. Periods of more frequent or looser stools are accompanied by urgency. Minor fecal incontinence may be a problem.
- Spastic colon presents with pain and, predominantly, constipation. Periods of hard pellets or ribbon-like stool with infrequent defecation and straining at stool. A sense of incomplete bowel evacuation may result in frequent trips to the toilet.

Patients may also experience:

- Heartburn, dyspepsia, belching, and nausea. Nausea is a common complaint.
- Fatigue, lassitude, and lethargy.
- Headache, palpitations.
- Dyspareunia, urinary frequency, and urgency.
- Backache. Colonic pain can also be referred to the thigh.

The clinical dilemma created by irritable bowel syndrome is to differentiate between this chronic benign functional disorder and organic disease. Six findings described as more prevalent in patients with irritable bowel syndrome than those with organic disease are recurrent complaints of:

- Abdominal pain relieved with bowel action.
- Frequent urgent defecation.

- Looser stools and/or more frequent stools coinciding with the onset of pain.
- Bloating, presenting either as tight clothing or visible distension.
- A frequently experienced sensation of incomplete evacuation.
- The passage of mucus.

Diagnostic criteria suggestive of irritable bowel are a history of at least 3 months of continuous or recurrent symptoms of:

- Abdominal pain that is:
  - relieved by defecation
  - associated with a change in the frequency of stool
  - associated with a change in the consistency of stool.
- Two or more of the following 25% of the time:
  - Altered stool frequency. More than three stools per day or less than three stools per week may be reported.
  - Altered stool form. Stools are described as lumpy, hard or loose, watery.
  - An altered stool passage. This includes straining, urgency, and a sensation of incomplete evacuation.
  - Mucus, no blood.
  - Bloating or a feeling of abdominal distension.

Danger signals which suggest that a diagnosis other than irritable bowel syndrome should be sought include:

- first presentation at 40 years of age or older
- recent onset of new symptoms, or a change in the pattern of existing symptoms
- nocturnal diarrhea or pain
- weight loss
- anemia
- rectal bleeding
- steatorrhea
- a palpable abdominal mass
- fever
- abnormal laboratory investigation (elevated erythrocyte sedimentation rate (ESR), lowered serum or cellular folate level).

IRRITABLE HIP

See: *Transient synovitis.*

KERATOACANTHOMA

This benign skin tumor resolves spontaneously, leaving a scar. It is found on sun-exposed areas and presents as:

- A rapidly growing mass. It reaches 20 mm within a few weeks, remains unchanged for a while, and then disappears within 6 months.
- A raised lesion with a central keratin plug.

KERATOCONJUNCTIVITIS SICCA

The clinical presentation is that of:

- dry, burning, itching eyes
- symptoms are aggravated by cigarette smoke, sun, and wind.

When keratoconjunctivitis sicca is found in association with a dry oral mucosa, the condition is known as *Sjögren's syndrome.*

Keratoconjunctivitis sicca is associated with:

- rheumatoid arthritis
- systemic lupus erythematosus
- scleroderma
- polymyositis
- lymphoma
- chronic hepatitis.

It should be noted that these conditions are believed to have an autoimmune component.

KLINEFELTER'S SYNDROME

Males with one or more extra X chromosome present with primary testicular failure. In this syndrome:

- the testes are small
- azoospermia is common
- gynecomastia is usual.

Other problems include:

- mental retardation
- diabetes mellitus
- a eunuchoid body.

KORSAKOFF PSYCHOSIS

See: *Psychosis.*

LABYRINTHITIS

Acute inflammation of the inner ear may follow a respiratory tract infection. Acute labyrinthitis presents with:

- intense vertigo
- marked tinnitus
- a staggering gait
- nystagmus
- sensory hearing loss.

In children with labyrinthitis, exclude mumps, measles, and influenza.

See: *Ménière's disease* (paroxysmal labyrinthine vertigo).

LACTASE DEFICIENCY

Lactase or disaccharidase intolerance, a particularly common form of dietary intolerance, may be:

- *Primary*. Deficiency of lactase, the enzyme which hydrolyzes the β 1–4 glycosidic bond, results in a milk intolerance that presents as osmotic diarrhea.
- *Secondary*. This occurs following repeated attacks of gastroenteritis. A diet rich in carbohydrates which encourages intestinal fermentation aggravates the problem. Symptoms usually occur 30 minutes after a lactose-rich meal. Disaccharide intolerance presents with any combination of:
  - frothy stools
  - flatus
  - abdominal pain
  - distension
  - recurrent abdominal pain.

Lactose intolerance can be clinically diagnosed using dietary testing. The diagnostic protocol for lactose intolerance is to:

- Eliminate other possible causes of gastric upset (e.g. viral or bacterial causes).
- Identify a direct correlation between lactose consumption and the onset of symptoms. Keep a food–symptom diary.
- Attempt to link specific foods with symptoms.
- Advise a low-lactose diet for 7–14 days, and then reassess.

If symptoms have resolved, lactose can be reintroduced to the patient's limit, usually up to 10 or 14 g/day. As lactase is deficient, rather than absent, children and adults can usually tolerate up to 300 ml of milk a day. Cheese is a good dairy source of calcium in lactose-intolerant persons. Fermented milk products are well tolerated, as lactose is catabolized by the fermenting micro-organisms. Yoghurt contains 3–5% lactose, cow's milk contains 4.4–5.2%, and dried skimmed milk contains 5.2% lactose.

Other diagnostic tests include:

- lactose breath hydrogen test
- lactose intolerance test
- duodenal biopsy for disaccharidase assay.

LARYNGITIS

Laryngitis is usually a mild, self-limiting condition that resolves within 3 weeks. Hoarseness may result from habitual voice abuse, alcohol, smoking, or inhalation of irritants. As most cases of acute laryngitis are viral, antibiotics are seldom required. Patients present with:

- Chronic hoarseness. Hoarseness is a harsh, husky, rough, or raspy dysphonia. Irritants such as tobacco, alcohol, dust, fumes, and vapors should be avoided.
- Vocal fatigue. Patients should limit communication to essential messages and not speak above a normal conversational tone in a good listening environment.
- Cough.
- Constant throat-clearing.

Although less than 2% of cases presenting in primary practice are attributable to a serious cause, cancer of the true vocal cords causes hoarseness early. Timely referral for radiotherapy or partial laryngectomy can result in cure. Indications for referring a patient with laryngitis are:

- Chronic hoarseness. This is hoarseness of more than 3 weeks' duration.
- Unexplained recurrent hoarseness.
- Painful hoarseness requiring analgesia.
- Hoarseness associated with any of the following:
  - hemoptysis
  - stridor
  - dysphonia
  - dysphagia
  - nontender cervical lymphadenopathy
  - a firm/hard localized thyroid enlargement.

LARYNGOTRACHEOBRONCHITIS

Laryngotracheobronchitis, or viral croup, occurs in young children (usually less than 24 months old). Viral croup is frequently caused by parainfluenzae viruses, but may also be caused by respiratory syncytial and influenza type A viruses. The presentation is one of:

- coryzal symptoms
- a harsh barking cough
- inspiratory stridor.

Indications for hospital referral include:

- Stridor on hyperventilation.
- Expiratory stridor (inspiratory stridor is not an indication for referral).

- Retraction of suprasternal tissues and/or the sternum.
- Lethargy and increasing tachycardia.
- Evidence of hypoxia, detected as:
  - tachypnea
  - tachycardia
  - restlessness.

LATERAL POPLITEAL PALSY

See: *Nerve entrapment.*

LEFT VENTRICULAR FAILURE

See: *Heart failure.*

LEUKEMIA

Leukemia is a malignancy of white cells. Disorders affecting the leukocyte series particularly impair humoral immunity; those affecting the lymphocyte series impair cell-mediated immunity. In general, the prognosis is better when more mature cells are involved. Blastic leukemias have a worse prognosis than cytic leukemias. Persons with chronic leukemia may be expected to live longer than those with acute leukemia.

Acute leukemia is definitively diagnosed on finding:

- blast cells on a blood film
- blast cells (> 30%) on bone marrow aspirate
- decreased erythrocytes, white cells, and platelets on blood count.

Depending on the blood picture, the diagnosis may be:

- *Acute lymphoblastic leukemia.* This form:
  - Is the most malignant of the lymphocyte/blast leukemias.
  - Is encountered in childhood (peak age 4 years).
  - Presents with: lymphadenopathy; moderate splenomegaly; bone tenderness; anemia is usually present.
- *Acute myeloblastic leukemia.* This form is most prevalent in middle-aged and older persons (peak age 70 years). Acute myeloblastic leukemia is characterized by:
  - pallor
  - petechiae
  - susceptibility to infection
  - bone tenderness
  - splenomegaly.

The blood picture also determines the type of *chronic leukemia*:

- *Chronic lymphatic leukemia.* This form of the disease is prevalent in late middle age and the elderly. Chronic lymphatic leukemia has an insidious onset characterized by:
  - lymphadenopathy
  - lymphocytosis
  - moderate hepatosplenomegaly
  - progressive anemia
  - recurrent chronic infections, including herpes
  - skin lesions (pruritus, erythroderma).
- *Chronic lymphoblastic leukemia* is characterized by:
  - splenomegaly
  - lymphocytosis.
- *Chronic myelocytic leukemia* presents with:
  - pallor
  - fever
  - lassitude
  - massive painless splenomegaly, moderate hepatomegaly, and slight lymphadenopathy.

Tooth extraction or trauma is followed by a prolonged bleeding time.

Infection also causes an increase in white cell numbers. This differs from leukemia in that:

- Only mature cells are involved.
- The infecting organism determines the dominant cellular response:
  - lymphocytosis in viral and fungal infections
  - leukocytosis (granulocytosis or neutrophilia) in bacterial infections
  - eosinophilia in parasitic infections and allergy.

LICE INFESTATION (pediculosis)

Human lice infestation may involve the head, body, or genital area.

Pediculosis capitis. This is caused by *Pediculosis humanis capitis.* The head louse lives among the hair on the head, and the condition presents with:

- severe itching
- moderate posterior cervical lymphadenopathy.

Small grayish-white nits are detected attached to the hair shaft of hair, usually of the scalp but also of the beard, eyelashes, and eyebrows. Unlike scales, nits cannot be detached from the hair. Lice may occasionally be detected behind the ears or the back of the head. Spread is by personal contact or by combs and hats.

Pediculosis pubis. This is caused by the crab louse (*Phthirus pubis*). The lice live in the genital region, and spread is by sexual contact. Patients present with itching in the anogenital region. Inspection of the genital area may detect:

- lice, on careful searching
- scattered minute dark specks of louse excreta
- eggs at the base of pubic hairs.

Pediculosis corporis. This is caused by *Pediculosis humanis corporis*. The lice live in the undergarments. Patients present with:

- itching, especially around the shoulders, abdomen, and buttocks
- red puncta (bite marks are often associated with areas of excoriation due to scratching).

Lice may be found in the seams of undergarments.

LIGAMENT TEARS

An *anterior cruciate ligament tear* is a serious injury which may cause residual instability. Patients present with:

- severe pain following injury
- immediate and gross effusion
- joint locking
- a positive pivot shift test in cases of instability.

A *posterior cruciate ligament tear* results from severe hyper-extension injury, which may result from a direct blow to the tibia in a patient with a flexed knee. Patients present with:

- popliteal pain, which radiates to the calf
- pain on running downhill
- posterior sag or recurvatum of the knee
- no or minimal swelling.

A *medial collateral ligament tear* may result from a lateral force applied to, or forced external rotation of, the knee. The presentation depends on the extent of the tear. In third-degree tears no end-point is detected on valgus stress testing. Patients present with:

- pain on the medial side of the knee
- localized medial swelling
- pain that is aggravated by twisting
- hamstring strain, which causes pseudolocking.

LIPOMA

This benign tumor of fatty tissue is found subcutaneously. Its clinical characteristics are that it is:

- soft, smooth, and lobulated
- painless
- rubbery, occasionally fluctuant.

LUMBAR OSTEOARTHRITIS

Lumbar spondylitis or degenerative osteoarthritis is more common in older age groups. It presents with:

- Low back stiffness that is:
  - worst on waking
  - aggravated by immobility.
- Low backache that:
  - Presents with acute episodes of back pain superimposed on a constant nagging ache.
  - Is aggravated by: heavy or intense activity; prolonged standing or sitting.
  - Relieved by: lying straight; gentle exercise.
- Restriction of spinal movement.

LUMBOSACRAL LESION

See: *Spinal dysfunction.*

LUNG ABSCESS

Obstruction of bronchial drainage, suppression of the cough reflex, aspiration of infected material, pneumonia, and pulmonary infarction all predispose to abscess formation. Lung abscesses present with:

- Fever and sweating.
- A cough. Although often nonproductive, when productive a foul-smelling, gray sputum is produced. Coughing is often sudden in onset.
- A definite area of lung consolidation. An abscess should be suspected when a previously diagnosed pneumonia fails to resolve on appropriate antibiotic treatment.
- Weight loss.
- Clubbing.
- Anemia.
- Central radiolucency and a fluid level indicate cavitation on the chest radiograph.

Complications of a lung abscess include hemoptysis, empyema, and pyopneumothorax.

LUNG CANCER

Lung cancer is an important cancer in smokers. The disease presents late. The earliest clinical clues are:

- A persistent cough (present in 80% of patients).
- Sputum which is:
  - blood streaked, in adenocarcinoma (single or repeated hemoptysis occurs in 70% of patients)
  - profuse and watery, in alveolar cell cancer.
- Dyspnea.
- Chest pain.
- Weight loss in the absence of anorexia.

Late findings include:

- Those due to localized obstruction:
  - persistent localized wheeze
  - recurrence of treated pneumonia
  - atelectasis.
- Metastatic lesions, often with pressure effects, may present as:
  - Supraclavicular lymphadenopathy.
  - Pancoast's syndrome. Cases of carcinoma of the apical bronchus may present with: shoulder/arm pain; ipsilateral Horner's syndrome (cervical sympathetic paralysis). The latter presents with: a small pupil/mild ptosis; partial ptosis; enophthalmos; lack of sweating on the ipsilateral half of the head and neck.
  - Recurrent laryngeal nerve palsy, which presents with: hoarseness; a nonexplosive cough.
  - Superior vena cava obstruction, which presents as: facial edema and plethora; dysphagia, stridor; a brassy cough, headaches, and blackouts.
  - Bone pain.
  - Bloody pleural effusion.
- Biochemical/endocrine changes. This may result in:
  - clubbing
  - myasthenia gravis
  - motor and sensory neuritis
  - Cushing's syndrome
  - hypercalcemia (squamous cell carcinomas secrete parathormone, prostaglandins, and steroids)
  - hypocalcemia (adenocarcinomas secrete calcitonin)
  - gynecomastia.

LYMPHEDEMA

Lymphedema results from impaired lymph drainage. It may be congenital or acquired. It usually presents with:

- Painless swelling of one or both lower extremities.
- A brawny edema. Although initially pitting, with time the edema becomes nonpitting.
- In contrast to venous obstruction, the absence of:
  - stasis pigmentation
  - ulceration
  - varicosities.

LYMPHOGRANULOMA VENEREUM

Chlamydia trachomatis causes this sexually transmitted disease, which presents with penile or labial lesions. After an incubation of 3–42 days (usually 14 days), the patient presents progressively with:

- an eroded papule or a small painless ulcer
- a fleeting or transient ulcer
- a single lesion, which is often missed
- moderate tender lymphadenopathy (this appears after the skin lesion has resolved)
- a bubo (lymphadenopathy progresses to a tender fluctuant abscess)
- a positive groove sign (lymphadenopathy causes a 'crease' in the region of the inguinal ligament)
- a positive complement-fixation test.

LYMPHOMA

Malignant lymphadenopathies are collectively categorized as the lymphomas. Disorders of the lymphoid series predominantly affect cell-mediated immunity. Malignant lymphomas, or the reticuloses, should be excluded in any patient who presents with malaise, fever, sweating, and weight loss of unknown origin.

Lymphoma may present as:

- An asymptomatic lump. Local lymphadenopathy may be the only finding.
- Generalized lymphadenopathy, including splenomegaly.
- Constitutional symptoms:
  - fatigue
  - weight loss (involuntary loss of more than 10% of body weight is suspect)
  - fever
  - night sweats.
- Incidentally detected peripheral blood lymphocytosis.

In all instances the definitive diagnosis is made on lymph-node biopsy.

The exact terminology of the lymphoma is determined by the histological characteristics of the lesion.

Hodgkin's disease. This is the most prevalent of the malignant lymphomas. In Hodgkin's disease the histological diagnostic criteria require:

- partial or complete destruction of nodal architecture
- the presence of abnormal reticulum cells
- the presence of Reed–Sternberg cells.

Hodgkin's disease is staged according to the number of anatomical regions involved and whether the spleen and other extranodal reticuloendothelial tissue has undergone neoplastic change. The more localized the lesion, the better the prognosis.

Non-Hodgkin's lymphomas. These are among the five leading causes of death from cancer in young people. Staging of the disease is used to evaluate the extent of the disease and provide a basis upon which to determine prognosis and treatment. In general, follicular lymphomas tend to remain localized and have a relatively better prognosis, while the diffuse lymphomas of lymphosarcoma and reticulum cell sarcoma often have a worse prognosis. The reticulum cell sarcoma is characterized by more local infiltration, while lymphosarcomas usually spread to involve regional nodes and viscera.

MACULAR DEGENERATION

Senile macular degeneration, or age-related maculopathy, presents with:

- insidious bilateral central scotoma
- mottling and altered pigmentation in the macular area on ophthalmoscopy.

MALARIA

Malaria is a protozoan infection spread by the anopheles mosquito. The clinical presentation and prognosis vary depending on the species of *Plasmodium* involved. The clinical features of malaria are:

- Paroxysmal attacks of:
  - Chills, which last 15–60 minutes, as the parasites are released from red blood cells.
  - Fever (the temperature may reach 40°C).
  - Sweating.
- Episodes of fever, which occur at intervals of:
  - 72 hours with *Plasmodium malariae* infection
  - 48 hours with *P. vivax*, *P. ovale*, and *P. falciparum* infection.

- Anemia and hemolytic jaundice.
- Splenomegaly.
- Delirium and coma.

Parasites in thick and thin blood smears confirm the diagnosis.

Death due to renal failure may occur in *P. falciparum* malaria. Without treatment the infection may persist for:

- 40 years in the case of *P. malariae* infection
- 5 years in *P. vivax* or *P. ovale* infection
- 8 months in the case of *P. falciparum* infection.

MALIGNANT MELANOMA

Melanoma is a neoplasm of the pigmented cells of the skin and eye. The Australian incidence of malignant melanoma is 30 melanomas per 100 000 people per year.

Skin changes suggestive of malignant melanoma include:

- a history of change in color, shape, or size
- a mild intermittent itch
- spontaneous bleeding or bleeding following minor trauma
- a family history of dysplastic nevi.

Immediate further investigation is indicated for lesions that:

- are asymmetrical
- have an irregular border
- are >5 mm in diameter
- are of variable color.

A high melanocytic nevi count correlates with a high risk of developing malignant melanoma. Persons with more than 200 nevi of 2 mm or more in diameter are at particular risk. Behaviors that correlate with a high count and increased risk are:

- more than 4 h/day of sun exposure
- a history of sunburn
- infrequent exposure of untanned skin to high doses of sunlight
- intermittent exposure of untanned skin to high doses of sunlight.

Other risk factors are age, light skin, and freckling.

Malignant melanoma is a common primary malignant neoplasm of the eye. Ocular malignant melanoma is usually found in middle-aged individuals. The clinical presentation includes:

- A gradual painless loss of vision in one eye.
- An absent red reflex.
- Ophthalmoscopy shows:
  - A pigmented tumor of the choroid that can be visualized through the retina as a dark oval mass.

– Secondary retinal detachment as a result of the malignant mass protruding into the vitreous.

MALIGNANT MYOPATHY

Muscle wasting and weakness may be associated with various malignancies.

MASTALGIA

Breast pain of clinical significance is suffered by 20% of women. Physiological changes can produce mild to moderate discomfort and swelling associated with the normal menstrual cycle. Mastalgia is known to be influenced by estrogens and is aggravated by consumption of methylxanthines, including caffeine, cola drinks, tea, chocolate, analgesics, and theophylline, and may be somewhat relieved by vitamin B_6 (50–100 mg/day), evening primrose oil, and diuretics taken 5–7 days premenstrually. The latter decrease tissue turgor.

The clinical spectrum of mastalgia includes:

- Unilateral or bilateral breast pain.
- Cyclical or noncyclical pain. In cyclical mastalgia, pain presents in the second half of the menstrual cycle, at ovulation, or 5–10 days before menstruation. In noncyclical mastalgia, pain of varying intensity persists throughout the cycle.
- Involvement of most, if not all, breast tissue. Focal pain implies separate pathology.

Only 10% of patients with breast cancer have pain, and the pain is localized.

Referral for exclusion of serious breast disease should be considered in patients with:

- focal or localized breast pain
- noncyclic tenderness and unilateral asymmetric thickening.

Women over 40 years of age should be referred for mammography.

MAST CELL TUMOR

The presentation is determined by the release of histamine in various tissues. Patients present with:

- urticaria pigmentosa (generalized, small to medium itchy brownish macules or papules are the most common clinical feature of this condition)

- secretory diarrhea
- weakness
- tachycardia
- headache
- rhinitis
- fever
- bone pain
- episodic flushing provoked by drinking alcohol
- weight loss.

MASTOIDITIS

Acute mastoiditis may result as a complication of chronic otitis media. It should be suspected when patients experience:

- persistent throbbing pain
- worsening discharge
- increasing deafness
- fever
- tenderness over the mastoid process
- inferolateral displacement of the pinna
- sagging of the roof of the canal near the pinna.

MEASLES

Measles, or rubeola, is a highly communicable viral disease spread by droplets. It has an incubation period of 8–13 days and may be transmitted from the beginning of the prodrome to 4 days after the appearance of the rash. Measles needs to be differentiated from roseola infantum in infants.

Measles presents clinically with:

- A prodrome of:
  - fever (temperature 38.5–40°C)
  - a dry barking cough
  - coryza, with an acute sore throat and nasal discharge
  - conjunctivitis and photophobia (ocular changes present late in the prodrome).
- Posterior cervical lymphadenopathy.
- Koplik spots. An enanthem of 1 mm, bluish white macules appears on the buccal mucosa opposite the molars, and the labial and gingival mucosa some 1–2 days before the skin rash.
- An exanthem. The rash of measles characteristically:
  - is a confluent, brick-red, blotchy maculopapular rash. The eruption fades on pressure
  - spreads from the face, starting at the hairline, to the trunk and, later, the extremities
  - lasts 4–7 days

- resolution with desquamation and temporary brown skin discoloration; desquamation lasts 2–3 days as the rash becomes fine and brown.

Fever is still present when the rash appears.

In older children and adults, measles is diagnosed in the presence of:

- a morbilliform rash
- a cough
- fever that is present at the time of onset of the rash.

Complications include bronchopneumonia, otitis media, chronic sinusitis, tracheobronchitis, encephalitis, and blindness. Malnourished children are most at risk of serious complications. Immunization is available.

MENIÉRÈ'S DISEASE

Ménière's disease, also known as paroxysmal labyrinthine vertigo, is characterized by:

- Episodic or intermittent attacks of vertigo.
- Attacks that:
  - last for a few hours
  - may be associated with nausea, vomiting, and profuse sweating.
- Progressive sensory neural hearing loss, often unilateral.
- Continuous tinnitus.

Acoustic neuroma is a less common cause of similar symptoms.

MENINGITIS

Bacterial infection of the meninges results in:

- Fever.
- The rapid onset of headache.
- A severe, steady, generalized headache.
- Pain that radiates to the neck.
- Neck rigidity. This is detected by:
  - Involuntary muscle spasm, which limits passive flexing of the neck. The patient cannot rest their chin on their chest.
  - A positive Kernig's sign. With the knee bent at 90°, passively flex the hip of the supine patient to 90°. Attempts to extend the knee produce hamstring spasm. This sign may also be found in a herniated disc.
  - A positive Brudzinski's sign. In the supine patient with extended legs, passive flexion of the neck causes flexion of the hips. This may also occur with a hip contracture.

- Generalized aches and pains.
- Photophobia.
- A skin rash.
- Nausea, vomiting.
- An altered level of consciousness, or coma.

MENISCAL INJURY

Meniscal tears result from twisting the knee. The medial meniscus tears with abduction and external rotation of the leg on the femur. The lateral meniscus tears with adduction and internal rotation of the leg on the femur. Meniscal tears present with:

- Knee pain:
  - during and after activity
  - on hyperextension of the knee
  - on hyperflexion of the knee
  - on rotation of the lower leg.
- Locking of the knee.
- Effusion.
- Localized tenderness over the joint line.
- Weakened or atrophied quadriceps.

Signs and symptoms are most pronounced medially in cases of medial tears, and laterally in cases of lateral meniscus tears.

MENOPAUSE

Menopause is a physiological phenomenon that leaves women in a state of estrogen deprivation. The nature and intensity of menopausal symptoms varies in different women and is related to estrogen fluctuations:

- high-estrogen months are characterized by breast pain and heavy periods
- low-estrogen months are associated with hot flushes, irritability, minimal breast discomfort, and light periods.

The clinical presentation of menopause includes:

- Symptoms secondary to irregular ovulation:
  - irregular vaginal bleeding (this may occur over 2–5 years)
  - a shortening of the cycle from 28 to 21 days (this is often the sign of the climacteric)
  - missed periods (this usually indicates that the last period is near).
- Vasomotor instability. Symptoms occur in 17% of healthy menstruating women over the age of 42 years. Menopausal women experience:

  - hot flushes (flushing persists in 35% of women for 5–10 years postmenopausally)
  - night sweats
  - palpitations
  - insomnia
  - dizziness
  - headaches/migraine.
- Urogenital atrophy. Symptoms are noticed months to years after menopause and persist for life. They include:
  - atrophic vaginitis, which results in dyspareunia, vaginal dryness, and vulvovaginal itch
  - dysuria, frequency, urgency
  - incontinence
  - decreased libido.
- Psychological changes are probably largely attributable to reduced cerebral blood flow. Symptoms, which peak 3 years prior to the cessation of menses and persist for indefinite periods, include:
  - irritability
  - mood swings
  - depression
  - anxiety
  - poor concentration
  - poor memory
  - lethargy and fatigue
  - insomnia (sleep disturbance is present even in the absence of hot flushes).
- Dry skin and hair.
- Joint and limb pains.
- Formication. Women experience a sensation of insects running over the skin.

Withdrawal of estrogen is associated with a lifelong increase in serum cholesterol levels and an increased risk of osteoporosis.

MERALGIA PARESTHETICA

See: *Nerve entrapment.*

MESENTERIC ADENITIS

Mesenteric adenitis is easily confused with acute appendicitis. Mesenteric adenitis presents with:

- right iliac fossa or midline pain
- a history of an upper respiratory tract infection or tonsillitis
- facial flushing
- markedly raised temperature

- tenderness in the right iliac fossa, with minimal guarding and no rigidity.

MESENTERIC ARTERY OCCLUSION

Occlusion of the mesenteric artery leads to bowel ischemia, which precipitates functional bowel obstruction and, as the intestinal wall necroses, peritoneal irritation. Patients present with:

- the sudden onset of severe abdominal pain
- vomiting
- diarrhea (patients with mesenteric ischemia experience diarrhea some 30 minutes after eating)
- shock
- peritonitis.

Mesenteric artery occlusion may also occur due to an embolus in patients with atrial fibrillation.

MIGRAINE

Migraine is a common problem in primary practice. Migraine patients complain of headaches that are:

- Slow to rapid in onset.
- Unilateral and throbbing in nature.
- Severe.
- Last for 4–6 hours and occur weekly or less frequently.
- Aggravated by glare, hypoglycemia, and foods rich in vasoactive amines.
- Relieved by sleep.
- Exacerbated by head-low positions and exertion.
- Sometimes associated with prodromal symptoms such as:
  - visual disturbances
  - gastrointestinal upsets
  - palsy of specific cranial nerves (e.g. third, seventh)
  - central nervous system changes associated with site of vasospasm.

The International Headache Society recognizes two variations: migraine with and without aura. For diagnosis of either of these variants, the patient should have five or more attacks in the absence of any other medical problem.

Migraine without aura is characterized by:

- Attacks that last 4–72 hours.
- The presence of at least two of the following:
  - unilateral pain

  - pulsating pain
  - moderate to severe pain
  - pain aggravated by movement.
- The presence of at least one of the following:
  - nausea
  - photophobia or phonophobia.

Migraine with aura is characterized by:

- Two or more attacks per month.
- The presence of at least three of the following:
  - one or more reversible aura symptoms representing cortical or brainstem dysfunction
  - one aura symptom developing gradually over more than 4 minutes, *or* two successive aura symptoms
  - an aura, which is often visual or sensory (scintillation or light flashes which move across the visual field are found in migraine; stationary flashes are found in epilepsy)
  - symptoms lasting for less than 60 minutes
  - headache following the aura within 60 minutes.

Some 90% of migraine patients have a family history of the condition.

Another variant is *facial migraine*. This presents with:

- pain located in the facial region
- attacks of pain similar to that experienced in classical migraine
- nausea
- visual disturbances.

An attempt should be made to manage an acute migraine attack with rest in a quiet darkened room, and physical and mental relaxation. Aspirin (600–900 mg) repeated after 2 hours or paracetamol (1000 mg) may be helpful.

MISCARRIAGE

See: *Abortion*.

MOLLUSCUM CONTAGIOSUM

After a 2- to 6-week incubation period, this common benign viral skin disorder presents with multiple umbilicated papules that:

- are pearly to flesh colored
- are 2–6 mm in diameter
- are found on an erythematous base
- have a central white curd-like core or plug.

Lesions are found in the groin and genitalia in adults, and on the face, trunk, and extremities in children.

The disorder can be spread by direct contact, including scratching and sexual contact.

MORTON'S NEUROMA

This is a common cause of pain over the ball of the foot. Development of a neuroma on a plantar interdigital nerve results in:

- Metatarsalgia. Initially, a mild ache or burning in the area of the head of the metatarsal. When the third plantar interdigital nerve is involved, burning is experienced over the head of the fourth metatarsal. With time, the burning may become constant and pain may radiate to the tips of the toes.
- A sensation similar to a pebble inside a shoe over the ball of the foot.
- Wincing when thumb pressure is exerted between the heads of the third and fourth metatarsals.

MOTION SICKNESS

Excess stimulation of the vestibular apparatus due to movement associated with sea, air, or land travel may result in:

- nausea, preceded by yawning, hyperventilation, salivation, and pallor
- cyclic nausea and vomiting
- symptoms aggravated by poor ventilation and emotional factors.

With prolonged exposure to motion, the individual may adapt. Symptoms recur if motion is increased.

MOTOR NEURON DISEASE

Motor neuron disease is characterized by progressive degeneration of the corticospinal tract and anterior horn cells. Patients present with:

- late and generalized motor involvement
- muscle weakness
- muscle fasciculations
- retained sensory function.

In *amyotrophic lateral sclerosis*:

- weakness starts in the hands and spreads to the forearms and legs
- spasticity, exaggerated tendon reflexes, and a Babinski response are present.

In *progressive spinal muscular atrophy*, anterior horn cell involvement dominates and patients present with:

- marked muscle wasting and weakness, starting in the hands and involving the limbs
- fasciculations are marked and may involve the tongue.

In *progressive bulbar palsy* the focus is on cranial nerves and the corticobulbar tract, and patients present with difficulty in:

- swallowing
- chewing
- talking
- emotional control.

MULTIPLE SCLEROSIS

Patchy demyelination of the nerves and spinal cord results in exacerbations and remission of diverse neurological signs and symptoms depending on the site of the lesion. Middle-aged women are most commonly affected. Presentations include:

- Brainstem involvement:
  - paresthesia on one side of the face (fifth cranial nerve)
  - facial weakness (seventh cranial nerve)
  - diplopia
  - slurred speech
  - difficulty swallowing.
- Spinal cord involvement:
  - clumsiness
  - transient weakness (mono-, para-, or quadraparesis)
  - paresthesia.
- Ocular involvement:
  - visual disturbances (retrobulbar neuritis with pain and partial blindness in one eye, scotomas, or diplopia)
  - blindness (atrophy of one or more optic nerve).
- Cerebellar involvement:
  - nystagmus (in ataxic nystagmus the abducting eye shows coarse and the adducting eye fine nystagmus; nystagmus that affects each eye differently is central in origin)
  - slurred speech
  - unsteady gait.
- Unusual fatiguability of one limb.
- Difficulty with bladder control, impotence.
- Cerebral involvement (emotional lability, confusion, dementia).

Any neurological finding may be encountered singly or in combination.

MUMPS

Mumps is a viral disease spread by droplets. The virus has an incubation period of 2–3 weeks. The disease is transmissible 6 days prior to and for 9 days after the appearance of parotid swelling. Mumps may be subclinical and last for 5 days.

Mumps presents clinically with:

- A prodrome of:
  - malaise
  - anorexia
  - headache
  - earache (described as pain behind the ear on chewing or swallowing).
- Parotid swelling, which presents with:
  - an elevated earlobe
  - swelling obscuring the angle of the mandible
  - pain in the parotid, precipitated by sour foods
  - swelling that lasts for less than 7 days.
- The orifices of the salivary glands, located opposite the second molar, are red and puffy.
- Persistent malaise, headache, and anorexia.
- At 7–10 days after parotid swelling, inflammation of other organs may result in:
  - abdominal pain, which is usually attributable to pancreatitis (oophoritis is usually asymptomatic)
  - meningoencephalitis
  - orchitis, with painful swelling of the testis (mumps is a concern in adult males, as swelling of the testis within the inflexible tunica vaginalis may result in pressure necrosis and infertility)
  - polyarthritis
  - encephalitis, with headache, stiff neck, vomiting, and fever (in 50% of cases, asymptomatic mumps encephalitis is present).

Prevention by immunization is desirable in males.

MUSCLE CONTRACTION HEADACHES

Muscle contraction headaches may be primary (see: *Tension headache*) or secondary.

Secondary muscle contraction headaches present with pain which:

- Is a nagging dull ache.
- Is mild to moderate.
- May be occipital, semicranial, or frontal.

- Occurs each day and lasts several hours.
- Is worst in the morning and improves as the day progresses.
- Is aggravated by initiating neck movements, but improves with exercise.
- Is relieved by muscle relaxation, heat, massage, or spinal adjustment.
- Is associated with:
  - paresthesia
  - neck stiffness
  - vertigo, tinnitus
  - dysphagia.
- May be attributable to one of the following underlying lesions:
  - cervical osteoarthritis/spondylosis
  - malocclusion of the temporomandibular joint with: limited mouth opening; temporomandibular joint crepitus; deviation of the mandible
  - cervical discogenic lesions
  - chronic mastoiditis.

MUSCULAR DYSTROPHY

Muscle dystrophy occurs in a group of conditions that are inherited and are associated with progressive muscle degeneration.

Duchenne dystrophy. Patients present with:

- symmetrical relentlessly progressive weakness of the hip and shoulder girdle
- muscle weakness accompanied by enlargement of the muscles.

The condition is clinically apparent before the age of 5 years and few patients survive beyond the age of 25 years. Benign pseudohypertrophic dystrophy starts in older children and has a slower course.

Myotonic dystrophy. Patients demonstrate:

- Weakness of the face, which presents with:
  - ptosis
  - drooping of the lower lip
  - sagging of the jaw.
- Slow muscle relaxation following strong muscle contraction.
- Hypersomnia.
- Intellectual impairment.
- Hormonal abnormalities.

Fascioscapularhumeral dystrophy. This is a relatively mild disorder. It involves:

- shoulder girdle and proximal arm weakness
- facial weakness, causing an expressionless face
- foot drop and leg weakness, which make walking difficult.

MUSHROOM POISONING

The clinical presentation depends on the species involved.

In *muscarine poisoning* patients present within 2 hours of ingesting the mushroom with:

- lacrimation
- salivation
- sweating
- myosis
- vomiting and diarrhea
- abdominal cramps
- vertigo
- confusion and coma.

In *phalloidin poisoning* patients present within 6–24 hours of ingesting the suspect mushroom with:

- vomiting, diarrhea, and abdominal cramps
- oliguria and anuria
- jaundice.

Patients are more likely to die of phalloidin than muscarine poisoning.

MYASTHENIA GRAVIS

Myasthenia is an autoimmune disease associated with impaired transmission at the myoneural junction. It presents clinically with:

- fluctuating symptoms
- painless muscle weakness
- muscle weakness that worsens as muscles fatigue.

Various muscle groups are involved, resulting in:

- ocular weakness (ptosis, diplopia)
- bulbar weakness (dysphagia, dysarthria)
- respiratory problems (dyspnea)
- limb weakness (generalized weakness).

MYELOFIBROSIS

Replacement of bone marrow with fibrous tissue and compensatory extramedullary hemopoiesis in the liver and spleen presents with:

- anemia
- splenomegaly
- hepatomegaly in 50% of cases
- increased risk of thrombosis.

MYELOMA

Multiple myeloma is a malignancy of plasma cells. The clinical presentation is:

- progressive anemia
- bone pain due to pathological fractures, osteolytic lesions, and osteomalacia
- Bence–Jones proteinuria
- hyperglobulinemia due to production of abnormal or excessive antibodies and susceptibility to infection
- bleeding due to thrombocytopenia
- neuropathy
- hyperuricemia, hypercalcemia.

The definitive diagnosis is made on bone marrow biopsy.

MYOCARDIAL INFARCTION

Myocardial infarction is a condition in which myocardial necrosis results from occlusion of a single branch of the coronary artery. Myocardial infarction may be precipitated by complete occlusion of a partially obstructed coronary artery by vascular spasm, thrombosis, or embolization from an ulcerating proximal plaque. It is recognized clinically by:

- Chest pain that:
  - is constricting and substernal (the pain is often described by holding a tight fist over the midchest)
  - may occur only in the epigastrium
  - radiates to the jaw, neck, arms and, occasionally, the back (interscapular area)
  - is usually severe, but may be painless (a silent infarct)
  - is not relieved by rest and may start in a resting patient
  - lasts for more than 20 minutes and more than 60 minutes in most cases.

One in five patients with myocardial infarction has no pain. A silent infarct is most likely to occur in the elderly or in persons with diabetes and/or hypertension. Neither the intensity nor the radiation of the pain correlates with the extent of myocardial ischemia.

- Evidence of circulatory failure:
  - a thready rapid pulse or a slow weak pulse
  - a drop in blood pressure (the blood pressure may remain raised above normal in hypertensive patients)
  - confusion.

Circulatory failure may be aggravated by any conduction defect (e.g. atrial fibrillation).

- Associated autonomic signs
  - sweating
  - weakness
  - nausea, vomiting
  - pallor.
- Auscultatory evidence of mild heart failure:
  - distant heart sound
  - S4 (fourth heart sound), S3 (third heart sound)
  - gallop rhythm
  - basal crackles.

The clinical diagnosis is confirmed by electrocardiogram (ECG) changes, particularly with respect to the Q wave and the ST segment, and raised cardiac enzymes:

- A positive rapid cardiac troponin T (cTnT) assay result obtained within 4–8 hours of the start of chest pain is a highly sensitive marker for myocardial infarction. A positive assay within 0–2 hours after the onset of chest pain increases the probability of a diagnosis of myocardial infarction six-fold. The sensitivity of this test is 33% and the specificity 86% when done within 2 hours, rising to 86% and 100%, respectively, when done in 8 hours.
- Creatine phosphokinase, the myocardial isomer (CPK-MB) starts to rise 4–8 hours after interruption of perfusion, peaks at 24–48 hours, and remains elevated for 3–5 days. CPK is raised in all cases of myocardial infarction within 48 hours of the episode. CPK-MB subform is usually able to detect myocardial infarction within 6 hours.
- Other enzymes which are elevated but are not specific for cardiac necrosis include SGOT and LDH.

Myocardial infarction may be fatal due to:

- Cardiogenic shock. Up to 6 weeks after infarction, ventricular rupture may occur as the damaged ventricular wall heals by producing granulation tissue. Between 6 and 13 weeks a cardiac aneurysm may form by stretching the damaged, incompletely repaired, myocardium. After 3 months death may result from progressive failure of an incapacitated organ.
- Congestive heart failure.
- Embolization of mural thrombi, which form on the endocardium lining underlying the inflamed myocardium.
- Cardiac arrhythmias. Cardiac asystole, heart block, and ventricular and atrial (supraventricular) arrhythmias may result from necrotic tissue impeding cardiac conduction. Arrhythmias may result in sudden death.

Patients with a history of myocardial infarction should be investigated and referred, as necessary, if they develop:

- an irregular pulse
- unstable angina

- evidence of cardiac failure
- a markedly displaced left ventricle
- worsening of cardiovascular symptoms.

MYOCARDITIS

Inflammation of the myocardium presents with:

- Tachycardia.
- A soft first heart sound.
- Changing systolic murmurs.
- Arrhythmias.
- An enlarged heart (cardiomyopathy).
- Evidence of cardiac failure:
  - a gallop rhythm
  - pulsus alternans
  - raised jugular venous pressure
  - hepatomegaly.

MYRINGITIS

Myringitis is inflammation of the tympanic membrane due to viral or bacterial infection. Patients present with:

- the sudden onset of earache, which persists for 24–48 hours
- vesicles on the eardrum
- pain cycles (pain is relieved by bleb rupture).

Fever and hearing loss suggest bacterial otitis media.

MYXEDEMA

See: *Thyroid disease.*

NEPHROBLASTOMA

This is a renal neoplasm of childhood. The patient presents with:

- flank pain
- hypertension
- an abdominal mass (this is usually an incidental discovery)
- occasionally, hematuria.

NEPHROTIC SYNDROME

The patient presents with:

- severe generalized edema
- marked proteinuria

- hypoalbuminemia
- lipiduria
- hypercholesterolemia
- occasionally, hematuria.

NERVE ENTRAPMENT

Pressure on a nerve which passes through a narrow rigid compartment results in:

- a sharp burning pain
- pain at rest
- pain is variously affected by activity, depending on the nerve and movement involved
- clearly demarcated pain (the distribution is consistent with the area supplied by the compressed nerve)
- tenderness over the nerve.

In the lower limb, nerves that are prone to entrapment are the sciatic, lateral femoral cutaneous, lateral popliteal, and posterior tibial nerves. In the upper limb, the ulnar, posterior interosseous, and median nerves deserve consideration.

In *tarsal tunnel syndrome* (*posterior tibial nerve entrapment*):

- Burning pain extends from the toes to the sole. The heel is rarely affected.
- Retrograde pain radiates to the leg.
- Discomfort is:
  - experienced on lying down at night
  - worst after standing.
- Numbness is a late symptom.
- Paresthesia may be reproduced by:
  - an ankle tourniquet
  - tapping the nerve inferoposterior to the medial malleolus (Tinel's test).

Causes include ankle dislocation and inflammation of structures in the tunnel (e.g. tenosynovitis, rheumatoid arthritis).

In *meralgia paresthetica* (*lateral femoral cutaneous nerve entrapment*) patients present with:

- a burning pain
- numbness and tingling
- symptoms localized to the lateral thigh.

The lateral femoral cutaneous nerve is most prone to entrapment in pregnancy, obesity, or by local restrictions such as belts, corsets, or trusses.

In *peroneal nerve* (*lateral popliteal*) *entrapment*:

- pain and sensory changes occur in the anterolateral leg and dorsum of the foot

- foot drop results from weakness of foot dorsiflexion and eversion.

Symptoms may follow trauma in the vicinity of the fibula.

Sciatica differs from other nerve entrapments in that pressure occurs at the level of the nerve root, in the spinal canal, or the intervertebral foramen, rather than in the body of the nerve. Sciatica is characterized by findings attributable to pressure on one or more of the nerve roots from L3 to S1. The clinical distribution of findings depends on the nerve roots that are trapped, varying within the total area supplied by the sciatic nerve. Common findings are:

- a loss of ankle jerk
- weak extension of the ankle joint
- calf wasting
- variable loss of sensation in the lower leg and foot.

Ulnar nerve entrapment presents as:

- pain beneath the medial epicondyle
- weakness in the little and ring fingers
- weakness of intrinsic muscles of the hand.

In posterior interosseous nerve compression:

- an aching elbow pain is referred down the forearm
- symptoms are reproduced by extension of the middle finger against resistance.

Carpal tunnel syndrome (*median nerve entrapment*) presents with:

- 'Pins and needles' or paresthesia:
  - In the pulps of the thumb, index, middle, and half of the ring finger. Sensory deficit may develop in the palmar aspect of the first three digits.
  - May be reproduced by tapping the median nerve over the wrist crease (Tinel's test).
- Pain, which may radiate from the wrist up the arm.
- Disturbed sleep. Patients wake from sleep at night with 'pins and needles' in their middle fingers, which subside on shaking the hand.
- Symptoms which may be reproduced by palmar flexion of the wrist for 1 minute (Phelan's test).

Damage to the *radial nerve* presents with:

- wrist drop due to weakness of wrist extensors
- weakness of triceps
- sensory loss on the radial side of the hand.

NERVE-ROOT PAIN (radiculopathy/neuropathy)

In addition to the prevalent nerve-root syndromes of the lower limb, collectively called sciatica, nerve roots C5 to T1 are frequently associated with nerve-root syndromes of the upper limb (Table III).

Table III
Pain referral patterns of vertebral lesions

Level of lesion	Pain referral pattern
C1–C2	Neck pain radiating to the top of the head
C3–C4	Neck pain radiating to the shoulder
C5–C6	Neck, shoulder, arm pain
C7–T2	Arm, infrascapular pain
T3–T11	Midback pain can radiate to the chest
T12–L1	Groin pain radiating to the genitals
L2	Low backache, pain upper thigh
L3	Low backache, upper and external thigh, knee
L4–L5	Low backache, pain below the knee
S1–S2	Sacral, posterior thigh, and popliteal fossa pain
S3–S5	Sacral, gluteal, and perineal pain

Pressure on the nerve root, usually by a prolapsed disc, results in:

- pain, paresthesia, or anesthesia in the dermatome supplied by the nerve root involved
- motor weakness and/or fatigue in the myotome supplied by the nerve root involved
- fatigue or reduced amplitude of reflexes, hyporeflexia
- pain in the distal limb that is more pronounced than pain in the back or neck.

Pressure on L3 results in:

- pain over the anterior aspect of the knee and leg and the anterior and inner thigh
- weak knee extension
- sensory changes over the anterior thigh
- a diminished or absent knee jerk.

Pressure on L4 results in:

- pain over the anterior aspect of the thigh extending to the knee
- weak knee flexion and foot inversion
- sensory changes in the inferolateral aspect of the thigh and knee and the medial aspect of the big toe
- a diminished or absent knee jerk.

Pressure on L5 results in:

- pain in the lateral leg and dorsum of the foot and big toe
- weak dorsiflexion of the big toe
- sensory changes over the dorsum of the foot, the first three toes, and the anterolateral aspect of the leg.

Pressure on S1 results in:

- pain over the buttock, back of the thigh and leg, and the lateral aspect of the ankle and foot
- weak foot eversion and ankle plantar flexion
- sensory changes over the lateral aspect of the ankle and foot
- a diminished or absent ankle jerk.

Pressure on C5 results in:

- sensory loss in the outer arm
- weak arm abduction
- a weak deltoid
- a diminished biceps jerk.

Pressure on C6 results in:

- sensory loss in the outer forearm, thumb, and index finger
- weak elbow flexion and wrist extension
- a weak biceps
- a diminished biceps and brachioradialis reflex.

Pressure on C7 results in:

- sensory loss in the hand and the middle and ring fingers
- weak elbow extension
- a weak triceps
- a diminished triceps jerk.

Pressure on C8 results in:

- sensory loss in the little finger and inner forearm
- a weak grip
- weakness of the long finger flexors and long thumb extensors.

Pressure on T1 results in:

- sensory loss in the inner arm
- weak finger spread
- weak interossei.

NERVOUS DIARRHEA

Nervous diarrhea presents with:

- the frequent passage of a loose stool
- diarrhea that is most troublesome during periods of stress

- the absence of blood in the stool
- the absence of mucus in the stool.

NERVOUS DYSPEPSIA

Persons with nervous dyspepsia may complain of:

- postprandial fullness and early satiety
- anorexia and nausea
- vomiting (this may be a dominant feature of the presentation, but seldom lasts for more than 48 hours)
- irritability
- anxiety
- tachycardia and sweating
- attacks of weakness
- insomnia.

NEURALGIA

Cranial neuralgia may present as:

- Trigeminal neuralgia, with:
  - a distinct stabbing pain, like an electric shock
  - pain triggered by touch, talking, chewing, and drinking
  - pain localized to distribution of and confined to one division of the fifth cranial nerve.
- Glossopharyngeal neuralgia, with:
  - a distinct stabbing pain
  - pain triggered by talking or swallowing
  - pain in the distribution of the ninth cranial nerve to the tongue, throat, tonsil, and ear.
- Occipital neuralgia with:
  - a distinct stabbing pain
  - spontaneous pain
  - pain triggered by pressure over the occiput.
- Postherpetic neuralgia, with:
  - a burning constant pain
  - a history of herpes (cold sore or a corneal ulcer).

NEURASTHENIA

Neurasthenia is a condition devoid of signs and diagnostically helpful laboratory findings. Patients with this functional condition complain of:

- Fatigue that is:
  - Selective. Fatigue is most marked on certain occasions or in particular circumstances, and can evaporate when the patient is engaged in an interesting pursuit.

  - Physical. Patients complain of listlessness.
  - Mental. Poor concentration is a common problem.
- Accomplishing little.
- Unrefreshing sleep.
- Various aches and pains.
- Being upset by minor emotional setbacks.

See: *Stress*.

NEUROFIBROMA

These benign tumors may be solitary or multiple. Multiple neurofibromas are found associated with café au lait spots as part of an inherited condition, von Recklinghausen's disease. A neurofibroma is:

- a firm, occasionally soft, subcutaneous mass
- aligned along the long axis of the limb associated with the peripheral nerve sheaths
- usually nontender (if put under pressure, tenderness may be experienced, along with paresthesia, in the distribution of the nerve)
- more mobile side-to-side than along the long axis of the limb.

NEURONITIS

See: *Bell's palsy* (neuronitis of seventh nerve); *Vestibular neuronitis*.

NEUROPATHY

Guillain–Barré syndrome, or postinfectious polyneuropathy, presents as an acute, predominantly motor, neuropathy. It is frequently ascending and is believed to involve autoimmune sensitization to the myelin nerve sheath. It may follow infection, trauma, or surgery. The patient presents with:

- Symmetrical weakness, which develops rapidly over 7–10 days. Weakness, which predominantly involves proximal muscles, then plateaus and decreases over weeks and months.
- Myalgia.
- Paresthesia.
- Bilateral facial paralysis.
- Slowly progressive dyspnea.
- Bulbar involvement may cause difficulty in speaking and swallowing.

Polyneuropathy may also result from a metabolic disorder. The distribution of polyneuropathy of diabetes mellitus is characteristically of the glove and stocking type.

NEUROSIS

Individuals:

- Experience generalized anxiety.
- Acquire maladaptive behavior patterns. The behaviors reduce anxiety in the short term, but are ultimately counterproductive. By avoiding social situations, sociophobics avoid anxiety in the short term, but in the long term suffer isolation due to social withdrawal.

The individual has insight into the problem but requires help such as psychological counseling or behavioral conditioning.

NOISE-INDUCED HEARING LOSS

Any noise louder than 85 decibels damages hearing. Patients present with:

- gradually progressive sensorineural hearing loss
- high-frequency tinnitus.

OBESITY

Obesity is diagnosed when an individual meets any of the following criteria:

- body fat over 25% in males or over 30% in females
- a triceps plus subscapular skinfold thickness of over 45 mm in males or over 69 mm in females
- a body mass index (BMI) of 30 kg/m^2 or greater (an individual's BMI is calculated by dividing their weight in kilograms by their height in meters squared: BMI = weight (kg)/height^2 (m^2))
- a relative body weight more than 20% above the upper limit for height on the Metropolitan Life Insurance Company and/or Fogarty tables
- a waist circumference of 102 cm or more in men and 88 cm or more in women.

Obesity is an important indication of an increased disease risk. The excess mortality in obese adults is attributable to an increased incidence of diabetes, biliary disease, appendicitis, liver cirrhosis, and accidents. Body fat and its pattern of distribution are recognized markers of cardiovascular risk factors such as high blood pressure, plasma lipids, and insulin resistance. Although management is met with varying degrees of success, obesity is a treatable condition. Detection of obesity and successful intervention can reduce an individual's risk of developing a variety of disorders.

OBSESSIVE–COMPULSIVE NEUROSIS

The individual is primarily concerned with keeping control of their life situation. They are often conscientious, intelligent, and predictable people with:

- constantly recurring thoughts (obsessions)
- repetitive actions (compulsions).

Anxiety is relieved by ritualistic behaviors. They have insight into their problem and recognize that their recurring thoughts and behavior are counterproductive.

OBSTRUCTIVE AIRWAYS DISEASE

In obstructive airways disease the underlying pathogenesis involves irritation of:

- Alveoli, leading to activation of proteases with destruction of alveolar tissue, loss of elastic recoil, and alteration of surface tension. This characterizes emphysema.
- Bronchi, with mucus hypersecretion by goblet cells and mucous glands. Excess secretion leads to the production of mucous plugs and a productive cough. This is characteristic of chronic bronchitis. The mucous plugs predispose the individual to respiratory infection.
- Bronchioles, with inflammatory generation of mucous plugs and fibrosis, resulting in expiratory obstruction to air flow. Chronic obstructive airways disease may show all the above features.

The level of the respiratory tree targeted determines the clinical presentation. The clinical presentation of chronic obstructive airways disease invariably involves:

- gradually progressive dyspnea
- chronic productive cough
- wheezing and prolonged expiration
- early inspiratory crackles (late in disease)
- varying degrees of emphysema and chronic bronchitis.

Spirometry shows a reduced vital capacity (VC) and a diminished peak flow rate (forced expiratory volume in 1 second (FEV_1)), a prolonged expiration resulting in a reduced FEV_1/ FVC ratio. The residual volume is increased in obstructive lung disease.

Referral is indicated for patients with:

- Evidence of respiratory distress.
- A very low peak expiratory flow rate (< 150 l/min).

- Previously uninvestigated or worsening:
  - cyanosis
  - use of accessory muscles
  - dyspnea at rest.

See Table IV.

Table IV
Differences between COAD (chronic bronchitis/emphysema) and asthma

	Asthma	Chronic bronchitis	Emphysema
Age of onset	Childhood	> 40 years	> 40 years
Common association	Allergy	Smoking	–
Presenting symptom	Episodic wheeze	Persistent productive cough	Breathlessness
Auscultatory impression	Wheezes during attacks	Noisy, persistent rhonchi	Silent chest
Exercise tolerance	Normal between attacks	Reduced	Poor
Infective episodes	Variable	Common	Occasional
Cor pulmonale	Absent	Occurs early	Occurs late
Central cyanosis	Only severe attack	Common, late stages	Pink early

OCULOMOTOR PALSY

Patients present with:

- diplopia
- divergent strabismus
- ptosis
- pupillary dilatation, except if diabetes is the cause
- pain, if aneurysm or a structural lesion is the cause.

OPTIC ATROPHY

Optic atrophy presents clinically with:

- The insidious onset of visual impairment.
- Ophthalmoscopic changes including:
  - a pale optic disc
  - clear disc margins in cases of: preceding retrobulbar neuritis and pressure on the optic nerve
  - blurred disc margins following papilledema.

Atrophy may be secondary to:

- pressure on the optic nerve due to a tumor, an aneurysm, or Paget's disease

- increased intraocular pressure, as in glaucoma
- increased intracranial pressure, as in papilledema
- inflammation, as in optic neuritis.

OPTIC NEURITIS

Optic neuritis may present as papillitis or retrobulbar neuritis. It may result from:

- ischemia
- multiple sclerosis
- toxins (e.g. methyl alcohol, tobacco, lead)
- diabetes mellitus
- vitamin B_{12} deficiency.

The clinical presentation of optic neuritis is:

- a large central scotoma
- poor visual acuity
- eye pain, but only with eye movement.

Ophthalmoscopy in cases with papillitis shows:

- a raised optic disc (may be unilateral)
- loss of the physiological cup
- hyperemia
- a pale disc (as time progresses, atrophy of the optic nerve leads to a pale disc).

Ophthalmoscopy in cases with retrobulbar neuritis shows:

- no visible lesion until late in the disease
- a pale disc (this occurs late in the disease).

ORAL CANCER

Patients present with:

- a persistent mass
- superinfection and ulceration
- halitosis
- pain (the distribution of pain is determined by the site of the lesion and the nerves involved).

ORBITAL CELLULITIS

Patients present with:

- swollen eyelids (sudden swelling of an eyelid and signs of infection are an indication for urgent referral)

- severe orbital pain
- exophthalmos
- impaired eye movement
- conjunctival infection, chemosis
- fever.

ORGANIC BRAIN DISORDER

See: *Cerebral tumors.*

OSTEOARTHRITIS

Osteoarthritis is a degenerative disease of cartilage. It is a common condition, encountered in every second person over the age of 60 years. Persons with osteoarthritis experience:

- slowly developing joint pain
- pain that follows use of the joint and is worst at the end of the day
- morning stiffness (this lasts for about 15 minutes after getting up)
- a decreased range of motion
- tenderness is usually absent, except along the joint margin in synovitis
- hard body swellings (osteophytes on joint margins or in ligamentous attachments and altered shapes of bone ends on radiography are detected)
- crepitation (this is a late sign)
- an absence of systemic signs
- radiography shows joint-space narrowing, with sclerosis and cystic areas in subchondral bone.

All synovial joints may be involved.

Primary osteoarthritis is a symmetrical condition affecting numerous joints, including:

- knees
- the metatarsophalangeal joints of the big toe and thumb
- the interphalangeal joints of the fingers
- the acromioclavicular joints
- small joints of the spine.

Secondary osteoarthritis is asymmetrical and affects weight-bearing joints such as the knee, hips, and intervertebral joints.

Overall, the joints most frequently found to be osteoarthritic are the carpometacarpal joint of the thumb, the first metatarsophalangeal joint of the big toe, and the distal interphalangeal joints of the hand. The knees, hips, and facet joints of the lumbar and cervical spine are also very frequently involved.

OSTEOID OSTEOMA

This benign bone tumor is particularly prone to occur in adolescent males. With the exception of the cranium, any bone can be involved. Patients present with pain that:

- occurs at night
- is relieved by aspirin
- is aggravated by alcohol.

OSTEOMYELITIS

Osteomyelitis is bone infection. The patient presents with:

- the sudden onset of bone pain or a vague pain
- point tenderness over the affected bone
- restriction of movement (e.g. a limp)
- a sharp increase in temperature in children (in adults this may be absent)
- a raised erythrocyte sedimentation rate (ESR).

OSTEOPOROSIS

Primary osteoporosis is a major public health problem in the western world and found in at least 25% of women of 60 years of age. Type 1 osteoporosis is linked to estrogen deprivation at menopause and is responsible for one-third of women aged over 65 years having one or more vertebral fractures. Type 2 or senile osteoporosis is found in both sexes and is related to a chronic negative calcium balance and advancing age. Over a number of years of steady bone demineralization, bones become porous and fragile and are prone to fracture after minimal trauma. The condition is asymptomatic until a significant amount of bone mass has been depleted.

Common clinical presentations for osteoporosis include:

- Fractures after no or minor trauma. Common sites are the:
  - Spine: a crush or wedge fracture of the spine may present as loss of height, the development of a dowager hump, or backache.
  - Forearm: a Colles fracture may be found.
  - Femur: the neck of the femur is particularly at risk in senile osteoporosis.
- Normal laboratory tests. Alkaline phosphatase and serum calcium and phosphate are usually within normal limits.
- Reduced bone mass measurements using:
  - single-photon absorptiometry of the distal forearm
  - dual-photon absorptiometry
  - computed tomography.

- An imbalance of markers of:
  - bone formation (i.e. alkaline phosphatase and serum osteocalcin)
  - bone resorption (i.e. hydroxyproline and urinary calcium).

Predisposition to osteoporosis is 75% genetically determined. Screening for variations in gene receptors for vitamin D by blood tests can determine if an individual has this gene variant.

Secondary osteoporosis is usually characterized by the underlying disorder. Secondary osteoporosis may result from:

- Osteomalacia. The patient presents with:
  - bone pain
  - skeletal deformity (e.g. kyphosis)
  - muscle weakness
  - low serum calcium and phosphorus
  - a raised alkaline phosphatase.
- Hyperparathyroidism. Patients present with:
  - Thirst.
  - Polyuria.
  - Constipation.
  - Renal colic, if renal calculi are present.
  - On laboratory investigation: a high serum calcium; low serum phosphate; elevated serum immunoreactive parathyroid hormone; elevated urinary cyclic adenosine monophosphate (cAMP).
- Glucocorticoid excess. Cushing's syndrome is often iatrogenically induced as a result of prolonged steroid therapy. The patient presents with:
  - wasted extremities
  - a round red face
  - a large abdomen and trunk.
- Thyrotoxicosis. Patients present with:
  - weight loss, despite a hearty appetite
  - fine skin and hair
  - heat intolerance and diarrhea
  - a bounding pulse
  - muscle weakness.
- Multiple myeloma. Patients present with:
  - bone pain
  - an elevated erythrocyte sedimentation rate (ESR)
  - Bence–Jones proteinuria.
- Immobilization. Prolonged immobilization and/or weightlessness are associated with bone mineral loss. It is important for skeletal health that bone be weight bearing.

OTIC BAROTRAUMA

Otic barotrauma is the result of damage to the middle ear due to ambient pressure changes. People are at greatest risk when the eustachian tube is malfunctioning. Persons with upper respiratory tract infections or allergy should avoid flying or diving. The presentation of otic barotrauma is:

- acute ear pain
- conduction deafness
- drum retraction and possible perforation
- bleeding into the middle ear.

OTITIS EXTERNA

Otitis externa may be diffuse or furuncular. Findings that suggest the need for intervention are:

- infected pierced ears
- pain on moving the pinna in patients with otitis externa
- a furuncle of the external ear.

Diffuse otitis externa presents with:

- Itching.
- Pain aggravated by chewing or moving the tragus.
- Pain on moving the pinna. This suggests cartilage involvement.
- A scanty discharge. Discharge varies with the cause. It is:
  - creamy in *Pseudomonas* infection
  - cheesy in fungal otitis externa
  - often absent in dermatitis.
- The canal may be:
  - red or scaly in mild cases
  - edematous in severe cases.

Furuncular otitis externa presents with:

- severe pain
- marked tenderness on compression of the tragus
- pre- and postauricular lymphadenopathy
- a boil may be visualized and swelling around the ear noted.

OTITIS INTERNA

Disorders of the inner ear affect hearing and balance. Persons undertaking high-impact aerobics or activities that involve repetitive jarring motions may develop inner ear problems such as:

- vertigo, dizziness, or balance dysfunction
- tinnitus or an ear-muffling sensation
- hearing loss, especially in the high-frequency range.

High-impact aerobics should be stopped or not be undertaken for more than 20 minutes at a time.

OTITIS MEDIA

Inflammation of the middle ear may result from eustachian tube occlusion or be attributable to infection.

Serous otitis media (glue ear). Opening the eustachian tube by swallowing equalizes the pressure in the middle ear with atmospheric pressure. In conditions in which the eustachian tube is occluded absorption of air in the middle ear creates a negative pressure, with consequent serous fluid accumulation. Infants are at particular risk, due to their shorter, wider, and more horizontal eustachian tubes. The natural history for the condition is one of fluctuation, with recurrences and remissions. There is a strong tendency to resolve over time. An asymptomatic nonpurulent effusion that persists for less than 3 months usually need not be referred.

The clinical presentation includes:

- Conduction deafness.
- Stuffiness of the involved ear(s).
- Transient pain. However, the presentation is rather one of painless hearing loss.
- A tympanic membrane which:
  - is dull or blue
  - suggests apparent shortening of the handle of the malleus
  - has red vessels radiating from the malleus and/or umbo
  - is immobile on pneumatic otoscopy.
- Bubbles or an amber fluid level in the middle ear.

Decongestants, antihistamines, mucolytics and nonsteroidal anti-inflammatory agents are ineffective in the treatment of serous otitis media. Antibiotics are recommended when:

- the duration of effusion is unclear
- symptomatic hearing loss is present.

Antibiotics, and possibly steroids, should be considered prior to surgical referral for insertion of a grommet. Grommets ventilate the middle ear and reverse the associated epithelial metaplasia. They do, however, tend to become blocked after about 10 months.

Referral is recommended if there is:

- hearing impairment
- delayed speech development
- repeated middle ear infection
- retraction of the tympanic membrane.

Acute otitis media. Diagnosis of acute otitis implies a duration of less than 3 weeks. The presentation varies depending on the age of the patient:

- A 3–5-year-old may present with:
  - fever

  - mouth-breathing
  - a runny nose.
- Older children present with:
  - earache
  - hearing loss.
- Infants may present with:
  - vomiting
  - diarrhea.

The clinical spectrum of acute otitis media includes:

- Fever, lethargy, and irritability.
- Headache.
- Throbbing earache, which subsides in 6–9 hours.
- Earache aggravated by swallowing/belching.
- Painful conduction hearing loss.
- Pain relieved upon rupture of the eardrum.
- Auricular discharge.
- An eardrum that progressively:
  - shows dullness
  - develops increased vascularity and redness around the malleus
  - is red and inflamed
  - loses its light reflex
  - bulges
  - ruptures, leaving a small perforation (due to antibiotics this is uncommon today).

Suspect viral infections in patients with:

- watery rhinitis
- a pink drum.

Suspect bacterial infection in patients with:

- fever
- marked irritability
- an acutely tender ear
- a bulging red drum.

Predisposing factors include coryza.

Recurrent acute otitis media. Some 17% of children experience three or more episodes of acute otitis media by the age of 12 months, and 74% experience three or more episodes by 7 years of age. Recurrent episodes of acute otitis media with effusion lead to hearing impairment and learning disability.

Acute suppurative otitis media. Severe or untreated acute otitis media leads to accumulation of a purulent exudate. Resolution follows drainage.

Chronic otitis media. A perforated drum with a discharge that persists for more than 1 month is considered chronic. Patients may present with:

- A central perforation of the eardrum and a mucoid discharge.

- A small anterior perforation and minimal hearing loss.
- A marginal perforation associated with:
  - atticoantral disease
  - an offensive purulent discharge
  - cholesteatoma formation.
- Ossicular pathology with severe hearing loss of up to 60 decibels.
- Mastoiditis.
- Complications:
  - A cholesteatoma. These wax-like sacs of epithelial tissue, which grow as cells are shed, may destroy the ossicles and cause cerebral abscess or meningitis.
  - Suppuration: meningitis; cerebral abscess formation; lateral sinus thrombosis; extra- and subdural abscesses; osteomyelitis.

OTOSCLEROSIS

This is a familial condition in which the footplate of the stapes undergoes ankylosis. Patients present with a:

- conductive hearing loss
- normal tympanic membrane.

OVARIAN CYSTS

Tubo-ovarian, pedunculated, or chocolate cysts may present with:

- a scanty vaginal discharge
- deep dyspareunia
- tenderness on vaginal examination
- occasional backache.

OVARIAN MALIGNANCY

Suspect ovarian malignancy in a postmenopausal woman who has:

- A pelvic mass.
  or
- Any combination of:
  - unexplained weight gain
  - increased abdominal girth
  - nonspecific minor bowel problems.
- Ascites may be the first sign of ovarian cancer.

OVARIAN PROLAPSE

Prolapse of the ovary can cause:

- pelvic pain, occasional backache
- dyspareunia (this is especially noticeable at ovulation and menstruation).

OVARIAN TORSION

Torsion of the ovary impairs blood supply and presents with:

- Abdominal pain that:
  - starts suddenly
  - is sharp and stabbing
  - is often located in one iliac region
  - may radiate to the lower back.
- A tender abdominal or pelvic mass.

OVERUSE SYNDROMES

Overuse of the lower limbs, usually by keen sportspersons, may cause repetitive trauma. Rest usually relieves the pain.

Patients may present with:

- Acute groin pain due to tendonitis and tendoperiostitis.
- Knee pain due to tendonitis and peritendonitis (see: *Patellofemoral pain syndrome*):
  - jogger's knee, due to patellofemoral pain
  - jumper's knee, due to patellar tendonitis
  - runner's knee, due to iliotibial band tendonitis (the deep ache on the lateral aspect of the knee is aggravated by running downhill).
- Lower leg pain due to:
  - Stress fractures. Pain over the tibia is diagnosed by bone scans.
  - Muscle tears. 'Tennis' leg is caused by rupture of the medial head of gastrocnemius and presents with a sudden sharp calf pain and localized tenderness. The individual walks on tip toes and cannot put their heel on the ground.
  - Tendonitis. Achilles tendonitis presents with pain that is aggravated by walking on the toes. The leg is stiff and sore on rising, but improves with exercise.
- Elbow pain (see: *Tennis elbow*).
- Hand (see: *Tenosynovitis*).

OVULATION SYNDROME

Mittelschmerz presents with:

- Pain that may be experienced in the:
  - iliac fossa
  - flank
  - suprapubic area
  - central abdomen
  - over the sacrum.

- Pain at the midpoint of the menstrual cycle.
- Suprapubic or iliac fossa tenderness.
- Breast tenderness following ovulation in 10% of women.

PAGET'S DISEASE

Paget's disease is the result of localized disorganized bone remodeling. It presents with:

- Bone pain.
- Skeletal deformity – enlargement and bowing of long bones, frontal bossing of the skull, vertebral compression fractures.

The risk of osteosarcoma and high output cardiac failure are increased.

In asymptomatic individuals an isolated raised serum alkaline phosphatase is suggestive as is elevated urinary hydroyproline, a marker of bone resorption. X-ray findings are diagnostic with plain X-rays showing expansion and deformity of bones with characteristic lytic and sclerotic lesions.

PANCREATIC CANCER

Cancer of the pancreas may be located in the head (70%), body, or tail. Diagnosis is late, with over 80% being diagnosed after local invasion and metastasis have occurred. Patients present with:

- Impaired digestion, resulting in:
  - fatty food intolerance
  - anorexia
  - steatorrhea
  - emaciation.
- Progressive jaundice. Jaundice is a late sign, and is associated with dark urine and pale stools. Jaundice is intermittent, due to sloughing of tumor, when the cancer is periampullary.
- Pain, which may:
  - present at a late stage
  - present as a dull, continuous ache in the epigastric region
  - radiate to the back (slight relief may be achieved by leaning forward).
- A palpable gallbladder. Cancer of the head of the pancreas may obstruct bile flow, causing back-pressure on the gallbladder, which enlarges. In patients with a history of gallstones, fibrosis, due to chronic irritation of the gallbladder, prevents such enlargement.

- Migratory thrombophlebitis.
- Diabetes. Elderly patients who present for the first time with diabetes should have pancreatic cancer excluded.
- Serum amylase may be raised and occult blood may be detected in the stool.

PANCREATITIS

Acute pancreatitis may be precipitated by alcohol (50% of cases), gallstones (34%), viral infections (e.g. mumps, coxsackie), trauma, or drugs (e.g. steroids). Acute pancreatitis is characterized by:

- Epigastric pain, which:
  - is sudden in onset, developing over 60–180 minutes
  - is severe and constant
  - persists for days
  - radiates to the back
  - is precipitated by alcohol
  - is aggravated by vomiting, lying supine, or walking
  - is relieved by leaning forward or crouching (kneeling forward)
  - is associated with visceral autonomic findings (e.g. nausea, vomiting).
- Jaundice. Edema of the head of the pancreas may partially obstruct the bile duct, precipitating a tinge of jaundice.
- Paralytic ileus. Peritoneal irritation results in abdominal distension, tenderness, and guarding.
- Fever may be present.
- Serum and urinary amylase are raised.

Chronic pancreatitis is usually found in males with a history of alcohol ingestion. Chronic pancreatitis presents with:

- recurrent episodes of abdominal pain
- recurrent jaundice
- steatorrhea (malabsorption results from pancreatic exocrine failure)
- diabetes (hyperglycemia results from pancreatic endocrine failure).

Both acute and chronic pancreatitis may relapse if the precipitating cause persists. Intervention is to remove the precipitating cause and refer the patient for medical monitoring.

PANHYPOPITUITARISM

Decreased pituitary function presents with:

- Weakness.
- Easy fatiguability.

- Failure to develop, or regression of, secondary sexual characteristics (e.g. pubic and axillary hair).
- Impaired resistance to stress and cold.
- Low blood pressure.
- Visual field defects. This occurs in cases when a pituitary lesion causes pressure on the optic chiasma.
- Laboratory findings include:
  - low thyroid-stimulating hormone (TSH) and T4
  - low luteinizing hormone (LH), follicle-stimulating hormone (FSH), and urinary 17-ketosteroids
  - low hydroxycorticosteroids.

PANIC DISORDERS

The clinical presentation of panic disorders may mimic hypoglycemia, hyperthyroidism, and/or pheochromocytoma. Consider a panic attack when laboratory tests are normal in a patient complaining of at least four of the following symptoms during at least one attack:

- dyspnea or smothering sensations
- dizziness, faintness, unsteady feelings
- palpitations or tachycardia
- trembling or shaking
- sweating
- choking
- nausea or abdominal distress
- depersonalization or derealization
- paresthesia or numbness.

Before diagnosing a panic attack, the following criteria should also be met:

- the attack should be unexpected, not the result of being the center of attention
- four attacks should occur within a 4-week period, or one or more attacks should be followed by at least 1 month during which the patient experiences a persistent fear of another attack.

PARALYTIC ILEUS

See: *Intestinal obstruction.*

PARAPHIMOSIS

Paraphimosis is a retracted foreskin which cannot be reduced over the glans. The tip of the patient's penis is:

- cherry red
- tender
- swollen.

PARATHYROID DISEASE

The parathyroid glands secrete a hormone that influences calcium metabolism. Excess parathyroid hormone secretion results in hyperparathyroidism (see: *Hyperparathyroidism*). Decreased parathyroid hormone secretion results in hypoparathyroidism (see: *Hypoparathyroidism*).

PARKINSON'S DISEASE

Degeneration of dopaminergic neurons in the substantia nigra results in Parkinson's disease. Patients are usually between 40 and 70 years of age and present with:

- A resting tremor (5 Hz). A pill-rolling tremor of the hands, in which movement of the finger and the metacarpophalangeal joints is combined with movements of the thumb, is characteristic. The tremor spreads to the legs, face, and tongue. Some patients also develop a faster action tremor.
- Bradykinesis. This presents with:
  - slowness in initiating movements
  - poverty of movement
  - a mask-like facies (loss of facial expression is frequently found)
  - paucity of blinking
  - slow, monotonous speech.
- Rigidity. This may present as:
  - cogwheel rigidity (this contrasts with the claspknife, sudden release, rigidity of an upper motor neuron lesion)
  - lead-pipe rigidity, manifest as sustained resistance or stiffness.
- An abnormal posture. Patients may demonstrate:
  - progressive flexion of the trunk (a stooped posture is characteristic)
  - elbow flexion.
- An abnormal gait. Patients walk with:
  - no arm swinging
  - shuffling
  - start hesitation
  - small steps
  - a festinating gait (as the speed of forward propulsion increases, gait becomes festinating and patients may fall).
- Autonomic symptoms. These include:
  - constipation
  - postural hypotension.

- Myalgia (muscle aches and cramps).

Intellectual deterioration only occurs in advanced cases. Sensation, power, and reflexes are normal.

PARONYCHIA

Acute paronychia is due to infection of the nail bed. This results in the lateral nail fold and mantle of the nail becoming:

- swollen
- red
- painful.

Pressure on the nail causes exquisite tenderness once pus has formed.

Staphylococci and herpes (whitlow) are both causes of paronychia.

Chronic paronychia is painless and is a traumatic nail dystrophy. Damage to the cuticle may lead to secondary infection with candida.

PAROXYSMAL ATRIAL (SUPRAVENTRICULAR) TACHYCARDIA

This is a disorder of unknown etiology found in apparently healthy adults. Paroxysmal atrial tachycardia presents with:

- a regular pulse
- a rapid pulse of more than 120 beats/min
- the sudden onset of palpitations
- dyspnea
- a history of a previous attack
- copious amounts of urine being passed after an attack.

Predisposing factors in susceptible individuals include:

- anxiety
- tension
- smoking.

An attack may be terminated by vagal stimulation. In certain cases the problem may be alleviated by normalizing spinal function. In the absence of organic heart disease, dysfunction of the upper thoracic spine (especially T4 and T5) has been linked with paroxysmal supraventricular tachycardia.

PATELLOFEMORAL PAIN SYNDROME

Chondromalacia patellae is the result of overuse of the knee. Patients present with:

- Deep knee pain or pain behind the patella.
- Pain is aggravated by weight-bearing activities involving knee flexion:
  - squatting
  - prolonged sitting
  - climbing stairs
  - walking downhill.
- Stretching the knee provides some relief. Patients select aisle seats so that they can stretch their leg out when seated for prolonged periods in planes and theaters.
- Crepitus may be detected around the patella.

PELVIC FLOOR TENSION MYALGIA

This condition is defined as pain in the pelvic floor muscles and their points of attachment. Patients present with one or more of:

- chronic pelvic pain
- dyspareunia
- pain on defecation.

Variations of this condition include piriformis syndrome and proctalgia fugax.

PELVIC INFLAMMATORY DISEASE

Gonococci, anaerobes, chlamydia, and/or mycoplasma are frequently encountered in this multibacterial disease. The patient presents with:

- Recurrent bilateral pelvic pain (this is found in 50% of patients).
- Increased vaginal discharge. Half of patients with pelvic inflammatory disease have a purulent discharge that may be offensive.
- Irregular heavy periods are found in one-third of patients.
- Congestive dysmenorrhea.
- Dyspareunia.
- Pyrexia (one-third of patients have a temperature over 38°C).
- Palpation findings, such as:
  - lower abdominal tenderness
  - adnexal tenderness
  - cervical motion tenderness
  - palpable adnexal mass (present in 50% of cases).
- Infertility.
- Right upper quadrant pain in severe cases.

Ectopic pregnancy should always be actively excluded.

Chronic salpingitis is a variant of pelvic inflammatory disease in which the focus of the infection is the fallopian tubes. This disease has an insidious onset and presents with:

- Chronic recurring pain. Common problems are:
  - backache
  - lower abdominal pain.
- Dyspareunia.
- Congestive dysmenorrhea. The pain is worst just before and during periods.
- A vaginal discharge.

The cervix and tubes are tender to palpation. Ectopic pregnancy and infertility are major complications.

Acute salpingitis may follow recent abortion, parturition, or venereal disease. It presents with:

- abdominal pain
- vaginal discharge
- intense pain on moving the cervix
- fever.

In *parametritis*, cellulitis of the posterior sacrouterine ligaments results in:

- backache
- lower abdominal pain.

PEPTIC STRICTURE

See: *Benign peptic stricture.*

PEPTIC ULCER DISEASE

At any one time some 4% of the adult population in an industrialized country has an active ulcer; one-quarter of these may be asymptomatic. Peptic ulcer disease is a condition characterized by relapses and remissions. The presentation of peptic ulcer syndrome includes:

- In nine out of ten patients:
  - Symptom periodicity. The history is one of symptom-free periods interrupted by attacks.
  - Abdominal pain: a well-localized epigastric pain is experienced by three out of four cases; a gnawing or aching pain in the right hypochondrium (this is suggestive of a duodenal ulcer); backache, usually in the region of T5–T8, suggests severe ulceration.
- In eight out of ten cases:
  - Symptomatic relief following food or alkali ingestion.

- A relationship between the onset of pain and food ingestion: in gastric ulcers the pain is initiated shortly after eating; in duodenal ulcers the pain is delayed for 1–2 hours after eating (the patient associates the pain with hunger rather than with food ingestion).
- Epigastric tenderness.

- Dyspepsia:
  - Heartburn. A burning retrosternal sensation following meals.
  - Waterbrash. A clear fluid in the back of the throat unassociated with the muscular effort of retching or the food content of vomitus. Waterbrash is often found in persons with duodenal ulcers.
  - Flatulence. This usually presents as belching and abdominal distension.
- A psychoemotional profile of:
  - high ambition
  - extreme hard working
  - conscientiousness and reliability
  - immaturity
  - passive dependence
  - rigidity and impaired adaptability.
- Chemical exposures such as:
  - cigarette smoking
  - aspirin and nonsteroidal anti-inflammatory drugs (NSAIDs). NSAIDs damage the mucosa via inhibition of prostaglandin synthesis (the same mechanism via which they achieve pain relief). About 30% of NSAID users have chronic gastric ulceration, and 5% have duodenal ulceration.
- *Helicobactor pylori* infection. This organism is found in over 95% of patients with duodenal ulcers and in 70% with gastric ulcers.

Peptic ulcer syndrome may be regarded as a spectrum of conditions. The spectrum includes the following.

Ulcer dyspepsia. This is the mildest form of the peptic ulcer syndrome. Patients present with:

- epigastric discomfort
- a history of previous attacks interspersed with symptom-free periods
- a family history
- the absence of an ulcer crater on barium meal and/or gastroscopy.

Ulceration is the major complication.

Gastric ulcers. These present with:

- Ulcer dyspepsia.
- Vomiting.
- Pain within an hour of eating.

- Weight loss (this results from avoiding eating for fear of precipitating pain).
- A gastric ulcer crater on barium meal or gastroscopy.
- Complications include:
  - Hemorrhage.
  - Penetration.
  - Perforation:
  - Sudden onset of severe abdominal pain starting in the epigastric region and spreading to involve the flanks, back, and shoulders.
  - Constant abdominal pain aggravated by movement or deep respiration.
  - Abdominal rigidity and the subsequent diminution and absence of peristaltic sounds.
- Carcinomatous change:
  - constant weight loss
  - excessive vomiting
  - vomiting old food (i.e. food eaten some time previously)
  - indigestion which fails to remit with treatment
  - daily symptomatology
  - anorexia
  - anemia
  - an abdominal mass
  - a positive occult blood test and/or raised ESR
  - evidence of metastatic disease. A hard nodular liver or enlarged supraclavicular lymph nodes are a late development.

Duodenal ulcers. The prevalence peaks in females by the age of 40 years, and in males by the age of 50 years. Patients present with:

- Ulcer dyspepsia.
- Waterbrash.
- Pain relief attributed to eating.
- A tendency to wake with pain between midnight and two in the morning.
- Complications include:
- - hemorrhage
  - perforation (see: *Gastric ulcers*)
  - penetration
  - fibrosis with stricture formation: persistent vomiting; a succussion splash
  - penetration of the pancreas: severe persistent backache.

Ulcer patients at low risk of ulcer complications:

- are less than 60 years old
- have no previous ulcer complications
- are not on NSAIDs
- have no concomitant serious medical condition
- have no more than two relapses annually
- have gradual development of symptoms with each episode.

Referral should be considered in patients:

- Who have not been previously diagnosed and whose symptoms persist despite having stopped smoking, drinking alcohol, or taking self-prescribed salicylates.
- Who despite at least two weeks of treatment have:
  - persistent symptoms
  - persistent vomiting
  - severe abdominal pain
  - develop melena.
- Over 40 years of age who have been diagnosed but have not been investigated to exclude cancer of the stomach.
- With complications. Patients at high risk of the complications from peptic ulceration:
  - are elderly
  - have coexisting medical conditions
  - have previous ulcer complications
  - are on NSAIDs (NSAID-induced ulcers can be asymptomatic, causing serious complications without prior warning)
  - continue to smoke
  - have frequent relapses.
- With an indication for surgery such as:
  - failure of primary healing (this is rarely an indication)
  - relapse despite maintenance therapy
  - a rapid recurrence after ceasing medical treatment
  - frequent ulcer relapse in a younger patient.

PERFORATED EARDRUM

Patients present with:

- conduction deafness
- a perforation of the drum.

Obligatory aural hygiene in these patients includes:

- Not putting anything in the ear, including no eardrops or syringing.
- A plug may be necessary for those working in a dusty environment.
- Not swimming/putting the head under water for 4 weeks or until the drum is healed.
- Keeping water out of the ear canal by one of the following methods:
  - cotton wool plus petroleum jelly
  - Blu Tack
  - silicone ear putty
  - tailor-made ear plugs or doc plugs (available in six sizes).

The ear must be checked weekly and immediate referral made if:

- signs of infection are present
- the tear has not healed in 4 weeks.

Findings on presentation which suggest that referral may be prudent, regardless of the cause, are:

- Evidence of a foreign body in the ear.
- Persistent bleeding from the ear.
- Possible cerebrospinal fluid leak from the nose or ear.
- Vertigo: either episodic over several days or persisting.
- Facial nerve palsy.
- Evidence of sensorineural deafness.
- No sign of healing after 6 weeks.
- Acute trauma (e.g. cleaning the ear with matchsticks, a blow to the ear, or head injury) resulting in:
  - pain
  - deafness
  - tinnitus
  - a tear in the eardrum, with or without bleeding.

PERIANAL ABSCESS

Patients present with:

- throbbing anal discomfort
- pain that disturbs sleep
- a tender inflamed mass in the perianal region
- a discharge, which may be bloodstained
- a sinus or fistula following discharge.

PERIANAL HEMATOMA (thrombosed external pile)

Patients present with:

- the acute onset of painful defecation
- a smooth tense lump at the anal margin which is bluish in color
- a history of the problem having occurred when straining at stool.

PERICARDITIS

Inflammation of the outer lining of the heart presents with:

- Precordial pain. Pericarditis associated with uremia, myocardial infarction, or malignancy is usually painless. In viral pericarditis, pain:
  - is either a steady crushing (occasionally burning) or stabbing retrosternal pain, or both
  - radiates to the neck, shoulder, and back in the flank area

- may be aggravated by coughing, deep inspiration, or swallowing
- is somewhat relieved on sitting up and leaning forward
- persists for hours and days
- may be synchronous with the heart beat.

- A pericardial friction rub. The superficial scratching sound is best heard to the left of the sternum in the precordial area.
- A pericardial effusion. This should be suspected when the following are detected:
  - dysphagia
  - increased cardiac dullness
  - dyspnea that is somewhat relieved by sitting up and leaning forward.
- Obstruction to venous return. Cardiac tamponade and constrictive pericarditis present with:
  - distended neck veins, hepatomegaly, ascites, and edema
  - a low pulse pressure and tachycardia
  - decreased cardiac output, with fatigue and weakness
  - pulsus paradoxus and progressive dyspnea
  - increased cardiac dullness and soft heart sounds.
- Electrocardiogram (ECG) changes.

PERIODONTITIS

Patients present with:

- halitosis
- spongy gums
- congested gums (gums may bleed if teeth are brushed vigorously)
- malodorous material between the teeth (this can be removed by flossing)
- gum recession.

PERIPHERAL VASCULAR DISEASE

See: *Arterial occlusion/insufficiency.*

PERITONITIS

Peritonitis is usually the result of an inflamed intra-abdominal organ. The onset is gradual as inflammation spreads through the wall of the inflamed viscus to involve the serous abdominal lining. The sudden onset of peritonitis suggests perforation of a viscus, with spilling of abdominal contents into a normally sterile peritoneal cavity. Peritonitis is an indication for urgent referral. Peritonitis should be suspected in patients with:

- Well-localized abdominal pain.
- Abdominal guarding and rigidity.
- Hyperesthesia of the skin overlying the affected area.
- Pyrexia, tachycardia, leukocytosis.
- Irritation of adjacent organs may result in:
  - paralytic ileus (patients have a silent abdomen and absolute constipation, passing neither feces nor flatus, due to the absence of peristalsis)
  - mucous diarrhea
  - vomiting
  - jaundice due to edema of the common bile duct
  - dysuria and frequency due to irritation of the urinary bladder.

PERITONSILLAR ABSCESS (quinsy)

Quinsy is a complication of a streptococcal throat. Patients present with:

- fever
- sore throat
- cervical lymphadenopathy
- unilateral pain that radiates to the ear on swallowing
- enlargement in the region of the tonsil and soft palate.

PERNICIOUS ANEMIA

See: *Anemia* (vitamin B_{12} deficiency anemia).

PERTHES' DISEASE

Children with avascular necrosis of the femoral head present with:

- a limp
- an aching hip
- limited abduction and internal rotation.

Diagnosis is made on detecting a subchondral fracture and pebble stone epiphysis on the radiograph. Children between 4 and 8 years of age are at greatest risk.

PHARYNGITIS

Acute viral pharyngitis presents with:

- a sore throat
- malaise

- fever
- a red hyperemic throat.

When patients have the above presentation plus:

- rhinorrhea and sneezing, diagnose coryza (the common cold)
- an exudate, diagnose acute exudative tonsillitis
- nasal speech, diagnose acute exudative adenoiditis.

The condition lasts for 5–10 days.

Functional pharyngitis is characterized by:

- a mentally tired or depressed patient
- a sore or relaxed throat, which occurs in the evenings
- a red throat (injection of the fauces is an unreliable sign, as many healthy throats are red)
- the absence of fever
- symptoms that persist for about a week.

Patients may continually clear their throat when anxious.

PHEOCHROMOCYTOMA

This is a tumor of the adrenal medulla, and is characterized by:

- Paroxysms of:
  - headache
  - hypertension
  - vasomotor instability
  - visual blurring
  - profuse sweating
  - anxiety.
- Occasionally, sustained hypertension.
- Weight loss.
- Postural tachycardia, and hypotension and palpitations.
- Hypermetabolism.
- Confirmatory laboratory findings include:
  - raised serum and urinary catecholamines and their metabolites
  - normal thyroxine levels.

PINWORM INFESTATION

Enterobius vermicularis is the most common intestinal parasite infecting children in temperate climates. The female worm migrates to the perianal region and deposits her eggs. Ova survive for up to 21 days. Transmission occurs by transfer of the eggs from the perianal area to fomites. Eggs may be:

- Ingested by direct contract.
- Inhaled. Airborne eggs, as results from shaking bed linen, may be inhaled and swallowed. In view of this spread, both the patient and the rest of the family usually require treatment.

Patients are often asymptomatic, but may present with perianal:

- itching
- excoriation
- ova.

Diagnosis is made by microscopic identification of the ova. Ova are collected by patting the perianal skin with transparent adhesive tape. The best time for collecting ova is before the child gets up in the morning.

PIRIFORMIS SYNDROME

Patients present with pain and paresthesia in the distribution of the sciatic nerve. Patients experience:

- Pain:
  - in the buttock which is poorly defined and described as a deep boring pain
  - which radiates to the posterolateral thigh and calf.
- A burning sensation in the region of the:
  - hip
  - over the greater trochanter (patients are unable to lie on their side).
- Limited internal rotation of the thigh. When supine, external rotation of the thigh is noted.
- Local burning when pressure is placed on trigger points around the insertion of piriformis into the greater trochanter. Trigger points are detected through the belly of gluteus.
- Pain radiation along the route of the sciatic nerve when pressure is placed on trigger points in the belly of piriformis.

PITUITARY TUMOR

Patients present with:

- headaches
- visual disturbances, with initial loss in the upper outer visual field
- varying degrees of hormonal disturbance (see: *Panhypopituitarism*).

PITYRIASIS ROSEA

This mild acute inflammatory skin condition is not contagious. It presents with:

- a herald patch, which precedes the eruption by 7–14 days
- oval scaly macules

- fawn-colored eruptions on the trunk and proximal extremities
- exfoliation, which starts in the center of the lesion and produces a crinkly scale. This occurs within 6 weeks. Patients occasionally complain of pruritus.

PITYRIASIS VERSICOLOR

This superficial infection is caused by a yeast, *Malassezia furfur*. The patient presents with:

- Patches that are:
  - red-brown and slightly scaly
  - hypopigmented and do not tan.
- Lesions that are predominantly found on the upper trunk extending to the neck and upper arm. The face and groin are less commonly involved.

PLANTAR FASCIITIS

This condition is related to the strain of weight bearing. Plantar fasciitis presents with pain:

- On the plantar surface of the heel
- Which is experienced on getting out of bed but is relieved after walking
- Which becomes worse:
  - towards the end of the day
  - on walking after sitting
- Tenderness that is either:
  - localized to the region of the medial tuberosity

  or
  - widespread on firm palpation of the inner border of the plantar fascia with the foot maximally flexed.

Individuals who are required to stand for prolonged periods are at most risk.

PLEURAL EFFUSION

A pleural effusion results for fluid in the pleural cavity. The fluid may be a transudate or an exudate. An exudate differs from a transudate in that it is rich in protein (> 2 g/100 ml). Exudates are found in patients with:

- underlying pneumonia
- malignancy
- pulmonary infarction
- a subphrenic abscess
- collagen disease.

Transudates occur in persons with cardiac, renal, or liver failure. Infection of an exudate or transudate results in empyema (pus in the pleural cavity). Regardless of its nature, a pleural effusion presents with:

- dyspnea, which may be acute or progressive depending on the size and rapidity with which the effusion develops
- stony dullness on percussion over the effusion
- local reduction of chest movement
- reduced breath sounds
- a pleural rub may be present
- tracheal deviation (in large effusions the trachea is moved away from the side of the lesion).

PLEURISY

The pleura is pain sensitive. Chest pain of respiratory origin is invariably attributable to pleural irritation. Pleurisy presents with:

- Pain that is:
  - sharp and stabbing
  - aggravated by coughing and deep inspiration.
- A pleural friction rub may or may not be present.

PNEUMOCONIOSIS

This is a group of conditions in which interstitial lung fibrosis results from occupational dust exposure. Persons exposed to silica, asbestos, bauxite, beryllium, iron, and coal dust are all at risk of progressive pulmonary insufficiency. The clinical presentation is influenced by the duration and extent of exposure. The typical clinical picture of interstitial fibrosis includes:

- dyspnea on exertion
- a dry cough, which may become productive as the disease progresses
- recurrent respiratory infection
- cor pulmonale.

A chest radiograph shows bilateral pulmonary fibrosis and hilar lymphadenopathy.

PNEUMOCYSTIS

See: *Pneumonia*.

PNEUMONIA

Pneumonia may be caused by various organisms. The clinical picture differs depending on the nature of the causative organism. The fundamental clinical changes associated with this lower respiratory disease are:

- Dyspnea.
- A productive cough.
- Fever.
- Signs of consolidation:
  - dullness to percussion
  - bronchial breathing
  - crackles (these are most pronounced early and late in the natural history of the disease, as consolidation develops and then resolves)
  - local reduction of chest movement.

Pneumonia in the elderly often has an atypical presentation, including:

- Coughing, sputum production, breathlessness, and/or sweating in 50% of patients.
- Deterioration of mentation, presenting as confusion.
- A loss of functional control:
  - ataxia and falls
  - incontinence
  - lethargy and diminished activity
  - anorexia.
- Worsening of a chronic condition: congestive cardiac failure, arrhythmias, chronic obstructive airways disease, diabetes, or renal insufficiency.

The elderly are three times as likely to die of pneumonia as a young adult.

Variations of pneumonia include the following.

Primary atypical pneumonia (viral pneumonia). This presents with:

- a gradual onset
- a low-grade fever
- production of scanty mucoid sputum
- minimal signs of consolidation on examination.

The chest radiograph shows the disease is more extensive than suggested by the clinical picture.

Mycoplasma pneumonia. This presents with:

- a persistent nonproductive cough
- fever and lethargy
- headache
- anorexia

- a sore throat
- crackles, especially basally
- antibodies to mycoplasma.

Pneumocystis pneumonia. This presents in patients with immune deficiencies (e.g. the acquired immune deficiency syndrome (AIDS), acute lymphatic leukemia) on immunosuppressive therapy. Patients present with:

- dyspnea
- fever
- a dry cough
- cyanosis
- increasing pulmonary infiltration with crackles.

Bacterial pneumonias.

- *Bronchopneumonia* presents with:
  - an insidious onset
  - a cough productive of purulent sputum
  - a slowing rising fever
  - patchy consolidation.
- *Lobar pneumonia* presents with:
  - an abrupt onset
  - rusty sputum (*Streptococcus pneumoniae* is the causative organism)
  - high fever and chills
  - consolidation confined to a lobe of the lung.
- *Klebsiella pneumonia* presents with:
  - red mucoid sputum
  - a very ill or toxic patient
  - pulmonary consolidation.

Factors predisposing to this Gram-negative pneumonia are:

- debility
- alcohol abuse
- malnourishment.

- *Staphylococcal pneumonia* presents with:
  - a prodrome of sore throat, laryngitis, or tracheobronchitis
  - bronchopneumonia
  - pleural effusion and/or empyema.

Referral is recommended in cases in which there is suspicion of:

- bacterial pneumonia
- pneumonia in an elderly patient.

Indications for specialist/hospital referral in a patient with pneumonia are:

- a respiratory rate of over 29 breaths/min
- low diastolic blood pressure
- atrial fibrillation

- fever, when the temperature is over 38.3°C
- age, when the patient is over 60 years
- confusion or altered consciousness
- extrapulmonary disease (e.g. meningitis, septic arthritis).

PNEUMOTHORAX

The presence of air in the pleural cavity is termed a pneumothorax. In 90% of cases a pneumothorax occurs spontaneously. In silicosis, tuberculosis, or emphysema, rupture of a lung bullus may cause a pneumothorax secondary to lung disease.

A pneumothorax presents with:

- Pain, which varies from a vague discomfort to the abrupt onset of pleuritic pain.
- Pain may be experienced in the anterior and posterior chest wall and be referred to the shoulder or arm.
- The acute onset of dyspnea.
- A tympanic percussion note.
- Diminished breath sounds on auscultation.

Should the lung act as a ball valve permitting air to enter but not leave the pleural cavity, a *tension pneumothorax* develops. As a tension pneumothorax develops there is:

- rapid escalation of pain
- rapidly progressive dyspnea (trapped air compresses lung tissue and impairs cardiopulmonary function)
- tracheal displacement (trapped air under pressure causes a mediastinal shift away from the side with the lesion).

Bleeding into the pleural cavity results in a *hemopneumothorax*.

POLYARTERITIS NODOSA

This disorder involves segmental inflammation of medium-sized arteries and results in tissue ischemia. Underlying hypersensitivity is suspected. Depending on the arteries involved, patients present with:

- fever
- abdominal pain
- peripheral neuropathy
- weakness
- weight loss
- myalgia, arthralgia
- headache
- renal involvement, which manifests as hypertension, edema, hematuria, proteinuria, and oliguria

- skin lesions, including purpura, petechiae, urticaria, ulcers, and subcutaneous nodules.

POLYCYSTIC KIDNEYS

This congenital disease may be discovered at any age. Patients present with:

- persistent, recurrent hematuria
- bilateral palpable kidneys
- hypertension.

POLYCYSTIC OVARIES

Patients complain of:

- amenorrhea
- hirsutism
- obesity.

The ovaries are palpable.

POLYCYTHEMIA

An increase in red cells may result from:

- An erythropoietic response to hypoxia (e.g. as in emphysema).
- Erythropoietin-producing tumors (e.g. certain renal and cerebellar tumors).
- As part of a myeloproliferative disorder (e.g. as in polycythemia vera). In this instance there is overproduction of all three cell lines. Pruritus and headache are common presenting complaints in this group.

Patients present with:

- A ruddy complexion.
- A tendency to thrombotic episodes (an increased risk of transient ischemic attacks, stroke, and/or myocardial infarction).
- Cyanosis without hypoxia. Cyanosis results from the increased circulating levels of deoxygenated hemoglobin in a patient with high hemoglobin levels.
- Retinal vein engorgement.

POLYMYALGIA RHEUMATICA

Painful restriction of movement of shoulder and hip girdle is common in polymyalgia rheumatica, a condition most prevalent in older people. Patients complain of intense muscle ache and stiffness that is:

- symmetrically distributed
- worst on waking, may disappear later in the day
- aggravated by inactivity.

Systemic symptoms include weight loss, malaise, anorexia, and depression. A raised erythrocyte sedimentation rate (ESR), usually over 100 mmHg, is an important diagnostic criterion.

POLYMYOSITIS

This is an inflammatory condition of skeletal muscle. Patients may present with one of the following:

- Primary idiopathic polymyositis. This insidiously progressive condition presents with:
  - proximal muscle weakness, which is noted initially as difficulty with squatting, climbing stairs, or combing of the hair
  - aching tender muscles are present in some patients.
- Primary idiopathic dermatomyositis presents as:
  - myositis
  - skin changes, including: local or diffuse erythema; exfoliative dermatitis; scaling dermatitis; maculopapular eruptions; a lilac-colored heliotrope rash.
- Polymyositis or dermatomyositis with a malignancy.
- Polymyositis or dermatomyositis with vasculitis.
- Polymyositis or dermatomyositis with a connective tissue disorder.

POLYPS

Polyps are benign tumors which may:

- Increase mucus production. Nasal polyps cause rhinorrhea.
- Bleed:
  - unilateral epistaxis in nasal polyps
  - occult blood in the feces in intestinal polyps.
- Cause obstruction. Nasal polyps are a cause of snoring.
- Undergo malignant change. Evidence supporting the notion that the majority of large bowel cancers arise from preexisting benign polyps includes:
  - Early bowel cancer specimens show contiguity between benign and malignant tissue. Over time the benign adenoma may be replaced by malignant tissue.
  - The incidence of adenomatous polyps paralleling the incidence of bowel cancer in any given population.

- The coincidental finding that adenomas increasing in size with time and the incidence of malignant change increases with increased size.
- The clinical observation that a significant proportion of benign adenomatous polyps followed over a long period undergo malignant change. Early cancers arising in flat mucosa are very rare.

Routine sigmoidoscopy and removal of adenomas may reduce the likelihood of rectal and low sigmoid cancer by 85% over a 20-year period. Villous adenomas have the highest risk of neoplastic change followed by tubular adenomas. Metaplastic polyps are not considered a cancer risk.

PORTAL HYPERTENSION

Pressure in the portal vein rises due to:

- Extrahepatic portal vein obstruction.
- Increased liver blood flow.
- Increased resistance to hepatic blood outflow. Transmission of hepatic arterial pressure to the portal system is a frequent complication of liver cirrhosis, in which fibrosis and regeneration of liver lobules disrupts the hepatic architecture.

Portal hypertension presents with:

- Liver cirrhosis.
- Congestion of the gastrointestinal tract manifests as:
  - flatulence
  - anorexia and nausea
  - vomiting.
- Splenomegaly.
- Ascites.
- Development of a collateral circulation, which may present as:
  - esophageal varices (these may present as hematemesis and/or melena)
  - caput medusa, visible as periumbilical veins
  - hemorrhoids.

Evidence of hepatic failure should also be sought.

POSITIONAL VERTIGO

Benign positional vertigo is characterized by:

- short attacks, usually less than 60 seconds
- attacks only occurring on head movement
- nystagmus.

Nausea or vomiting is rare. The condition resolves spontaneously within several weeks.

POSTERIOR COLUMN DYSFUNCTION

The posterior columns carry touch, two-point discrimination, and proprioceptors from the muscle tendons and joints. Patients with posterior column lesions present with:

- Ataxia. As persons with posterior column defects use vision to provide information about the position of their limbs, unsteadiness is aggravated by closing the eyes or in darkness. Romberg's sign is positive (i.e. individuals are unable to stand without swaying for 5 seconds with their feet together and their eyes closed).
- Loss of position sense (i.e. loss of the ability to recognize limb position without visual assistance).
- Astereognosis.
- Loss of two-point discrimination.
- Loss of vibration sense.

POSTERIOR FOSSA LESIONS

Tumors of the cerebellum and fourth ventricle present with:

- Early symptoms of raised intracranial pressure, including:
  - gradually progressive headache
  - a headache that is worst on waking
  - vomiting (this is characteristically projectile)
  - papilledema.
- Evidence of cerebellar dysfunction:
  - ataxic gait
  - intention tremor
  - dysdiadochokinesia, past pointing.

POSTINFECTIOUS POLYNEUROPATHY

Postinfectious polyneuropathy is also known as Guillain–Barré syndrome. (See: *Neuropathy*.)

POSTNASAL DRIP

Sinusitis and chronic rhinitis may be associated with a discharge passing into the respiratory passages. Patients with a postnasal drip may complain of a:

- chronic cough
- sore throat
- the symptoms of chronic rhinitis or sinusitis.

POST-TRAUMATIC STRESS

Acute and chronic psychological distress following trauma presents with:

- A history of a traumatic event that would evoke distress in almost anybody.
- Re-experience of the traumatic event by recurrent recollections, dreams, or feeling as if the event were recurring.
- Numbing of responsiveness, or withdrawal.
- The presence of two or more of the following:
  - an exaggerated startle response, or hyperalertness
  - a sleep disturbance
  - guilt about having survived
  - memory impairment or difficulty concentrating
  - intensification of symptoms when exposed to triggers resembling the traumatic event
  - avoidance of activities that trigger recollection of the traumatic event.

PREGNANCY

Some 4–8 weeks after conception, women present with:

- Missed menstrual period(s), amenorrhea.
- Morning sickness, nausea.
- Breast changes:
  - increased vascularity, resulting in a heavy, almost tender, sensation
  - increased pigmentation of and around the nipple
  - prominence of abortive accessory lactiferous ducts.
- Urinary frequency.

The pregnancy test becomes positive within the first 4 weeks.

PREMENSTRUAL SYNDROME

The premenstrual syndrome (PMS) is described as a constellation of psychological, behavioral, and somatic symptoms that have a regular relationship to the menstrual cycle. Symptoms present during the luteal phase of the menstrual cycle and are absent for at least 1 week in the cycle. Theories proposed to explain the phenomenon vary from it being biologically based to psycho-social causes. Symptoms occur in most cycles and remit after menstruation. Some 150 symptoms have been reported. Symptom severity is difficult to ascertain, and exact timing of symptoms is unclear.

Major clinical findings include:

- fatigue
- mood swings, depression, and irritability
- difficulty concentrating
- breast swelling and tenderness
- headaches
- sleep disturbances.

An attempt to subcategorize and differentially manage according to subcategory has been made. There are overlaps between these subcategories. Below, the dominant clinical characteristics of each of these syndromes is described and a discrete pathogenesis postulated.

PMT-A. The major impact is on mood, with:

- anxiety
- irritability
- mood swings
- tension.

Type A premenstrual tension (PMT-A) is thought to be attributed to estrogen excess.

PMT-C. This is dominated by manifestations similar to hypoglycemia:

- sugar craving/increased appetite
- headache
- fatigue
- dizziness/fainting
- palpitations.

PMT-C is linked to increased carbohydrate tolerance and PGE_1 deficiency.

PMT-D. These patients present with:

- depression
- crying
- forgetfulness
- confusion
- insomnia.

PMT-D has been attributed to low estrogen and high progestogen levels.

PMT-H. These patients are particularly troubled by fluid retention, leading to:

- weight gain in excess of 3 kg
- breast tenderness
- swollen extremities
- abdominal bloating.

PMT-H has been linked to aldosterone excess.

PRESBYCUSIS

This is normal age-related hearing loss. Patients present with sensorineural hearing loss. The higher frequencies are affected first.

PRICKLY HEAT (miliaria)

Sweat is trapped in the epidermis or dermis, and presents with:

- prickling skin irritation
- if superficial, minute pruritus vesicles
- if deep, red skin discoloration.

Miliaria is usually encountered in hot sticky weather, but may be found in cool climates in overdressed patients.

PROCTALGIA FUGAX

Proctalgia fugax is caused by uncontrolled spasm of the levator ani, the muscles of the pelvic floor. Rectal pain is an isolated complaint. The clinical presentation includes rectal pain that is:

- severe
- fleeting, lasting minutes to several hours
- may occur at night and wake the patient
- recurs over a number of years
- sometimes precipitated on stretching the puborectalis muscle on rectal examination.

The condition is exacerbated by stress. Systemic examination is noncontributory. In cases in which severe puborectalis spasm obstructs defecation, neoplasm must be excluded.

Management includes reassurance, stress reduction, and increased intake of fiber and fluid to stretch the puborectalis muscle. Massage or dilatation of puborectalis may be helpful.

PROSTATE CANCER

Prostate cancer is a common malignancy in males, second only to lung cancer. Prostatectomy is second only to cataract removal as the most common operation in men.

Screening for prostate cancer by digital rectal examination is recommended annually for males over the age of 50 years. When combined with testing for prostate-specific antigen, digital rectal examination is almost as effective a screening tool as routine transurethral ultrasound. A diet low in fat and rich in soy protein may prevent and slow the progression of prostate cancer. In 95% of cases the cancer is an adenocarcinoma, and the periphery of the gland is often involved. Prostate cancer often coexists with prostatic hypertrophy, although the two do not appear to be causally linked.

Patients with prostate cancer are often asymptomatic, but may present with:

- Prostatism.
- Acute urinary retention.
- Chronic low backache due to spinal metastases.
- Terminal hematuria.
- Nocturia, uremia.
- A hard irregular nodular prostate with an obliterated median sulcus.
- An increase of 0.75 µg/l or more of prostate-specific antigen per annum (specificity 90%); serum acid phosphatase is also elevated.
- Signs and symptoms suggestive of metastasis include:
  - weight loss
  - anemia
  - bone pain, pathological fracture (metastasis to pelvic bones, spine, femur, and ribs are common)
  - neurological signs attributable to cord compression, including urinary retention
  - pelvic pain
  - pedal edema due to lymphatic obstruction
  - palpable nodes in the neck, groin, and/or abdomen.

PROSTATIC HYPERPLASIA (benign prostatic hypertrophy)

Some 50–70% of men are ultimately affected. Benign prostatic hypertrophy may result from an imbalance between cell growth and cell death, or be the result of increased connective tissue proliferation. Exposure of prostatic tissue to estrogens primes the prostate to be more responsive to androgens. Current thinking suggests that 5-hydroxytestosterone has a permissive rather than causative role in benign prostatic hypertrophy.

Patients with prostatic hypertrophy present with

- prostatism (see: *Prostatism*)
- an enlarged firm prostate, which is convex and has a smooth lateral border.

The size of the prostate correlates poorly with the severity of the clinical picture.

It is important to establish baseline creatinine and urinalysis data. Surgical referral is indicated in patients with:

- Distressing symptoms of nocturia, frequency, and decreased urinary stream. Patients should be referred if they are unable to achieve satisfactory control of their symptoms by:
  - voiding frequently
  - allowing sufficient time to void completely
  - avoiding drinks before going to bed
  - avoiding decongestants
  - phytosterol therapy.
- Compromised renal function.
- Recurrent urinary tract infections.
- Chronic urinary retention with hydronephrosis.
- Acute urinary retention.
- Recurrent urinary tract infection with large residual urine.
- Recurrent hematuria.
- Bladder stones.

Complications of prostatectomy include sexual dysfunction, urinary infection, incontinence, and bleeding.

PROSTATISM

Prostatism results from compression or obstruction of the urethra by an enlarged prostate. Patients present with:

- Obstructive symptoms. As the enlarging prostate increasingly obstructs the urethral lumen, the patient progressively experiences:
  - Hesitancy (there is a delay in starting micturition).
  - A weak intermittent urinary stream (passing urine is somewhat easier when seated).
  - Prolonged micturition due to a flow rate of less than 10 ml/s (the urinary flow rate normally exceeds 20 ml/s).
  - Straining. In contrast to urethral stricture, the strength of the urinary stream is not improved by straining.
  - Postmicturition or terminal dribbling.
  - Urinary retention. Acute urinary retention may be precipitated should the contractility of the bladder muscle be compromised by chronic fecal impaction, alcohol, social inhibition of voiding, or taking drugs such as diuretics or tricyclic antidepressants.
  - Paradoxical or overflow incontinence.
- Irritative symptoms. Once the obstruction reaches a point when the detrusor muscle can no longer adequately compensate for the resistance to outflow, partial urinary retention persists and the bladder is prone to infection. In addition to obstructive symptoms, the patient with prostatism may present with any combination of the following irritative symptoms:
  - urgency
  - frequency

- nocturia
- urge incontinence
- small voided volume
- suprapubic pain
- dysuria.

Signs of obstruction with or without irritative symptoms may be found in benign prostate hypertrophy, prostate cancer, urethral or meatal stricture, bladder cancer, and/or bladder neck hypertrophy.

PROSTATITIS

Men aged 30–50 years are most susceptible. Inflammation of the prostate may result in the following.

Acute prostatitis. The clinical presentation of acute prostatitis includes:

- pain in the perineum, low back, and suprapubic area
- irritative urinary symptoms of dysuria, nocturia, and frequency
- fever and chills
- variable symptoms of obstructive uropathy
- an exquisitely tender, swollen, indurated prostate.

Chronic prostatitis. The clinical presentation of chronic bacterial prostatitis includes:

- a long history of prostate tenderness
- recurrent urinary tract infections
- recurrent symptoms of urinary irritation
- perineal discomfort
- macroscopic hematuria
- hematospermia (a bloodstained ejaculate).

Chronic nonbacterial prostatitis. This presents with:

- pain referred to the low lumbar region
- pain on prostate palpation
- symptoms are relieved by prostate massage
- prostatic fluid containing over 15 pus cells per high-power field
- negative culture of prostatic fluid (viral or chlamydial infection is likely).

Nonbacterial prostatitis is more common than bacterial prostatitis.

PROSTATODYNIA

Prostatic pain may be experienced in bacterial prostatitis, nonbacterial prostatitis, and in patients with urethral sphincter spasm. A diagnosis of prostatodynia is made when:

- the prostate is painful
- symptoms are relieved by prostate massage
- there are no polymorphs in prostatic fluid
- urinary and prostatic fluid culture is negative
- prostatic rectal examination is normal.

PROTEIN-LOSING ENTEROPATHY

Excessive loss of protein into the intestinal lumen may result from increased mucosal permeability, inflammatory exudation, excess cell desquamation, or lymphatic obstruction. Protein-losing enteropathy is encountered in lymphoma, gastric cancer, allergic gastroenteropathy, and inflammatory small bowel disease. Patients present with:

- hypoproteinemia
- generalized edema
- frequent loose stools.

PSEUDOMEMBRANOUS COLITIS

See: *Antibiotic diarrhea.*

PSOAS SPASM

Patients present with:

- low back pain
- a fixed forward flexion and increased lumbar lordosis
- occasionally, inguinal pain
- a discrepancy in arm length when the arms are extended above the head.

Suspect either psoas spasm or a fixed flexion contracture if the extended leg is raised off the table when the patient lies in a supine position with one knee flexed and the other extended.

PSORIASIS

Psoriasis is a chronic disorder with skin and joint lesions. There is little correlation between joint and skin activity. Although the etiology is unknown, psoriasis has been postulated to be associated with a disorder of arachidonic acid metabolism. Certainly a diet rich in fish appears to improve the skin manifestations. The clinical presentation of psoriasis includes:

- Skin lesions with a recurrent history of exacerbations and remissions may present as:
  - Erythematous dry scaly patches, found especially on the extensor surfaces of the knees and elbows.
  - Silvery scales on red plaques.
  - Discoid lesions or plaques, commonly found on the scalp, trunk, and limbs.
  - Pustular variants, usually confined to one area (e.g. palms, soles).
  - Moist lesions in flexures (these are more common in the elderly).
  - Nails that are pitted, with transverse ridging and yellowing nail destruction.
- Arthritis. Few joints are involved, but large or small joints may be affected. Psoriatic arthritis presents with:
  - distal interphalangeal joint inflammation and pitted nails
  - systemic polyarthropathy, similar to that seen in rheumatoid arthritis
  - asymmetric spondylitis and sacroiliitis
  - destructive resorptive arthritis.

PSYCHOGENIC CHEST PAIN

Patients with psychogenic chest pain need to have serious causes of chest pain excluded before this diagnosis is made. Clinical features consistent with psychogenic chest pain are pain that is:

- described as continuous, sharp, or pricking pain
- lasts several hours or days
- rarely radiates
- often found over the left submammary region, although the location may vary
- unchanged with exercise
- aggravated by tiredness or anxiety.

Associated findings suggest underlying stress and include:

- air hunger
- hyperventilation (this may lead to paresthesia or a tingling numbness)
- headaches
- dry mouth.

Like angina, pain may be relieved by nitroglycerine.

PSYCHOGENIC VOMITING

Vomiting can be present for many years and is of little concern to the patient. Psychogenic vomiting presents with vomiting:

- in the early morning, on rising, or after breakfast
- which typically occurs after meals and may be self-induced
- which can be suppressed if necessary.

There may occasionally be associated weight loss.

PSYCHOSIS

Psychosis presents as disorders of thought and feeling either due to a primary abnormality of cerebral mechanisms or be secondary to metabolic disturbances. Psychosis is characterized by:

- being out of touch with reality (psychotics lack insight into their problem)
- delusions, which vary from grandiose to paranoid delusions
- hallucinations, which may be auditory, visual, olfactory, or tactile.

Alcoholics may develop psychotic symptoms, including:

- Delirium tremens. In response to alcohol withdrawal, alcoholics develop:
  - extreme confusion and agitation
  - vivid hallucinations, which may be tactile, visual, or auditory
  - delusions
  - autonomic hyperactivity (sweating, tachycardia, hypertension)
  - tremors and shaking.
- Korsakoff's psychosis. Malnourished alcoholics, especially those with deficiencies of the B group of vitamins, particularly thiamine, may present with:
  - gross disturbances of recent memory
  - confabulation to conceal memory defects (confabulations or false descriptions are created to fill in the memory gaps).

PULLED ELBOW

This occurs when sudden traction is applied to the extended and pronated forearm of a child. The head of the radius can be pulled through the round radioulnar ligament. The tearful child:

- refuses to use the involved arm
- holds the arm limp by the side
- holds the elbow slightly flexed and the forearm in midposition or pronated
- has a tender elbow region.

No bruising or deformity is present.

PULMONARY ATELECTASIS

Complete bronchial obstruction can result in massive collapse of a lung or lobe. Pulmonary atelectasis may result from bronchial obstruction due to an inhaled foreign body, bronchospasm superimposed upon tenacious secretions, or a hemorrhage into a protruding bronchial cancer. The clinical presentation of atelectasis is:

- Marked dyspnea.
- Cyanosis.
- Chest pain.
- On the side of the collapsed lung or lobe:
  - reduced chest movement
  - narrowing of the intercostal spaces
  - dullness to percussion
  - decreased or absent breath sounds
  - upward displacement of the diaphragm.
- A mediastinal shift. Chest contents may deviate towards the side of the lesion. Palpable structures, which move to the affected side, include the trachea and maximum cardiac impulse.

PULMONARY EDEMA

Pulmonary edema may present as a result of:

- increased capillary pressure, due to left-sided heart failure
- increased capillary permeability, due to inhalation of noxious gases or uremia
- decreased plasma oncotic pressure, as in hypoalbuminemia
- lymphatic obstruction.

In addition to the underlying disease, the clinical presentation includes the features of pulmonary edema, which are:

- dyspnea that is worst on lying (both orthopnea and paroxysmal nocturnal dyspnea may be present)
- frothy sputum
- cyanosis
- basal crackles.

PULMONARY EMBOLISM

Approximately 75% of all thrombotic emboli arise from the lower limbs. Pulmonary emboli are an important and potentially fatal complication of venous disorders. The clinical presentation, depending on the size of the embolus, may be:

- Sudden death. About 20% of cases of sudden death are attributable to a large pulmonary embolus.

- Chest pain. The sudden onset of chest pain aggravated by coughing is suggestive of pulmonary embolism.
- Gradually progressive dyspnea. Patients may insidiously develop respiratory failure as small emboli lodge in the pulmonary vasculature and functional lung tissue is replaced by fibrous tissue.

An embolus that lodges in a large pulmonary artery presents with:

- acute right heart failure
- syncope and shock
- dyspnea and cyanosis
- sudden death.

An embolus that lodges in a medium-sized artery presents with:

- the sudden onset of dyspnea
- pleuritic pain
- hemoptysis
- tachycardia
- a widely split second heart sound
- signs of ventricular failure
- adventitious breath sounds (crackles, wheezes).

Emboli that lodge in terminal arteries may present with:

- A dry cough.
- Fever.
- A pleural friction rub.
- Gradually progressive dyspnea. Multiple small emboli lodging in the lung over a long period progressively impair pulmonary function. Progressive fibrosis follows repeated minor embolic infarcts. These patients may be asymptomatic until dyspnea results from depletion of functional lung tissue.
- Cor pulmonale. Progressive pulmonary fibrosis leads to right-sided cardiac enlargement and failure.

PULMONARY FIBROSIS

Fibrosis of lung tissue results in an imbalance of ventilation and perfusion and/or reduced gaseous diffusion. Depending on the cause and extent of pulmonary fibrosis, the patient may present with:

- progressive dyspnea
- cyanosis
- progressive respiratory impairment.

The major types of fibrosis are:

- *Interstitial fibrosis*, in which the fibrosis is diffuse and bilateral. Conditions predisposing to interstitial fibrosis include allergic fibrosis, sarcoidosis, and lung fibrosis associated with connective tissue disorders. (See: *Fibrosing (allergic) alveolitis.*)

- *Focal fibrosis*, in which the fibrosis is widespread. (See: *Pneumoconiosis.*)
- *Replacement fibrosis* differs from the other forms of fibrosis in that it may be localized or diffuse and depends on the underlying condition. It is encountered following destruction of lung tissue in tuberculosis or pulmonary infarction. (See: *Pulmonary embolism.*)

PYELONEPHRITIS

See: *Urinary tract infection.*

RAYNAUD'S DISEASE AND PHENOMENON

Raynaud's disease. This is a primary condition and is more common in women than men. Clinically, Raynaud's disease presents with:

- The presence of peripheral pulses.
- Attacks of vasoconstriction, characterized by:
  - pallor of the extremities
  - followed by cyanosis of the fingers
  - followed by skin flushing, throbbing pain, and slight swelling (this is attributed to vasodilatation)
  - precipitated by cold or emotion
  - spontaneous termination or by warming the hand.
- Extremities are bilaterally involved.

Gangrene, if present, is limited to the fingertips. This symptom complex must be present for at least 2 years before a diagnosis of Raynaud's disease is made. The disease improves spontaneously in 15% of cases.

Raynaud's phenomenon. This phenomenon occurs secondary to:

- A connective tissue disorder, such as scleroderma, rheumatoid arthritis, or polymyositis. In scleroderma, 90% of patients have Raynaud's phenomenon, and in 30% it is the presenting symptom.
- Drugs.
- Neurovascular compression, which may present as the thoracic outlet syndrome.
- Hematological problems, particularly polycythemia.
- Occupational use of vibrating tools.

Raynaud's phenomenon occurs in an older age group and may affect 30% of females in certain geographical areas. The clinical presentation includes:

- the signs and symptoms of Raynaud's disease
- possible atrophy of the terminal fat pad
- possible digital skin ulceration and gangrene.

RECTAL CANCER

See: *Colorectal cancer.*

RECTAL PROLAPSE

Patients present with:

- a history of straining at stool
- mucosa protruding through the anus (concentric lines on the mucosa are diagnostic)
- mucous soiling
- perianal pruritus.

REFLEX SYMPATHETIC DYSTROPHY SYNDROME

Also known as Sudek's atrophy and shoulder–hand syndrome, this condition may develop following local trauma, peripheral nerve injury, myocardial infarction, or stroke. The patient presents with discomfort, usually of the hand or foot, which progressively demonstrates:

- Vasomotor instability detected as a:
  - burning pain, which is aggravated by movement and heat
  - throbbing pain, which is worst at night.
- Trophic skin changes. Clinical features are:
  - initially, red swollen hands and a warm dry skin
  - later, cold cyanosed mottled hands and a moist skin.
- Atrophy with:
  - shiny stiff fingers
  - small-muscle wasting
  - flexion contractures in a cold painful arm.
- Bone demineralization. Patchy bone decalcification is detected on radiographs.

Early recognition and treatment, with exercise and pain relief, can prevent disability.

REFLUX ESOPHAGITIS

See: *Esophageal reflux.*

REFRACTIVE ERROR

Patients present with:

- A mild headache.
- Impaired vision that is corrected using the pinhole test. (Punch a 1-mm hole in a sheet of paper using a pen or large pin and ask the patient to look at the Snellen chart through the pinhole. If vision improves, suspect a refractive error. If vision is unchanged or deteriorates, refer for management of vitreous or retinal disease.)

REITER'S SYNDROME

The clinical characteristics of this syndrome are:

- nonspecific urethritis, which may result in hematuria and sterile pyuria
- recurrent conjunctivitis and/or uveitis
- symmetrical subacute arthritis, with or without tenosynovitis
- buccal ulcers
- circinate balanitis.

RENAL CARCINOMA (adenocarcinoma/hypernephroma)

Hypernephroma usually occurs in patients aged 55 years or older. Patients present with:

- painless persistent or intermittent hematuria
- fatigue/malaise
- anemia
- weight loss
- fever
- flank pain
- an abdominal mass
- lung, liver, bone and, occasionally, brain metastases.

RENAL COLIC

See: *Urolithiasis.*

RENAL FAILURE

Persons with early renal failure may be asymptomatic. Screening for renal disease is therefore recommended in any patient suspected of having:

- Nocturia.
- Polyuria: the passage of more than 2500 ml urine in 24 hours.
- Oliguria: the passage of less than 400 ml urine in 24 hours.
- Anuria: the passage of less than 100 ml urine in 24 hours. As anuria may result from bladder obstruction, bladder percussion is an integral component of patient assessment.

Urinalysis includes:

- Phase contrast microscopy of fresh urine. This may show casts or dysmorphic red cells, indicating bleeding from the glomerulus.
- Specific gravity. Isosthenuria, a fixed specific gravity, is indicative of renal functional impairment.
- Proteinuria of more than:
  - 2 g/day suggests significant renal impairment
  - 3 g/day indicates probable glomerular disease
  - 5 g/day, or more than 3.5 g/day plus a serum albumin of less than 3.0 g/dl, is diagnostic of the nephrotic syndrome.
- Examination of the urinary sediment:
  - red-cell casts suggest glomerulonephritis
  - white-cell casts are found in pyelonephritis or interstitial nephritis
  - oval fat bodies (lipiduria) are found in the nephrotic syndrome.

Renal failure is progressive, resulting in a sequential series of clinical changes as renal function is increasingly impaired. When renal reserves are decreased by:

- 50%, or the glomerular filtration rate (GFR) is greater than 60 ml/min and serum creatinine is less than 0.26 mmol/l, the patient is:
  - susceptible to dehydration.
- 50–70%, or the GFR is 25–60 ml/min, the patient complains of:
  - headaches
  - hypertension
  - leg cramps.
- 80–90%, or the GFR is 10–25 ml/min and the serum creatinine up to 0.6 mmol/l, the patient experiences:
  - anorexia, nausea, and diarrhea
  - oral ulceration
  - pallor, due to both occult bleeding and bone marrow suppression
  - impaired glucose tolerance
  - edema
  - acidosis.
- >90% and creatinine exceeds 2.0 mmol/l, the patient presents with:
  - restless legs due to sensory and motor neuropathy
  - lethargy, confusion, drowsiness

- pruritus
- bone pain
- muscle twitching, convulsions
- urochrome pigmentation.

In all cases the blood chemistry will show varying degrees of azotemia/uremia and acidosis.

Compared with chronic renal failure, in *acute renal failure*:

- symptoms are more severe
- fluid retention is more pronounced
- hyperkalemia is more common
- acidosis is more severe
- anemia is symptomatic
- pruritus is less common.

RESTRICTIVE LUNG DISEASE

This group of conditions all demonstrate a loss of functional lung tissue. Immunological destruction of lung tissue as in the pneumoconioses (dust exposure – silica, asbestos, coal, bauxite), connective tissue disorders (lupus, rheumatoid arthritis, polyarteritis), allergic alveolitis, or sarcoidosis), thoracic cage abnormalities (ankylosing spondylitis, kyphoscoliosis), and pleural abnormalities (pneumothorax, pleural effusion) may all cause loss of functional lung tissue.

The clinical presentation suggestive of chronic restrictive lung disease attributable to immunological destruction is typified by interstitial fibrosis, which presents with:

- gradually progressive dyspnea
- dyspnea on exertion
- cough
- fever
- late inspiratory crackles that are unchanged by coughing
- cyanosis
- weight loss
- clubbing.

Spirometry shows a reduced vital capacity (VC) and a diminished peak flow rate (forced expiratory volume in 1 second (FEV_1)). As restrictive lung disease has a reduced total lung capacity, the FEV_1/forced FVC ratio is normal (70–80%). The residual volume is normal.

(See: *Fibrosing (allergic) alveolitis*; *Pneumoconiosis*; *Sarcoidosis*.)

RETINAL DETACHMENT

Detachment of the retina from the underlying choroid and associated blood supply usually follows trauma. Myopic patients are particularly at risk.

The clinical presentation includes:

- A painless loss of vision.
- Unilateral symptoms.
- Detachment, which is often preceded by:
  - Photopsia. Flashing lights may be attributed to cortical or retinal lesions. Retinal tears are suggested by brief flashes of light which: last for seconds (cortical flashes (scintillations) last for minutes); are confined to the periphery of the retinal field; are provoked by head movement.
  - Blurred vision.
  - Scotoma.
  - Showers of spots (this indicates vitreous hemorrhage).
  - Blue bubbles of light (this indicates traction on a retinal break).
- An advancing dark area or area of 'blindness' covering the field of vision.
- Loss of the red reflex over the detached area (it is normal elsewhere).
- A fold of pale detached retina in which the initiating tear may be visible on ophthalmoscopy.

RETROPERITONEAL LESION

Hemorrhage or abscess formation in the retroperitoneal area presents with:

- Pain:
  - in the abdomen or flank
  - in the hip, leg, or knee, from psoas muscle involvement
  - on hip extension.
- Evidence of infection (e.g. fever) in cases of abscess formation.
- Evidence of blood loss in cases of hemorrhage.

RHEUMATIC FEVER

Some 3 weeks after a streptococcal sore throat the patient may present with a nonsuppurative, probably immunologically mediated, condition. Rheumatic fever is diagnosed in the presence of two major, or one major and two minor, criteria (Duckett–Jones criteria).

Patients present with *major criteria* such as:

- Carditis detected as:
  - changing heart murmurs
  - heart failure
  - arrhythmias
  - pericarditis.
- Migratory polyarthritis, usually of the large joint. Monoarticular involvement may occur.

- Chorea, presenting with involuntary, rapid, purposeless, non-repetitive movements. Voluntary movements are abrupt and coordination is impaired.
- Transitory painless subcutaneous nodules. These are most commonly found on the extensor surfaces of large joints.
- Erythema marginatum. Circinate, transitory, painless areas of erythema are found.

Minor criteria include:

- evidence of inflammation (e.g. a raised erythrocyte sedimentation rate (ESR), C-reactive protein)
- a raised antistreptolysis O titer
- fever
- arthralgia
- electrocardiographic changes, such as a prolonged P–R interval.

RHEUMATIC HEART DISEASE

Atherosclerotic coronary heart disease, hypertension, and rheumatic heart disease are the three most common causes of heart disease. Rheumatic fever is the most common cause of heart disease in persons under the age of 50 years.

Patients present with valvular lesions:

- Aortic stenosis. Auscultatory findings are:
  - an ejection systolic murmur, which radiates up to the neck. An ejection click may also be heard as the valve opens
  - a murmur, which is best heard on expiration over the second intercostal space using the diaphragm of the stethoscope.
- Aortic incompetence. Auscultatory findings are:
  - a blowing diastolic murmur (the valvular incompetence causes a wide pulse pressure or collapsing pulse)
  - a murmur best heard on expiration over Erb's point using the diaphragm of the stethoscope.
- Mitral stenosis. Auscultatory findings are:
  - a rumbling diastolic murmur confined to the apex. A loud first heart sound and an opening snap may be present as the fibrosed valve opens and closes
  - a murmur best heard on expiration at the apex of the heart using the bell of the stethoscope.
- Mitral incompetence. Auscultatory findings are:
  - a pansystolic murmur which radiates to the axilla
  - a murmur best heard on expiration at the apex of the heart using the diaphragm of the stethoscope.

Pulmonary and tricuspid valvular lesions may also occur. The auscultatory findings are similar, except that the murmurs are loudest on inspiration when the negative thoracic pressure enhances blood flow through the right side of the heart.

Patients also have an increased risk of:

- Heart failure.
- Endocarditis. Subacute bacterial endocarditis is a particular risk in patients with valvular distortion.

RHEUMATOID ARTHRITIS

Rheumatoid arthritis is a chronic inflammatory polyarthritis affecting two to three persons in every hundred. Prevalence peaks between 30 and 55 years of age. The pain of rheumatoid arthritis is persistent, and joint involvement is widespread and symmetrical, especially in the fingers and the upper and lower limbs. Rheumatoid arthritis is also present as a monoarticular arthritis of the knee. Joint pain is relieved by activity, and rest encourages stiffness. Rheumatoid arthritis is a systemic condition.

A diagnosis of rheumatoid arthritis is probable if three signs are present, definite if five are present, and classical if seven signs are detected. To meet these criteria, asterisked (*) signs only score if they are present continuously for 6 weeks or longer. Diagnostic signs are:

- Morning joint stiffness.* This is present in two-thirds of cases and can last for hours.
- Joint tenderness* or pain precipitated by movement* affecting one or more joints.
- Soft-tissue thickening* or effusion of one (score 1) or more (score 2) joints.
- Symmetrical joint swelling,* except for distal interphalangeal joint swelling.
- Subcutaneous nodules.
- Serology is positive for rheumatoid factor.
- Synovial fluid demonstrates poor mucin clotting.
- Characteristic histological changes of synovium.
- Characteristic histological changes in subcutaneous nodule(s).
- Typical radiographic changes. Radiographs are usually normal in the early stages of the disease. The four characteristic radiographic signs of rheumatoid arthritis that develop later in the disease are:
  - fusiform soft-tissue swelling
  - periarticular osteopenia
  - diffuse loss of interosseous space
  - marginal erosion of bone.

Other nonspecific findings include:

- lethargy
- anorexia and weight loss
- lymphadenopathy
- anemia

- muscle weakness
- inflammatory manifestations (vasculitis, pleuritis, pancarditis, raised erythrocyte sedimentation rate (ESR), and C-reactive protein).

RHINITIS

Rhinitis is irritation of the nasal mucosa. Chronic rhinitis without objective evidence of allergy may be due to immunodeficiency. Patients with poor sleep habits, snoring, and rhinitis are more likely to have a chronic upper airway allergy than a sleep disorder. Rhinitis may be allergic, atrophic, iatrogenic, or vasomotor in origin.

Allergic rhinitis ('sneezers and runners'). One in 10 people are affected. Seasonal (hay fever) and perennial variants are found. Seasonal symptoms are usually found in spring and early summer, and are associated with grass, weed, or tree pollen. Perennial allergens include dust mites, molds, and animals. Clinical features include:

- Rhinorrhea:
  - persistent sniffing
  - thin watery discharge.
- Nasal obstruction or congestion, presenting with:
  - pronounced nasal stuffiness
  - mouth-breathing
  - a nasal mucosa that is swollen, pale, and turgid
  - a blocked eustachian tube.
- Nasal irritation and itchiness, leading to:
  - frequent, violent sneezing
  - an 'allergic salute'
  - nose-twitching
  - nasal and palatal pruritus.
- Other evidence of allergy, including:
  - anorexia, lassitude
  - dark bags under the eyes
  - watery, itching eyes with conjunctival hyperemia
  - loss of taste and smell
  - eosinophilia and a low or normal erythrocyte sedimentation rate (ESR).

Atrophic rhinitis. This presents with:

- mild or minimal nasal stuffiness
- halitosis
- crusted nasal mucosa.

Iatrogenic rhinitis. This is the result of persistent use of hypotensive drugs (α-adrenergic agents, methyldopa, reserpine), estrogens (the contraceptive pill), aspirin, cocaine, and/or decongestants. Patients present with:

- chronic watery discharge
- a boggy mucosa
- nasal stuffiness.

Vasomotor rhinitis ('blockers'). Patients present with:

- pronounced nasal stuffiness, congestion, or obstruction
- a scant thick seromucoid nasal discharge
- a red nasal mucosa with mildly enlarged turbinates
- occasional paroxysmal sneezing.

Further evidence of autonomic nervous system imbalance is obtained by the condition being precipitated by changes in temperature, emotion, or humidity. Decongestants may be helpful.

ROSACEA

This chronic facial disorder is encountered in middle-aged people. The patient presents with:

- facial flushing and burning on alcohol ingestion
- facial erythema
- telangiectasia
- an aciniform component (papules, pustules, and seborrhea are found)
- a glandular component, which results in hyperplasia of the soft tissue of the nose.

The periorbital and perioral areas are usually spared.

ROSEOLA INFANTUM

Roseola infantum is not highly contagious and is common in children under 12 months. Roseola is characterized by:

- distinct rose-pink maculopapules
- a rash which appears first on the trunk and lasts 2 days.

Roseola infantum is associated with febrile convulsions. The fever drops before the rash appears.

ROSS RIVER VIRUS INFECTION (epidemic polyarthralgia)

The patient has little or no fever or constitutional symptoms, and presents with:

- joint pains
- a maculopapular rash of variable distribution and appearance.

RUBELLA

German measles, or rubella, is a mild viral disease with no prodrome. The virus is spread by droplets and has an incubation period of 2–3 weeks. The patient is infectious (i.e. the virus can be transmitted) during the last week of incubation and for 4 days after the appearance of the rash.

Rubella presents clinically with:

- a mild fever
- malaise
- coryza
- a fine maculopapular rash, which starts at the face and spreads rapidly within 24 hours to involve the trunk and the extremities
- posterior cervical and postauricular lymphadenopathy (the lymphadenopathy develops before the rash and may persist for several weeks after its resolution)
- arthralgia (this is common in young women).

Fetal infection with rubella virus may result in fetal malformations including blindness, heart defects, and deafness. Only fetuses of women without antibodies to the virus are at risk. Fetal abnormalities can be prevented by immunization of women prior to pregnancy.

SACROILIAC SYNDROME

Sacroiliac dysfunction may either result from simple joint locking or be complicated by compensatory hypermobility in adjacent articulations. Patients present with:

- Local pain which presents as:
  - a dull ache
  - unilateral buttock pain.
- Radiating pain causing heavy aching:
  - in the groin and thigh anteriorly
  - in the thigh, calf, ankle, and foot posteriorly.
- Referred pain to the L5, S1, and S2 dermatomal area. No other sensory changes, such as paresthesia or numbness, are present.
- Pain on pelvic compression.

SALMONELLA

Salmonella is a Gram-negative bacillus transmitted by food and water. Depending on the species of salmonella, the patient may present with:

- *Gastroenteritis.* Within 48 hours of eating contaminated food patients develop:
  - diarrhea, which lasts less than 24 hours
  - fever
  - mild abdominal pain.
- *Typhoid. Salmonella typhi* causes:
  - fever and bradycardia
  - headache
  - malaise
  - a sore throat
  - constipation early, and diarrhea later, in the disease
  - abdominal pain and tenderness
  - rose spots, which emerge in crops and blanch on pressure
  - splenomegaly
  - delirium and stupor
  - intestinal hemorrhage and/or perforation (this may be fatal).

SALPINGITIS

See: *Pelvic inflammatory disease.*

SARCOIDOSIS

Sarcoidosis is often asymptomatic and, although it usually resolves spontaneously, it may be fatal. The clinical picture includes:

- An asymptomatic period during the early stages.
- Late development of dyspnea.
- Late development of a cough.
- Lymphadenopathy.
- Radiographic findings of lung infiltration and hilar lymphadenopathy.
- Blood tests show hypercalcemia, hypergammaglobulinemia, and a raised erythrocyte sedimentation rate (ESR).
- Skin shows a positive Kveim test.
- Systemic findings include:
  - iridocyclitis
  - polyarthritis
  - skin lesions.
- Complications are pulmonary hypertension and cor pulmonale.

SCABIES

The mite *Sarcoptes scabiei* burrows into the skin. After an incubation period of 14–28 days, the patient presents with:

- crawling pruritus or itching, which is worst at night when the patient is warm
- multiple pruritic nodules
- lesions with an erythematous base
- disseminated skin lesions, which usually include the:
  - wrists
  - finger webbing
  - axillae
  - crotch
- mild or absent lymphadenopathy.

SCARLET FEVER

See: *Tonsillitis syndrome.*

SCHIZOPHRENIA

This group of psychiatric illnesses, usually first diagnosed in young people, is characterized by:

- Disorders of thinking:
  - delusions, a disorder of thought content
  - poverty of thinking
  - woolly thinking
  - impaired communication.
- Disorders of emotion:
  - inappropriate feelings or expression of emotion
  - blunting of feeling.
- Perceptual disorders:
  - hallucinations, especially auditory.
- Lack of motivation:
  - apathy
  - social withdrawal
  - personality deterioration
  - work deterioration.
- Slow movements.

SCLERITIS

Scleritis is frequently encountered in patients with connective tissue disorders with a positive rheumatoid factor, destructive joint disease, and cutaneous nodules. Scleritis presents with:

- unilateral focal redness of the sclera
- impaired visual acuity
- pain, which starts in the eye and radiates around the head.

SCLERODERMA

The basic lesion of this multisystem disorder is fibrosis and vascular obliteration. Patients present with:

- Raynaud's phenomenon
- skin fibrosis
- telangiectasia
- esophageal hypomobility
- arthritis and arthralgia
- pulmonary fibrosis.

SCOMBROID

Histamine intoxication resulting from fish spoilage due to storage under nonchilled conditions may result in scombroid. Fish frequently involved are anchovies, mackerel, sardines, tuna, and pilchards. Shortly after eating, patients present with:

- headache
- hypotension
- bronchoconstriction
- nausea
- abdominal pain.

SCURVY

Inadequate vitamin C intake presents with:

- fatigue
- progressive weakness
- pallor due to anemia
- spongy bleeding gums
- follicular hyperkeratosis and perifollicular hemorrhages (the skin is rough and dry)
- petechiae, ecchymoses, and hematomas
- epiphysial enlargement with joint pain.

SEBORRHEIC DERMATITIS

Seborrheic dermatitis is a chronic inflammatory skin condition characterized by:

- Erythematous patches.
- Dry or greasy yellowish scales.
- Dandruff. Dry scales are found on the scalp. Alopecia does not result.

- Seborrheic blepharitis. Greasy scales along the margin of the eyelid are associated with burning eyes and some loss of eyelashes.

Eyebrows, the nasolabial fold, the axillae, the central chest, and the areas behind the ears are other commonly involved sites.

SEBORRHEIC KERATOSIS (senile warts)

Seborrheic keratosis, a benign lesion, needs to be differentiated from melanoma. Lesions begin to appear in people over 20 years of age and are commonly found on the neck, flexures, face, and trunk. Clinical features include:

- Lesions which:
  - are found in light- and nonlight-exposed areas, particularly along the hair lines and in flexures
  - recur: increase with age; are completely asymptomatic; have an elevated or 'stuck on' appearance.
- Lesions of variable appearance, including:
  - classical warty lesions
  - brown slightly waxy lesions with discrete edges
  - pale, flesh colored, flat scaly lesions. Scales may be: greasy or dry; yellowish; point outwards.

SEIZURES

Patients present with loss of consciousness, which:

- Has an abrupt onset.
- May be associated with cyanosis.
- Is accompanied by stertorous respiration.
- Is commonly associated with:
  - convulsions
  - urinary incontinence
  - postictal confusion.
- Is occasionally associated with focal neurological abnormalities.

SEPTIC ARTHRITIS

Patients of any age can present with:

- The acute onset of monoarticular arthritis. Occasionally, more than one joint is involved. Wrist and weight-bearing joints are most commonly affected.
- A prodrome of migratory polyarthralgia. This may be present and is often seen in gonococcal arthritis.

- Intense joint pain.
- A hot swollen joint.
- Fever, chills.

Joint aspiration is diagnostic.

SEPTICEMIA

Patients with a symptomatic bacteremia present with:

- Fever.
- Chills and rigors.
- A positive blood culture.
- Any combination of:
  - skin eruptions, especially petechiae and purpura
  - nausea, diarrhea, vomiting
  - delirium.
- Possible complications including:
  - secondary infection such as meningitis or endocarditis
  - metastatic abscess formation
  - septic shock.

SEXUALLY TRANSMITTED DISEASES

See: *AIDS*; *Chancroid*; *Chlamydia*; *Donovanosis*; *Gonorrhea*; *Herpes*; *Lymphogranuloma venereum*; *Molluscum contagiosum*; *Syphilis*; *Viral hepatitis* (hepatitis B, C, and D); *Warts* (venereal warts).

SHIGELLOSIS (bacillary dysentery)

Infection with this Gram-negative bacterium results in a condition that varies from mild watery diarrhea to dysentery. Children and the elderly are most at risk. Spread is by direct contact, and symptoms present 7 days after exposure. Patients present with:

- The sudden onset of:
  - fever
  - abdominal pain.
- Stools which are:
  - frequent
  - passed with straining (tenesmus)
  - contain mucus and, later, blood.
- Weight loss. Emaciation may result in severe or chronic cases.

SHOCK

Shock is characterized by inadequate tissue perfusion. This may be attributable to impaired cardiac output due to pump failure, or peripheral circulatory failure due to an inadequate circulatory volume or increased vessel capacity. Dizziness, confusion, and syncope are common findings. The clinical presentation depends on the cause.

Cardiogenic shock is attributable to failure of the heart (pump) (e.g. myocardial infarction). It presents with:

- decreased cardiac output
- low blood pressure
- weak thready pulse
- raised central venous pressure.

Oligemic shock is attributable to loss of circulating volume, as in hemorrhage or peritoneal burns. It is initially characterized by intense sympathetic stimulation in order to restore an adequate circulating volume. It presents with:

- tachycardia
- raised blood pressure
- cold extremities (monitor the temperature of the tip of the nose)
- sweating and a clammy skin
- hypotension in the late stages.

The urgency of referral depends on the volume of blood lost. In cases of acute blood loss, emergency referral is required if placing the patient at an angle of 75° for 3 minutes causes the pulse to increase by more than 25 beats/min and/or the blood pressure to drop by 20–30 mmHg. Immediate hospital referral is also indicated in patients who have two or more of the following criteria:

- a blood pressure of 100 mmHg or less
- a pulse that exceeds 100 beats/min
- a postural blood pressure drop of over 10 mmHg
- a hemoglobin of less than 10 g/dl
- age in excess of 59 years.

Detection of any one of the above findings indicates the need for the patient to be monitored, and referred should further evidence of shock develop.

Anaphylactic shock occurs when an immunological reaction results in widespread histamine-induced vasodilatation. The patient presents with:

- sudden faintness or syncope
- low blood pressure
- a pale, clammy skin.

Septic shock is encountered in Gram-negative septicemia when release of bacterial toxins causes vasodilatation of the capillary bed, increasing the capacitance of the vasculature. The patient presents with:

- low blood pressure
- low central venous pressure
- a congested skin.

(See: *Toxic shock syndrome.)*

Neurocardiogenic syncope, or a *vasovagal attack*, occurs in otherwise healthy people when there is an interruption to the normal sympathetic tone. Increased vagal activity presents as:

- Bradycardia.
- Low blood pressure.
- Fainting.
- Premonitory symptoms include:
  - sweating
  - epigastric queasiness
  - pallor
  - light-headedness
  - visual blurring
  - tinnitus.
- Bladder and bowel control are never lost.

(See: *Syncope*.)

SINUS BRADYCARDIA

The clinical presentation of bradycardia includes:

- A slow regular pulse. Conduction passes through the atrioventricular node, and therefore the beat is regular. The rate is around 40 beats/min.
- Responsiveness to autonomic nervous system stimulation. Exercise, through sympathetic stimulation, increases the heart rate.

Circumstances in which this arrhythmia may arise at the sinoatrial node include:

- jaundice
- myxedema
- hypothermia
- raised intracranial pressure
- a fit athlete
- drugs (e.g. digitalis).

SINUSITIS

The minimal diagnostic criteria for sinusitis include:

- maxillary toothache
- a poor response to nasal decongestants
- a history of a colored nasal discharge
- purulent nasal secretions
- tenderness on palpation over involved sinuses
- abnormal transillumination of sinuses.

Sinusitis is excluded if none of the above are present. If four of the listed criteria are detected, the likelihood of sinusitis is 3:2.

Acute sinusitis presents with:

- Deep-seated aching facial pain, which is worst:
  - on bending
  - in the morning.
- Tenderness on pressure over the involved sinus. Tenderness should be differentiated from nonsinus bone pressure by palpating the temporal bones or zygomatic arch. Facial tenderness is elicited by putting firm pressure over the anatomical site of the sinus:
  - in frontal sinusitis, above the orbit
  - in maxillary or antral sinusitis, below the orbit
  - in ethmoidal sinusitis, medial to the orbit.

In *sphenoidal sinusitis* the area above the posterior nasal space cannot be palpated. It is characterized by headache and pain radiation. The location of the pain depends on the sinus involved:

- *Frontal sinusitis* is unusual before the age of 10 years. Pain:
  - is felt over the eyebrows
  - presents as a frontal headache. (Vacuum headaches result from air absorption in a sinus with a blocked osteum. Positive pressure headaches are experienced when the sinus fills with pus and drainage cannot occur.)
- *Maxillary sinusitis* is unusual before the age of 6 years. Pain:
  - refers to the teeth
  - presents as a frontal headache
  - is associated with a sensation of fullness over the cheek (drainage is on the superior surface of the sinus).
- *Anterior ethmoidal sinusitis* is rare before the age of 1 year. Patients:
  - frequently grasp the bridge of the nose
  - complain of a retro-orbital headache.
- *Posterior ethmoidal sinusitis* is rare before the age of 1 year. Pain is referred:
  - retro-orbitally
  - to the temple.

- *Sphenoidal sinusitis* presents with diffuse pain which may involve the:
  - retro- and periorbital regions
  - the temple
  - the vertex and occiput.

In addition to headache and pain radiation:

- Changes in position may aggravate or relieve the pain.
- Alcohol frequently worsens sinus pain.
- Nasal congestion (this may be reflex congestion or attributable to the underlying cause).
- A colored nasal discharge.
- Respiratory infection of longer than 7 days.
- Additional findings in adults are:
  - a sore throat (the result of a postnasal drip)
  - halitosis
  - voice changes
  - epiphora (tearing).
- Additional findings in children are:
  - a persistent cough
  - purulent nasal discharge which persists for more than 10–14 days.

Recurrent acute sinusitis presents with:

- recurrent episodes
- symptom-free intervals.

Acute-on-chronic sinusitis presents with continuous symptoms for more than 3 months. Sinusitis may be associated with:

- halitosis
- eustachian tube dysfunction.

Persons with *chronic sinusitis* are at increased risk of bronchiectasis.

Half of the cases of acute sinusitis resolve spontaneously. Indications suggesting the need for more active intervention are:

- Pyrexia.
- Associated dental infection.
- Suspected complications. Urgent attention is required if there is:
  - a suspicion of cellulitis of the orbit (see: *Orbital cellulitis*).
  - edema over a sinus
  - osteomyelitis
  - cavernous sinus thrombosis
  - evidence of intracranial involvement.
- Failure to improve within 72 hours on a therapeutic regimen (see below).

The aim of a therapeutic regimen may be to correct predisposing factors, such as those:

- affecting the ciliary function (cigarette smoking, pollution, foreign bodies, viral infection)
- affecting the mucus blanket (dehydration, antihistamines, immunodeficiency syndromes, cystic fibrosis)
- causing obstruction (overuse of nasal decongestants, adenoids, deviated nasal septum, nasal polyps/tumors, allergy, viral infections).

Alternatively, a therapeutic regimen may be aimed at providing symptomatic relief by means of symptomatic intervention:

- *Steam inhalation.* The patient is instructed to:
  - Pour boiling water into a pan or basin placed on a low table.
  - Create a steam funnel by sitting at the table with a towel draped over the head, shoulders, and pan.
  - Hold the nose a few inches above the water and breathe through the nose for about 10 minutes. Menthol or eucalyptus oil is often added to the boiling water.
- *Nasal lavage.* Three to five saline drops may be dropped into the nostrils every 4 hours.
- *Drug intervention.* This ranges from pain relief with paracetamol to topical decongestants such as phenylephrine or oxymetazoline. These drugs may initially relieve congestion, but their persistent use results in rebound mucosal swelling. Systemic decongestants are also available. Antihistamines and corticosteroids may be used to relieve stuffiness.

SINUS TACHYCARDIA

The clinical presentation of tachycardia includes:

- A fast regular pulse. Conduction passes through the atrioventricular node, and therefore the beat is regular. The rate is 100–150 beats/min.
- Responsiveness to autonomic nervous system stimulation. Vagal stimulation slows a tachycardia. The vagus may be stimulated by:
  - carotid sinus massage (carotid sinus massage is contraindicated in persons over 75 years of age, in those with a carotid bruit, and those with hemodynamic instability or with possible digitalis toxicity)
  - exerting pressure on the eyeballs
  - retching
  - gagging
  - breath-holding.

Conditions associated with arrhythmias arising at the sinoatrial node include:

- hyperdynamic circulation
- congestive cardiac failure
- hypovolemic shock
- emotion
- stress
- fever
- exercise.

SJÖGREN'S SYNDROME

Associated with connective tissue type disorders, this syndrome includes:

- dry eyes
- a dry mouth
- arthritis.

SLEEP DISORDERS

An unfavorable change in the amount and/or quality of sleep can result in fatigue. A sleep cycle lasts for about 90 minutes. Sleep consists of two phases:

- Non-REM (rapid eye movement) sleep, which has four stages. Slow waves are present in stages 3 and 4. Non-REM sleep dominates the first third of the night.
- REM sleep, during which the brain uses as much oxygen and glucose as it does during waking. During this phase there are eye movements, vivid dreams, and inhibition of the motor system. It appears that REM sleep is involved in brain plasticity and is associated with learning and establishing connections. REM sleep decreases greatly in the elderly. REM sleep occurs mostly in the last third of the night. With sleep deprivation there is a rebound of REM sleep. REM sleep is affected by antidepressants.

Three typical sleep disorder problems are:

- *Insomnia*, which may be acute or chronic. Acute stress and environmental disturbances are the most common causes of transient and short-term insomnia. About 5% of adults have chronic insomnia. Chronic insomnia is often associated with:
  - psychiatric disorders (e.g. depression, personality disorder)
  - persistent psychophysiologic disorders such as learned or conditioned insomnia and inadequate sleep hygiene. (Alcohol, caffeine, and nicotine all disrupt sleep. Alcohol, although a depressant which initially reduces sleep latency and decreases arousals, causes increased waking in the

second half of the night. Alcohol promotes fragmentation of normal sleep.)
  - drug dependence
  - restless legs syndrome.
- *Abnormal sleep behavior.*
- *Excessive daytime sleepiness.* Likely diagnoses include:
  - obstructive sleep disorder
  - narcolepsy. Sleepiness is temporarily but rapidly reversed by brief naps of a few minutes.

Recognized syndromes associated with sleep disturbance include the following.

Conditioned insomnia. Conditioned insomnia follows acute stress-related insomnia and is maintained by negative associations and anxiety regarding sleep initiation. Two of the following must be present for a diagnosis of conditioned insomnia:

- excessive worry regarding sleep
- a significant effort to fall asleep
- the ability to fall asleep when not in the bedroom (e.g. in front of television)
- paradoxical improvement away from home (i.e. away from the usual anxiety-provoking sleep setting)
- difficulty with sleeping begins during the stressful period but persists after the stress has abated.

The patient may spend excessive time in bed trying to sleep. In order to ensure 6 hours of sleep the individual may spend 9 hours in bed. A handy therapeutic tip is to appropriately shorten the time spent in bed, no naps should be taken within 6–8 hours of going to bed, and coffee, caffeine, and alcohol should be avoided 8–10 hours before going to sleep.

Shift work. Shift workers suffer insomnia as a result of disruption of their circadian rhythm. The impact of this disruption can be minimized by rotating shifts in a clockwise direction and not more than once in 3 days. When workers get off work they should use very dark glasses when outdoors and sleep in darkened, quiet surroundings. Work should be done in bright light.

Delayed sleep phase syndrome. Prevalent in adolescence, delayed sleep phase syndrome sufferers present with:

- chronic tiredness
- a delay in sleep onset (sufferers go to sleep very late)
- a normal quantity and quality of sleep (society permitting)
- a delay in wake-up time (sufferers wake up very late).

Advanced sleep phase syndrome. In contrast to delayed sleep phase syndrome, advanced sleep phase syndrome is more common in the elderly who demonstrate:

- early bedtime
- early waking
- late afternoon fatigue.

Sleep apnea. Sleep apnea occurs more commonly in males (10 : 1) and involves repetitive upper airways obstruction, resulting in oxygen desaturation and/or sleep fragmentation. Patients at particular risk are obese, middle-aged males with a short neck. Patients present with:

- Nocturnal findings including:
  - Snoring. Obstruction is most severe when apnea of more than 10 seconds is followed by a snort.
  - Sleep fragmentation. If an individual is awake for less than 2 minutes, there is no memory of having woken. Patients may therefore say they slept well but awoke unrefreshed.
  - Restlessness.
  - Gastroesophageal reflux.
  - Cardiac arrhythmias. These are prone to occur when oxygen saturation falls to less than 70%.
  - Nasal obstruction. This may be due to an edematous pharynx.
- Daytime findings including:
  - tiredness which is gradual in onset
  - inappropriate daytime somnolence
  - forgetfulness (decreased concentration span and impaired short-term memory)
  - weight gain
  - reduced work performance
  - personality change, irritability.

Narcolepsy. REM sleep intrudes into the boundary between sleep and waking. People with narcolepsy fall asleep within 5 minutes in sleep latency tests. Narcolepsy is characterized by:

- Excessive daytime somnolence, characterized by:
  - increased frequency of daytime sleep episodes
  - decreased vigilance or automatic behavior.
- Cataplexy. A sudden loss of muscle strength is precipitated by emotional stimulation or stress.
- Disrupted nocturnal sleep.
- Hypnagogic hallucinations between sleep and waking (i.e. awake dreaming).
- Sleep paralysis. On waking, sufferers may be unable to move for short periods or until gently shaken.

Nearly 100% of Caucasians with narcolepsy have the HLA-DR2 antigen.

Nocturnal myoclonus. Nocturnal myoclonus or periodic limb movement disorder occurs during sleep and causes multiple brief arousals. Patients present with:

- Periodic brief movements of the feet or legs at 30-second intervals.
- Movements typically include:
  - extension of the big toe
  - dorsiflexion of the ankle
  - flexion of the hip and/or knee.

Restless legs syndrome. Restless legs syndrome affects 5% of the population. It presents with:

- Unpleasant sensations in the leg(s), which may be described as aching, tingling, crawling, pulling, or itching.
- A need to move. The patient gets up and paces.
- Symptoms which occur when awake, day and night.

Conditions associated with this syndrome include: renal failure, chronic lung disease, peripheral neuropathy, anemia, iron deficiency, leukemia, diabetes, rheumatoid arthritis, pregnancy, and drug withdrawal (valium, barbiturates).

Chronic rhinosinusitis. Chronic upper airways obstruction results in:

- drowsiness and fatigue
- nasal stuffiness
- mouth-breathing
- snoring
- poor sleep habits.

Iatrogenic fatigue. Fatigue, drowsiness, and lethargy are common side-effects associated with treatment involving:

- antihypertensives: beta blockers (propranolol), methyldopa, reserpine, clonidine
- long-acting night sedatives and minor tranquilizers
- antidepressants, particularly amitriptyline, doxepin, and trazodone
- diuretics causing hypokalemia and/or hypotension
- steroid withdrawal
- antihistamines.

A recent review of prescription medication includes the following as drugs reported to cause insomnia: α-methyldopa, propranolol, xanthine derivative, β-adrenergic agonists, catecholamine blocking agents, antiarrhythmic drugs, oral contraceptives, thyroid hormones, and stimulant antidepressants (e.g. fluoxetine). Drugs that are lipid soluble and cross the blood–brain barrier may influence neurotransmitters. Antihistaminics cause drowsiness; anticholinergics, adrenergic blockers, GABA system stimulants, and serotonergics all cause sedation. Drugs that penetrate the central nervous system need to be considered as possible causes of fatigue.

Patients with hypertension, angina pectoris, cardiac arrhythmias, migraine or thyrotoxicosis are all potential candidates for therapy with beta blockers.

- *Rebound insomnia.* Rebound insomnia occurs following termination of therapy with short and intermediate benzodiazepines.
- *Drug dose problems.* The half-life of a drug is the time it takes for the serum level of that drug to reach 50% of its peak plasma concentration. Drugs with a long half-life accumulate if taken too frequently. In order to avoid daytime sleepiness, a

drug with a short or medium half-life should be used to treat insomnia. Drugs with a half-life of more than about 6 hours are likely to accumulate and cause daytime drowsiness.

SLIPPED UPPER FEMORAL EPIPHYSIS

As avascular necrosis is a potential complication, early diagnosis and treatment are essential. Patients, usually teenagers, present with:

- a limp
- knee pain
- hip discomfort on movement
- limitation of all hip movement, especially internal rotation
- on hip flexion, external rotation occurs.

Radiography of both hips is recommended in teenagers who develop hip pain and a limp.

SOLAR KERATOSIS

Solar keratosis has a very low risk of malignant change (1/1000/year), but is a risk factor for nonmelanotic skin cancer. It is a premalignant condition:

- which occurs on light-exposed areas
- which comes and goes, often clearing in winter
- with erythematous dysplastic scaly lesions
- which stings if picked at.

In persons with solar keratosis check for:

- squamous cell carcinoma, by stretching the skin to detect an everted edge
- basal cell carcinoma, by stretching the skin to detect the pearly edge.

SPINAL CANAL STENOSIS

Patients present with:

- A long history of backache.
- Burning or numbing pain. If pain is cramping, think of vascular claudication.
- Paresthesia of the buttock.
- Burning or tingling which later descends down the lower limb.
- Pain provoked by:
  - walking

  - prolonged standing
  - lumbar extension.
- Pain is relieved within 20 minutes after:
  - assuming a flexed spinal position, as in squatting
  - lying down.
- Bladder and bowel symptoms may be present.

SPINAL DYSFUNCTION

Mechanical back pain can present with varying degrees of dysfunction of the facet joints and internal disruption of the intervertebral disc. Possible progressively more serious presentations include the following.

Facet dysfunction. Facet dysfunction responds well to spinal manipulation and presents with:

- a dull ache
- pain relieved by rest
- pain aggravated by activity
- localized tenderness (in the case of low back pain L4–S1 are usually involved).

Disc disruption. Internal disc disruption may produce intrinsic pain with apophyseal joint dysfunction, presenting with:

- protective muscle spasm
- pain in the corresponding segment
- normal function and radiographic appearance.

Extrinsic pain may result from pressure on surrounding structures. Pain may be radicular or nonradicular.

Disc disruption that responds to conservative care presents with:

- Deep backache punctuated with episodic stabbing pain.
- Distal paresthesia. Pain may be referred to the arms and shoulders from cervical lesions; to the arms, anterior and posterior chest wall, and abdomen in thoracic lesions; to the groin, lower limb, and foot in lumbar lesions; and to the back of the lower limb and foot in sacral lesions.
- Loss of the normal spinal curvature (e.g. the lumbar lordosis is lost in cases with lumbar disc problems).
- Restricted movement.

Disc protrusion. Disc protrusion requires surgery. Patients present with unilateral signs of:

- motor weakness (e.g. foot drop)
- loss of reflexes
- paresthesia.

The pain of an acute disc prolapse is aggravated by sitting.

Spinal cord compression. In cases with spinal cord compression, emergency referral is required. Patients present with bilateral signs, including:

- upper and lower motor neuron lesions
- distal anesthesia
- limb weakness.

The presentation of spinal dysfunction is also influenced by the level of the spine involved. Lesions of the cervical spine may present with:

- A dull ache in the neck.
- Radiation of pain in upper cervical lesions to:
  - the head (muscle-contraction headache or migraine may result)
  - the face, especially the temple
  - the periauricular region, resulting in earache.
- Radiation of pain in lower cervical lesions to the:
  - scapular and subscapular area
  - anterior chest
  - arm and hand.
- Neck movement, impairment, including:
  - stiffness
  - a tendency to lock with specific movements, especially rotation
  - variable restriction of movement.
- Local neck tenderness.
- Dizziness.
- Visual dysfunction.
- Normal radiograph.

SPINAL FRACTURE

Patients usually present following injury. However, osteoporotic individuals and persons with spinal metastasis may present with a pathological fracture. Pathological compression fractures should always be excluded in patients who develop acute backache in the absence of trauma. Clinical manifestations of spinal fracture include:

- Spinal pain. This is:
  - aggravated by activity, standing, coughing, sneezing, and straining
  - relieved by rest.
- Intense muscle spasm. This is associated with:
  - marked restriction of movement
  - deformity.
- The nature of the fracture is influenced by the injury. For example:

- a compression fracture results from flexion injury or a compression force applied to the spine
- a transverse or spinous process fracture may follow a violent twisting force
- a coccygeal fracture may result from falling in the seated position.

- Unstable fracture. Unless immediately immobilized, irreparable neural damage with paralysis may occur. Unstable fractures are associated with:
  - burst or shearing fractures
  - pain is rapidly relieved by lying down and recurs on standing.

Patients should have their cervical spine supported and immobilized until radiographs can exclude a fracture.

SPONDYLOLISTHESIS

Spondylolisthesis is forward displacement of one vertebra on another. This congenital abnormality may or may not cause backache. Pain is thought to occur when stretching of the interspinous ligaments or nerve roots is associated with disc degeneration. When symptomatic, spondylolisthesis presents with:

- Low dull backache.
- Bilateral or unilateral pain radiation into the buttocks, hips, thighs, and feet. Paresthesia may be experienced in the legs.
- Pain is worst on standing and walking; stiffness occurs after exercise.
- Pain is relieved by sitting.
- Patients have a stiff waddling gait and a lumbar lordosis.

SPONDYLOSIS

The presentation of degenerative spinal osteoarthritis varies depending on the site of the lesion. (See: *Cervical spondylosis (osteoarthritis)*; *Lumbar osteoarthritis*.)

SPRAINED ANKLE

A sprain is a complete or partial ligamentous injury and usually occurs following trauma or twisting injuries. The most common ankle injury occurs with the foot plantar flexed and forcibly inverted. The presenting complaint includes:

- a sensation of the ankle giving way (this usually follows landing awkwardly after a jump or while walking on uneven ground)

- mild to severe discomfort
- difficulty with weight bearing
- swelling and bruising.

Intervention depends on the extent of ligament laxity. A fracture should always be excluded.

SQUAMOUS CELL CARCINOMA

Squamous cell carcinoma is a malignant tumor of the epidermis which tends to arise in sun-exposed areas. The hands, forearms, head, and neck are at particular risk. The cancer can arise de novo or in areas of skin trauma such as solar keratosis. The presentation of squamous cell carcinoma depends on the stage of the disease:

- The initial lesion:
  - is a progressive scaly erythematous patch on a sun-exposed area
  - undergoes cycles of macular and scaly erythematous lesions (the scaly lesions have a sandpaper texture on palpation)
  - is often found in sun-damaged areas.
- In advanced cases, the lesion is a:
  - hard enlarging flesh colored nodule
  - an ulcerated nodule with an everted edge and crusts.

The tumor can metastasize.

STAPHYLOCOCCAL DISEASES

Staphylococcus aureus may cause various skin lesions:

- Folliculitis, which presents with:
  - superficial pustules surrounding a hair follicle
  - hairs are easily removed
  - new papules tend to develop.
- Furunculoses (boils), which present with:
  - acute, tender perifollicular nodules
  - the nodule becomes a pustule with an area of central necrosis
  - the pustule discharges a sanguineous purulent exudate.
- Carbuncles are clusters of furuncles. They present with:
  - fever
  - subcutaneous infection, suppuration, and sloughing
  - predisposing factors are diabetes mellitus, debility, and old age.

In addition, the organism causes:

- Food poisoning.

- Osteomyelitis:
  - fever, chills
  - pain, tenderness
  - limitation of joint movement
  - diagnosis based on a culture of the lesion or blood.
- Pneumonia.
- Impetigo.
- Paronychia.

Methicillin-resistant *Staph.* are a serious problem, especially in hospitals.

STERNALIS SYNDROME

Patients present with:

- central chest wall pain
- tenderness over the manubriosternal junction (synchondrosis) or overlying muscles.

Symptoms last for days and weeks.

STEVENS–JOHNSON SYNDROME

Clinical features of this syndrome include:

- fever and constitutional symptoms
- ocular lesions, such as conjunctivitis, uveitis, and corneal ulcers
- genital lesions, including urethritis, balanitis, or vulvovaginitis
- oral bullae and hemorrhagic crusting
- skin lesions such as erythema multiforme.

STOMACH CANCER

Stomach cancer is asymptomatic during the early stages of the disease. Stomach cancer should therefore always be excluded in:

- Middle-aged patients who present with dyspepsia of recent onset.
- Patients with a changing clinical picture after a long history of:
  - gastric ulcer
  - pernicious anemia.

The clinical presentation includes:

- Recent onset of upper gastrointestinal symptoms in a patient over 40 years of age.
- Dyspepsia that fails to respond to treatment.
- Epigastric fullness.

- Anorexia, nausea.
- Belching.
- Late signs include:
  - vomiting of 'old' food
  - anemia
  - an abdominal mass
  - supraventricular lymphadenopathy
  - weight loss.

STRESS

Stress, or 'burn-out', may result from an incapacity to cope with psychosocial stressors. Stress is largely related to the individual's perception of change as loss or threat. Patients with burn-out are frequently anxious and depressed, suffer from insomnia, and fail to experience self-actualization. Stress has physical, emotional, and cognitive repercussions:

- Physical evidence of stress is an anxious patient who may experience:
  - trembling hands
  - stomach butterflies
  - tightness in the shoulders, head, and lower back
  - restlessness (the stressed individual cannot relax; foot tapping or key jiggling are often noted)
  - an exaggerated startle response (the person is continually vigilant and, therefore, is also easily fatigued)
  - stuttering or falling over their words (people under stress speak quickly)
  - frequent minor ailments
  - sleep problems
  - hatband headache
  - back pain
  - loss of libido
  - stomach upsets.
- Emotional lability may present as:
  - tearfulness
  - impulsive behavior
  - irritability, short temperedness
  - hostility, aggressiveness
  - feelings of being a failure
  - feelings of frustration
  - feeling apathetic or agitated
  - sadness or depression
  - withdrawal and disinterest
  - emotional outbursts with little provocation
  - significant interpersonal conflict, argumentative.

- Cognitive evidence of stress is evidenced by:
  - memory problems, forgetfulness
  - indecisiveness
  - flitting from one idea or activity to another
  - a tendency to make mistakes or get muddled
  - mental blocks
  - foggy, disorganized thinking
  - procrastination (an inability to plan ahead or manage time)
  - working longer hours
  - an inability to relax and/or find time for enjoyment.
- Evidence of failure to cope with persistent stress presents as:
  - rigid inflexibility (this is the individual's effort to maintain control)
  - needing sleeping tablets or tranquilizers
  - needing alcohol or other drugs
  - losing contact with your friends
  - flare-up of stress-related illnesses: asthma, psoriasis, irritable bowel, ulcers, headaches
  - depression
  - persistent anxiety
  - over-eating or loss of appetite, with weight changes.

STRESS FRACTURE

Stress fractures may affect the tarsals or metatarsals. Patients present with:

- Podalgia, which may:
  - gradually develop
  - be sudden in onset.
- An aching pain.
- Examination and radiographs are often negative.
- A bone scan is diagnostic.
- Stress fracture of the:
  - navicular (this is suspected when runners present with poorly localized midfoot pain)
  - forefoot (a stress fracture may involve the neck of the second or third metatarsal after marching)
  - base of the fifth metatarsal (this may be caused by a severe ankle sprain with muscle spasm).

Stress fractures require rest for at least 6 weeks. Strong supportive footwear is recommended.

STROKE

Strokes are the third most common cause of death in Australia, and about one-third of stroke patients die within 1 month. A stroke presents as a focal neurological deficit lasting longer than 24 hours, and is caused by a vascular phenomenon.

Strokes may be preceded by a history of:

- Transient ischemic attacks. A reversible ischemic neurological deficit lasts for less than 24 hours. (See: *Transient ischemic attack*.)
- A stroke-in-evolution. The neurological deficit persists for several hours and continues to worsen. The enlarging neurological deficit, presumably due to infarction, increases over 24–48 hours.

The presentation and progression of a stroke is influenced by its cause. Strokes may result from:

- *Thrombosis in cerebral vessels*. Strokes attributable to thrombosis cause focal lesions and present with:
  - gradually developing symptoms
  - stepwise progression of the disorder
  - retention of consciousness
  - gradual improvement over a number of weeks.

Patients with a cerebral thrombosis often have underlying atherosclerosis, arteritis, a hypercoagulable state, or carotid artery trauma.

- *Emboli to the brain*. In cerebral embolism the presentation is:
  - a sudden onset
  - rapid improvement after the initial attack
  - the absence of prodromal symptoms.

Cerebral embolism is most prevalent in patients with atrial fibrillation and/or valvular disease.

- *Cerebral hemorrhage*. A history of hypertension or trauma may be present. Cerebrovascular accidents attributable to hemorrhage present with:
  - an abrupt onset
  - loss of consciousness
  - insidious loss of function, which progresses unremittingly
  - rapid deterioration
  - a stiff neck and positive Babinski sign
  - prodromal symptoms, including severe headache and dizziness.

  Associated findings are:
  - a slow bounding pulse
  - deep, stertorous respiration
  - localizing neurological signs.

While thrombosis, embolus, or hemorrhage are all associated with a particular progression, the outcome and precise clinical picture are determined by the anatomical, and therefore functional, area of the brain involved. A lesion of the:

- anterior cerebral artery results in hemiparesis of the opposite side of the body (the arm and face are spared)
- the vertebrobasilar artery may present with ipsilateral facial involvement, contralateral paralysis/paresthesia of the body, cranial nerve lesions, ataxia, vertigo, and hearing loss.

An alternate approach focuses on the type of cerebral infarction:

- *Lacunar syndromes* occur when there is in situ small-vessel disease. Possible clinical presentations include:
  - pure motor hemiparesis (this is the most common outcome; the infarct is usually in the internal capsule)
  - ataxic hemiparesis (ataxia of the upper or lower limbs in excess of that expected from muscle weakness)
  - dysarthria, clumsy hand syndrome (profound dysarthria and clumsiness confined to the upper limb)
  - pure sensory stroke
  - sensory–motor stroke.

A lack of cortical signs due to the confined nature of the lesion is a common feature. Prognosis is usually good.

- *Cortical-type syndrome.* This may result from cardioembolic disease or from large-vessel disease. In the former, underlying cardiac pathology needs to be identified; in the latter, infarction results from emboli transmitted from artery to artery. The clinical presentation is:
  - dysphasia in the left hemisphere
  - visual or sensory neglect in the right hemisphere
  - constructional/dressing dyspraxia in the right hemisphere
  - long-tract involvement.

Fifty percent of cases are preceded by transient ischemic attack.

STYE (external hordeolum)

A stye is an acute abscess involving the gland or follicle of an eyelash. Patients present with:

- redness of the lid margin
- a tender swelling on the lid margin, usually on the medial side
- pustule formation.

SUBACROMIAL BURSITIS

Patients may require hospital admission for pain control. Subacromial bursitis presents with:

- intense constant pain
- limitation of all shoulder movements, especially rotation (patients have a frozen shoulder)

- difficulty in dressing
- marked tenderness below the acromion over the deltoid (this is a reliable sign).

SUBARACHNOID HEMORRHAGE

The clinical features of a subarachnoid hemorrhage are:

- Head pain that is:
  - sudden in onset
  - moderate to severe
  - steady or persistent
  - often precipitated by straining
  - often initially localized to the occipital region and neck, and later becomes generalized.
- Signs of meningismus, including:
  - neck stiffness
  - a positive Brudzinski's sign
  - photophobia.
- The presence of focal neurological defects.
- An altered level of consciousness:
  - small leaks lead to confusion but no loss of consciousness
  - large bleeds present with vomiting, confusion, and coma.

Other prevalent findings are an extensor plantar response, bradycardia, or hypertension.

Subarachnoid hemorrhages are most prevalent in middle-aged persons.

SUBCAPITAL FRACTURE

Elderly patients are at particular risk of a subcapital fracture. Patients present with:

- a history of either a painful fall or report that the hip just 'gave way'
- a painful hip
- no obvious deformity.

Impacted subcapital femoral fractures permit weight bearing. It is therefore obligatory to radiograph all elderly patients with hip pain. A bone scan or computed tomography may also be indicated.

SUBCONJUNCTIVAL HEMORRHAGE

Patients with a subconjunctival hemorrhage present with:

- a painless red eye

- a unilateral focal homogeneous redness with a definite posterior margin.

If no posterior margin can be seen and there is a history of trauma, an orbital fracture should be suspected.

Blood pressure evaluation is recommended in all cases where there is no history of trauma.

SUBDURAL HEMATOMA

Rupture of cortical veins as they cross the subdural space may occur spontaneously or following trauma. A latent period of days or months may occur before symptoms develop. A chronic subdural hematoma presents with:

- Fluctuating symptoms that change from day to day.
- Evidence of increased intracranial pressure (see: *Intracranial pressure*).
- A fluctuating level of consciousness.
- Evidence of an intracranial space-occupying lesion, with localizing signs such as:
  - hemiparesis
  - third cranial nerve lesions.
- A history of trauma. Trauma may often be minor, and forgotten.

SUDEK'S ATROPHY

See: *Functional arterial disorders*; *Reflex sympathetic dystrophy syndrome*.

SUNBURN

Ultraviolet radiation damage to the skin resulting in release of leukotrienes and histamine presents with either:

- mild erythema
- moderate erythema followed by redness, heat, and pain
- severe erythema with heat, pain, and swelling followed by vesicles and desquamation.

SUPRASPINATUS TEAR

A *partial* tendon tear which leaves the rotator cuff intact presents with:

- Pain referred to the insertion of the deltoid. There is no local tenderness.

- Active elevation of the arm at 90° abduction is:
  - painless up to 60°
  - causes excruciating pain beyond 60°.
- Tenderness is detected at the tip of the acromion.

A *complete* tendon tear is associated with some rotator cuff tearing. Patients present with:

- active elevation of the arm at 90° abduction is restricted to less than 40°
- passive movement to 180° is free and painless
- crepitus on palpation of the shoulder while the arm is moved forward.

SUPRASPINATUS TENDONITIS

Inflammation of the supraspinatus tendon is the most common shoulder problem encountered in primary practice. Patients present with:

- Shoulder pain that is worst over the deltoid insertion.
- Pain which:
  - radiates to the elbow
  - is throbbing
  - is constant
  - is aggravated by heat, lying on the shoulder, or putting on a blouse.
- Arm abduction is painful:
  - between 60° and 120°
  - when resisted.

In *chronic supraspinatus tendonitis* tenderness can be elicited between the greater and lesser tubercles of the humerus or beneath the tip of the acromion. There is no tenderness at the insertion of the deltoid.

SYNCOPE

Syncope is a transient loss of consciousness. It may be categorized as:

- *Vasomotor syncope.* Autonomic imbalance following emotional or physical stress results in a fall in blood pressure and decreased cerebral perfusion. Reflex syncope is found in:
  - carotid sinus stimulation
  - vasovagal attack
  - micturition syncope associated with emptying a very full bladder after significant alcohol ingestion.
- *Cardiac syncope.* Cardiac arrhythmia and valvular disease may cause syncope due to:

- A slow ventricular rate. Asystole or ventricular fibrillation may lead to inadequate cerebral perfusion, with loss of consciousness. Recovery is accompanied by flushing as the peripheral vessels, dilated by anoxia, are perfused. A variant of this is *carotid sinus syncope*, in which elderly people faint as a result of slight carotid sinus stimulation. Head positions that facilitate light carotid sinus touch, such as turning the head while wearing a collar, precipitate vagal stimulation.
- A fast ventricular rate. When the rate of ventricular contraction is so rapid as to not permit adequate filling of the ventricle, the stroke volume drops and the cardiac output may fail to achieve adequate cerebral perfusion.
- Postural syncope. Orthostatic hypotension occurs when the sympathetic response to changes in position is dampened with drugs (e.g. antihypertensive agents, nitrate) or disorders of the autonomic nervous system (e.g. diabetic neuropathy). Micturition syncope occurs as a result of the combination of peripheral vasodilatation and increased intrathoracic pressure due to straining.

- *Anoxic syncope*. A drop in oxygen saturation due to paroxysms of coughing may result in fainting due to interference with venous return as a result of the increased intrathoracic pressure associated with coughing.
- *Cerebral syncope*. This may be associated with the onset of cerebral embolism or thrombosis. Ischemia may be due to neurological or metabolic disease, including:
  - transient ischemic attacks in patients with underlying atherosclerosis
  - vertebrobasal ischemia
  - subclavian steal syndrome
  - cerebral vasospasm
  - hypoglycemia.

The clinical features of syncope are a transient loss of consciousness which is:

- Often gradual in onset.
- Of short duration (loss of consciousness lasts from a few seconds to less than 3 minutes).
- Followed by quick recovery.
- Commonly related to posture.
- Accompanied by shallow respiration.
- Associated with:
  - sweating
  - pallor.
- A variable prodrome of presyncopal symptoms is common. This includes:
  - giddiness, light-headedness, or faintness
  - nausea
  - fading hearing

- feeling hot or cold
- blurred vision.

SYPHILIS

Treponema pallidum is the spirochete responsible for syphilis. Serology is positive.

Primary syphilis has an incubation period of 2–4 weeks and presents with:

- a painless indurated raised chancre, usually found on the penis, labia, or cervix
- an indolent ulcer with a clean base and a raised edge
- nontender discrete rubbery lymphadenopathy.

Secondary syphilis presents with:

- a pink nonpruritic skin rash on the trunk and extremities
- infectious, moist, pink or gray patches (condylomata lata) in the intertriginous areas
- mucous patches in the mouth or on the genitalia, that are painless gray erosions with a red periphery.

Tertiary syphilis is rare since the introduction of penicillin. It presents as:

- Meningovascular syphilis with:
  - headache
  - vertigo
  - insomnia
  - psychological changes.
- General paralysis of the insane with:
  - memory problems
  - hyperreflexia.
- Tabes dorsalis, with demyelinization of the posterior column, resulting in:
  - an ataxic broad-based gait
  - bladder disturbances
  - trophic joint degeneration.
- Cardiovascular syphilis, with:
  - aortitis
  - an aortic arch aneurysm.

SYSTEMIC LUPUS ERYTHEMATOSUS

This inflammatory connective tissue disorder may present as systemic lupus erythematosus (SLE) or discoid lupus erythematosus, primarily affecting the skin. The presence of autoantibodies such as antinuclear antibodies and lupus erythematosus (LE) cells suggests this is an autoimmune condition. The condition is characterized by exacerbations and remissions. Virtually any organ system can be involved. SLE presents with any combination of the following:

- fatigue, malaise, and weight loss
- fever, which may be acute in onset or episodic
- joint pains, varying from intermittent arthralgia to polyarthritis
- myositis
- photosensitivity
- an erythematous rash, characteristically with a butterfly facial distribution
- anemia, neutropenia, thrombocytopenia
- lymphadenopathy, splenomegaly
- pleuritis, pneumonitis, vasculitis, pericarditis, and nephritis
- psychosis and seizures.

TEMPORAL ARTERITIS

Temporal arteritis is caused by immunogenic inflammation of extracranial vessels. Elderly patients (>50 years) are at most risk. The condition responds to steroids. Temporal arteritis presents with:

- Pain:
  - of recent onset which becomes constant
  - which presents as: a unilateral, often mild, headache; jaw claudication.
- Tenderness over the:
  - scalp (patients cannot brush their hair)
  - local tenderness over the temporal artery and temples (patients cannot wear a hat).
- Anemia.
- Fatigue.
- Weight loss.
- A high erythrocyte sedimentation rate.

Complications include irreversible partial or complete loss of vision due to ischemic optic neuropathy.

TEMPORAL LOBE TUMOR

See: *Cerebral tumors.*

TEMPOROMANDIBULAR DISEASE

Patients may present with malocclusion of the temporomandibular joint and a joint lesion. Similar findings may be encountered in anxious patients without joint disease who grind

PART THREE

their teeth or have developed tension-related jaw clenching habits. Patients may present with:

- Pain causing:
  - unilateral aching in the preauricular area
  - a nagging dull occipital headache.
- Pain may radiate to the:
  - temporal region
  - anteromedial area of the pinna
  - angle of the jaw
  - the occiput.
- Tenderness over:
  - the joint
  - the muscles used for mastication.
- Costen's syndrome:
  - earache
  - tinnitus
  - mild deafness is sometimes present.
- Occasionally, popping or clicking sounds over the joint.

TENDONITIS

Patients present with:

- Pain which:
  - is a dull ache
  - becomes acute and sharp on squeezing the affected tendon.
- A friction rub may be felt or auscultated on movement of the tendon in its sheath.

TENNIS ELBOW

Overuse or overload of the forearm muscles may lead to epicondylitis or tennis elbow. Two varieties are: lateral, or backhand, tennis elbow; and medial, or forehand, tennis elbow.

Lateral tennis elbow is due to excess strain on the forearm extensors from wrist extension. Patients present with:

- No elbow swelling or limitation of movement.
- Pain:
  - at the outer elbow
  - referred down the forearm
  - aggravated by hand movements (e.g. unscrewing bottles, taps), passively stretching the wrist, resisted wrist extension.
- Rest and night pain in severe cases.
- Localized tenderness over the lateral epicondyle.

Medial tennis elbow, or golfer's elbow, presents with:

- pain on the inner side of the elbow
- localized tenderness on palpation of the medial epicondyle
- pain and resisted flexion of the wrist.

TENOSYNOVITIS

Patients present with:

- pain over the involved area
- tenderness along the involved tendon sheath
- swelling in the affected area
- crepitus on moving the relevant tendon in acute nonsuppurative tenosynovitis.

De Quervain's tenosynovitis (washerwoman's sprain) is a work-induced condition of stenosing tenosynovitis of the first dorsal extensor compartment tendons. Patients present with:

- Pain:
  - at and proximal to the wrist on the radial side
  - on thumb and wrist movement
  - on pinch grasping
  - increased or produced on rotating the wrist in the ulnar direction with the thumb palmed in the fist of the involved side.
- Just proximal to the radial styloid:
  - tenderness to palpation
  - a firm localized swelling.

Trigger finger or thumb, or *stenosing flexor tenosynovitis*, presents with:

- painless finger/thumb flexion
- a sharp painful snap on finger/thumb re-extension.

Pain may be referred to the dorsum of the hand.

TENSION HEADACHE

Primary muscle-contraction or tension headaches are frequently encountered in primary practice. The history, and physical and neurological examination do not suggest any underlying disease. Tension headaches:

- are continuous daily headaches
- worsen as the day progresses
- are relieved by alcohol
- are associated with stress or tension (anxious patients may hyperventilate and develop light-headedness).

Two broad diagnostic categories have been identified, *episodic tension-type headaches* and *chronic tension type headaches.* In both cases at least two of the following pain characteristics are present:

- constricting, pressing, tightening, or hatband type pain
- mild or moderate intensity
- bilateral headache
- no aggravation on routine physical activity.

In addition, episodic tension-type headaches:

- occur no more than 15 times per month or 180 times per year
- last 30 minutes to 7 days
- have neither, or no more than one, of photophobia or phonophobia
- are not associated with nausea or vomiting.

Before labeling patients as episodic tension headache sufferers, they should have fulfilled the above criteria on at least 10 previous occasions.

Clinical features of chronic tension-type headaches are:

- the absence of vomiting
- not more than one of: nausea, photophobia, or phonophobia
- an occurrence rate of at least 15 times per month for 6 months or longer.

Overuse of analgesics, opiates, or ergotamine may be an important contributing factor to the development of a chronic tension-type headache.

(See: *Muscle contraction headaches.*)

TESTICULAR CANCER

Although testicular cancer is extremely rare before the age of 20 and after the age of 60 years, it is the most common cancer in males aged 15–40 years. The lifetime risk of developing the disease is 1:300; the lifetime risk of dying of the disease is 1:10 000. The clinical presentation of a testicular tumor is:

- a hard or firm nontender mass, distinct from cord structures, in the body of the testis
- a painless mass (hemorrhage into the tumor causes pain)
- loss of testicular sensation
- scrotal heaviness.

One of the reasons why this is a very curable form of cancer is that it can be detected and removed when the disease is localized to the testis.

Periodic testicular self-examination may enhance the chances of early diagnosis and treatment. As in most cases only one testis is affected, treatment by removal of that testis does not impair sexual function.

TESTICULAR MALPOSITION

Testis not located in the scrotum may be:

- *Undescended.* An undescended testis is one that has stopped in the normal path of descent to the scrotum and cannot be manipulated into the bottom of the scrotum.
- *Retractile.* The testis can be drawn down to the bottom of the scrotum. Retractile testis are usually found in the scrotum when warm but retract on exposure to cold.
- *Ascending.* The testis has descended into the scrotum but has been drawn back into the groin due to failure of the spermatic cord to elongate adequately.
- *Ectopic.* An ectopic testis fails to follow the normal route to the scrotum and can be found in the groin, upper thigh, base of the penis, or anterior abdomen.

Testes located outside of the scrotum run an increased risk of:

- dysplasia and infertility
- malignant change
- trauma.

TESTICULAR TORSION

Torsion of the testis is largely a problem of childhood and adolescence, but may occur in young adults. Twisting of the testis compromises the blood supply and testicular gangrene results unless the blood supply is restored within 4 hours. Torsion of the testis presents with:

- the sudden onset of increasingly severe pain
- an exquisitely tender testis
- nausea and vomiting
- the involved testis lying high and transverse in the scrotum (a testis with a horizontal lie on the uninvolved side strengthens the diagnosis)
- an enlarged edematous red scrotum
- an absent cremasteric reflex.

Lifting the testis does not ease the pain in these afebrile patients.

THIRD NERVE PALSY

See: *Oculomotor palsy.*

THORACIC OUTLET SYNDROME

Compression of the brachial plexus and subclavian artery presents with:

- Pain and paresthesia:
  - in the arm, especially in the ulnar region of the hand and forearm
  - which is aggravated at night and by prolonged use of the hand.
- Weakness and atrophy, especially of the small muscles of the hand.
- Cold, blue hands.
- Diminished ulnar and radial pulses.

THROMBASTHENIA

Thrombasthenia results from a functional defect in platelets. Such platelet dysfunction can be induced by nonsteroidal anti-inflammatory drugs (NSAIDs), which are particularly effective at inhibiting platelet aggregation. Aspirin irreversibly acetylates cyclooxygenase and, as this inhibitory effect lasts the lifetime of the platelet, aspirin is often used to reduce the risk of thrombosis.

Persons with a functional platelet deficiency may present with:

- bleeding into skin and mucous membranes
- petechiae, purpura
- epistaxis
- menorrhagia
- immediate postoperative oozing
- a normal platelet count, but abnormal platelet function tests (e.g. bleeding time).

THROMBOCYTOPENIA

Thrombocytopenia indicates a decreased number of platelets. Platelet numbers may be reduced as a result of:

- bone marrow disorders
- immunological lysis of platelets
- excessive splenic destruction of platelets
- exaggerated utilization of platelets, as in disseminated intravascular coagulopathy.

Persons with a platelet deficiency present with:

- bleeding into skin and mucous membranes
- petechiae, purpura
- epistaxis

- menorrhagia
- immediate postoperative oozing
- a reduced platelet count (a platelet count is helpful in establishing the presence, but not the cause, of thrombocytopenia).

Thrombasthenia has a normal platelet count, but presents with a similar clinical picture due to a qualitative defect in platelets.

THROMBOPHLEBITIS

See: *Venous thrombosis.*

THYROID DISEASE

Persons at increased risk of thyroid disease and suitable for screening include:

- those with a strong family history of thyroid disease
- the elderly
- postpartum women (4–8 weeks after delivery)
- persons with autoimmune disease.

In diagnosing thyroid disease it is necessary to ascertain:

- the physical condition of the gland
- the cause of thyroid dysfunction
- the hormonal status of the patient (this is ascertained at a clinical and laboratory or biochemical level).

The gland may be diffusely enlarged or may contain one or more nodules. Thyroid enlargement may cause pressure on surrounding structures. Diffuse enlargement of the gland is encountered in:

- *Graves' disease.* This autoimmune condition is associated with increased hormone secretion.
- *Thyroiditis.* Whether of immunological or infectious origin, thyroiditis usually presents as a diffusely enlarged, sometimes painful, hypofunctioning thyroid.

Nodules are found in:

- *Multinodular or simple goiters.* Goiters may be found in iodine-deficient areas and are usually hypofunctioning glands.
- *Single nodules.* Scans have found that 70–80% of single nodules are cold (hypofunctioning), 5–10% are warm (normal tracer uptake), and 10–20% are 'hot' (increased uptake). Single hot nodules are indicative of autonomous function and a malignancy is unlikely.

Thyroid enlargement may be benign or malignant. There is an equal risk of malignancy in cold and warm nodules. Findings suggestive of malignancy include:

- hoarseness
- vocal cord paralysis
- a single firm dominant nodule
- enlarged lymph nodes and distant metastases
- previous neck irradiation
- elevated serum calcitonin
- failure to regress on thyroxine therapy.

Children, young adults, and men are at greater risk than older women.

Thyroid malignancy may present as:

- *Papillary carcinoma.* These are not usually clinically palpable and are the most common type encountered. Excision is curative provided the malignancy has not spread beyond the thyroid capsule.
- *Follicular carcinoma.* The prognosis is good.
- *Anaplastic carcinoma.* Anaplastic carcinoma is usually fatal within 8 months. It may present as a single nodule or a bulky thyroid.
- *Medullary cancer.* The malignancy of medullary cancers vary.

Benign solitary nodules include follicular adenomas, cysts, and focal thyroiditis.

The thyroid hormone status of the patient largely determines the clinical presentation. Altered thyroid hormone levels affect many organ systems:

- menorrhagia (amenorrhea may also sometimes be found in hyperthyroidism)
- altered bowel function
- weight changes
- increased sensitivity to heat or cold
- skin changes
- mood changes
- abnormal thyroid function tests.

The nature of the clinical changes in any one patient is a consequence of either increased or decreased thyroid hormone circulation. A variety of factors alter thyroid binding globulin levels. As only the free hormone is active, evaluation of thyroid function is undertaken by requesting free thyroxine (FT4) and free triiodothyronine (FT3) levels.

Graves' disease, toxic multinodular goiter, toxic adenoma, and subacute thyroiditis may all be associated with thyrotoxicosis. Thyrotoxicosis or hyperthyroidism should be suspected in patients who complain of:

- anxious exhaustion, the inability to relax
- irritability
- a good appetite, weight loss, loose stools
- tachycardia, palpitations

- atrial fibrillation
- heat intolerance and sweating
- warm, moist fine skin
- a stare characterized by lid lag, lid retraction, and infrequent blinking
- a fine tremor and hyperkinesis
- proximal muscle weakness
- laboratory tests show a:
  - low TSH
  - high FT4 and/or FT3.

In addition to the above, patients with Graves' disease present with:

- exophthalmos
- proptosis and an associated disorder of eye movement
- chemosis, corneal damage
- infiltrative dermopathy presenting as localized pretibial myxedema.

In the elderly, evidence of hypermetabolism may be minimal. Elderly patients may present only with apathy and/or cardiac failure. In older patients check for thyrotoxicosis with laboratory tests in cases presenting with:

- unexplained cardiac failure
- cardiac arrhythmias
- weight loss
- diarrhea.

In all cases the clinical diagnosis is confirmed on laboratory investigation.

Myxedema, or hypothyroidism, is a condition of reduced thyroid hormone function. In adults reduced thyroid function presents with:

- fatigue, weakness, muscle aches and pains
- slowing of mental and physical activity, including speech
- cold intolerance
- menorrhagia
- hoarseness
- constipation (an empty rectum suggests colonic inertia)
- a decreased sense of taste and smell
- modest weight gain
- dry, cold, flaky, coarse skin and pruritus
- thin brittle nails
- thinning of hair
- puffy face and eyelids
- bradycardia
- delayed deep tendon reflexes
- a predisposition to carpal tunnel syndrome.

In children, cretinism, a congenital condition of hypothyroidism, presents with:

- dwarfism
- mental retardation
- a 'pot' belly and possible umbilical hernia
- dry cold skin, brittle hair
- large tongue
- cold extremities, cold sensitivity
- delayed bone age
- epiphysial 'stippling'
- mental and physical sluggishness.

Laboratory findings that confirm thyroid hypofunction include:

- an elevated thyroid stimulating hormone (TSH)
- reduced free thyroxine (T4)
- raised serum cholesterol.

A decrease in free serum thyroxine and a raised serum sensitive thyrotropin confirm a diagnosis of hypothyroidism due to thyroid gland failure.

In patients who are not on thyroxine, useful diagnostic combinations include:

- Autonomous thyroid function: low TSH, normal FT3 and FT4.
- Multinodular or diffuse goiter: normal TSH, normal FT4 in the presence of a goiter.
- Subclinical/compensated hypothyroidism: high TSH, normal FT4.
- Sick euthyroid or, rarely, hypothyroidism due to pituitary failure: normal TSH, borderline/low FT4.
- In the absence of thyroid disease, serum FT4 is normal or raised in mild to moderate illness, TSH is normal. The more severe the illness, the greater the degree of abnormality found in tests of thyroid function.

Special investigation and management is required in persons with thyroid disease or suspected thyroid disease and:

- Diagnostic uncertainty.
- Heart disease.
- Eye disease.
- Pregnancy.
- Suspected malignancy suggested by:
  - recent onset or enlarging nodule
  - very hard irregular mass
  - cervical lymphadenopathy
  - metastases to bone, lungs, brain.
- Local obstructive symptoms manifest as:
  - dysphagia
  - a persistent cough

- shortness of breath
- a sensation of pressure or pain in the neck
- facial engorgement due to venous obstruction or superior vena cava obstruction.

- A retrosternal thyroid gland or mass.
- Thyrotoxicosis.
- Cosmetic concerns.
- A history of neck irradiation.
- Recurrent disease.
- Drug therapy:
  - dopamine
  - glucocorticoids
  - high dose frusemide
  - phenytoin
  - lithium.

TINEA

The terminology used to describe dermatophyte infections varies with the area involved. This fungal infection may present as:

- *Tinea capitis* presents with:
  - scaly round patches on the scalp
  - bald patches with clumps of broken hairs.
- *Tinea corporis* (ringworm) presents with red round macules and patches, with:
  - clearing in the center
  - a well-defined erythematous advancing edge
  - a scaly or vesicular edge
  - moderate to intense pruritus.
- *Tinea pedis* (athlete's foot) presents with:
  - scaling, vesicular soggy lesions between the toes
  - scaly vesicular rash on the dorsum of the foot
  - mild itching
  - foot odor.
- *Tinea unguium* presents with:
  - mild yellow-brown discoloration at the distal portion of the nail
  - white spots on the nail
  - crumbling of the nail, which starts at the outer edge and spreads to the base.
- *Tinea cruris* presents with:
  - circinate spreading lesions in the groin
  - lesions with a clear center
  - mild pruritus.

In all instances, vesicles may be found on the hands and feet. This is the Id (phenomenon) reaction, an allergic response to dermatophyte infection.

Kerion formation, an inflamed boggy mass, may result when the host has had an exaggerated immune response to a geophilic or zoophilic fungus.

TINEA VERSICOLOR

See: *Pityriasis versicolor.*

TONSILLITIS SYNDROME

Acute tonsillitis is characterized by:

- a sore throat
- marked focal pharyngeal erythema
- fever
- nasal speech
- cervical lymphadenopathy.

Acute tonsillitis may result from bacterial or viral infection.

Streptococcal pharyngitis (pharyngotonsillitis). In susceptible patients this throat infection carries a risk of rheumatic fever and/or acute glomerulonephritis. As the clinical features correlate poorly with the etiology, and therefore the prognosis, referral should be determined on the basis of the severity of illness and psychosocial factors that may influence disability and outcome. Infection by *Streptococcus pyogenes* causes exudative tonsillitis and presents with:

- inflammation, which is greatest over the tonsillar region
- follicles, detected as large white to gray patches on the tonsil
- severe dysphagia
- tender cervical lymphadenopathy
- pyrexia
- earache
- headache
- malaise.

In children under 4 years of age:

- the onset is gradual
- a nasal discharge is present
- otitis media is common.

In children aged 4–15 years:

- the onset is sudden
- fever is prominent
- the pharynx is edematous, inflamed, and painful.

In adolescents (>16 years) common findings are:

- a sore throat
- dysphagia
- earache
- headache.

Complications of streptococcal pharyngotonsillitis include:

- Quinsy. A peritonsillar abscess is likely to have developed in cases with odynophagia and drooling.
- Sinusitis.
- Otitis media.
- Septic arthritis.
- Rheumatic fever.
- Scarlet fever. Infection of *Strep. pyogenes* by a bacteriophage leads to production of an erythrogenic toxin responsible for the clinical features of scarlet fever. In addition to the presentation and potential complications of streptococcal pharyngotonsillitis, patients present with:
  - a diffuse pink-red macular rash
  - a flushed skin which blanches on pressure
  - dark red lines in the creases of skin folds
  - circumoral pallor (the face is flushed with pallor around the mouth)
  - a strawberry tongue (the inflamed beefy tongue has red papillae protruding through a white coating)
  - skin desquamation.

Viral pharyngitis. A diversity of viral infections may give rise to a sore throat. Viral pharyngitis does not carry the potentially serious immunological complications of a streptococcal sore throat.

Adenovirus pharyngitis presents with:

- a very sore throat
- dysphagia
- pharyngeal hyperemia (an exudate may be present)
- conjunctivitis
- associated findings which may be present include fever, malaise, chills, dizziness, myalgia, and headache.

Upper respiratory viral infections also present with a *nonspecific viral syndrome* characterized by a sore throat and any of the following:

- fever, malaise
- headache, arthralgia, myalgia
- cough
- nausea, vomiting, diarrhea
- a skin rash.

Herpangina, a condition caused by Coxsackie A virus, presents with:

- fever
- painful ulcers in the region of the tonsils, uvula, and soft palate (the lesions heal in 7 days).

In contrast, *herpes stomatitis* affects the anterior tongue and gums.

TORTICOLLIS

Torticollis, or acute wry neck, is usually a self-limiting disorder associated with muscle spasm. Patients present with:

- acute neck pain
- a lateral flexion deformity associated with slight flexion rotation
- lateral flexion is away from the painful side
- a loss of extension
- the absence of neurological signs.

TOXIC SHOCK SYNDROME

Toxic shock syndrome, originally diagnosed in young menstruating women using tampons, is now recognized as a multisystem disease resulting from infection by a toxigenic strain of *Staphylococcus aureus*. It can occur at any age and in both sexes.

When five of the following criteria are met, a diagnosis of toxic shock syndrome is made:

- Fever in excess of 38.8°C.
- A diffuse macular rash.
- Hypotension.
- Desquamation, particularly of the palms or soles, 7–14 days after the onset of the illness.
- Three or more of the following:
  - diarrhea or vomiting
  - myalgia (creatine phosphokinase (CPK) is twice the normal level)
  - hyperemia of mucous membranes
  - raised urea or serum creatinine
  - raised bilirubin or abnormal liver function tests
  - disorientation
  - a platelet count of less than 100 000/ml.

TRACHEITIS

The patient presents with:

- a barking cough
- stridor (there is a harsh whistling with inspiration)

- mild hoarseness
- mild cyanosis in severe cases
- a normal white cell count
- subglottic narrowing on an anteroposterior film.

Respiratory arrest is a rare complication in 3–36-month-olds. It is nonetheless prudent to refer children if symptoms progress. *Staphylococcus aureus* is frequently involved.

TRACHEOBRONCHITIS

Viral tracheobronchitis presents with:

- cough
- retrosternal burning pain
- hoarseness.

TRACHOMA

Chlamydia trachomatis infection may infect the eye and spreads to involve both eyes. Trachoma presents with:

- A tearing, itching red eye.
- Photophobia.
- Papillae and white follicles on the palpebral conjunctiva. This is detected on everting the eyelid.
- The gradual development of a pannus. A vascularized infiltrate extends over the upper palpebral conjunctiva and involves the cornea.
- Scarring of the eyelid, resulting in:
  - ectropion (an everted eyelid)

  or
  - entropion (an inverted eyelid).
- Corneal damage due to:
  - scarring from the eyelashes, in entropion
  - drying, in ectropion.

TRANSIENT GLOBAL AMNESIA

This is a rare condition occasionally encountered in middle-aged or elderly people. Epilepsy or vascular problems (e.g. vertebrobasilar ischemia) may cause:

- Attacks characterized by:
  - the abrupt loss of the ability to form new memories
  - retrograde amnesia for both events and people, including personal identity
  - confusion and bewilderment.

- Episodes may last for hours.
- Amnesia for events during the attack.

TRANSIENT ISCHEMIC ATTACK

A transient ischemic attack (TIA) is a focal short-lived neurological deficit that disappears within 24 hours. Attacks that last:

- Less than an hour (usually 7–10 minutes) are often associated with severe stenosis or occlusion of main arteries.
- Longer than an hour are often associated with intracranial embolism. Most TIAs are thought to be related to cardiogenic or artery-to-artery embolism.

Symptoms suggestive of a TIA are:

- weakness or clumsiness of a single limb on one side of the body or face, or bilaterally
- an unsteady gait
- slurred speech
- difficulty swallowing
- an altered or loss of sensation of a single limb on one side of the body or face, or bilaterally
- a loss of vision in one eye, or half or the whole of the visual field in both eyes
- dizziness
- difficulty with the expression or understanding of verbal or written language.

Carotid (anterior circulatory) TIAs account for 4 out of 5 attacks seen clinically. The most common presentation is either:

- Transient monocular blindness, which usually lasts less than 15 minutes. Amaurosis fugax is sudden blindness in one eye.
  or
- A transient hemisphere attack, which may present with:
  - unilateral motor loss
  - unilateral sensory symptoms
  - homonymous hemianopia
  - aphasia
  - dysphagia.

Occasionally, dysarthria and cerebellar ataxia are found.

Vertebrobasilar (posterior circulatory) TIAs may result in:

- transient global amnesia and confusion, which lasts for hours
- bilateral motor loss
- crossed sensory symptoms
- bilateral blindness or blurring of vision
- cerebellar ataxia
- dysarthria
- diplopia

- vertigo
- drop attacks.

Aspirin (100–300 mg/day) has been shown to reduce the risk of a subsequent stroke in patients with a TIA by about 20–25%. The addition of 400 IU of vitamin E per day will decrease the risk of vascular occlusions resulting in stroke by a further 25%.

TRANSIENT SYNOVITIS

Most commonly encountered in children between 4 and 8 years of age, transient synovitis presents with the sudden onset of:

- a limp
- hip pain
- limited hip movement, especially on abduction and internal rotation.

Blood tests and radiographs are normal.

TRAVELER'S DIARRHEA

Traveler's diarrhea is diagnosed when the patient presents with diarrhea within 14 days of arriving in a new, usually underdeveloped, country. The watery diarrhea syndrome lasts 3–5 days and is usually self-limiting. Rest and rehydration are important. Traveler's diarrhea can be divided into three types:

- *Watery diarrhea syndrome. Escherichia coli* is a Gram-negative bacterium found in the human bowel. It is used as an index organism for detecting fecal contamination of water. It is a frequent cause of traveler's diarrhea. Enteropathogenic *E. coli* infection presents with:
  - acute diarrhea 1–3 days after ingesting contaminated food or water
  - vomiting, in some cases
  - recovery within 1–3 days.

Enterotoxin produced by the organism stimulates adenyl cyclase and causes an outpouring of water and electrolytes. This is the classical form of traveler's diarrhea.

- *Dysentery with bloody diarrhea, pain, mucus, and fever.* Infection with invasive *E. coli* damages the bowel mucosa and presents with dysentery. Symptoms occur 1–3 days after ingesting infected food or water. Other causes include *Shigella dysenteriae*, a Gram-negative bacillus, which is spread by direct contact.
- *Chronic persistent diarrhea.* This may be attributable to:
  - giardiasis (the patient has bulky offensive loose stools)

- amebic dysentery (the patient has a fever and feels unwell)
- other noninfective causes.

TRICHOMONAS VAGINITIS

Trichomonas vaginalis infection is often asymptomatic in men. The prostate acts as a reservoir of infection. Women present with:

- a profuse yellow to green vaginal discharge
- an offensive frothy discharge
- intense vaginal inflammation
- dysuria.

Both partners require treatment.

TROCHANTERIC BURSITIS

Patients present with hip pain that:

- Is experienced over the lateral side of the hip.
- May radiate down the lateral aspect of the thigh.
- Tends to occur at night. This helps to differentiate bursitis from gluteus medius tendonitis, which occurs after prolonged activity and has a tender point immediately above the superior aspect of the greater trochanter.

TUBERCULOSIS

Mycobacterium tuberculosis is a slow-growing acid-fast bacillus, spread by droplets, and is responsible for tuberculosis. The clinical presentation of pulmonary tuberculosis is:

- a chronic cough
- hemoptysis
- weight loss
- night sweats
- malaise, lassitude, easy fatiguability
- clinical evidence of involvement of the lung apex
- radiological evidence of fibrosis or cavitation in the lung apex, with associated hilar lymphadenopathy.

Acid-fast bacilli are detected in the sputum using the Ziehl–Neelsen stain.

Immunological tests include:

- An interferon tuberculosis blood test. This test replaces the skin Mantoux test and ascertains cell-mediated immunity to tuberculosis by testing for the production of interferon-γ released by the patient's lymphocytes. Overnight incubation of the patient's blood is required.

- A positive Heaf, Mantoux, or tine test for hypersensitivity to tuberculin.

Neither adults nor children with tuberculosis infection (i.e. a positive Mantoux test) without disease (i.e., no signs and symptoms) are contagious. Because of the increased risk of disease among infected children, preventive therapy is nonetheless recommended for all asymptomatic children and adolescents who are Mantoux positive. For exposed children under 5 years of age, preventive therapy is recommended irrespective of Mantoux status.

Tuberculosis should always be excluded in adults who present with persistent cough, fatigue, weight loss, fever and night sweats, and hemoptysis. Close contacts of adults with pulmonary tuberculosis must be screened. Childhood tuberculosis disease is rarely contagious, except in older adolescents with adult-type cavitative disease or, less commonly, with laryngeal tuberculosis.

ULCERATIVE COLITIS

See: *Inflammatory bowel disease.*

UPPER RESPIRATORY TRACT INFECTION

Viral upper respiratory tract infections may present with:

- coryza (see: *Coryza (common cold)*)
- rhinitis (see: *Rhinitis*)
- pharyngitis (see: *Pharyngitis*)
- laryngitis (see: *Laryngitis*)
- tracheobronchitis (see: *Tracheobronchitis*).

URETHRAL CARUNCLE

Urethral caruncles occur at any age, but are most common in postmenopausal women. They may be asymptomatic, but more frequently present with:

- dysuria
- tenderness
- dyspareunia
- vaginal bleeding
- leukorrhea.

Complications include vaginitis, urethritis, and ulceration.

URETHRITIS

This presents with:

- dysuria
- initial hematuria
- a bloodstained discharge independent of micturition.

(See: *Chlamydia*; *Gonorrhea.*)

Important causes of non-gonococcal urethritis are chlamydia and T-mycoplasma.

URINARY TRACT INFECTION

Recurrent urinary tract infections are believed to carry a risk of renal impairment. This risk may be reduced by good urinary hygiene such as:

- a fluid intake of at least 2 liters/day
- complete bladder emptying, especially before going to bed and after sexual intercourse
- females avoiding the use of the diaphragm as a means of contraception.

Acute urethral syndrome, or nonbacterial dysuria, is encountered in young sexually active women with a sterile urine or urinalysis of less than 10^5 organism/ml who complain of:

- frequency
- dysuria.

Cystitis, or infection of the bladder, presents with:

- dysuria
- urgency
- nocturia
- frequency
- suprapubic tenderness, in some patients
- cloudy or 'smelly' urine, in some instances
- slight, if any, fever
- pyuria on urinalysis. (This is diagnostic. If dysuria is present without pyuria suspect urethritis or vulvovaginitis.)

In men the differential diagnosis of dysuria always includes *acute urethritis* and *prostatitis*.

Pyelonephritis, or kidney infection, presents with:

- Malaise.
- Anorexia.
- Abdominal pain:
  - unilateral backache including flank and lumbar pain is characteristic
  - which may radiate to the suprapubic area.

- Loin tenderness.
- Frequency, nocturia, enuresis.
- Pyuria.
- Headache, malaise.
- Fever, chills, and vomiting may be present.

White cell casts on urinalysis helps to differentiate renal involvement from cystitis. Women with a clinical picture of acute pyelonephritis without pyuria should be investigated for appendicitis or salpingitis.

Microscopy, culture, and sensitivity are required to definitively diagnose urinary tract infection. Indications for urine culture include:

- Relapsing or recurrent infection.
- Suspected pyelonephritis.
- An uncertain history with a positive dipstick test for either nitrites and/or leukocytes. The following urinary culture results are diagnostic of a urinary tract infection:
  - a urinary culture $\geq 10^5$ colony forming units/ml
  - a colony growth of 10^2–10^4 of a single pathogen in a symptomatic patient
  - a carefully voided midstream specimen with a colony count of > 1000 colony forming units/ml of a potential pathogen in a symptomatic female.

Complications of urinary tract infections include:

- renal papillary necrosis
- urolithiasis
- chronic pyelonephritis, with impaired renal function.

In view of these complications referral for investigation is indicated when:

- Gross or microscopic hematuria is detected.
- Obstruction or abnormal urine flow due to reflux, congenital structural abnormalities, stones, prostatic hypertrophy, or pregnancy is suspected. Cases suitable for referral include:
  - Those with obstructive symptoms.
  - Children after their first urinary tract infection.
  - Males who have recurrent urinary tract infections. In males, due to a longer urethra and prostatic secretion with its antibacterial effect, urinary tract infection suggests some other underlying abnormality. In women, contamination of the distal portion of their short urethra creates an environment in which turbulent urine flow can introduce organisms into a normally sterile area.
- Relapses or recurrent infections occur in:
  - Diabetics (glycosuria provides a good culture medium).
  - Women whose symptoms persists despite antibiotic therapy. Sodium citrate will neutralize an acid urine and reduce

burning, but neutralization of urine in the absence of antibiotic cover masks the condition and encourages multiplication of organisms. Citra soda should consequently only be used in association with a urinary antiseptic.

UROLITHIASIS

Urinary stones result from crystallization of urinary solutes. Predisposing factors are:

- Increased concentrations of urinary crystalloids (e.g. calcium salts, uric acid, cystine).
- Changes in urinary pH affecting crystalloid solubility. Uric acid solubility increases six-fold between a pH of 5 and 6. Acidic urine predisposes to urate and cystine stones. Alkaline urine predisposes to calcium and magnesium–ammonium stones.
- Reduced urine flow. A low urinary volume is associated with an increased solute concentration.
- Variations in poorly identified inhibitors or promoters of stone formation.
- Chronic urinary tract infections. Organisms and sloughed cells can provide a focus for solute precipitation.

Renal stones may be asymptomatic. When symptomatic, renal or ureteric colic is the most usual overt manifestation of ureteric calculi. *Renal colic* presents with:

- The abrupt onset of pain, which may present as:
  - intense, unilateral loin-to-groin pain which waxes and wanes
  - a relatively constant ache in the loin.
- Pain may radiate to the groin, testicles, labia, and/or suprapubic area:
  - penile-tip pain is reported in patients with bladder stones which abut on the vesicourethral junction
  - testicular pain is experienced with distension of the ipsilateral upper ureter
  - scrotum pain occurs with distension of the ipsilateral lower ureter.
- Costovertebral angle tenderness.
- Abdominal distension due to an associated reflex ileus.
- Hematuria. This is often microscopic, but is always present, except in cases of complete kidney obstruction.
- Dysuria and urinary frequency.
- A restless patient who cannot get comfortable.
- Autonomic evidence of severe pain:
  - sweating, tachycardia, tachypnea
  - nausea and vomiting.

More than 90% of stones pass without complication within 3–7 days of presentation. Spontaneous passage usually occurs when stones are less than 5 mm in diameter. However, once an individual has produced a urinary calculus, he or she is at increased risk of further stone formation. Seven out of 10 cases of urolithiasis will suffer a recurrence within the next 5 years.

While the clinical manifestations of acute urinary lithiasis are similar, the previous history and radio-opacity of the current stone provide a clue to the type of stone formed.

- Uric acid stones are radiolucent; calcium stones are densely radio-opaque.
- The most common type of stone encountered in western countries is calcium oxalate; this is followed in prevalence by calcium phosphate.
- Cystine stones are faintly radio-opaque and are usually found in persons with a family history of the condition.
- Magnesium ammonium phosphate (staghorn) calculi are moderately radio-opaque, are precipitated in alkaline urine, and are usually associated with urinary infections.

The crystalline nature of the stone is important, as recent studies suggest that nutritional intervention, in at least some cases of urinary stones, may prevent future recurrences.

Patients with suspected urolithiasis should be referred if they have:

- persistent pain
- recurrent pain
- worsening obstruction.

Urgent referral is indicated if there is evidence of:

- stone obstruction
- infection
- a solitary functioning kidney
- bilateral calculus obstruction.

Urologist referral is indicated if there is:

- ongoing pain
- evidence of infection
- a stone larger than 5 mm in diameter
- a stone less than 5 mm in diameter which is failing to pass (as shown on serial plain radiographs)
- staghorn calculus
- hydronephrosis of intravenous pyelogram.

Less than 5% of patients whose stones do not pass spontaneously require surgery, the remainder have the stone removed by lithotripsy, percutaneous nephrolithotomy, or an endourological procedure.

URTICARIA

Urticaria is an immunoglobulin E (IgE) type hypersensitivity. Precipitating factors include drugs (aspirin, codeine), food (nuts, strawberries, seafood), insect bites, emotional stress, and systemic disorders, including Hodgkin's disease and collagen-type disorders. Urticaria is characterized by:

- transient itchy, edematous plaques and papules (wheals)
- wheals, which are initially white but later become red
- vesicles (these are only occasionally formed)
- an onset within minutes of exposure
- symptoms peaking in 1–3 days and lasting 7–21 days.

Urticaria may be:

- superficial, involving the dermis (hives)
- deep, affecting subcutaneous tissue (angioneurotic edema).

UTERINE CANCER

Cancer may affect the body of the uterus or the cervix. (See: *Cervical carcinoma*.) Cancer of the body of the uterus may present with:

- abnormal vaginal bleeding
- low backache.

The risk of endometrial cancer is increased in women with a body mass index of 28–30 and those on unopposed estrogen hormone-replacement therapy.

UTERINE DISPLACEMENT

Uterovaginal prolapse (procidentia) presents with:

- a dull sacral or low backache
- discomfort that is aggravated by walking and standing
- stress incontinence (this is often a problem).

Multiple pregnancies predispose to uterovaginal prolapse. The patient should be reassured and advised to eat a high-fiber diet, to avoid straining at stool, and to lose weight if necessary.

A retroverted uterus presents with:

- a dragging ache
- discomfort which is worst prior to menstruation.

VAGINITIS

Inflammation of the vaginal area may result from infection or chemical irritation (e.g. deodorants, scented condoms, tampons). Clinical features are:

- external dysuria
- vaginal discharge
- vulvovaginal irritation.

(See: *Candidiasis (moniliasis)*; *Menopause*; *Trichomonas vaginitis*.)

VARICOCELE

Varicoceles are usually asymptomatic. The characteristic presentation of symptomatic varicoceles is:

- Scrotal heaviness, rather than pain
- Varicosities, which present as a soft bunch of vessels on the left side and collapse when:
  - the patient lies down
  - the testis is elevated.
- Subfertility.

Patients should be referred to exclude malignant obstruction to venous drainage if their varicocele is:

- on the right side
- of recent onset
- the patient is an older male.

VARICOSE VEINS

Varicose veins are abnormally dilated, tortuous veins, usually encountered in the superficial veins of the lower limb. The superficial veins are poorly supported and subject to tortuosity if exposed to high venous back-pressure. Primary varicose veins are attributable to incompetence of the valves in the superficial veins or in the veins communicating between the deep and superficial systems. Women, particularly pregnant and multiparous women, are at increased risk. Secondary varicose veins result from deep vein thrombosis or vein compression by pelvic or abdominal tumors.

Varicose veins are often asymptomatic, but may present clinically as a:

- dull aching heaviness
- discomfort aggravated by standing
- an ache that is improved by walking or elevating the leg.

A characteristic of varicose veins is rapid venous filling on returning an elevated leg to the dependent position. The level of the incompetent perforator can be identified by exerting digital pressure. Digital pressure over the incompetent perforator prevents back-flow of blood, and the venous filling time reverts to normal for as long as this pressure is maintained.

Complications include:

- Rupture. Bleeding may be controlled by elevating the leg and applying pressure over the area.
- Thrombosis. Superficial thrombophlebitis presents:
  - as a tender subcutaneous cord in the leg
  - with localized edema.
- Minimal skin changes. Eczema, ulceration, and squamous cell carcinoma may occur.
- Calcification.

VASCULAR INSUFFICIENCY

Arterial insufficiency is usually the result of atherosclerosis causing peripheral vascular disease. Venous insufficiency may result from impaired perfusion due to deep vein thrombosis. (See Table V.)

VASOSPASM

See: *Functional arterial disorders.*

VASOVAGAL ATTACK

Anxiety or pain may cause reflex inhibition of sympathetic and enhanced parasympathetic activity, resulting in:

- bradycardia
- peripheral vasodilatation with hypotension
- syncope, with transient loss of consciousness.

VENOUS THROMBOSIS

Venous occlusion may result from thrombosis in an inflamed vein (*thrombophlebitis*) or from a predisposition to coagulation in a noninflamed vein (*phlebothrombosis*). The clinical presentation of thrombophlebitis and phlebothrombosis is similar:

- a dull ache in the region of the vein
- local tenderness, redness, induration
- late development of a firm cord due to the thrombosed vein.

Table V
The clinical presentation of venous and arterial insufficiency

	Arterial insufficiency	Chronic venous insufficiency
Predisposing factors	Arteriosclerosis Advanced age Diabetes Hypertension Smoking	History of DVT Valvular incompetence in the perforating veins Obesity Immobility
Associated changes in the leg	Thin, shiny, dry skin Thickened, slow-growing nails Absence of hair growth Pallor on elevation, dependency rubor Limb may be cool Diminished pulses	Firm (brawny) edema Venous eczema Hardened indurated skin, areas of atrophic skin Dilated and tortuous superficial veins Limb may be warm Ankle flare (dilated venules medial malleolus) Reddish-brown pigmentation
Ulcer location	Between toes or on tip of toes Over phalangeal heads Above lateral malleolus (for diabetes) over metatarsal heads on side of sole or foot	Gaiter region (i.e. lower third of leg including medial and lateral malleoli)
Ulcer characteristics	Well-demarcated edges Black or necrotic tissue Dry base Punched out Poor-quality granulation in base May involve deep fascia Surrounding skin pale Pale	Uneven, sloping, ragged edges Ruddy granulation tissue Moist exudative base with slough Superficial Surrounding skin pigmented Pinkish edge
Prevalence of chronic ulcers	25%	50%
Pain	Exceedingly painful Paresthesia, numbness Intermittent claudication Pain at rest, relieved by lowering leg to a dependent position Worse at night	Moderate to minimal pain Burning feet Heavy, aching legs Discomfort relieved by elevation of leg Pitting edema often present Restless legs
Surrounding area	May have neuropathy Limb is dusky-red/pink on dependency and turns pale on elevation	Venous eczema may cause pruritus Leaking edema may result in maceration
Pulses	Diminished or absent in foot and leg	Normal in foot and leg

The pathogenesis and prognosis of the two conditions is, however, very different. Superficial thrombophlebitis may serve as a marker of a serious underlying condition. Thrombophlebitis migrans is a condition in which superficial thrombosis successively affects veins in diverse parts of the body. Thrombophlebitis migrans is found in patients with:

- Occult malignancy, especially cancer of the stomach, pancreas, bronchus, and female genital tract.
- Buerger's disease (thromboangiitis obliterans). In this condition perfusion of the lower limbs is progressively impaired. Patients with Buerger's disease experience rest pain due to arterial insufficiency, and amputation is a predictable outcome. The condition is aggravated by smoking.

Patients with superficial thrombophlebitis can be managed using aspirin as an anticoagulant in a dose of 150 mg/day for 30 days.

Pulmonary embolism is a significant hazard during the early phases of phlebothrombosis. As the vessel wall becomes increasingly involved in the inflammatory process, the risk of embolization decreases. Conditions predisposing to phlebothrombosis are those predisposing to thrombosis:

- stasis
- hypercoagulable states
- intimal damage.

(See: *Deep vein thrombosis.*)

VENTRICULAR ARRHYTHMIAS

In general, referral is a safe option in patients with ventricular arrhythmias.

Ventricular extrasystoles or multiple ventricular extrasystoles present with:

- The patient experiencing an isolated thump followed by a pause. The tap test in which the heart beat is tapped out with a finger is used to demonstrate this rhythm.
- A pause in pulse followed by normal rhythm. The ectopic impulse arises earlier than normal beat.

Ventricular extrasystoles are dangerous if the frequency exceeds 5–6/min. They may be associated with: ischemic heart disease, thyrotoxicosis, myocarditis, cardiomyopathy, electrolyte imbalance, drugs (e.g. coffee, tea, smoking, digitalis).

Ventricular tachycardia presents with:

- a rapid pulse of up to 200 beats/min
- a first heart sound of varying intensity (this sound is often split)

- tachycardia that does not respond by slowing on vagal stimulation
- a heart rate that is unchanged by exercise.

This is a sinister life-threatening arrhythmia. Impaired filling of the ventricle at the end of diastole due to ventricular contractions can lead to inadequate perfusion. Sustained ventricular tachycardia is usually associated with left ventricular dysfunction and heart failure. All cases should be referred for evaluation and appropriate management.

Ventricular fibrillation and/or flutter present with:

- an irregular pulse
- inefficient ventricular contractions, resulting in impaired perfusion.

This is the most serious of ventricular arrhythmias. It is frequently fatal. Ventricular fibrillation or flutter require urgent referral.

VERTEBRAL DYSFUNCTION

Vertebral dysfunction of the lower cervical or upper thoracic region results in:

- a dull aching pain referred to the anterior chest wall (the pain follows a nerve root distribution) (See: *Nerve root pain (radiculopathy/neuropathy)*.)
- localized spinal tenderness
- restriction on motion palpation
- pain that is aggravated by exertion, deep inspiration, and certain movements.

The prognosis is good.

VERTEBROBASILAR INSUFFICIENCY

See: *Transient ischemic attack.*

VESTIBULAR DYSFUNCTION

Vestibular dysfunction is characterized by:

- Nystagmus. Jerking nystagmus affects both eyes due to an imbalance of labyrinthine stimuli. Nystagmus is most marked on looking in the direction of the quick phase. The first phase of nystagmus is towards an irritative lesion and away from a paralytic lesion.
- Nausea.

- Vomiting.
- Vertigo.
- Ataxia.

VESTIBULAR NEURONITIS

Vestibular neuronitis tends to occur in epidemics. It may follow a respiratory tract infection in an otherwise healthy adult. The initial attack is often severe but subsequent attacks become progressively less severe and of shorter duration. Vestibular neuronitis is a benign disorder in which viral infection of the vestibular nerve presents with a single attack of severe vertigo which may result in unsteadiness for up to 6 weeks. Vertigo is:

- abrupt in onset (the patient experiences a sense of whirling, which reaches a peak in 24–48 hours)
- initially constant and later paroxysmal
- associated with:
  - nausea and vomiting
  - nystagmus with the rapid component away from the lesion
  - incapacity (raising the head precipitates vertigo, and therefore the patient may remain lying down in bed for several days).

There is no associated hearing loss or tinnitus.

VIRAL HEPATITIS

A number of different viruses may cause hepatitis. The clinical presentation and prognosis depends on the nature of the particular virus.

Hepatitis A. Infectious hepatitis is caused by the fecal–oral spread of an RNA virus. Infection is acquired through contaminated food or water or close contact with infected persons, including sexual anal–oral contact. Hepatitis A virus can survive temperatures of 56°C for 30 minutes, remains infectious after storage at −18°C for several years, and is more resistant to chlorine than many bacteria found in drinking water. It is inactivated on heating at 98°C for 1 minute.

The incubation lasts between 2 and 6 weeks, during which time the virus multiplies in the liver and is excreted in the bile. Fecal excretion of the virus starts some 2–3 weeks before the onset of clinical illness, and ceases within 3–10 days of the appearance of jaundice.

After a prodrome of malaise, the patient presents complaining of the abrupt onset of:

- Anorexia, nausea, and vomiting.
- A dislike of fatty foods and cigarette smoke.

- Fever.
- Aches and pains.
- Jaundice (this is present in 50% of cases).
- Serology changes include raised:
  - immunoglobulin M (IgM) antibody levels, indicating recent infection
  - immunoglobulin G (IgG) antibody, indicating past infection and lifelong immunity.
- Leukopenia and lymphocytosis.

Hepatitis A causes a mild to moderate illness. Children and young adults are most commonly infected. It is usually subclinical in children, and half of adults become symptomatic. The severity of the condition increases with age. Most patients recover completely, but up to 20% may relapse. Complications are rare. Patients who present with severe vomiting, abdominal pain, or whose jaundice persists for more than 10 days should be referred.

Active immunization using killed vaccines is now available, this providing protection for about 10 years after a three-injection course. Passive (γ-globulin) immunization against hepatitis A is also available.

Hepatitis B. Serum hepatitis is spread in blood and body fluids. Hepatitis C and D are also spread in body fluids, and sexual transmission is a consideration. The incubation period for hepatitis B is 4 weeks to 6 months. The acute infection is often subclinical. The illness varies from mild to severe, with half of infected adults becoming symptomatic. Infected babies often appear healthy but demonstrate liver disease 30–40 years later. Hepatitis B can become integrated into the genome of the hepatocyte.

The condition has an insidious onset and is characterized by:

- a prodrome of joint pains and skin rashes
- malaise
- anorexia and nausea
- polyarthritis
- jaundice (this is present in 33% of cases).

Complications are:

- Chronic liver disease. (See: *Cirrhosis*.)
- A chronic carrier state. Some 5–10% of infected persons will become chronic carriers. All chronic carriers are a potential source of infection to others and have a high personal risk of developing chronic hepatitis and liver cancer later in life. Serology is helpful in the diagnosis and prognosis.
- HBcAg (core antigen) stimulates anti-HBc antibodies:
  - IgM is detectable within weeks of infection and remains raised for about 10 months after acute infection. IgM antibodies to HBcAg are used to diagnose acute hepatitis B infection.

  - IgG is detected several weeks after infection and persists indefinitely. IgG antibodies to HBcAg are used to diagnose past and chronic infections and chronic carriers.
- HBsAG (surface antigen) is indicative of infectious serum. It is detected in acute and chronic hepatitis and in carriers. Antibodies to HBsAg indicate good immune status. Persons successfully immunized against hepatitis B are anti-HBs positive.
- HBeAg in serum indicates active hepatitis and is a good predictor of the infectivity of blood and body fluids. The level of HBeAg usually falls within a few weeks of infection. If HBeAg is positive in carriers there is a risk of liver disease. HBe antibody usually only rises after HBeAg has been cleared.

Both active and passive (γ-globulin) immunization against hepatitis B are available. Immunoprophylaxis using hepatitis B immunoglobulin provides protection after needlestick injuries with infected blood. Immunoglobulin with a high level of hepatitis B virus (HBV) surface antigen is required. Appropriate use of hepatitis B immunoglobulin and vaccine can prevent vertical transmission of the organism in pregnancy. Routine immunization of children against hepatitis B is under consideration.

Hepatitis C. Acute hepatitis C is asymptomatic in up to 75% of cases. It does, however, carry an almost 50% risk of indolent, insidious chronic hepatitis. Carrier states are a complication in 50–80% of cases. About 20% of those infected will have a persistent illness, and less than 5% of these will have serious consequences some 20–30 years later. The 'window period', i.e. the time during which an individual is infectious but has not yet developed antibodies, which can be detected by screening, is up to 6 months. The incubation period is 6 weeks to 6 months. The ability of the virus to vary its antigenic structure combined with its poor propensity to induce interferon facilitates viral persistence.

The organism is primarily a blood-borne virus. Overall, the sexual and/or transplacental transmission of the virus is low compared with that of hepatitis B.

When symptomatic, hepatitis C has an insidious onset and presents with:

- Anorexia and nausea.
- Tiredness.
- Right upper quadrant discomfort.
- Jaundice (this is present in 25% of cases).
- A raised alanine aminotransferase level. This may be detected in persons with chronic hepatitis but, as aminotransferase is only slightly raised and the level fluctuates around normal, the test must be repeated at least three times in a 6-month period before liver involvement can be excluded.

A positive HVC antibody test is found in 9 out of 10 cases some 3–6 months after infection.

The severity of the acute illness is mild to moderate, and is often subclinical. Chronic hepatitis may take the form of:

- A relatively benign chronic persistent hepatitis. This is the case in 50% of cases.
- Chronic active hepatitis with complications developing over the next 10–30 years. Cirrhosis develops at around 10 years and hepatoma at around 30 years. It is estimated that 10% of cases will resolve, and 20% of patients will develop liver cirrhosis, some of whom will develop hepatocellular cancer. Progression to cirrhosis is enhanced by hepatotoxic drugs (e.g. alcohol) and concurrent hepatitis B infection. Hepatitis C and alcohol are associated with a bad prognosis.

Hepatitis D. This is spread by blood and blood products and is only encountered in persons infected with hepatitis B. The hepatitis D particle is a defective RNA virus that can only replicate if it coats itself in a layer of hepatitis B surface antigens. It predisposes to severe liver damage.

Hepatitis E. This has a fecal–oral, mainly waterborne, spread. The incubation period is 2–9 weeks and, like hepatitis A and D, it has an acute onset. Patients present with nausea and vomiting. One in five patients is jaundiced.

VITREOUS HEMORRHAGE

Retinal hemorrhaging may occur in diabetes, hypertensive retinopathy, or as a result of blood dyscrasias. If sufficiently severe, blood may erupt into the vitreous cavity. The clinical presentation includes:

- Loss of vision which:
  - is sudden
  - is painless
  - is unilateral
  - may be preceded by 'seeing' a shower of spots.
- On ophthalmoscopy:
  - blood is detected in the posterior chamber
  - the red reflex is poor or absent.

WARTS

Human papilloma virus invades the skin through small abrasions and causes abnormal skin masses, which usually resolve spontaneously over months or years. The average incubation period is 4 months and the peak prevalence is in adolescence.

Common warts (verruca vulgaris). These present:

- as skin-colored masses
- as tumors with a rough surface
- on the fingers, knees, and elbows.

Plane warts. These present:

- as linear clusters along scratch lines
- as skin-colored flat lesions
- on the face and limbs.

Digitate warts. These present:

- with finger-like projections
- on the scalp.

Filiform warts. These present:

- with fine, elongated fronds
- on the face and neck.

Plantar warts. These present with:

- a raised area
- tender, hyperkeratotic skin lesions in areas of pressure (e.g. the sole)
- multiple bleeding pinpoints within a sharply circumscribed area on paring.

Senile warts (See: *Seborrheic keratosis.*)

Venereal warts (condyloma acuminata). These present as:

- thin flexible papules
- cauliflower lesions, when growth is confluent
- painless, benign infections of the papilloma virus.

These viral lesions should not be confused with *condyloma lata*, the flat coppery wart of secondary syphilis.

WHIPLASH

Whiplash usually occurs due to hyperextension of the neck followed by recoil hyperflexion. Although most patients experience symptoms within 6 hours, delayed symptoms with the patient feeling no pain until 24–96 hours later are possible. Patients present with:

- Neck stiffness.
- Pain in the neck and upper shoulders.
- Pain radiates:
  - suboccipitally
  - to between the shoulder blades
  - down the arms.
- Headache is:
  - usually occipital, but may be temporal or ocular
  - persistent (it may last for months).

- Paresthesia to the little finger.
- Nausea.
- Dizziness.

Complications include depression and asymptomatic osteoarthritis becoming symptomatic.

WHOOPING COUGH

Whooping cough has an incubation period of 7–10 days and is communicated for 1 week before and 3 weeks after the onset of paroxysms of coughing. The disease is spread by droplets. Immunization against whooping cough (*Bordetella*) is available. Whooping cough has three phases:

- The catarrhal phase, with:
  - mild fever
  - rhinitis
  - sneezing
  - lacrimation
  - an irritating cough.
- The whooping/paroxysmal phase lasts 2–6 weeks, during which:
  - A staccato coughing is followed by a post-tussive inspiratory gasp. The patient coughs repeatedly during one expiration, which is followed by a sudden deep crowing inspiration, the 'whoop'.
  - Paroxysms of coughing occur.
  - Apneic episodes are followed by vomiting. This is attributable to hypoxia.
  - Paroxysms may be precipitated by eating.
  - Tenacious clear mucus may be produced.
- Convalescence:
  - a habit pattern of coughing may persist for weeks.

Complications include: pneumonia, atelectasis, emphysema, and bronchiectasis. Children are at increased risk of complications. Infants and children who have not been immunized may require referral. Evidence of anoxia, such as whooping complicated by convulsions, is an indication for referral.

In adults, whooping cough may present as a dry cough which persists for 2–14 weeks. Cough suppressants should not be used.

Patients who present with recurrent 'whooping cough' probably have an adenovirus infection. Onset is sudden and the household attack rate is high. These patients present with:

- a persistent whoop
- retrosternal discomfort
- moderate fever
- myalgia
- rhinorrhea
- a sore throat.

WINTER ITCH

Winter itch is a common cause of generalized pruritus. Patients present with:

- dry scaly, chapped skin
- pruritus.

The cause is a cold windy climate.

XIPHOIDALGIA

Patients present with:

- Spontaneous pain in the anterior chest which radiates deep into the chest, back, shoulder, and epigastrium.
- Pain which is aggravated by bending, stooping, and twisting.
- Xiphisternal pressure reproduces local discomfort and pain radiation.
- Tenderness of the xiphoid sternum.

The syndrome persists for weeks or months and then resolves spontaneously.

YERSINIA ENTEROCOLITIS

Patients infected with *Yersinia enterocolitica*, after an incubation period of 3–8 hours following ingestion of infected food, often milk, present with:

- fever
- diarrhea
- abdominal cramps.

Diarrhea may persist for months.

ZINC DEFICIENCY

Zinc deficiency is a common problem as the soil of many countries is zinc deficient. Zinc is required for nucleic acid and protein synthesis. In zinc deficiency the cells with the most rapid turnover (red blood cells and the intestinal epithelium) are, therefore, likely to be the first to demonstrate abnormalities. The zinc tally taste test is a good indicator of clinical zinc status.

Acute zinc deficiency (*acrodermatitis enteropathica*) leads to:

- hair loss
- diarrhea
- pustular dermatitis.

Chronic zinc deficiency presents clinically with:

- anorexia
- anosmia (loss of smell)
- hypogeusia and dysgeusia (diminished taste)
- cold extremities
- slow healing
- skin disorders, including acne and white spots on the nails
- hypogonadism
- impaired immunity, including lymphopenia and reduced T-cell function.

In pregnancy, zinc deficiency is associated with retardation of growth and fetal development.

FURTHER READING

General

Goroll A H, May L A, Mulley A G 1995 Primary care medicine, 3rd edn. J B Lippincott, Philadelphia, PA

Griffith H W, Dambro M R 1994 The 5 minute clinical consult. Lea & Febiger, Philadelphia, PA

Kasper D et al 2005 Harrison's principles of internal medicine, 16th edn. McGraw Hill, New York

Murtagh J 2005 General Practice Series, 3rd edn. McGraw Hill, Sydney

Schroeder S A, Krupp M A, Tierney L M 1998 Current medical diagnosis and treatment, 37th edn. Prentice Hall, Englewood Cliffs, NJ

Acne

Layton A M 2006 A review on the treatment of acne vulgaris. International Journal of Clinical Practice 60:64–72

Alcoholism

Luggen A S 2006 Alcohol and the older adult. Advances in Nursing Practice 14:47–52

Yost D 1996 Alcohol withdrawal syndrome. American Family Physician 54:657–664

Arrhythmias

Murtagh J 1992 Palpitations. Australian Family Physician 21:475–482

Arthritis

Cohen M L, Richter M B 1994 Can we manage our arthritis patients without NSAIDs? Current Therapeutics 35:10–13

Machold K P, Nell V, Stamm T, Aletaha D, Smolen J S 2006 Early rheumatoid arthritis. Current Opinion in Rheumatology 18(3):282–288

Asthma

Behbehani N, Fitzgerald J M 2006 The assessment and management of patients with acute asthma. International Journal of Tuberculosis and Lung Disease (Paris) 10(4):356–364

Berlow B A 1997 Eight key questions to ask when your patient with asthma doesn't get better. American Family Physician 55:183–189

Fitzgerald D, Callahan L A 1996 Office evaluation of pulmonary function: beyond the numbers. American Family Physician 54:525–534

Breast cancer

Crea P 1995 Breast cancer: a GP's guide to detection and treatment options. Modern Medicine 38:20–34

Fruscalzo A, Lelle R J, Calcagno A, Driul L, Damante G, Marchesoni D 2006 Management of gynecological tumors associated with BRCA1 and BRCA2 germline mutations. Case report and literature review. Minerva Ginecologica (Torino) 58(2):171–175

Morra M E, Blumberg B D 1991 Women's perceptions of early detection in breast cancer: how are we doing? Seminars in Oncology Nursing 7:151–160

Smith P E 1993 Breast cancer prevention and detection update. Seminars in Oncology Nursing 9:150–154

Caffeinism

Abbott P J 1986 Caffeine: a toxicological overview. Medical Journal of Australia 145:518–521

Harris S S, Dawson-Hughes B 1994 Caffeine and bone loss in healthy postmenopausal women. American Journal of Clinical Nutrition 60:573–578

Silverman K, Evans S, Strain E C, Griffiths R R 1992 Withdrawal syndrome after double blind cessation of caffeine consumption. New England Journal of Medicine 327:1109–1114

Celiac disease

Pham T H, Barr G D 1996 Coeliac disease in adults. Australian Family Physician 25:62–65

Westerberg D P, Gill J M, Dave B, DiPrinzio M J, Quisel A, Foy A 2006 New strategies for diagnosis and management of celiac disease. Journal of the American Osteopathic Association 106(3):145–151

Chronic fatigue syndrome

Epstein K R 1995 The chronically fatigued patient. Medical Clinics of North America 79:315–328

Holmwood C, Shanon C 1992 Chronic fatigue syndrome. Australian Family Physician 21:278–285

Loblay R H 1993 Allergic to the 20th century. Australian Family Physician 22:1992–1997

Murdoch J C 1992 Chronic fatigue syndrome. Australian Family Physician 21:1205–1206

Staines D R 2006 Postulated vasoactive neuropeptide autoimmunity in fatigue-related conditions: A brief review and hypothesis. Clinical Development in Immunology 13(1):25–39

Walls R S 1995 How to investigate the patient with chronic fatigue. Modern Medicine, Australia 38:115–120

Colorectal cancer

Cowen A E 1984 A clinical approach to improving survival in colorectal cancer. Australian Family Physician 13:406–413

Giovannucci E, Egan K M, Hunter D I et al 1995 Aspirin and the risk of colorectal cancer in women. New England Journal of Medicine 333:609–614

Martinez S R, Young S E, Hoedema R E, Foshag L J, Bilchik A J 2006 Colorectal cancer screening and surveillance: Current standards and future trends. Annals of Surgical Oncology

Meagher A, Ward R 1997 Advances in the treatment of colorectal cancer. Modern Medicine 40(5):22–29

Vines G 1994 Bananas keep cancer at bay. New Scientist 142:9

Cushing's disease

Sambrook P, Birmingham J, Kelly P et al 1993 Prevention of corticosteroid osteoporosis: a comparison of calcium, calcitriol and calcitonin. New England Journal of Medicine 328:1747–1752

Diabetes

Best J D, O'Neal D 1993 Diabetes and vascular disease. Australian Family Physician 22:1563–1571

Borkman M, Campbell L V 1993 Non insulin dependent diabetes mellitus. Australian Family Physician 22:1549–1560

Campbell L V 1995 Preserving diabetic feet for a lifetime: a team effort. Modern Medicine, Australia 38:74–83

Chapman L, Zimmet P 1995 The role of the GP in the prevention of diabetes complications. Modern Medicine, Australia 38:104–108

Collett P 1992 Investigation of a patient with proteinuria by dipstick testing. Modern Medicine, Australia June:131–133

Cooper M E 1995 Microalbuminuria. Current Therapeutics 2:16–18

Kohl H W, Gordon N F, Villegas J A, Blair S N 1992 Cardiorespiratory fitness, glycaemic status and mortality risk in men. Diabetes Care 15:184–192

Lording D W 1993 The impact of diabetes on the lower limb. Australian Family Physician 22:1583–1590

O'Day J, Harper A 1995 Systemic disease and the eye. Modern Medicine, Australia 38:34–43

Phillipov G, Alimat A, Phillips P J, Drew A C 1995 Screening for diabetic retinopathy. Medical Journal of Australia 162:518–520

Popplewell P 1995 Type 2 diabetes and cardiovascular disease. Modern Medicine, Australia 38:92–102

Popplewell P, Phillips P 1994 Diabetes in older people. Australian Family Physician 23:1307–1318

Saaddine J B, Cadwell B, Gregg E W et al 2006 Improvements in diabetes processes of care and intermediate outcomes: United States, 1988–2002. Annals of Internal Medicine 144(7):465–474

Sanchez-Torres R J, Delgado-Osorio H 2005 The metabolic syndrome and its cardiovascular manifestations. Boletin-Asociacion Medica de Puerto Rico 97(4):271–280

Fibromyalgia

Bennett R M 1993 Fibromyalgia and the facts. Rheumatic Disease Clinics of North America 19:45–60

Block S R 1993 Fibromyalgia and the rheumatisms. Rheumatic Disease Clinics of North America 19:61–78

Burckhardt C S 2006 Multidisciplinary approaches for management of fibromyalgia. Current Pharma 12(1):59–66

Crofford L J, Pillemer S R, Kalogeras K T et al 1994 Hypothalamic–pituitary–adrenal perturbations in patients with fibromyalgia. Arthritis and Rheumatism 37:1583–1592

Edwards R R, Bingham C O 3rd, Bathon J, Haythornthwaite J A 2006 Catastrophizing and pain in arthritis, fibromyalgia, and other rheumatic diseases. Arthritis and Rheumatism 55(2):325–332

Kaplan K H, Goldenberg D L, Galvin-Nadeau M 1993 The impact of a meditation-based stress reduction program on fibromyalgia. General Hospital Psychiatry 15(5):284–289

Lorenzen I 1994 Fibromyalgia: a clinical challenge. Journal of Internal Medicine 235(3):199–203

Meggs W J 1995 Neurogenic switching: a hypothesis for a mechanism for shifting the site of inflammation in allergy and chemical sensitivity. Environmental Health Perspectives 103(1):54–56

Moldofsky H 1989 Sleep and fibrositis syndrome. Rheumatic Disease Clinics of North America 15(1):91–103

Ozgocmen S 2006 New strategies in evaluation of therapeutic efficacy in fibromyalgia syndrome. Pharmaceutical Design 12(1):67–71

Triadafilopoulos G, Simms R W, Goldenberg D L 1991 Bowel dysfunction in fibromyalgia syndrome. Digestive Disease Science 36(1):59–64

Veale D, Kavanagh G, Fielding J F, Fitzgerald O 1991 Primary fibromyalgia and the irritable bowel syndrome: different expressions of a common pathogenetic process. British Journal of Rheumatology 30(3):220–222

Wigers S H, Stiles T C, Vogel P A 1996 Effects of aerobic exercise versus stress management treatment in fibromyalgia. A 4.5 year prospective study. Scandinavian Journal of Rheumatology 25(2):77–86

Gastroesophageal/intestinal motility disorders

Abell T L, Werkman R F 1996 Gastrointestinal motility disorders. American Family Physician 54:895–902

Australian Gastroenterology Institute 1997 Gastro-oesophageal reflux disease in adults. Modern Medicine, Australia 40(1):61–69

Mendelsohn M 1995 Throat symptoms: can it be gastroesophageal reflux? Modern Medicine, Australia 38:86–90

Talley N J, Hu W, Holtmann G 1995 Symptoms, investigation and treatment of gastroparesis. Modern Medicine, Australia 38:27–32

Gout

Lee S J, Terkeltaub R A, Kavanaugh A 2006 Recent developments in diet and gout. Current Opinion in Rheumatology 18(2):193–198

Mikuls T R, Saag K G 2006 New insights into gout epidemiology. Current Opinion in Rheumatology 18(2):199–203

Heart failure

Saraiva R M, Hare J M 2006 Nitric oxide signaling in the cardiovascular system: implications for heart failure. Current Opinion in Cardiology 21(3):221–228

Hypertension

Adcock B B, Ireland R B 1997 Secondary hypertension: a practical diagnostic approach. American Family Physician 55:1263–1270

Angeli F, Verdecchia P, Gattobigio R, Sardone M, Reboldi G 2005 White-coat hypertension in adults. Blood Pressure Monitoring 10(6):301–305

Ryan M P 1996 How to investigate the patient with hypertension. Modern Medicine, Australia 39:96–98

Incontinence

Hahn I, Milson I, Fall M et al 1993 Long term results of pelvic floor training in female stress urinary incontinence. British Journal of Urology 72:421–427

Inflammatory bowel disease

Bui A 1996 Surgical choices in colitis care. The Practitioner 240:178–182

Gibson P R, Iser J 2005 Inflammatory bowel disease. Australian Family Physician 34(4):233–237

Pavli P 1994 The inflammatory bowel diseases. General Practitioner 2:204–207, 213–215

Ramchandani D, Schindler B, Katz J 1994 Evolving concepts of psychopathology in inflammatory bowel disease. Medical Clinics of North America 78:1321–1329

Irritable bowel syndrome

Australian Gastroenterology Statement 1994 Irritable bowel syndrome. Modern Medicine, Australia 37:90–98

Barnes J 1996 When to investigate and treat IBS symptoms. The Practitioner 240:184–187

Dalton C B, Drossman D A 1997 Diagnosis and treatment of iritable bowel syndrome. American Family Physician 55:875–880

Lynn R B, Friedman L S 1995 Irritable bowel syndrome: managing the patients with abdominal pain and altered bowel habits. Medical Clinics of North America 79:373–390

Prior A, Holdsworth C D 1990 Irritable bowel syndrome. Medicine International 3263–3268

Leukemia

De Boer R, Grigg A 1994 Adult leukaemia – making the diagnosis. Australian Family Physician 23:1508–1518

Szer J 1994 Current thinking in the management of leukaemia. Australian Family Physician 23:1500–1505

Vowela M R 1994 Common presentations and management of leukaemia in childhood. Australian Family Physician 23:1519–1526

Lymphoma

Flecknoe-Brown S 1993 Malignant lymphoma: a clinicopathological approach. General Practitioner 1:125–129

Wolf M 1994 Non-Hodgkin's lymphoma – diagnosis and management. Australian Family Physician 23:1491–1497

Melanoma

Dixon A J, Hall R S 2005 Managing skin cancer–23 golden rules. Australian Family Physician 34(8):669–671

Westerahl J, Olsson H, Ingvar C 1994 At what age do sunburn episodes play a crucial role for the development of malignant melanoma? European Journal of Cancer 30A:1647–1654

Menopause

Hammond C B 1997 Management of menopause. American Family Physician 55:1667–1673

O'Neill S 1995 Presentation of menopausal problems. Current Therapeutics 36:25–31

Obesity

Kannel W B, D'Agostino R B, Cobb J L 1996 Effect of weight on cardiovascular disease. American Journal of Clinical Nutrition 63:419S–422S

Lean M E J, Han T S, Morrison C E 1995 Waist circumference as a measure for indicating need for weight management. British Medical Journal 311:158–161

Mason J E, Willett W C, Stampfer M J et al 1995 Body weight and mortality among women. New England Journal of Medicine 333:677–685

Meisler J G, St Jeor S 1996 Foreward. American Journal of Clinical Nutrition 63(suppl): 409S–411S

Reynolds K, He J 2005 Epidemiology of the metabolic syndrome. American Journal of the Medical Sciences 330(6):273–279

Otitis

Blomgren K, Pitkaranta A 2005 Current challenges in diagnosis of acute otitis media. International Journal of Pediatric Otorhinolaryngol 69(3):295–299

Briggs R J S 1995 Otitis externa. Australian Family Physician 24:1859–1864

Vandeleur T J 1997 An update on glue ear. Modern Medicine, Australia 40(6):108–112

Prostate disorders

Arnold E P 1986 Benign prostatic hypertrophy. Patient Management 10:11–23

Buck A C 1996 Phytotherapy for the prostate. British Journal of Urology 78:325–336

Carter H B, Pearson J D, Metter E J et al 1992 Longitudinal evaluation of prostate specific antigen levels in men with and without prostate disease. Journal of the American Medical Association 267:2215–2220

Fitzpatrick J M 2006 The natural history of benign prostatic hyperplasia. BJU Int 97(Suppl 2):3–6

Holmes A B 1993 Carcinoma of the prostate. Australian Family Physician 22:1375–1384

Johnson W 1993 Benign prostate hyperplasia: a complete guide to modern management. Modern Medicine, Australia 36:14–25

Mahon S M 2005 Screening for prostate cancer: informing men about their options. Clinical Journal of Oncology Nursing 9(5):625–627

Sladden M, Dickinson J 1993 Effectiveness of screening for prostate cancer. Australian Family Physician 22:1385–1392

Psoriasis

Bittiner S B, Tucker W F G, Cartwright I, Bleehen S S 1988 A double-blind randomized, placebo-controlled trial of fish oil in psoriasis. Lancet 1(8582):378–380

Donaldson L, Douglas W 1997 Current thinking on psoriasis. The Practitioner 241:66–72

Healy P J, Helliwell P S 2005 Classification of the spondyloarthropathies. Current Opinion in Rheumatology 17(4):395–399

Rhinitis

Scadding G 1996 Rhinitis: common, debilitating and treatable. The Practitioner 240:48–53

Walls R S 1995 Allergic and nonallergic rhinitis: diagnosis and management. Modern Medicine, Australia 37:74–86

Shock

Hoffman N E 1994 Gastrointestinal bleeding. Current Therapeutics 1:18–20

Sinusitis

Slack R 1996 A realistic view of sinusitis. The Practitioner 240:54–57

Sleep disorders

Farney R J, Walker J M 1995 Office management of common sleep wake disorders. Medical Clinics of North America 79:391–414

Pagel J F 2005 Medications and their effects on sleep. Primary Care 32(2):491–509

Stroke

Crimmins D S, Pokorny C S 1995 How to investigate the patient with TIA. Modern Medicine, Australia 39:71–75

Gorelick P B 1995 Stroke prevention. Archives Neurology 52:347–355

Joffe R 1994 Diagnosis and treatment of transient ischaemic attacks. Modern Medicine, Australia 37:18–23

Thompson D W, Furlan A J 1996 Clinical epidemiology of stroke. Neurology Clinics 14:309–315

Syncope

Waterston J 1993 Unexplained syncope: keys to target the cause. Modern Medicine, Australia 36:16–22

Testicular cancer

Albers P, Albrecht W, Algaba F et al 2005 Guidelines on testicular cancer. European Urology 48(6):885–894

Sladden M, Dickinson J 1993 Testicular cancer. How effective is screening? Australian Family Physician 22:1350–1356

Thyroid disease

Delbridge L 1994 Thyroid lumps: which ones need the surgeon's knife? Modern Medicine, Australia 37:38–43

Guirguis-Blake J, Hales C M 2005 Screening for thyroid disease. American Family Physician 71(7):1369–1370

Henessey J V 1996 Diagnosis and management of thyrotoxicosis. American Family Physician 54:1315–1324

Houston M S, Hay I D 1990 Practical management of hyperthyroidism. American Family Physician March:909–916

Surks M I 1990 American thyroid association guidelines for use of laboratory tests in thyroid disorders. Journal of the American Medical Association 16:1529–1532

Surks M I, Chopra I J, Mariash C N et al 1990 American thyroid association guidelines for the use of laboratory tests in thyroid disorders. Journal of the American Medical Association 263:1529–1532

Wood W E A 1988 Clinical pitfalls in testing thyroid function. Modern Medicine, Australia 31(6):103–105

Urinary disorders

Becker G J 1992 Renal stones: avoiding surgery and preventing recurrence. Modern Medicine, Australia April:104–112

Costello A 1992 Lithotripsy for kidney stones. Australian Family Physician 21:438–440

Curhan G C, Willet W C, Kimm E B et al 1993 Stones. New England Journal of Medicine 328:833–838

Morgan T 1984 Renal colic. Australian Family Physician 13:399–401

Wise K A 1992 Urinary tract infection. Modern Medicine, Australia December:16–22

Viral hepatitis

Batey R G 1994 Hepatitis B immunization. Current Therapeutics 35:11–13

Chou R, Clark E C, Helfand M; U.S. Preventive Services Task Force 2004 Screening for hepatitis C virus infection: a review of the evidence for the U.S. Preventive Services Task Force. Annals of Internal Medicine 140(6):465–479

Lang S A 1993 A vaccine for hepatitis A. Current Therapeutics 34:9–13

Mills P, McPeake J, McCruden E 1996 Rational approach to hepatitis C. The Practitioner 240:172–176

Statement of the Australian Gastroenterology Institute 1992 What do I need to know about hepatitis C? Modern Medicine, Australia, March:88–91

Tasman-Jones C 1994 Chronic hepatitis B and C: the role of interferon. Current Therapeutics 35:17–20

Glossary

Glossary

This glossary has been prepared to link patients' complaints with professional terms.

Patient's complaint	Professional term
pain	
breast pain	mastalgia
burning upper abdominal pain	pyrosis
cramping abdominal pain	colic: may be renal or intestinal
cramping leg pain	claudication
joint pain	arthralgia
joint pain plus signs of inflammation	arthritis
muscle pain	myalgia
pain on passing urine	dysuria
painful sexual intercourse	dyspareunia
period/menstrual pain	dysmenorrhea
bleeding	
bleeding into a joint	hemarthrosis
bleeding into the skin	purpura: small – petechiae; large – ecchymoses
bleeding into tissue	hematoma
blood in the urine	hematuria
coughing blood	hemoptysis
dark blood passed in the stool	melena
heavy period	menorrhagia
nose bleed	epistaxis
vaginal bleeding between periods	metrorrhagia
vomiting blood	hematemesis
bad-smelling breath	halitosis
blue discoloration of skin/mucous membrane	cyanosis
breathlessness	dyspnea
difficulty swallowing	dysphagia
indigestion	dyspepsia
itch	pruritus
pale fatty malodorous stool that floats	steatorrhea
pins and needles	paresthesia
runny nose	rhinorrhea
stone	lithiasis: cholelithiasis (gallstones); urolithiasis (kidney stones)
tortuous distended veins	varicosity
yellow discoloration of sclera, skin	jaundice

Patient's complaint	Professional term
inflammation of the:	*...itis*
eyelid	blepharitis
deep subcutaneous tissue	cellulitis
bladder	cystitis
cornea	keratitis
voice box	laryngitis
inflamed/infected lymph node	lymphadenitis
serosal lining of the heart/pericardial sac	pericarditis
throat	pharyngitis
serosal lining of the lung	pleuritis
nasal mucosa	rhinitis
vertebral joint inflammation	spondylitis
joint lining	synovitis
urethra	urethritis
vagina	vaginitis
high/low	*hyper-/hypo-*
high/low blood glucose	hyper/hypoglycemia
increased/decreased depth, rate breathing	hyper/hypoventilation
excess/inadequate levels thyroid hormone	hyper/hypothyroidism
enlargement of the:	*...megaly*
heart	cardiomegaly
liver	hepatomegaly
spleen	splenomegaly
a localized area of pus	abscess
appendages. Uterine adnexae: ovaries, fallopian tubes, uterine ligaments	adnexae
bowel sounds	borborygmia
sound of blood running through a distorted vessel	bruit
a destructive sore, often raised	chancre
short adventitious lung sound similar to crushing dry leaves	crackle
intellectual deterioration	dementia
episode characterized by the plentiful production of urine	diuresis
a disorder of articulation	dysarthria
disorder (usual reference is to a blood dyscrasia)	dyscrasia
painful menstruation/period pain	dysmenorrhea
painful sexual intercourse	dyspareunia
difficulty with swallowing	dysphagia
disorder in use of symbols of communication (written, read, spoken, heard)	dysphasia
disorder of vocalization	dysphonia
breathlessness	dyspnea
painful urination/micturition	dysuria
material from a distal site which lodges in, and occludes, a smaller vessel	embolus
surgical incision into the perineum and vagina to facilitate childbirth	episiotomy
cause	etiology
breath out	expiration
irregular contraction of a heart chamber	fibrillation
a tract connecting two *epithelial* surfaces (e.g. bladder and vagina)	fistula
caused by the practitioner/doctor	iatrogenic
due to an unknown cause	idiopathic
uncontrolled leakage (e.g. of urine, feces)	incontinence
breath in	inspiration
a portion of bowel telescopes into the bowel lumen	intussusception
urine of constant specific gravity	isosthenuria
acidosis (i.e. excess accumulation of acidic metabolic end-products)	ketosis

Patient's complaint	Professional term
whitish viscid vaginal discharge	leukorrhea
filling of alveoli (air spaces) or a lobe of the lung	lobar consolidation
area of the low back	lumbosacral
enlarged lymph node(s)	lymphadenopathy
new growth, may be benign or malignant (e.g. cancer)	neoplasia
a series of rhythmic oscillations of the eye	nystagmus
breathlessness, which is worst on lying down	orthopnea
simulates peritonitis with a rigid abdomen	peritonism
air in the urine	pneumaturia
after sexual intercourse	postcoital
mental and physical	psychomotor
a discrepancy between heart and pulse rate	pulse deficit
an arterial pulse of varying amplitude due to a changing stroke volume	pulsus alternans
blood pressure fluctuation between inspiration and expiration > 15 mmHg	pulsus paradoxus
bruises (bleeding into the skin)	purpura
leathery sound of friction between inflamed serosal surfaces (pleural, pericardial)	rub
a congenital forward displacement of one vertebra upon another	spondylolisthesis
a congenital defect of the neural arch	spondylolysis
spinal osteoarthritis or degenerative back disease	spondylosis
joint injury involving incomplete rupture of supporting ligaments	sprain
deformation, overstretching and tearing of musculotendinous tissue	strain
straining at stool	tenesmus
a palpable cardiac murmur	thrill
a ringing/buzzing in the ears	tinnitus
spasm of the vaginal muscles	vaginismus
dizziness	vertigo
regurgitation of sour fluid	waterbrash
high-pitched musical note	wheeze

Index

Numbers in italic refer to flowcharts; numbers in bold refer to clinical conditions section.

A

B

D

E

H

Q

R

S

X

Y

Z

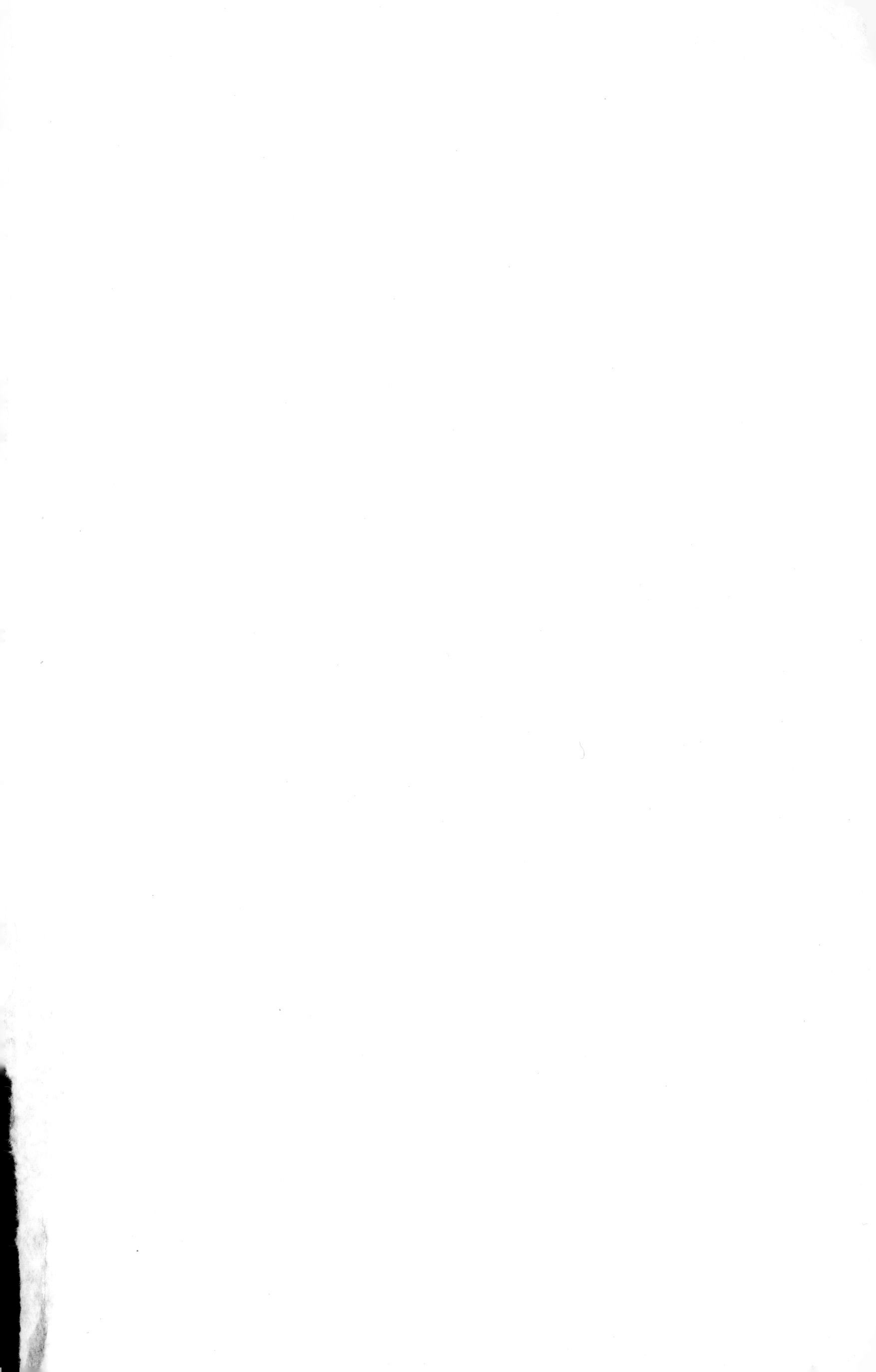